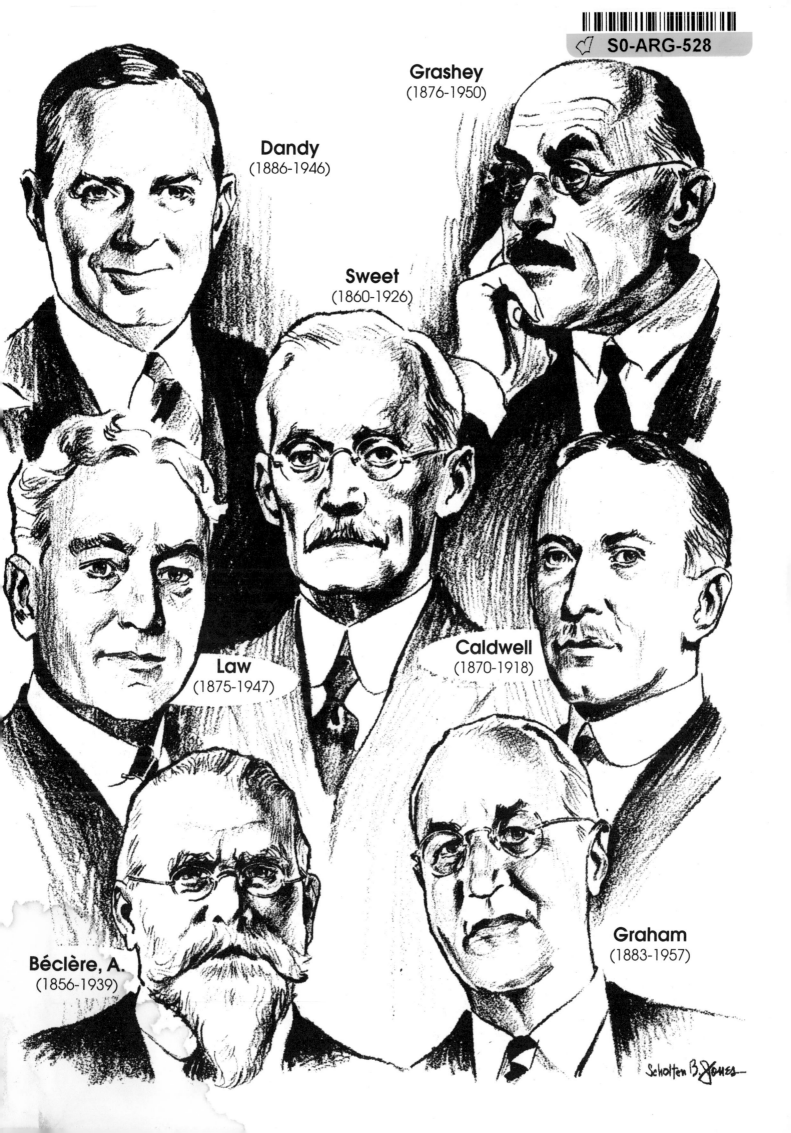

Grashey
(1876-1950)

Dandy
(1886-1946)

Sweet
(1860-1926)

Law
(1875-1947)

Caldwell
(1870-1918)

Béclère, A.
(1856-1939)

Graham
(1883-1957)

Scholten B. Jones

MERRILL'S ATLAS *of*

RADIOGRAPHIC POSITIONING & PROCEDURES

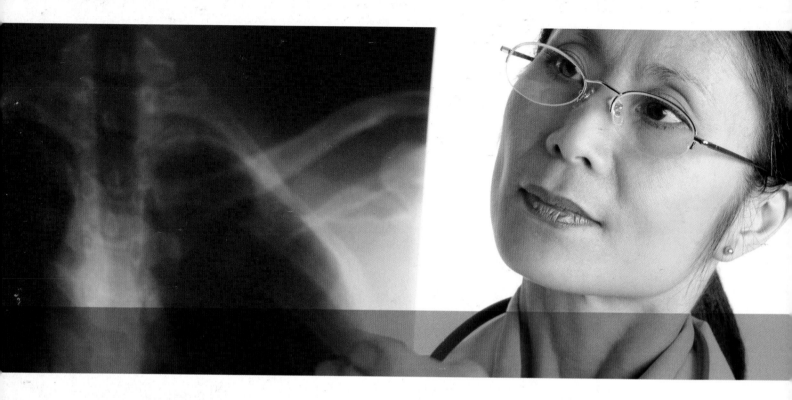

Twelfth Edition
Volume One

MERRILL'S ATLAS *of*

RADIOGRAPHIC POSITIONING & PROCEDURES

Eugene D. Frank, MA, RT(R), FASRT, FAEIRS
Retired Director, Radiography Program
Riverland Community College
Austin, Minnesota;
Assistant Professor of Radiology, Emeritus
Mayo Clinic College of Medicine
Rochester, Minnesota

Bruce W. Long, MS, RT(R)(CV), FASRT
Director and Associate Professor
Radiologic Imaging and Sciences Programs
Indiana University School of Medicine
Indianapolis, Indiana

Barbara J. Smith, MS, RT(R)(QM), FASRT, FAEIRS
Instructor, Radiologic Technology
Medical Imaging Department
Portland Community College
Portland, Oregon

ELSEVIER
MOSBY

ELSEVIER
MOSBY

3251 Riverport Lane
St. Louis, Missouri 63043

MERRILL'S ATLAS OF RADIOGRAPHIC POSITIONING AND PROCEDURES, EDITION 12

ISBN: 978-0-323-07321-9 (vol 1)
ISBN: 978-0-323-07322-6 (vol 2)
ISBN: 978-0-323-07323-3 (vol 3)
ISBN: 978-0-323-07334-9 (set)

Notices

Knowledge and best practice in this field are constantly changing. As new research and experience broaden our understanding, changes in research methods, professional practices, or medical treatment may become necessary.

Practitioners and researchers must always rely on their own experience and knowledge in evaluating and using any information, methods, compounds, or experiments described herein. In using such information or methods they should be mindful of their own safety and the safety of others, including parties for whom they have a professional responsibility.

With respect to any drug or pharmaceutical products identified, readers are advised to check the most current information provided (i) on procedures featured or (ii) by the manufacturer of each product to be administered, to verify the recommended dose or formula, the method and duration of administration, and contraindications. It is the responsibility of practitioners, relying on their own experience and knowledge of their patients, to make diagnoses, to determine dosages and the best treatment for each individual patient, and to take all appropriate safety precautions.

To the fullest extent of the law, neither the Publisher nor the authors, contributors, or editors, assume any liability for any injury and/or damage to persons or property as a matter of products liability, negligence or otherwise, or from any use or operation of any methods, products, instructions, or ideas contained in the material herein.

The Publisher

Library of Congress Cataloging-in-Publication Data

Frank, Eugene D.
  Merrill's atlas of radiographic positioning & procedures.—12th ed. / Eugene D. Frank, Bruce W. Long, Barbara J. Smith.
      p. ; cm.
  Merrill's atlas of radiographic positioning and procedures
  Atlas of radiographic positioning & procedures
  Includes bibliographical references and index.
  ISBN 978-0-323-07334-9 (set : hardcover : alk. paper)—ISBN 978-0-323-07321-9 (v. 1 : hardcover : alk. paper) -- ISBN 978-0-323-07322-6 (v. 2 : hardcover : alk. paper)—ISBN 978-0-323-07323-3 (v. 3 : hardcover : alk. paper)
  1. Radiography, Medical—Positioning—Atlases. I. Long, Bruce W. II. Smith, Barbara J.
III. Merrill, Vinita, 1905-1977. IV. Title. V. Title: Merrill's atlas of radiographic positioning and procedures. VI. Title: Atlas of radiographic positioning & procedures. [DNLM: 1. Technology, Radiologic—Atlases. 2. Diagnostic Imaging—Atlases. WN 17]
  RC78.4.F736 2012
  616.07'572--dc22

                                                    2010042965

Publisher: Jeanne Olson
Senior Developmental Editor: Linda Woodard
Publishing Services Manager: Catherine Jackson
Project Manager: Carol O'Connell
Cover Designer: Amy Buxton
Text Designer: Amy Buxton

Printed in the United States of America
Last digit is the print number: 9 8 7 6 5 4 3 2 1

PREVIOUS AUTHORS

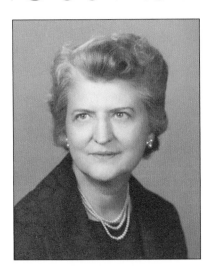

Vinita Merrill
1905-1977

Vinita Merrill was born in Oklahoma in 1905 and died in New York City in 1977. Vinita began compilation of Merrill's in 1936 while she worked as Technical Director and Chief Technologist in the Department of Radiology, and Instructor in the School of Radiography at the New York Hospital. In 1949, while employed as Director of the Educational Department of Picker X-ray Corporation, she wrote the first edition of the *Atlas of Roentgenographic Positions.* She completed three more editions from 1959 to 1975. Sixty-two years later Vinita's work lives on in the twelfth edition of *Merrill's Atlas of Radiographic Positioning & Procedures.*

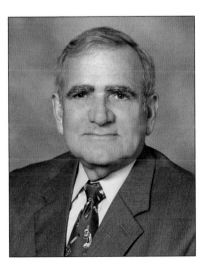

Philip W. Ballinger, PhD, RT(R), FAEIRS, FASRT, became the author of *Merrill's Atlas* in its fifth edition, which published in 1982. He served as author through the tenth edition, helping to launch successful careers for thousands of students who have learned radiographic positioning from *Merrill's.* Phil is now Assistant Professor Emeritus in the Radiologic Technology Division of the School of Allied Medical Professions at The Ohio State University. In 1995 he retired after a 25-year career as Radiography Program Director, and, after ably guiding *Merrill's Atlas* through six editions, he retired as *Merrill's* author. Phil continues to be involved in professional activities, such as speaking engagements at state, national, and international meetings.

THE MERRILL'S TEAM

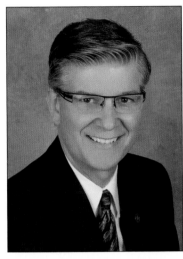

Eugene D. Frank, MA, RT(R), FASRT, FAEIRS, retired from the Mayo Clinic/Foundation in Rochester, Minnesota, in 2001, after 31 years of employment. He was Assistant Professor of Radiology in the College of Medicine and Director of the Radiography Program. He also served as Director of the Radiography Program at Riverland Community College, Austin, Minnesota, for six years before retiring in 2007. He is a Life Member in his state society and in the AEIRS. In addition to being coauthor of Merrill's, he is the coauthor of two radiography textbooks *(Quality Control in Diagnostic Imaging* and *Radiography Essentials for Limited Practice),* two radiography workbooks, and two chapters in other texts. The twelfth edition is Gene's fourth on the Merrill's team.

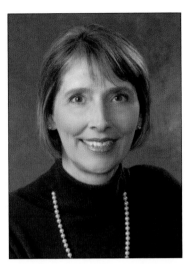

Barbara J. Smith, MS, RT(R)(QM), FASRT, FAEIRS, is an instructor in the Radiologic Technology program at Portland Community College, where she has taught for 26 years. The Oregon Society of Radiologic Technologists inducted her as a Life Member in 2003. She presents at state, regional, and national meetings and is involved in professional activities at these levels. Her publication activities include articles, book reviews, and chapter contributions. As coauthor, her primary role on the Merrill's team is working with the contributing authors and editing Volume 3. The twelfth edition is Barb's second on the Merrill's team.

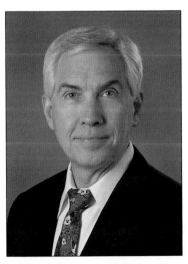

Bruce W. Long, MS, RT(R)(CV), FASRT, is Director and Associate Professor of the Indiana University Radiologic and Imaging Sciences Programs, where he has taught for 25 years. A Life Member of the Indiana Society of Radiologic Technologists, he frequently presents at state and national professional meetings. His publication activities include 28 articles in national professional journals and two books, *Orthopaedic Radiography* and *Radiography Essentials for Limited Practice,* in addition to being coauthor of the atlas. The twelfth edition is Bruce's second on the Merrill's team.

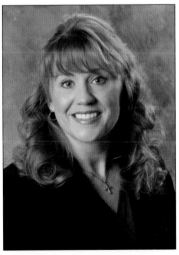

Jeannean Hall Rollins, MRC, BSRT(R)(CV), is an Associate Professor in the Medical Imaging and Radiation Sciences department at Arkansas State University, where she has taught for 18 years. She is involved in the imaging profession at local, state, and national levels. Her publication activities include articles, book reviews, and chapter contributions. Jeannean's first contribution to *Merrill's Atlas* was on the tenth edition as co-author of the trauma radiography chapter. Her primary role on the Merrill's team is writing the Workbook, Mosby's Radiography Online, and the Instructor Resources that accompany *Merrill's Atlas.* The twelfth edition is Jeannean's second on the Merrill's team.

ADVISORY BOARD

This edition of *Merrill's Atlas* benefits from the expertise of a special advisory board. The following board members have provided professional input and advice and have helped the authors make decisions about atlas content throughout the preparation of the twelfth edition:

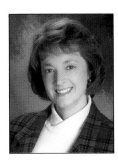

Andrea J. Cornuelle, MS, RT(R)
Professor, Radiologic Technology
Director, Health Science Program
Northern Kentucky University
Highland Heights, Kentucky

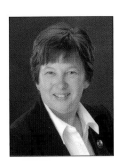

Lynn M. Foss, RT(R), ACR, DipEd, BHS
Instructor, Saint John School of
Radiological Technology
Horizon Health Network
Saint John, New Brunswick, Canada

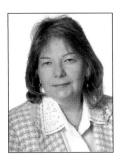

Diedre Costic, MPS, RT(R)(M)
Associate Professor Emeritus
Orange County Community College
Middleton, New York
Adjunct Faculty
Mount Aloysius College
DuBois, Pennsylvania

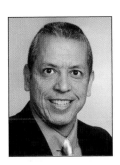

Joe A. Garza, MS, RT(R)
Associate Professor, Radiography
Program
Lone Star College—Montgomery
Conroe, Texas

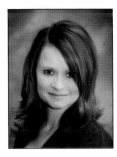

Tammy Curtis, MSRS, RT(R)
Associate Professor and Clinical
Coordinator
Radiologic Sciences
Northwestern State University
Shreveport, Louisiana

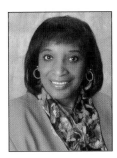

Ms. Johnnie B. Moore, MEd, RT(R)
Chair, Radiography Program—Retired
The former Barnes-Jewish College
of Nursing and Allied Health—
Mallinckrodt Institute of Radiology
St. Louis, Missouri

CONTRIBUTORS

Valerie F. Andolina, RT(R)(M)
Imaging Technology Manager
Elizabeth Wende Breast Care, LLC
Rochester, New York

Albert Aziza, MRT(R), MHSc, BHA, BSc
Manager, Imaging Guided Therapy, MRI, MEG
The Hospital for Sick Children
Toronto, Canada

Peter J. Barger, MS, RT(R)(CT)
Radiography Program Director
Southeast Missouri Hospital
College of Nursing and Health Sciences
Cape Girardeau, Missouri

Terri Bruckner, MA, RT(R)(CV)
Clinical Instructor and Clinical
   Coordinator
Radiologic Sciences and Therapy
   Division
The Ohio State University
Columbus, Ohio

Leila A. Bussman-Yeakel, MEd, RT(R)(T)
Director, Radiation Therapy Program
Mayo School of Health Sciences
Mayo Clinic College of Medicine
Rochester, Minnesota

Ellen Charkot, MRT(R)
Director, Diagnostic Imaging
The Hospital for Sick Children
Toronto, Ontario

Cheryl DuBose, MSRS, RT(R)(MR)(CT)(QM)
Assistant Professor
Program Director, MRI Program
Department of Medical Imaging and
   Radiation Sciences
Arkansas State University
Jonesboro, Arkansas

Michael L. Grey, PhD, RT(R)(MR)(CT)
Associate Professor
Radiologic Sciences Program
Southern Illinois University
Carbondale, Illinois

Steven C. Jensen, PhD
Director, Radiologic Sciences Program
Southern Illinois University
Carbondale, Illinois

Sara A. Kaderlik, RT(R), (VI), RCIS
Special Procedures Radiographer
St. Charles Medical Center
Bend, Oregon

Lois J. Layne, MSHA, RT(R)(CV)
Methodist Medical Center of Oak Ridge
Manager of Interventional Services
Oak Ridge, Tennessee

Eric P. Matthews, PhD, RT(R)(CV)(MR), EMT
Assistant Professor, Radiologic Sciences
   Program
Southern Illinois University
Carbondale, Illinois

Elton A. Mosman, MBA, CNMT, PET
Director, Nuclear Medicine Program
Mayo Clinic College of Medicine
Rochester, Minnesota

Sandra J. Nauman, MS, RT(R)(M)
Program Director, Radiography Program
Riverland Community College
Austin, Minnesota

Susanna L. Ovel, RT(R), RDMS, RVT
Sonographer, Clinical Instructor
Radiological Associates of Sacramento
Elk Grove, California

Paula Pate-Schloder, MS, RT(R)(CV)(CT)(VI)
Associate Professor, Medical Imaging
   Department
Misericordia University
Dallas, Pennsylvania

Bartram J. Pierce, BS, RT(R)(MR)
MRI Supervisor
Good Samaritan Regional Medical
   Center
Corvallis, Oregon

Jeannean Hall Rollins, MRC, BSRT(R)(CV)
Associate Professor
Department of Medical Imaging
   and Radiation Sciences
Arkansas State University
Jonesboro, Arkansas

Sharon R. Wartenbee, RT(R)(BD), CDT, FASRT
Senior Diagnostic and Bone
   Densitometry Technologist
McGreevy Clinic Avera
Sioux Falls, South Dakota

Kari J. Wetterlin, MA, RT(R)
Lead Technologist, General and Surgical
   Radiology
Mayo Clinic/Foundation
Rochester, Minnesota

Gayle K. Wright, BS, RT(R)(MR)(CT)
Instructor, Radiography Program
CT Program Coordinator
Portland Community College
Portland, Oregon

IN MEMORIAM

Sharon A. Coffee, MS, RT(R)

Contributing author Sharon Coffee of Houston, Texas, died in March 2007 at age 67 of kidney disease. She was an instructor in the radiography program at Houston Community College. Sharon cowrote the first text of the Trauma chapter with Jeannean Hall Rollins in 2003 and coauthored the chapter for two editions of the Atlas. Sharon was a nationally recognized trauma radiographer who had one of the most extensive collections of trauma radiographs, many of which are in *Merrill's*.

Joel A. Permar, RT(R)

Contributing author Joel Permar of Birmingham, Alabama, died in April 2008 at age 40 of colon cancer. Joel was a surgical radiographer at the University of Alabama Hospital in Birmingham. Joel cowrote the first text of the Surgical Radiography chapter in 2003 with Kari Wetterlin and coauthored the chapter for two editions of the *Atlas*.

PREFACE

Welcome to the twelfth edition of *Merrill's Atlas of Radiographic Positioning and Procedures.* The twelfth edition continues the tradition of excellence begun in 1949, when Vinita Merrill wrote the first edition of what has become a classic text. Over the last 62 years, *Merrill's Atlas* has provided a strong foundation in anatomy and positioning for thousands of students around the world who have gone on to successful careers as imaging technologists. *Merrill's Atlas* is also a mainstay for everyday reference in imaging departments all over the world. As the coauthors of the twelfth edition, we are honored to follow in Vinita Merrill's footsteps.

Learning and Perfecting Positioning Skills

Merrill's Atlas has an established tradition of helping students learn and perfect their positioning skills. After covering preliminary steps in radiography, radiation protection, and terminology in introductory chapters, the first two volumes of *Merrill's* then teaches anatomy and positioning in separate chapters for each bone group or organ system. The student learns to position the patient properly so that the resulting radiograph provides the information the physician needs to correctly diagnose the patient's problem. The atlas presents this information for commonly requested projections, as well as those less commonly requested, making it the only reference of its kind in the world.

The third volume of the atlas provides basic information about a variety of special imaging modalities, such as mobile, surgical, geriatrics, computed tomography, cardiac catheterization, magnetic resonance imaging, sonography, nuclear medicine technology, and radiation therapy.

Merrill's Atlas is not only a comprehensive resource for students to learn from but also an indispensable reference as they move into the clinical environment and ultimately into their practice as imaging professionals.

New to This Edition

Since the first edition of *Merrill's Atlas* in 1949, many changes have occurred. This new edition incorporates many significant changes designed not only to reflect the technologic progress and advancements in the profession but also to meet the needs of today's radiography students. The major changes in this edition are highlighted as follows.

WORKING WITH THE OBESE PATIENT

Many in the profession, especially students, requested that we include material on how to work with obese and morbidly obese patients. *Joe Garza* of our Advisory Board conducted initial research on the topic and prepared the master outline for a new section. With input from a wide variety of educators and practitioners, we are pleased to state that *Merrill's* now includes an extensive illustrated section in Chapter 1 on working effectively with this growing segment of the population.

DIGITAL RADIOGRAPHY COLLIMATION

With the expanding use of digital radiography (DR) and the decline in the use of plates and cassettes in Bucky mechanisms, concern was raised regarding the collimation sizes for the various projections. With collimation considered one of the critical aspects of obtaining an optimal image, especially with CR and DR, this edition contains the specific collimation sizes that students and radiographers should use when using manual collimation with DR in-room and DR mobile systems. The correct collimation size for projections is now included as a separate head.

ENGLISH/METRIC IR SIZES

English and metric sizes for image receptors (IRs) continue to challenge radiographers and authors in the absence of a standardized national system. With film/screen technology there was a trend toward metric for most of the cassette sizes. However, with computed radiography (CR) and digital radiography (DR) there has been a trend back to English sizes. Most of the DR x-ray systems use English for collimator settings. With this trend, the IR sizes and collimation settings for all projections are stated in English with metric in parentheses.

SECTIONAL ANATOMY CHAPTER

With the growing use of computed tomography (CT) and magnetic resonance imaging (MRI), the Sectional Anatomy chapter has been updated with new images and matching art. This revised chapter is comprehensive enough to learn all the essential aspects of cross-sectional anatomy.

CT AND MRI CHAPTERS

With CT slowly working its way into the curriculum, the CT chapter had been updated with the basic protocols for the most common examinations done. The CT and MRI chapters have been updated with many new images to reflect the current state-of-art images in these modalities.

INTEGRATION OF CT AND MRI

In the past two editions, both CT and MRI images have been included in the anatomy and projection pages. This edition continues the trend of having students learn cross-section anatomy with regular anatomy. Over 40 additional CT and MRI images are included in every chapter of this edition.

NEW ILLUSTRATIONS

Many who use *Merrill's* in teaching and learning have stated that the line art is one of the most useful aspects in learning new projections. Many new illustrations have been added to all chapters in this edition to enable the user to comprehend bone position, central ray (CR) direction, and body angulations.

REVISED VERTEBRAL ART

Learning cross-sectional anatomy as shown in CT and MRI images is now commonplace in radiography classrooms. CT and MRI anatomy is displayed in a very specific manner with the spine "down" and the anterior aspect of the body "up." To enable students to learn anatomy as seen in radiology department, the vertebral body art in Chapter 8 has been turned so that the spine is down instead of up. All anatomical art in the *Atlas* is standardized to CT and MRI imaging.

SIMPLIFIED SHOULDER GIRDLE CHAPTER

The projections in this chapter have been rearranged in a more user-friendly manner. All projections are now arranged by body part.

SIMPLIFIED DIGESTIVE SYSTEM CHAPTERS

The material in Chapter 16 is now focused exclusively on the abdomen, improving instructional delivery for educators and increasing learning for the radiography student. Chapter 17 now includes all material related to the digestive system, with the transfer of biliary system content to this chapter.

COMPENSATING FILTERS CHAPTER

This edition of *Merrill's* is the second in which the new Compensating Filters chapter has been included. We have added a new commonly used filter for the foot, with and without images, to help students understand the importance of the use of filters in positioning.

NEW PATIENT PHOTOGRAPHY

New patient positioning photographs are included in Chapters 10 and 22. These new photographs show positioning detail to a greater extent. In addition, the equipment in these photos is the most modern available and computed radiography plates are used. The use of electronic central ray angles enables a better understanding of where the central ray should enter the patient. Scott Slinkard, from the Southeast Missouri Hospital College of Nursing and Health Sciences, Cape Girardeau, Missouri, provided the photographs.

DIGITAL RADIOGRAPHY UPDATED

Because of the rapid expansion and acceptance of computed radiography (CR) and direct digital radiography (DR), either selected positioning considerations and modifications or special instructions are indicated where necessary. A special icon alerts the reader to digital notes. The icon is shown here:

COMPUTED RADIOGRAPHY

OBSOLETE PROJECTIONS DELETED

Projections identified as obsolete by the authors and the advisory board continue to be deleted. A summary is provided at the beginning of any chapter containing deleted projections so that the reader may refer to previous editions for information. Continued advances in CT, MRI, and ultrasound have prompted these deletions.

CHAPTERS DELETED OR MERGED

The Tomography chapter has been eliminated from the atlas beginning with this edition. Very few, if any, tomogram procedures are done in today's radiology department. Tomograms are done with some regularity for Intravenous Urography (IVU) and continue to be described in Chapter 18.

NEW RADIOGRAPHS

Nearly every chapter contains new and additional optimum radiographs, including many that demonstrate pathology. With the addition of new radiographic images, the twelfth edition has the most comprehensive collection of high-quality radiographs available to students and practitioners.

NEW PHOTOGRAPHY

Many new color anatomy, patient positioning, or procedure-related photographs have been added. These added or replacement photographs aid students in learning radiography positioning concepts.

Learning Aids for the Student
POCKET GUIDE TO RADIOGRAPHY

The new edition of *Merrill's Pocket Guide to Radiography* complements the revision of *Merrill's Atlas*. In addition to instructions for positioning the patient and the body part for all the essential projections, the new pocket guide includes information on digital radiography and exposure indexes for use with CR and DR. A new Collimation header had been added that state the exact sizings needed for the projections. Tabs have been added to help the user locate the beginning of each section. Space is provided for writing department techniques specific to the user.

RADIOGRAPHIC ANATOMY, POSITIONING, AND PROCEDURES WORKBOOK

The new edition of this workbook features extensive review and self-assessment exercises that cover the first 31 chapters in *Merrill's Atlas* in one convenient volume. The features of the previous editions, including anatomy labeling exercises, positioning exercises, and self-tests, are still available, but this edition features more image evaluations to give students additional opportunities to evaluate radiographs for proper positioning and more positioning questions to complement the workbook's strong anatomy review. The comprehensive multiple-choice tests at the end of each chapter help students assess their comprehension of the whole chapter. New exercises in this edition focus on improved understanding of essential projections and the necessity of appropriate collimated field sizes for digital imaging. Additionally, review and assessment exercises in this edition have been expanded for the Pediatrics, Geriatrics, Vascular and Interventional Radiography, Sectional Anatomy, and Computed Tomography chapters in Volume 3. Exercises in these chapters will help students learn the theory and concepts of these special techniques with greater ease.

Teaching Aids for the Instructor
EVOLVE INSTRUCTOR ELECTRONIC RESOURCES

This comprehensive resource provides valuable tools, such as lesson plans, power point slides, and an electronic test bank, for teaching an anatomy and positioning class. The test bank includes more than 1500 questions, each coded by category and level of difficulty. Four exams are already compiled within the test bank to be used "as is" at the instructor's discretion. The instructor also has the option of building new tests as often as desired by pulling questions from the Examview pool or using a combination of questions from the test bank and questions that the instructor adds.

Evolve may be used to publish the class syllabus, outlines, and lecture notes; set up "virtual office hours" and e-mail communication; share important dates and information through the online class Calendar; and encourage student participation through Chat Rooms and Discussion Boards. Evolve allows instructors to post exams and manage their grade books online. For more information, visit http://www.evolve.elsevier.com or contact an Elsevier sales representative.

MOSBY'S RADIOGRAPHY ONLINE

Mosby's Radiography Online: Anatomy and Positioning is a well-developed online course companion that includes animations with narration and interactive activities and exercises to assist in the understanding of anatomy and positioning. Used in conjunction with the *Merrill's Atlas* textbook, it offers greater learning opportunities while accommodating diverse learning styles and circumstances. This unique program promotes problem-based learning with the goal of developing critical thinking skills that will be needed in the clinical setting.

EVOLVE—ONLINE COURSE MANAGEMENT

Evolve is an interactive learning environment designed to work in coordination with *Merrill's Atlas*. Instructors may use Evolve to provide an Internet-based course component that reinforces and expands on the concepts delivered in class.

We hope you will find this edition of *Merrill's Atlas of Radiographic Positioning and Procedures* the best ever. Input from generations of readers has helped to keep the atlas strong through ten editions, and we welcome your comments and suggestions. We are constantly striving to build on Vinita Merrill's work, and we trust that she would be proud and pleased to know that the work she began 62 years ago is still so appreciated and valued by the imaging sciences community.

Eugene D. Frank
Bruce W. Long
Barbara J. Smith
and Jeannean Hall Rollins

ACKNOWLEDGMENTS

In preparing for the twelfth edition, our advisory board continually provided professional expertise and aid in decision making on the revision of this edition. The advisory board members are listed on p. vii. We are most grateful for their input and contributions to this edition of the *Atlas.*

Scott Slinkard, a radiography student from the College of Nursing and Health Sciences in Cape Girardeau, Missouri, and a professional photographer, provided many of the new photographs seen throughout the *Atlas.*

Reviewers

The group of radiography professionals listed below reviewed aspects of this edition of the *Atlas* and made many insightful suggestions for strengthening the *Atlas.* We are most appreciative of their willingness to lend their expertise.

Dennis Bowman, RT(R)
Community Hospital of Monterey
  Peninsula
Monterey, California

Timothy Daly, BS, RT(R)
Mayo Clinic Foundation
Rochester, Minnesota

Scott Davis, RT(R)(QM)
Providence St. Vincent Medical Center
Portland, Oregon

Patricia Duffy, MPS, RT(R)(CT)
Clinical Education Coordinator
SUNY Upstate Medical University
Syracuse, New York

Dan Ferlic, RT(R)
Ferlic Filters
White Bear Lake, Minnesota

M. Elia Flores, MEd, RT(R)
Program Director
Blinn College
Bryan, Texas

Henrique da Guia Costa, MBA, RT(R)
Radiographer
Radiography Consultant
Lisbon, Portugal

Susan Herron, AS, RT(R)
Wishard Memorial Hospital
Indianapolis, Indiana

James Johnston, MS, RT(R)
Midwestern State University
Wichita Falls, Texas

Robin Jones, MS, RT(R)
Indiana University Northwest
Gary, Indiana

Dimitris Koumoranos, MSc, RT(R)(CT) (MR)
Radiographer
General Hospital Elpis
Athens, Greece

Elise LeBlanc, BHSc, RT(R)
QEII Health Sciences Center
Halifax, Nova Scotia, Canada

Seiji Nishio, BA, RT(R)
Radiographer
Komazawa University
Tokyo, Japan

Ann Obergfell, JD, RT(R)
St. Catherine College
St. Catherine, Kentucky

Roger Preston, MSRS, RT(R)
Reid Hospital & Health Care Services
Richmond, Indiana

J. Louis Rankin, BS, RT(R)(MR)
St. Francis Hospital
Indianapolis, Indiana

Bill Ruskin
Instructor
Medical Diagnostics
Saskatchewan Institute of Applied
  Science and Technology
Saskatoon, Canada

Jennifer Stayner
Red River College
Winnepig, Manitoba, Canada

Andrew Woodward MA, RT(R)(CT) (QM)(ARRT)
Assistant Professor and Clinical
  Coordinator
University of North Carolina at Chapel
  Hill
Chapel Hill, North Carolina

Beth Vealé, MEd, RT(R)(QM)
Midwestern State University
Wichita Falls, Texas

CONTENTS

1

PRELIMINARY STEPS IN RADIOGRAPHY

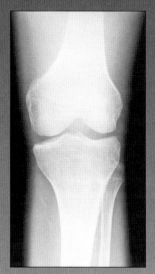
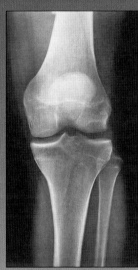
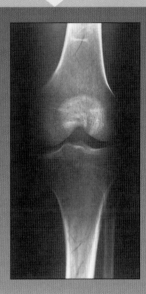

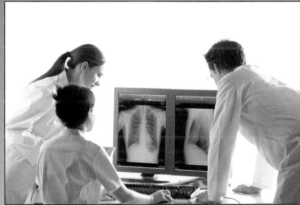

Ethics in Radiologic Technology

Ethics is the term applied to a health professional's moral responsibility and the science of appropriate conduct toward others. The work of the medical professional requires strict rules of conduct. The physician, who is responsible for the welfare of the patient, depends on the absolute honesty and integrity of all health care professionals to carry out orders and report mistakes.

The American Society of Radiologic Technologists (ASRT) developed the current code of ethics.[1] The Canadian Association of Medical Radiation Technologists (CAMRT) has adopted a similar code of ethics.[2] All radiographers should familiarize themselves with these codes.

AMERICAN SOCIETY OF RADIOLOGIC TECHNOLOGISTS CODE OF ETHICS

1. The radiologic technologist conducts himself or herself in a professional manner, responds to patient needs, and supports colleagues and associates in providing quality patient care.
2. The radiologic technologist acts to advance the principal objective of the profession to provide services to humanity with full respect for the dignity of humankind.
3. The radiologic technologist delivers patient care and service unrestricted by concerns of personal attributes or the nature of the disease or illness, and without discrimination, regardless of gender, race, creed, religion, or socioeconomic status.
4. The radiologic technologist practices technology founded on theoretic knowledge and concepts, uses equipment and accessories consistent with the purpose for which they have been designed, and employs procedures and techniques appropriately.
5. The radiologic technologist assesses situations; exercises care, discretion, and judgment; assumes responsibility for professional decisions; and acts in the best interest of the patient.
6. The radiologic technologist acts as an agent through observation and communication to obtain pertinent information for the physician to aid in the diagnosis and treatment management of the patient. He or she recognizes that interpretation and diagnosis are outside the scope of practice for the profession.
7. The radiologic technologist uses equipment and accessories; employs techniques and procedures; performs services in accordance with an accepted standard of practice; and demonstrates expertise in minimizing radiation exposure to the patient, self, and other members of the health care team.
8. The radiologic technologist practices ethical conduct appropriate to the profession and protects the patient's right to quality radiologic technology care.
9. The radiologic technologist respects confidence entrusted in the course of professional practice, respects the patient's right to privacy, and reveals confidential information only as required by law or to protect the welfare of the individual or the community.
10. The radiologic technologist continually strives to improve knowledge and skills by participating in educational and professional activities, sharing knowledge with colleagues, and investigating new and innovative aspects of professional practice.

CANADIAN ASSOCIATION OF MEDICAL RADIATION TECHNOLOGISTS CODE OF ETHICS

The CAMRT recognizes its obligation to identify and promote professional standards of conduct and performance. The execution of such standards is the personal responsibility of each member.

The code of ethics, adopted in June 1991, requires all members to do the following:

- Provide service with dignity and respect to all people regardless of race, national or ethnic origin, color, gender, religion, age, type of illness, and mental or physical challenges.
- Encourage the trust and confidence of the public through high standards of professional competence, conduct, and appearance.
- Conduct all technical procedures with due regard to current radiation safety standards.
- Practice only those procedures for which the necessary qualifications are held unless such procedures have been properly delegated by an appropriate medical authority and for which the technologist has received adequate training to an acceptable level of competence.
- Practice only those disciplines of medical radiation technology for which he or she has been certified by the CAMRT and is currently competent.
- Be mindful that patients must seek diagnostic information from their treating physician. In those instances where a discreet comment to the appropriate authority may assist diagnosis or treatment, the technologist may feel morally obliged to provide one.
- Preserve and protect the confidentiality of any information, either medical or personal, acquired through professional contact with the patient. An exception may be appropriate when the disclosure of such information is necessary to the treatment of the patient or the safety of other patients and health care providers or is a legal requirement.
- Cooperate with other health care providers.
- Advance the art and science of medical radiation technology through ongoing professional development.
- Recognize that the participation and support of our association is a professional responsibility.

Image Receptor

In radiography, the *image receptor* (IR) is the device that receives the energy of the x-ray beam and forms the image of the body part. In diagnostic radiology, the IR is one of the following five devices:

---

[1]Code of ethics, ASRT, February 2003.
[2]CAMRT, Approved, June 2008.

1. *Cassette with film:* A device that contains special intensifying screens that glow when struck by x-rays and imprints the x-ray image on film. The use of a darkroom, where the film is developed in a processor, is required. Afterward the radiographic film image is ready for viewing on an illuminator (Fig. 1-1, *A*).

2. *Image plate* (IP): A device, used for computed radiography (CR), similar to a conventional intensifying screen. The IP is housed in a specially designed cassette that contains special phosphorus to store the x-ray image. The IP is a component of the new "digital" imaging systems. The cassette is inserted into a reader device, which scans the IP with a laser. The radiographic image is converted to digital format and is viewed on a computer monitor or printed on film (Fig. 1-1, *B*).

3. *Solid-state detectors:* A flat panel thin-film transistor (TFT) detector or a charge-coupled device (CCD) used for direct digital radiography (DR). This type of digital imaging system is called "cassetteless" because it does not use a cassette or an IP. The flat panel detector or CCD built into the x-ray table or other device captures the x-ray image and converts it directly into digital format. The image is viewed on a computer monitor or printed on film (Fig. 1-1, *C*). This is the fastest processing system with images available in 6 seconds or less. The DR flat panel detector is a component of the new "digital" imaging systems.

4. *Portable digital radiography:* A portable, lightweight DR system that can be used for lateral and axial imaging of limbs and for trauma and bedside applications. Its 14 × 17 inches (35 × 43 cm) size is large enough for chest and abdomen images. The unit can be tethered to the computer via Ethernet, or the newest systems allow wireless transmission (Fig. 1-1, *D*).

5. *Fluoroscopic screen:* X-rays strike a fluoroscopic screen, where the image is formed and is transmitted to a television monitor via a camera. This is a "real-time" device in which the body part is viewed live on a television (Fig. 1-1, *E*).

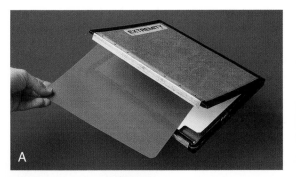
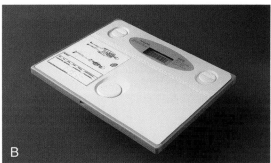
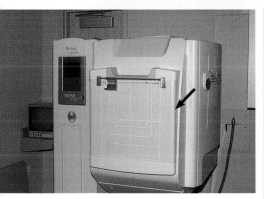
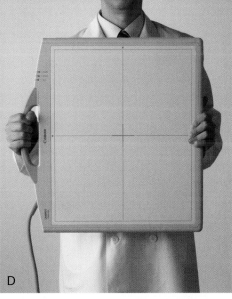
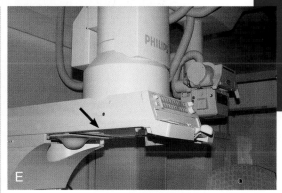

Fig. 1-1 Image receptors. **A,** Conventional radiographic cassette, opened and showing a sheet of x-ray film. **B,** CR cassette. This contains a storage-phosphor image plate that stores x-ray image. **C,** DR chest x-ray machine. A flat panel detector is located behind the unit (*arrow*) and stores x-ray image. **D,** Portable DR system is lightweight and can be carried anywhere for obtaining fast images. **E,** Fluoroscopic screen located under fluoroscopic tower (*arrow*) transmits x-ray image to a camera and then to a television for real-time viewing.

(**D,** Courtesy Canon USA, Inc.)

Radiograph

Each step in performing a radiographic procedure must be completed accurately to ensure that the maximal amount of information is recorded on the image. The information that results from performing the radiographic examination generally shows the presence or absence of abnormality or trauma. This information assists in the diagnosis and treatment of the patient. Accuracy and attention to detail are essential in each radiologic examination.

The radiographer must be thoroughly familiar with the radiographic attenuation patterns cast by normal anatomy structures. To develop the ability to analyze radiographs properly and to correct or prevent errors in performing the examination, the radiographer should study radiographs from the following standpoints:

1. *Superimposition:* The relationship of the anatomic superimposition to size, shape, position, and angulation must be reviewed.
2. *Adjacent structures:* Each anatomic structure must be compared with adjacent structures and reviewed to ensure that the structure is present and properly shown.
3. *Optical density* (OD): OD is known as degree of blackening when associated with radiographic film and as brightness when describing appearance on a digital display monitor. The OD must be within a "diagnostic range" to display all desired anatomic structures. Images with ODs outside the diagnostic range (too light or too dark) are primarily associated with screen-film radiography (Fig. 1-2), although they are possible with digital imaging. The primary controlling factor for screen-film OD is milliampere-second (mAs). For digital imaging, the OD of displayed images is primarily controlled by automatic rescaling, so mAs selection affects patient radiation dose and image noise.
4. *Contrast:* The contrast, or the difference in density between any two areas on a radiograph, must be sufficient to allow radiographic distinction of adjacent structures with different tissue densities. A wide range of contrast levels is produced among the various radiographic examinations performed (Fig. 1-3). A low-contrast image displays many density levels, and a high-contrast image displays few density levels. The primary controlling factor of radiographic contrast is kilovoltage peak (kVp).
5. *Recorded detail:* The recorded detail, or the ability to visualize small structures, must be sufficient to show clearly the desired anatomic part (Fig. 1-4). Recorded detail is primarily controlled by the following:
   - Geometry
   - Film
   - IP phosphor (digital)
   - Flat panel detector (digital)
   - Distance
   - Screen
   - Focal spot size
   - Motion

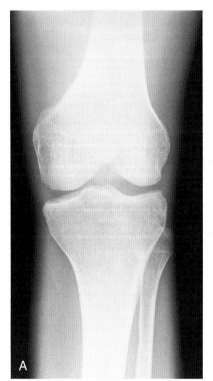 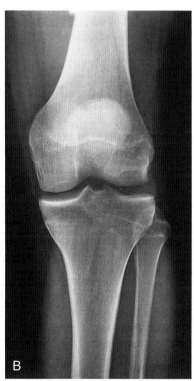 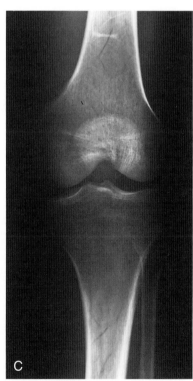

Fig. 1-2 Sufficient radiographic density is necessary to make a diagnosis. **A,** Radiograph of the knee with insufficient density. It is too light to make a diagnosis, and a repeat radiograph is necessary. **B,** Radiograph of the knee with proper density. All bony aspects of the knee are seen, including soft tissue detail around the bone. **C,** Radiograph of the knee with too much density—a diagnosis cannot be made, and a repeat radiograph is necessary.

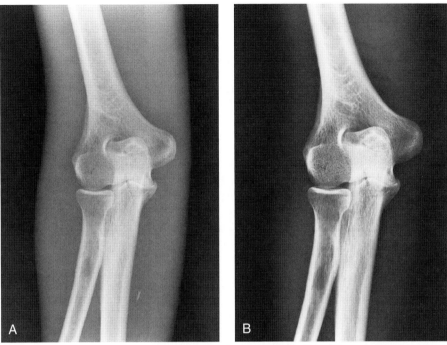

Fig. 1-3 Sufficient contrast is necessary to make a diagnosis. Two different scales of contrast are shown on the elbow. **A,** Long scale (low contrast). **B,** Short scale (high contrast).

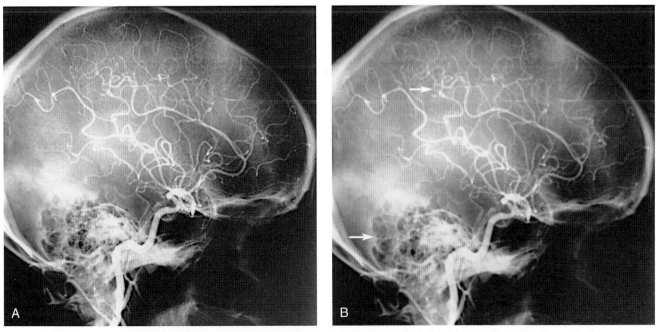

Fig. 1-4 Different levels of recorded detail. **A,** Excellent recorded detail is seen throughout this radiograph of the arteries in the head. **B,** Poor recorded detail. Note the fuzzy edges of the arteries and bony structures in this image (*arrows*).

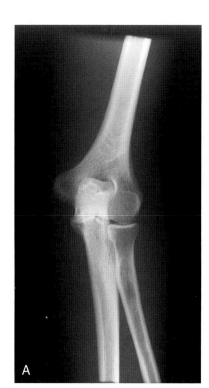
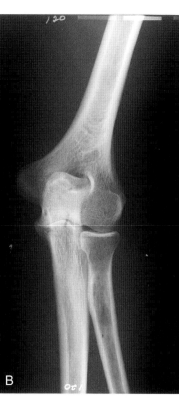

Fig. 1-5 Magnification of body part. **A,** AP projection of the elbow at normal magnification level. **B,** Same projection, with elbow magnified.

6. *Magnification:* The magnification of the body part must be evaluated, taking into account the controlling factors of *object–to–image receptor distance* (OID), or how far the body part is from the IR, and *source–to–image receptor distance* (SID), or how far the x-ray tube is from the IR. All radiographs yield some degree of magnification because all body parts are three-dimensional (Fig. 1-5).

7. *Shape distortion:* The shape distortion of the body part must be analyzed, and the following primary controlling factors must be studied:
   • Alignment
   • Central ray
   • Anatomic part
   • IR
   • Angulation

   An example of shape distortion is when a bone is projected longer or shorter than it actually is. *Distortion* is the misrepresentation of the size or shape of any anatomic structure (Fig. 1-6).

   A strong knowledge of anatomy and the ability to analyze radiographs correctly are paramount—especially to radiographers who work without a radiologist in constant attendance. In this situation, the patient's physician must be able to depend on the radiographer to perform the technical phase of examinations without assistance.

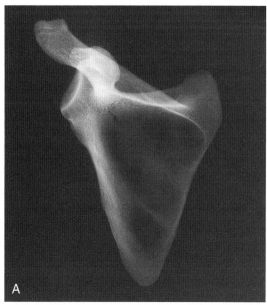
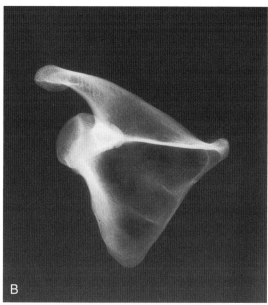

Fig. 1-6 Distortion of body part. **A,** Scapula bone nondistorted. **B,** Same bone projected shorter than in **A** and distorted.

DISPLAY OF RADIOGRAPHS

Radiographs are generally oriented on the display device according to the preference of the interpreting physician. Because methods of displaying radiographic images have developed largely through custom, no fixed rules have been established. The radiologist, who is responsible for making a diagnosis on the basis of the radiographic examination, and the radiographer, who performs the examination, follow traditional standards of practice, however, regarding the placement of radiographs on the viewing device. In clinical practice, the viewing device is commonly called a *viewbox,* or *illuminator,* for screen-film radiography and a display monitor for digital imaging.

ANATOMIC POSITION

Radiographs are usually oriented on the display device so that the person looking at the image sees the body part placed in the anatomic position. The *anatomic position* refers to the patient standing erect with the face and eyes directed forward, arms extended by the sides with the palms of the hands facing forward, heels together, and toes pointing anteriorly (Fig. 1-7). When the radiograph is displayed in this manner, the patient's left side is on the viewer's right side and vice versa (Fig. 1-8). Medical professionals always describe the body, a body part, or a body movement as though it were in the anatomic position.

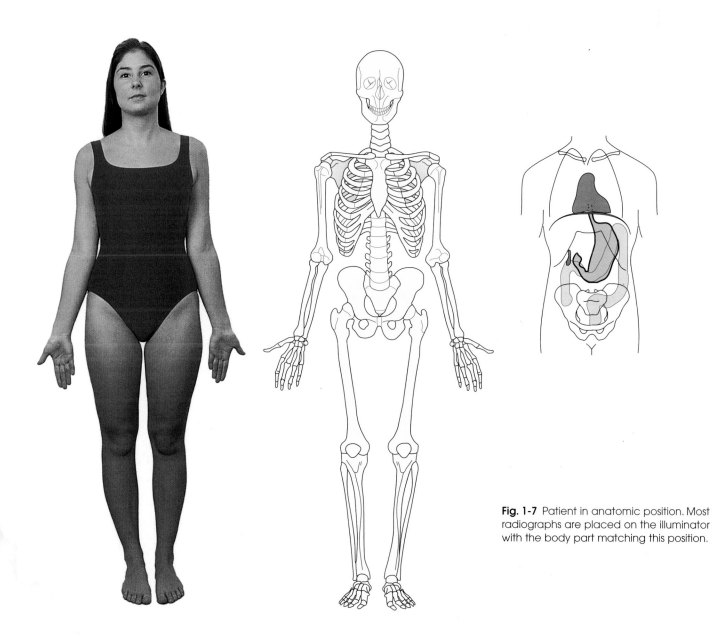

Fig. 1-7 Patient in anatomic position. Most radiographs are placed on the illuminator with the body part matching this position.

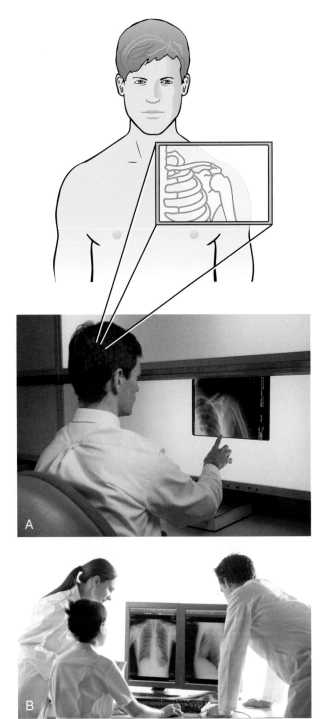

Fig. 1-8 A, Radiologist interpreting radiograph of a patient's left shoulder. Radiograph is placed on the illuminator with the patient's left side on the viewer's right side. The radiologist spatially pictured the patient's anatomy in the anatomic position and placed the radiograph on the illuminator in that position. **B,** Radiographs displayed correctly on a digital display. The same orientation rules apply to digital imaging.

(**B,** Courtesy Canon USA, Inc.)

Posteroanterior and anteroposterior radiographs

Fig. 1-9, *A*, illustrates the anterior (front) aspect of the patient's chest placed closest to the IR for a *posteroanterior* (PA) projection. Fig. 1-9, *B*, illustrates the posterior (back) aspect of the patient's chest placed closest to the IR for an *anteroposterior* (AP) projection. Regardless of whether the anterior or posterior body surface is closest to the IR, the radiograph is usually placed in the anatomic position (Fig. 1-10). (Positioning terminology is fully described in Chapter 3.)

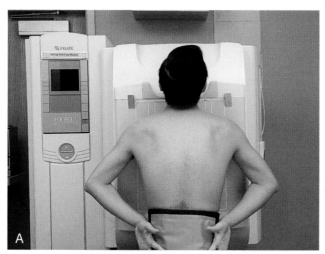
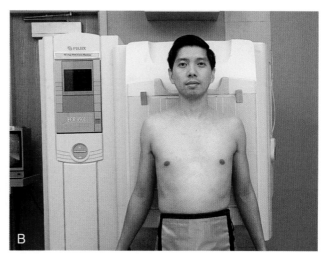

Fig. 1-9 A, Patient positioned for PA projection of the chest. Anterior aspect of the chest is closest to IR. **B,** Patient positioned for AP projection of the chest. Posterior aspect of the chest is closest to IR.

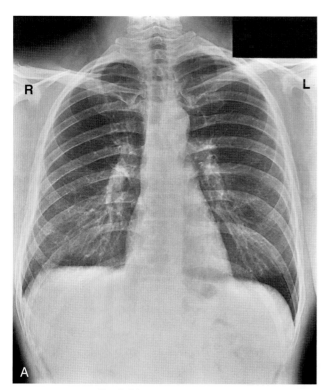
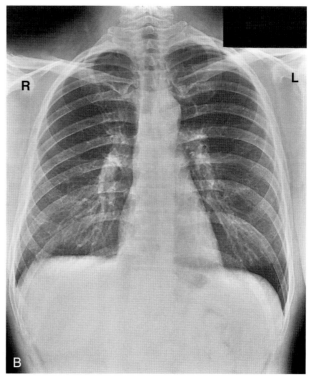

Fig. 1-10 A, PA projection of the chest. **B,** AP projection of the chest on the same patient as in **A.** Both radiographs are correctly displayed with the anatomy in the anatomic position even though the patient was positioned differently. Note the patient's left side is on your right, as though the patient were facing you.

Exceptions to these guidelines include the hands, fingers, wrists, feet, and toes. Hand, finger, and wrist radiographs are routinely displayed with the digits (fingers) pointed to the ceiling. Foot and toe radiographs are also placed on the illuminator with the toes pointing to the ceiling. Hand, finger, wrist, toe, and foot radiographs are viewed from the perspective of the x-ray tube, or exactly as the anatomy was projected onto the IR (Figs. 1-11 and 1-12). This perspective means that the individual looking at the radiograph is in the same position as the x-ray tube.

Lateral radiographs

Lateral radiographs are obtained with the patient's right or left side placed against the IR. The patient is generally placed on the illuminator in the same orientation as though the viewer were looking at the patient from the perspective of the x-ray tube at the side where the x-rays first enter the patient—exactly like radiographs of the hands, wrists, feet, and toes. Another way to describe this is to display the radiograph so that the side of the patient closest to the IR during the procedure is also the side in the image closest to the illuminator. A patient positioned for a left lateral chest radiograph is depicted in Fig. 1-13. The resulting left lateral chest radiograph is placed on the illuminator as shown in Fig. 1-14. A right lateral chest position and its accompanying radiograph would be positioned and displayed the opposite of that shown in Figs. 1-13 and 1-14.

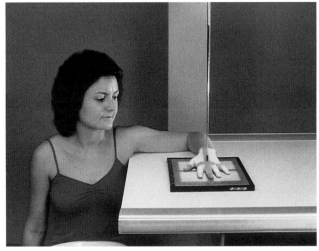

Fig. 1-11 Proper placement of patient and body part position for PA projection of the left hand.

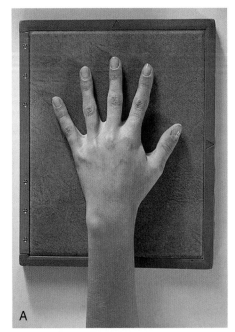 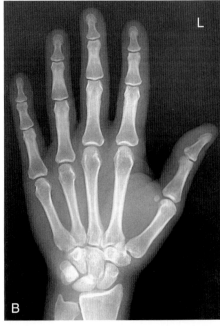

Fig. 1-12 A, Left hand positioned on IR. This view is from the perspective of the x-ray tube. **B,** Radiograph of the left hand is placed on illuminator in the same manner, with the digits pointed upward.

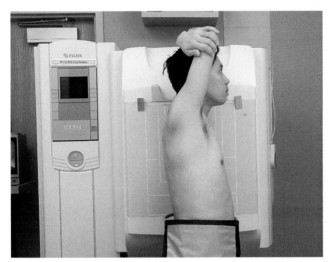

Fig. 1-13 Proper patient position for left lateral chest radiograph. The left side of the patient is placed against the IR.

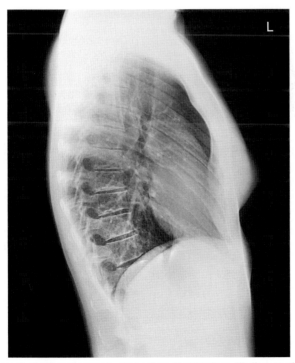

Fig. 1-14 Left lateral chest radiograph placed on illuminator with the anatomy seen from the perspective of the x-ray tube.

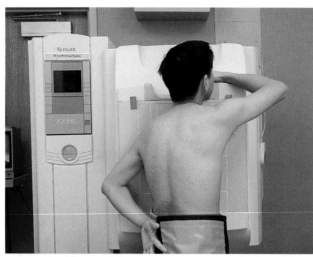

Fig. 1-15 A patient placed in left anterior oblique (LAO) position for PA oblique projection of chest.

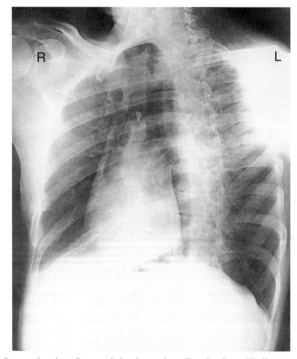

Fig. 1-16 PA oblique chest radiograph is placed on illuminator with the anatomy in the anatomic position. The patient's left side is on your right, as though the patient were facing you.

Oblique radiographs

Oblique radiographs are obtained when the patient's body is rotated so that the projection obtained is not frontal, posterior, or lateral (Fig. 1-15). These radiographs are viewed with the patient's anatomy placed in the anatomic position (Fig. 1-16).

Other radiographs

Many other less commonly performed radiographic projections are described throughout this atlas. The most common method of displaying the radiograph that is used in the radiology department and most clinical practice areas is generally either in the anatomic position or from the perspective of the x-ray tube; however, there are exceptions. Some physicians prefer to view all radiographs from the perspective of the x-ray tube rather than in the anatomic position. A neurosurgeon operates on the posterior aspect of the body and does not display spine radiographs in the anatomic position or from the perspective of the x-ray tube. The radiographs are displayed with the patient's right side on the surgeon's right side as though looking at the posterior aspect of the patient. What the surgeon sees on the radiograph is exactly what is seen in the open body part during surgery.

Clinical History

The radiographer is responsible for performing radiographic examinations according to the standard department procedure except when contraindicated by the patient's condition. The radiologist is a physician who is board certified to read, or interpret, x-ray examinations. As the demand for the radiologist's time increases, less time is available to devote to the technical aspects of radiology. This situation makes the radiologist more dependent on the radiographer to perform the technical aspects of patient care. The additional responsibility makes it necessary for the radiographer to know the following:

- Normal anatomy and normal anatomic variations so that the patient can be accurately positioned
- The radiographic characteristics of numerous common abnormalities

Although the radiographer is not responsible for explaining the cause, diagnosis, or treatment of the disease, the radiographer's professional responsibility is to produce an image that clearly shows the abnormality.

When the physician does not see the patient, the radiographer is responsible for obtaining the necessary clinical history and observing any apparent abnormality that might affect the radiographic result (Fig. 1-17). Examples include noting jaundice or swelling, body surface masses possibly casting a density that could be mistaken for internal changes, tattoos that contain ferrous pigment, surface scars that may be visible radiographically, and some decorative or ornamental clothing. The physician should give specific instructions about what information is necessary if the radiographer assumes this responsibility.

The requisition received by the radiographer should clearly identify the exact region to be radiographed and the suspected or existing diagnosis. The patient must be positioned and the exposure factors selected according to the region involved and the radiographic characteristics of the existent abnormality. Radiographers must understand the rationale behind the examination; otherwise, radiographs of diagnostic value cannot be produced. Having the information in advance prevents delay, inconvenience, and, more importantly, unnecessary radiation exposure to the patient.

With many institutions updating to electronic records, the radiographer may be using the computer system to enter information about the patient. In many of these information systems, the full patient' history may be accessed. The radiographer needs to observe rules of confidentiality.

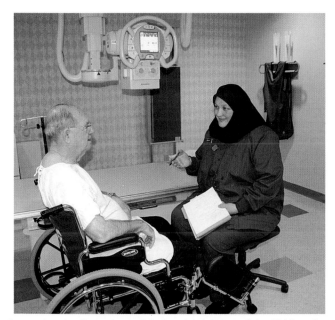

Fig. 1-17 Radiographer is often responsible for obtaining a clinical history from the patient.

Advanced Clinical Practice

In response to increased demands on the radiologist's time, a level of advanced clinical practice has developed for the radiographer. This advanced clinical role allows the radiographer to act as a "radiologist extender," similar to the physician assistant for a primary care physician. These radiographers take a leading role in patient care activities, perform selected radiologic procedures under the radiologist's supervision, and may be responsible for making initial image observations that are forwarded to the supervising radiologist for incorporation into the final report. The titles of *radiologist assistant* (RA) and *radiology practitioner assistant* (RPA) are currently used to designate radiographers who provide these advanced clinical services in the diagnostic imaging department. Requirements for practice include certification as a radiographer by the ARRT, pertinent additional education, and clinical experience under the supervision of a radiologist preceptor. RAs and RPAs also write advanced-level certification examinations.

Initial Examination

The radiographs obtained for the initial examination of each body part are based on the anatomy or function of the part and the type of abnormality indicated by the clinical history. The radiographs obtained for the initial examination are usually the minimum required to detect any demonstrable abnormality in the region. Supplemental studies for further investigation are made as needed. This method saves time, eliminates unnecessary radiographs, and reduces patient exposure to radiation.

Diagnosis and the Radiographer

A patient is naturally anxious about examination results and is likely to ask questions. The radiographer should tactfully advise the patient that the referring physician will receive the report as soon as the radiographs have been interpreted by the radiologist. Referring physicians may also ask the radiographer questions, and they should be instructed to contact the interpreting radiologist.

Care of the Radiographic Examining Room

The radiographic examining room should be as scrupulously clean as any other room used for medical purposes. The mechanical parts of the x-ray machine, such as the tableside, supporting structure, and collimator, should be wiped with a clean, damp (not soaked) cloth daily. The metal parts of the machine should be periodically cleaned with a disinfectant. The overhead system, x-ray tube, and other parts that conduct electricity should be cleaned with alcohol or a clean, dry cloth. Water is never used to clean electrical parts.

The tabletop should be cleaned after each examination. Cones, collimators, compression devices, gonad shields, and other accessories should be cleaned daily and after any contact with a patient. Adhesive tape residue left on cassettes and cassette stands should be removed, and the cassette should be disinfected. Cassettes should be protected from patients who are bleeding, and disposable protective covers should be manipulated so that they do not come in contact with ulcers or other discharging lesions. Use of stained or damaged cassettes is inexcusable and does not represent a professional atmosphere.

The radiographic room should be prepared for the examination before the patient arrives. The room should look clean and organized—not disarranged from the previous examination (Fig. 1-18). Fresh linens should be put on the table and pillow, and accessories needed during the examination should be placed nearby. Performing these preexamination steps requires only a few minutes but creates a positive, lasting impression on the patient; not performing these steps beforehand leaves a negative impression.

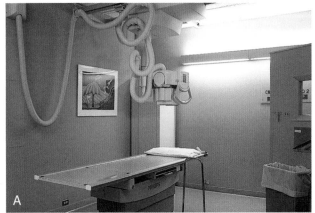 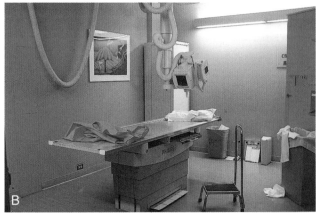

Fig. 1-18 A, Radiographic room should always be clean and straightened before any examination begins. **B,** This room is not ready to receive a patient. Note devices stored on the floor and previous patient's gowns and towels lying on the table. This room does not present a welcoming sight for a patient.

Standard Precautions

Radiographers are engaged in caring for sick patients and should be thoroughly familiar with *standard precautions*. They should know the way to handle patients who are on isolation status without contaminating their hands, clothing, or apparatus, and radiographers must know the method of disinfecting these items when they become contaminated. Standard precautions are designed to reduce the risk of transmission of unrecognized sources of blood-borne and other pathogens in health care institutions. Standard precautions apply to:

- Blood
- All body fluids
- Secretions and excretions (except sweat)
- Nonintact skin
- Mucous membranes

Handwashing is the easiest and most convenient method of preventing the spread of microorganisms (Fig. 1-19, *A*). Radiographers should wash their hands before and after working with each patient. Hands must always be washed, without exception, in the following specific situations:

- After examining patients with known communicable diseases
- After coming in contact with blood or body fluids
- Before beginning invasive procedures
- Before touching patients who are at risk of infections

As one of the first steps in aseptic technique, radiographers' hands should be kept smooth and free from roughness or chapping by the frequent use of soothing lotions. All abrasions should be protected by bandages to prevent the entrance of bacteria.

For the protection of the health of radiographers' and patients', the laws of asepsis and prophylaxis must be obeyed. Radiographers should practice scrupulous cleanliness when handling all patients, whether or not the patients are known to have an infectious disease. If a radiographer is to examine the patient's head, face, or teeth, the patient should ideally see the radiographer perform handwashing. If this is not possible, the radiographer should perform handwashing and then enter the room drying the hands with a fresh towel. If the patient's face is to come in contact with the IR front or table, the patient should see the radiographer clean the device with a disinfectant or cover it with a clean drape.

A sufficient supply of gowns and disposable gloves should be kept in the radiographic room to be used to care for infectious patients. After examining infectious patients, radiographers must wash their hands in warm, running water and soapsuds and rinse and dry them thoroughly. If the sink is not equipped with a knee control for the water supply, the radiographer opens the valve of the faucet with a paper towel. After proper handwashing, the radiographer closes the valve of the faucet with a paper towel.

Before bringing a patient from an isolation unit to the radiology department, the transporter should drape the stretcher or wheelchair with a clean sheet to prevent contamination of anything the patient might touch. When the patient must be transferred to the radiographic table, the table should be draped with a sheet. The edges of the sheet may be folded back over the patient so that the radiographer can position the patient through the clean side of the sheet without becoming contaminated.

A folded sheet should be placed over the end of the stretcher or table to protect the IRs when a non-Bucky technique is used. The IR is placed between the clean fold of the sheet, and with the hands between the clean fold, the radiographer can position the patient through the sheet. If the radiographer must handle the patient directly, an assistant should position the tube and operate the equipment to prevent contamination. If a patient has any moisture or body fluids on the body surface that could come in contact with the IR, a non–moisture-penetrable material must be used to cover the IR.

When the examination is finished, the contaminated linen should be folded with the clean side out and returned to the patient's room with the patient. There the linen receives the special attention given to linen used for isolation unit patients or is disposed of according to the established policy of the institution. All radiographic tables must be cleaned after patients have touched it with their bare skin and after patients with communicable diseases have been on the table (Fig. 1-19, *B*).

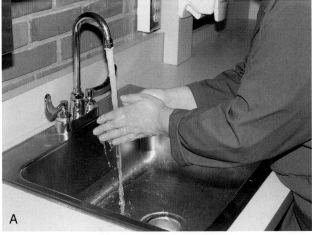
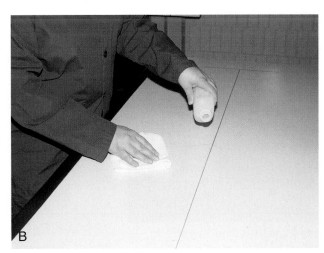

Fig. 1-19 A, Radiographers should practice scrupulous cleanliness, which includes regular handwashing. **B,** Radiographic tables and equipment should be cleaned with a disinfectant according to department policy.

Disinfectants and Antiseptics

Chemical substances that kill pathogenic bacteria are classified as *germicides* and *disinfectants* (e.g., dilute bleach is sometimes used as a disinfectant). Disinfection is the process of killing only microorganisms that are pathogenic. The objection to the use of many chemical disinfectants is that to be effective, they must be used in solutions so strong that they damage the material being disinfected. Chemical substances that inhibit the growth of but without killing pathogenic microorganisms are called antiseptics. Alcohol, which is commonly used for medical or practical asepsis in medical facilities, has antiseptic but not disinfectant properties. Sterilization, which is usually performed by means of heat or chemicals, is the destruction of all microorganisms.

BOX 1-1

Body fluids that may contain pathogenic microorganisms

Blood
Any fluid containing blood
Amniotic fluid
Pericardial fluid
Pleural fluid
Synovial fluid
Cerebrospinal fluid
Seminal fluid
Vaginal fluid
Urine
Sputum

Centers for Disease Control and Prevention

For the protection of health care workers, the U.S. Centers for Disease Control and Prevention (CDC)[1] has issued recommendations for handling blood and other body fluids. According to the CDC, all human blood and certain body fluids should be treated as if they contain pathogenic microorganisms (Box 1-1). These precautions should apply to all contacts involving patients. Health care workers should wear gloves whenever they come into contact with blood, mucous membranes, wounds, and any surface or body fluid containing blood. For any procedure in which blood or other body fluids may be sprayed or splashed, the radiographer should wear a mask, protective eyewear (e.g., eye shields, goggles), and a gown.

Health care workers must be cautious to prevent needle stick injuries. Needles should never be recapped, bent, broken, or clipped. Instead, they should be placed in a puncture-proof container and properly discarded (Fig. 1-20).

---

[1]www.cdc.gov.

Operating Room

Chapter 29 of this atlas contains comprehensive information about the radiographer's work in the operating room (OR). A radiographer who has not had extensive patient care education must exercise extreme caution to prevent contaminating sterile objects in the OR. The radiographer should perform handwashing and wear scrub clothing, a scrub cap, and a mask and should survey the particular setup in the OR before bringing in the x-ray equipment. By taking this precaution, the radiographer can ensure that sufficient space is available to do the work without the danger of contamination. If necessary, the radiographer should ask the circulating nurse to move any sterile items. Because of the danger of contamination of the sterile field, sterile supplies, and persons scrubbed for the procedure, the radiographer should never approach the operative side of the surgical table unless directed to do so.

After checking the room setup, the radiographer should thoroughly wipe the x-ray equipment with a damp (not soaked) cloth before taking it into the OR. The

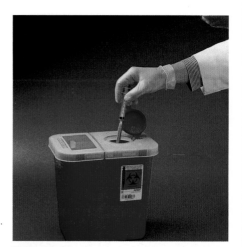

Fig. 1-20 All needles should be discarded in puncture-resistant containers.

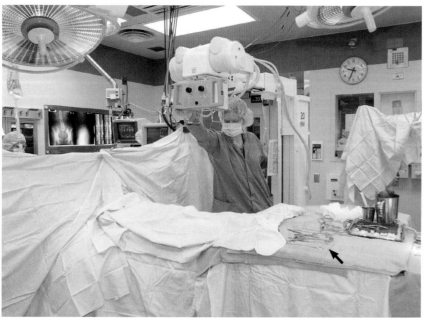

Fig. 1-21 Radiographer carefully positioning mobile x-ray tube during a surgical procedure. The sterile incision site is properly covered to maintain a sterile field. Note the sterile instruments in the foreground (*arrow*). The radiographer should never move radiographic equipment over uncovered sterile instruments or an uncovered surgical site.

radiographer moves the mobile machine, or C-arm unit, to the free side of the operating table—the side opposite the surgeon, scrub nurse, and sterile layout (Fig. 1-21). The machine should be maneuvered into a general position that makes the final adjustments easy when the surgeon is ready to proceed with the examination.

The IR is placed in a sterile covering, depending on the type of examination to be performed. The surgeon or one of the assistants holds the sterile case open while the radiographer gently drops the IR into it, being careful not to touch the sterile case. The radiographer may give directions for positioning and securing the cassette for the exposure.

The radiographer should make the necessary arrangements with the OR supervisor when performing work that requires the use of a tunnel or other special equipment. When an IR is being prepared for the patient, any tunnel or grid should be placed on the table with the tray opening to the side of the table opposite the sterile field. With the cooperation of the surgeon and OR supervisor, a system can be developed for performing radiographic examinations accurately and quickly without moving the patient or endangering the sterile field (Fig. 1-22).

Minor Surgical Procedures in the Radiology Department

Procedures that require a rigid aseptic technique, such as cystography, intravenous urography, spinal punctures, angiography, and angiocardiography, are performed in the radiology department (Fig. 1-23). Although the physician needs the assistance of a nurse in certain procedures, the radiographer can make the necessary preparations and provide assistance in many procedures.

For procedures that do not require a nurse, the radiographer should know which surgical instruments and supplies are necessary and how to prepare and sterilize them. Radiographers may make arrangements with the surgical supervisor to acquire the education necessary to perform these procedures.

Procedure Book

A procedure or protocol book covering each examination performed in the radiology department is essential. Under the appropriate heading, each procedure should be outlined and should state the staff required and duties of each team member. A listing of sterile and nonsterile items should also be included. A copy of the sterile instrument requirements should be given to the supervisor of the central sterile supply department to assist preparation of the trays for each procedure.

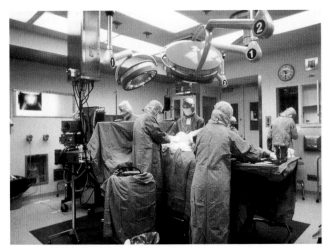

Fig. 1-22 Radiographer must exercise extreme caution to prevent contaminating sterile objects in OR.

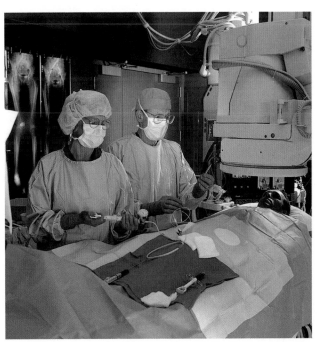

Fig. 1-23 Many radiographic procedures require strict aseptic technique, such as seen in this procedure involving passing a catheter into the patient's femoral artery.

Bowel Preparation

Radiologic examinations involving the abdomen often require that the entire colon be cleansed before the examination so that diagnostic-quality radiographs can be obtained. The patient's colon may be cleansed by one or any combination of the following:

- Limited diet
- Laxatives
- Enemas

The technique used to cleanse the patient's colon generally is selected by the medical facility or physician. The patient should be questioned about any bowel preparation that may have been completed before an abdominal procedure is begun. For additional information on bowel preparation, see Chapter 17.

Motion and Its Control

Patient motion plays a large role in radiography (Fig. 1-24). Because motion is the result of muscle action, the radiographer needs to have some knowledge about the functions of various muscles. The radiographer should use this knowledge to eliminate or control motion for the exposure time necessary to complete a satisfactory examination. The three types of muscular tissue that affect motion are the following:

- Smooth (involuntary)
- Cardiac (involuntary)
- Striated (voluntary)

INVOLUNTARY MUSCLES

The visceral (organ) muscles are composed of *smooth* muscular tissue and are controlled partially by the autonomic nervous system and the muscles' inherent characteristics of rhythmic contractility. By their rhythmic contraction and relaxation, these muscles perform the movement of the internal organs. The rhythmic action of the muscular tissue of the alimentary tract, called *peristalsis,* is normally more active in the stomach (about three or four waves per minute) and gradually diminishes along the intestine. The specialized *cardiac* muscular tissue functions by contracting the heart to pump blood into the arteries and expanding or relaxing to permit the heart to receive blood from the veins. The pulse rate of the heart varies with emotions, exercise, diet, size, age, and gender.

Involuntary motion is caused by the following:

- Heart pulsation
- Chill
- Peristalsis
- Tremor
- Spasm
- Pain

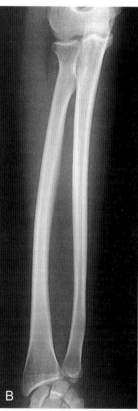

Fig. 1-24 A, Forearm radiograph of a patient who moved during the exposure. Note the fuzzy appearance of the edges of the bones. **B,** Radiograph of patient without motion.

Involuntary muscle control

The primary method of reducing involuntary motion is to control the length of exposure time—the less exposure time to the patient, the better.

VOLUNTARY MUSCLES

The voluntary, or skeletal, muscles are composed of *striated* muscular tissue and are controlled by the central nervous system. These muscles perform the movements of the body initiated by the individual. In radiography, the patient's body must be positioned in such a way that the skeletal muscles are relaxed. The patient's comfort level is a good guide to determine the success of the position.

Voluntary motion resulting from lack of control is caused by the following:

• Nervousness
• Discomfort
• Excitability
• Mental illness
• Fear
• Age
• Breathing

Voluntary muscle control

The radiographer can control voluntary patient motion by doing the following:

• Giving clear instructions
• Providing patient comfort
• Adjusting support devices
• Applying immobilization

Decreasing the length of exposure time is the best way to control voluntary motion that results from mental illness or the age of the patient. Immobilization for limb radiography can often be obtained for the duration of the exposure by having the patient phonate an *mmm* sound with the mouth closed or an *ahhh* sound with the mouth open. The radiographer should always be watching the patient during the exposure to ensure that the exposure is made during suspended respiration. Sponges and sandbags are commonly used as immobilization devices (Fig. 1-25, *A*). A leg holder is used to stabilize the opposite leg for lateral radiographs of the legs, knee, femur, and hip (Fig. 1-25, *B*). A thin radiolucent mattress, called a *table pad,* may be placed on the radiographic table to reduce movement related to patient discomfort caused by lying on the hard surface. These table pads should not be used when the increased OID would result in unacceptable magnification, such as in radiography of the limbs. If possible, radiographers should use table pads under the patient in the body areas where the projections are not made.

Patient Instructions

When an examination requires preparation, such as in kidney and gastrointestinal examinations, the radiographer must carefully instruct the patient. Although the particular examination or procedure may be repetitive to the radiographer, it is new to the patient. Frequently, what a radiographer interprets as patient stupidity results from lack of sufficiently explicit directions. The radiographer must ensure that the patient understands not only what to do, but also why it must be done. A patient is more likely to follow instructions correctly if the reason for the instructions is clear. If the instructions are complicated, they should be written out and verbally reviewed with the patient if necessary. Few patients know the way to give themselves an enema correctly, so the radiographer should question the patient and, when necessary, take the time to explain the correct procedure. This approach often saves film, time, and radiation exposure to the patient.

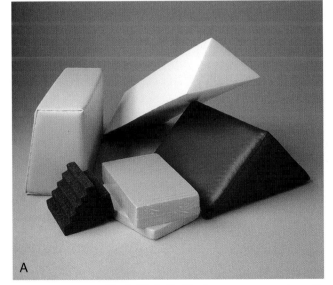
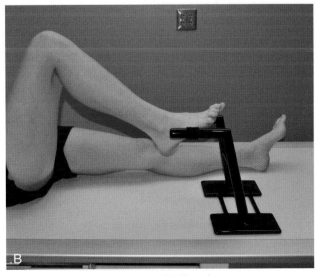

Fig. 1-25 A, Positioning sponges and sandbags are commonly used as immobilization devices. **B,** Ferlic leg holder and immobilization device.

(**B,** Courtesy Ferlic Filter Company, LLC, White Bear Lake, MN.)

Patient's Attire, Ornaments, and Surgical Dressings

The patient should be dressed in a gown that allows exposure of limited body regions under examination. A patient is never exposed unnecessarily; a sheet should be used when appropriate. If a region of the body needs to be exposed to complete the examination, only the area under examination should be uncovered while the rest of the patient's body is completely covered for warmth and privacy. When the radiographer is examining parts that must remain covered, disposable paper gowns or cotton cloth gowns without metal or plastic snaps are preferred (Fig. 1-26). If washable gowns are used, they should not be starched; starch is *radi-opaque,* which means it cannot be penetrated easily by x-rays. Any folds in the cloth should be straightened to prevent confusing densities on the radiograph. The length of exposure should also be considered. Material that does not cast a density on a heavy exposure, such as that used on an adult abdomen, may show clearly on a light exposure, such as that used on a child's abdomen.

Any radiopaque object should be removed from the region to be radiographed. Zippers, necklaces, snaps, thick elastic, and buttons should be removed when radiographs of the chest and abdomen are produced (Fig. 1-27). When radiographing the skull, the radiographer must make sure that dentures, removable bridgework, earrings, necklaces, and all hairpins are removed.

When the abdomen, pelvis, or hips of an infant are radiographed, the diaper should be removed. Because some diaper rash ointments are radiopaque, the area may need to be cleansed before the procedure.

Surgical dressings, such as metallic salves and adhesive tape, should be examined for radiopaque substances. If permission to remove the dressings has not been obtained or the radiographer does not know how to remove them and the radiology department physician is not present, the surgeon or nurse should be asked to accompany the patient to the radiology department to remove the dressings. When dressings are removed, the radiographer should always ensure that a cover of sterile gauze adequately protects open wounds.

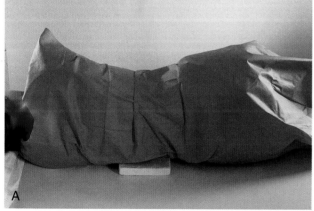 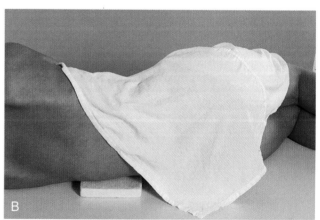

Fig. 1-26 A, A female patient wearing a disposable paper gown and positioned for a lateral projection of the lumbar spine. Private areas are completely covered. The gown is smoothed around the contour of the body for accurate positioning. **B,** The same patient wearing a traditional cloth hospital gown. The gown is positioned for maximal privacy.

Handling of Patients

Patients who are coherent and capable of understanding should be given an explanation of the procedure to be performed. Patients should understand exactly what is expected and be made comfortable. If patients are apprehensive about the examination, their fears should be alleviated. If the procedure will cause discomfort or be unpleasant, such as with cystoscopy and intravenous injections, the radiographer should calmly and truthfully explain the procedure. Patients should be told that it will cause some discomfort or be unpleasant, but because the procedure is a necessary part of the examination, full cooperation is necessary. Patients usually respond favorably if they understand that all steps are being taken to alleviate discomfort.

Because the entire procedure may be a new experience, patients usually respond incorrectly when given more than one instruction at a time. For example, when instructed to get up on the table and lie on the abdomen, a patient may get onto the table in the most awkward possible manner and lie on his or her back. Instead of asking a patient to get onto the table in a specific position, the radiographer should first have the patient sit on the table and then give instructions on assuming the desired position. If the patient sits on the table first, the position can be assumed with less strain and fewer awkward movements. The radiographer should never rush a patient. If patients feel hurried, they will be nervous and less able to cooperate. When moving and adjusting a patient into position, the radiographer should manipulate the patient gently but firmly; a light touch can be as irritating as one that is too firm. Patients should be instructed and allowed to do as much of the moving as possible.

X-ray grids move under the radiographic table, and with floating or moving tabletops, patients may injure their fingers. To reduce the possibility of injury, the radiographer should inform patients to keep their fingers on top of the table at all times. Regardless of the part being examined, the patient's entire body must be adjusted with resultant motion or rotation to prevent muscle pull in the area of interest. When a patient is in an oblique (angled) position, the radiographer should use support devices and adjust the patient to relieve any strain. Immobilization devices and compression bands should be used whenever necessary, but not to the point of discomfort. The radiographer should be cautious when releasing a compression band over the abdomen and should perform the procedure slowly.

When making final adjustments to a patient's position, the radiographer should stand with the eyes in line with the position of the x-ray tube, visualize the internal structures, and adjust the part accordingly. Although there are few rules on positioning patients, many repeat examinations can be eliminated by following these guidelines. (See Chapters 26 and 27 for handling instructions for pediatric and geriatric patients.)

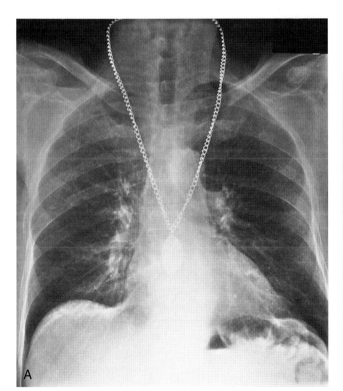
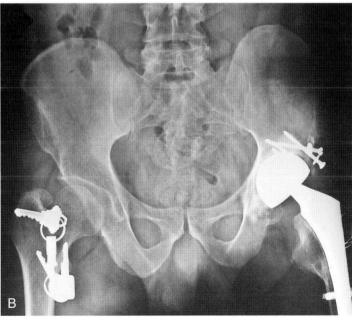

Fig. 1-27 A, A necklace was left on for this chest radiograph. **B,** Keys were left in the pocket of a lightweight hospital robe during the examination of this patient's pelvis. Both radiographs had to be repeated because the metal objects were not removed before the examination.

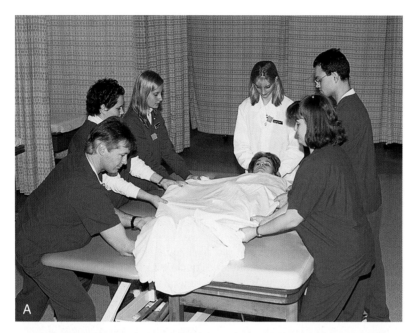

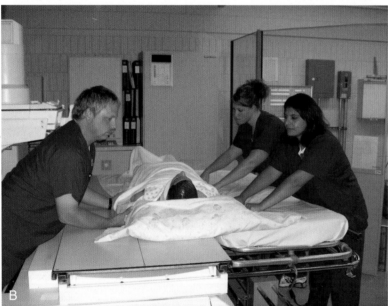

Fig. 1-28 A, Technique for a six-person transfer of a patient who is unable to move from a cart to the procedure table. Note the person holding and supporting the head. **B,** Three-person transfer of a patient back onto the cart. Note two people are always on the side that is pulling the patient, and one person is on the opposite side pushing the patient. Note also the backs of the three people are straight, following correct lifting and moving practices.

ILL OR INJURED PATIENTS

Great care must be exercised in handling trauma patients, particularly patients with skull, spinal, and long bone injuries. A physician should perform any necessary manipulation to prevent the possibility of fragment displacement. The positioning technique should be adapted to each patient and necessitate as little movement as possible. If the tube-part-imaging plane relationship is maintained, the resultant projection is the same regardless of the patient's position.

When a patient who is too sick to move alone must be moved, the following considerations should be kept in mind:

1. The patient should be moved as little as possible.
2. The radiographer should never try to lift a helpless patient alone.
3. To prevent straining the back muscles when lifting a heavy patient, one should flex the knees, straighten the back, and bend from the hips.
4. When a patient's shoulders are lifted, the head should be supported. While holding the head with one hand, one slides the opposite arm under the shoulders and grasps the axilla so that the head can rest on the bend of the elbow when the patient is raised.
5. When moving the patient's hips, the patient's knees are flexed first. In this position, patients may be able to raise themselves. If not, lifting the body when the patient's knees are bent is easier.
6. When a helpless patient must be transferred to the radiographic table from a stretcher or bed, he or she should be moved on a sheet by at least four and preferably six people. The stretcher is placed parallel to and touching the table. Under ideal circumstances, at least three people should be stationed on the side of the stretcher and two on the far side of the radiographic table to grasp the sheet at the shoulder and hip levels. One person should support the patient's head, and another person should support the feet. When the signal is given, all six people should *smoothly and slowly* lift and move the patient in unison (Fig. 1-28, *A*). Often, radiographers use the three-person move for patients who are not in a critical condition (Fig. 1-28, *B*).

Many hospitals now have a specially equipped radiographic room adjoining the emergency department. These units often have special radiographic equipment and stretchers with radiolucent tops that allow severely injured patients to be examined on the stretcher and in the position in which they arrive. A mobile radiographic machine is often taken into the emergency department and radiographs are exposed there. Where this ideal emergency setup does not exist, trauma patients are often conveyed to the main radiology department. There they must be given precedence over nonemergency patients (see Chapters 13 and 28).

Age-Specific Competencies

Age-specific competence is defined as the knowledge, skills, ability, and behaviors that are essential for providing optimal care to defined groups of patients. Examples of defined groups include neonatal, pediatric, adolescent, and geriatric patients. Appropriate staff competence in working with these diverse patient groups is crucial in providing quality patient care. The Joint Commission[1] requires that age-specific competencies be written for all health care personnel who provide direct patient care. Radiographers are considered direct patient care providers. The Joint Commission requires radiology departments to document that radiographers maintain competency in providing radio-

logic examinations to defined groups of patients.

Age-specific competence is based on the knowledge that different groups of patients have special physical and psychosocial needs. Different types and levels of competence are required for specific patient populations. A radiographer who is obtaining radiographic images on a neonatal or pediatric patient must be skilled at interpreting nonverbal communication. Working with a geriatric patient requires the radiographer to have the knowledge and skills necessary to assess and maintain the integrity of fragile skin.

Health care facilities that provide patient care may classify the different age groups for which age-specific competence is defined. Some hospitals may classify patients by *chronologic* age, some may use *functional* age, and others may use *life stage* groupings.[1,2] Specialty organizations, such as pediatric hospitals, veterans' hospitals, psychiatric hospitals, or long-term care facilities, might use institution-specific criteria, such as premature or newborn, Vietnam veteran, closed ward, or Alzheimer' disease.

The principle supporting age-related competencies is that staff involved in direct patient care who are not competent to provide care to patients in specific age or functional groups can alter treatment, increase patient complaints about care, make serious medical errors, and increase

operational costs. The Joint Commission looks for evidence of staff development programs that are effective and ongoing and serve to maintain and improve staff competence.

When the Joint Commission surveys organizations, it looks for evidence of competence assessment primarily in personnel records. The Joint Review Committee on Education in Radiologic Technology (JRCERT), the organization that accredits radiography programs, makes site visits of radiography programs and looks for evidence that students not only learn the basic theories supporting age-related competence, but also are competent. Table 1-1 shows a checklist that can be used in a radiography program to document that a student has shown basic competence in several different life stages. Box 1-2 provides examples of age-specific competencies that should be required of a radiographer. Health care facilities are required to prepare age-related competencies for all age groups, including neonates, infants, children, adolescents, adults, and geriatrics.

Merrill's Atlas essentially addresses the normal adult patient in the age group from about 18 to 60 years. Although an organization would have published age-specific competencies for this broad age group, this group could be considered the "standard group" for which radiologic procedures are standardized and written. Radiographers must learn the specifics of how to adapt and modify procedures for the extreme groups, such as neonates and geriatric patients, and those in between, such as adolescents.

[1]The Joint Commission, Oakbrook Terrace, IL.

[1]*Age-specific competence,* Oakbrook Terrace, IL, 1998, The Joint Commission.
[2]*Assessing hospital staff competence,* Oakbrook Terrace, IL, 2002, The Joint Commission.

TABLE 1-1

Age-specific criteria checklist

This planning tool is an example of a general checklist that can assist organizations in assessing age-specific competencies of staff

	Neonatal	Pediatric	Adolescent	Adult	Geriatric
Knowledge of growth and development					
Ability to assess age-specific data					
Ability to interpret age-specific data					
Possesses skills/ knowledge to perform treatments (i.e., medications, equipment)					
Age-appropriate communication skills					
Possesses knowledge of age-specific community resources					
Involves family or significant other, or both, in plan of care					

Used with permission from the Joint Commission, Oakbrook Terrace, Ill, 1998.

BOX 1-2

Age-specific competencies that should be required of a radiographer for two selected age groups

Neonate (1-30 days)
Explain examination to the parents if present.
Cover infant with a blanket to conserve body heat.
Cover image receptor with a blanket or sheet to protect the skin from injury.
Collimate to specific area of interest only.
Shield patient and any attendants.

Geriatric (68 years old)
Speak clearly and do not raise voice.
Do not rush examination.
Use positioning aids whenever possible.
Ensure that patient is warm owing to decreased circulation.
Do not leave patient unattended on the x-ray table.

Note: This list is not inclusive for the two age groups listed. Age-related competencies are prepared for other age groups as well.

Identification of Radiographs

All radiographs must include the following information (Fig. 1-29, *A*):

- Date
- Patient's name or identification number
- Right or left marker
- Institution identity

Correct identification is vital and should always be confirmed. Identification is absolutely vital in comparison studies, on follow-up examinations, and in medicolegal cases. Radiographers should develop the habit of rechecking the identification side marker just before placing it on the IR. Digital systems introduced in recent years use a computer in the radiography room. The radiographer inputs the patient's identification and other data directly on each radiograph via the computer (Fig. 1-29, *B* and *C*). Side markers should still be physically placed on the IR, however. The computer should not be used to place *right* and *left* markers on the image.

Other patient identification information includes the patient's age or date of birth, time of day, and the name of the radiographer or attending physician. For certain examinations, the radiograph should include such markings as cumulative time after introduction of contrast medium (e.g., 5 minutes postinjection) and the level of the fulcrum (e.g., 9 cm) in tomography. Other radiographs are marked to indicate the position of the patient (e.g., upright, decubitus) or with other markings specified by the institution.

Numerous methods of marking radiographs for identification are available. These methods include radiographing the identification information along with the part, "flashing" it onto the film in the darkroom before development, writing it on the film after it has been processed, perforating the information on the film, and attaching adhesive labels. Although most patient information is automatically added to digital images, additional information may be typed on the image after processing. This is commonly called *annotation.*

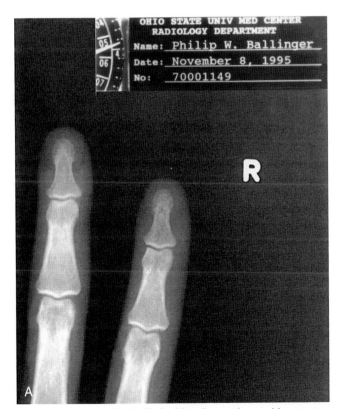

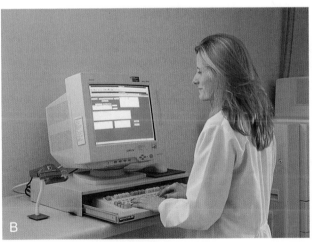

Fig. 1-29 A, All radiographs must be permanently identified and should contain a minimum of four identification markings. **B,** Radiographer using CR system and entering a patient's identification data into a computer in the radiography room. **C,** Resulting laser image showing the patient's information.

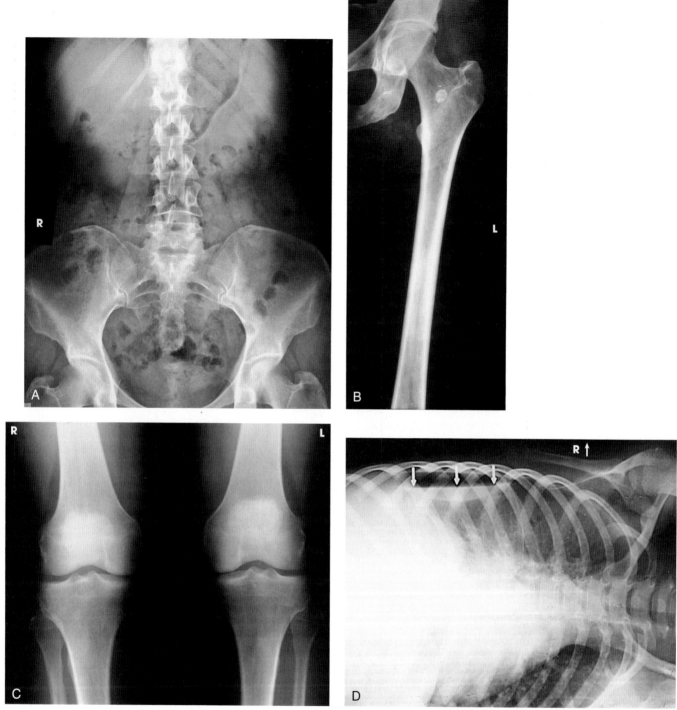

Fig. 1-30 A, AP projection of the abdomen showing right (*R*) marker. **B,** AP projection of the left limb showing left (*L*) marker on outer margin of the image. **C,** AP projection of the right and left knees on one image showing R and L markers. **D,** AP projection of the chest performed in the left lateral decubitus position showing R marker on the "upper" portion of IR.

Anatomic Markers

Each radiograph must include an appropriate marker that clearly identifies the patient's right (R) or left (L) side. Medicolegal requirements mandate that these markers be present. Radiographers and physicians must see them to determine the correct side of the patient or the correct limb. Markers are typically made of lead and placed directly on the IR or tabletop. The marker is seen on the image along with the anatomic part (Fig. 1-30). Writing the *R* or *L* by hand on a radiograph after processing is unacceptable. The only exception may be for certain projections performed during surgical and trauma procedures. Box 1-3 presents the specific rules of marker placement.

Basic marker conventions include the following:
- The marker should never obscure anatomy.
- The marker should never be placed over the patient's identification information.
- The marker should always be placed on the edge of the collimation border.
- The marker should always be placed outside of any lead shielding.
- R and L markers must be used with CR and DR digital imaging.

DIGITAL IMAGING

The development of digital imaging and the use of CR and DR have enabled an environment in which the R and L markers can be placed on the image electronically at the computer workstation. *This is not recommended* because of the great potential for error and legal implications; this is especially true when patients are examined in the prone position. Anatomic markers should be placed on the CR cassette or DR table similar to screen-film cassettes. Additionally, markers should never be placed on the body part.

BOX 1-3

Specific marker placement rules

1. For AP and PA projections that include R and L sides of the body (head, spine, chest, abdomen, and pelvis), R marker is typically used.
2. For lateral projections of the head and trunk (head, spine, chest, abdomen, and pelvis), always mark the side closest to IR. If the left side is closest, use L marker. The marker is typically placed anterior to the anatomy.
3. For oblique projections that include R and L sides of the body (spine, chest, and abdomen), the side down, or nearest IR, is typically marked. For a right posterior oblique (RPO) position, mark R side.
4. For limb projections, use appropriate R or L marker. The marker must be placed within the edge of the collimated x-ray beam.
5. For limb projections that are done with two images on one IR, only one of the projections needs to be marked.
6. For limb projections where R and L sides are imaged side by side on one IR (e.g., R and L, AP knees), R and L markers must be used to identify the two sides clearly.
7. For AP, PA, or oblique chest projections, marker is placed on the upper-outer corner so that the thoracic anatomy is not obscured.
8. For decubitus positions of the chest and abdomen, R or L marker should always be placed on the side up (opposite the side laid on) and away from the anatomy of interest.

Note: No matter which projection is performed, and no matter what position the patient is in, if R marker is used, it must be placed on the "right" side of the patient's body. If L marker is used, it must be placed on the "left" side of the patient's body.

Image Receptor Placement

The part to be examined is usually centered on the center point of the IR or to the position where the angulation of the central ray projects it to the center. The IR should be adjusted so that its long axis lies parallel with the long axis of the part being examined. Although a long bone angled across the radiograph does not impair the diagnostic value of the image, such an arrangement can be aesthetically distracting. The three general positions of the IR are shown in Fig. 1-31. These positions are named on the basis of their position in relation to the long axis of the body. The longitudinal IR position is the most frequently used position.

Although the lesion may be known to be at the midbody (central portion) of a long bone, an IR large enough to include at least one joint should be used on all long bone studies (Fig. 1-32). This method is the only means of determining the precise position of the part and localizing the lesion. Many institutions require that both joints be shown when a long bone is initially radiographed. For tall patients, two exposures may be required, one for the long bone and joint closest to the area of concern and a second to show the joint at the opposite end.

An IR just large enough to cover the region being examined should always be used. In addition to being extravagant, large IRs include extraneous parts that detract from the appearance of the radiograph and, more important, cause unnecessary radiation exposure to the patient. The exception to this rule is when using DR with a 17- × 17-inch (43- × 43-cm) IR built into the table. The radiographer has to collimate exactly to the body part size anywhere on the detector.

A standard rule in radiography is to place the object as close to the IR as possible. When obtaining lateral images of the middle and ring fingers, the radiographer increases the OID so that the part lies parallel with the IR. In some situations, this rule is modified. Although magnification is greater, less distortion occurs. The radiographer can increase the SID to compensate for the increase in OID, reducing magnification. In certain instances, intentional magnification is desirable and can

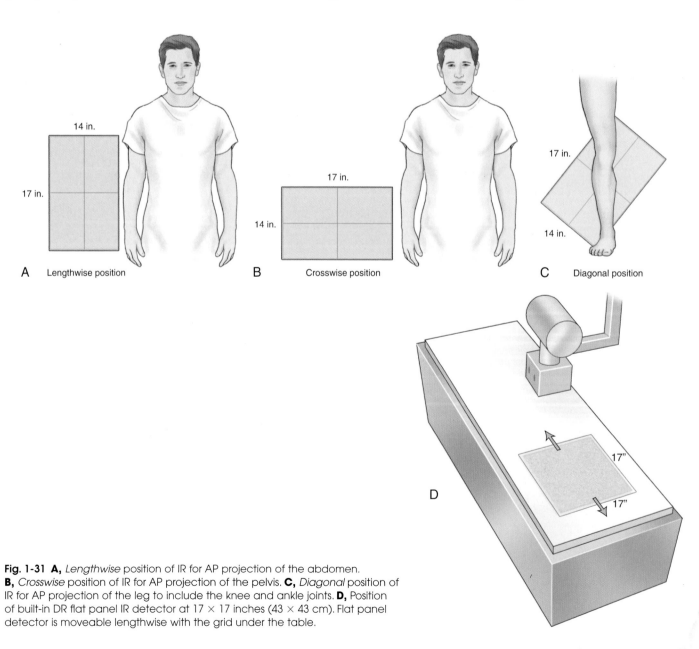

14 in.

17 in.

A Lengthwise position

17 in.

14 in.

B Crosswise position

17 in.

14 in.

C Diagonal position

17"

17"

D

Fig. 1-31 A, *Lengthwise* position of IR for AP projection of the abdomen. **B,** *Crosswise* position of IR for AP projection of the pelvis. **C,** *Diagonal* position of IR for AP projection of the leg to include the knee and ankle joints. **D,** Position of built-in DR flat panel IR detector at 17 × 17 inches (43 × 43 cm). Flat panel detector is moveable lengthwise with the grid under the table.

be obtained by positioning and supporting the object between the IR and the focal spot of the tube. This procedure is known as *magnification radiography*.

For ease of comparison, bilateral examinations of small body parts may be placed on one IR. Exact duplication of the location of the images on the film is difficult, however, if the IR is not marked accurately. Many IRs have permanent markings on the edges to assist the radiographer in equally spacing multiple images on one IR. Depending on the size and shape of the body part being radiographed, the IR can be divided in half either transversely or longitudinally. In some instances, the IR may be divided into thirds or fourths (Fig. 1-33).

Body parts *must* always be identified by right or left side and placed on the IR in the same manner, either facing or backing each other, according to established routines. The radiographer plans the exposures so that the image identification marker does not interfere with the part of interest.

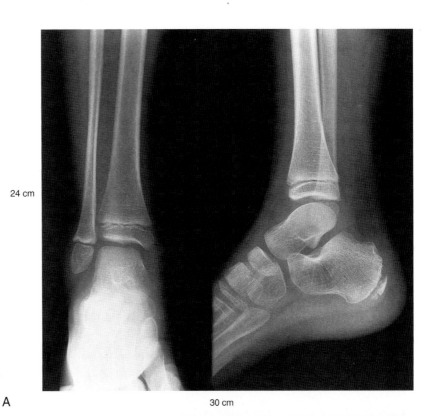

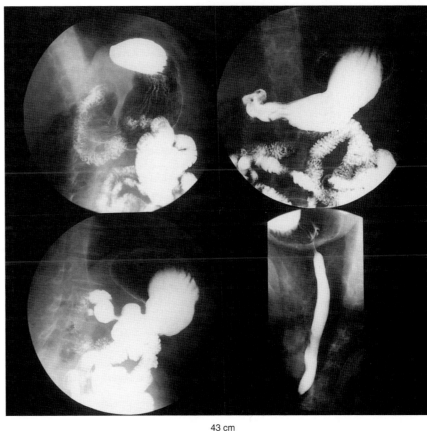

Fig. 1-33 Examples of multiple exposures on one film. **A,** AP and lateral projections of the ankle radiographically exposed side by side on 10- × 12-inch (24- × 30-cm) film. **B,** Four projections of the stomach directly imaged on 14- × 17-inch (35- × 43-cm) film.

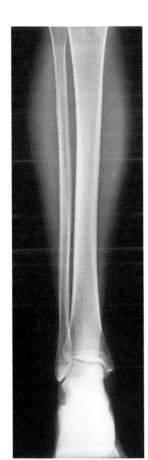

Fig. 1-32 AP projection of the leg showing the ankle joint included on the image. One joint should be shown on all images of long bones.

29

English-Metric Conversion and Film Sizes

Measures are the standards used to determine size. People in the United States and a few other countries use standards that belong to the customary, or English, system of measurement. Although this system was developed in England, people in nearly all other countries including England now use the metric system of measurement.

In the past couple of decades, efforts have been made to convert all English measurements to the world standard metric system. These efforts have not been particularly effective. Nevertheless, total conversion to the metric system most likely will occur in the future.

The following information is provided to assist the radiographer in converting measurements from the English system to the metric system and vice versa:
- 1 inch = 2.54 centimeters (cm)
- 1 cm = 0.3937 inch
- 40 inch SID = 1 meter (m) (approximately)

Radiographic film is manufactured in English and metric sizes. Most sizes used in the United States have more recently been converted to metric. (Table 1-2 lists the most common film sizes used in radiology departments in the United States along with their general usage.) Four of the 11 common sizes continue to be manufactured in an English size, however. The 24- × 30-cm size has replaced the 10- × 12-inch size. The 10- × 12-inch size continues to be manufactured for use in grid cassettes. Few, if any, English sizes are used outside the United States. Four of the former English film sizes are no longer manufactured. Several additional film sizes are used routinely in departments outside the United States, including the 30- × 40-cm and 40- × 40-cm sizes.

CR plates are generally manufactured in five sizes. Many departments use only the 10- × 12-inch (24- × 30-cm) and 14- × 17-inch (35- × 43-cm) plates for all routine images (Table 1-3).

FILM SIZES IN THIS ATLAS

Film or IR sizes recommended in this atlas are for *adults*. These sizes are subject to modification as needed to fit the size of the body part. Metric sizes are used in the atlas. The only exception is for the films that continue to be manufactured in English sizes.

TABLE 1-2

Most common radiology film sizes used in United States*

Current film sizes	Former film sizes†	Usage‡
18 × 24 cm		Mammography
8 × 10 inches		General examinations
24 × 24 cm	9 × 9 inches	Fluoroscopic spots
24 × 30 cm		General examinations and mammography
10 × 12 inches		General examinations (grid cassettes)
18 × 43 cm	7 × 17 inches	Forearms, legs
30 × 35 cm	11 × 14 inches	General examinations
35 × 35 cm		Fluoroscopic spots
35 × 43 cm	14 × 17 inches	General examinations
14 × 36 inches		Upright spine
14 × 51 inches		Upright hip-to-ankle

*In order of smallest to largest size.
†English sizes no longer in use.
‡Most common uses in United States. Outside United States, usage may differ.

TABLE 1-3

Most common computed radiography plate sizes*

Inches	Centimeters
8 × 10	18 × 24
10 × 12	24 × 30
14 × 14	35 × 35
14 × 17	35 × 43
14 × 36	35 × 91

*Some manufactures build in inches and some in centimeters.

Direction of Central Ray

The central or principal beam of rays, simply referred to as the *central ray* (CR), is always centered to the IR unless receptor displacement is being used. The CR is angled through the part of interest under the following conditions:

- When overlying or underlying structures must not be superimposed
- When a curved structure, such as the sacrum or coccyx, must not be stacked on itself
- When projection through angled joints, such as the knee joint and lumbosacral junction, is necessary
- When projection through angled structures must be obtained without foreshortening or elongation, such as with a lateral image of the neck of the femur

The general goal is to place the CR at right angles to the structure. Accurate positioning of the part and accurate centering of the CR are of equal importance in obtaining a true structural projection.

Source–to–Image Receptor Distance

SID is the distance from the anode inside the x-ray tube to the IR (Fig. 1-34). SID is an important technical consideration in the production of radiographs of optimal quality. This distance is a critical component of each radiograph because it directly affects magnification of the body part, the recorded detail, the radiographic density, and the dose to the patient. The greater the SID, the less the body part is magnified and the greater the recorded detail. SID of 40 inches (102 cm) traditionally is used for most conventional examinations. In recent years, the SID has increased to 48 inches (122 cm) in some departments.[1-6] SID must be established for each radiographic projection, and it must be indicated on the technique chart.

[1]Eastman TR: Digital systems require x-ray charts too, *Radiol Technol* 67:354, 1996.

[2]Eastman TR: X-ray film quality and national contracts, *Radiol Technol* 69:12, 1997.

[3]Gray JE et al: *Quality control in diagnostic imaging,* Rockville, MD, 1983, Aspen.

[4]Kebart RC, James CD: Benefits of increasing focal film distance, *Radiol Technol* 62:434, 1991.

[5]Brennan PC, Nash M: Increasing SID: an effective dose-reducing tool for lateral lumbar spine investigations, *Radiography* 4:251, 1998.

[6]Carlton RR, Adler AM: *Principles of radiographic imaging,* ed 4, Albany, NY, 2006, Thomson Delmar Learning.

For some radiographic projections, SID less than 40 inches (<102 cm) is desirable. In certain examinations, such as examination of the odontoid in the open-mouth position, a short SID of 30 inches (76 cm) may be used. Some textbooks state that images should not be done at SID less than 40 inches because of the dose to the patient. For some projections, the best image possible is obtained at SID 30 inches or less because it increases the field-of-view. Additionally, dose is not increased because the shorter SID prompts a lower mAs. To maintain density when going from a 40-inch SID to a 30-inch SID, the mAs can be reduced 44%, and there is an accompanying reduction in dose to the patient. The goal in these reduced SID images is to show the body part with one image and avoid a repeat or second projection.

Conversely, a longer than standard SID is used for some radiographic projections. In chest radiography, a 72-inch (183-cm) SID is the minimum distance, and in many departments a distance up to 120 inches (305 cm) is used. These long distances are necessary to ensure that the lungs fit onto the 14-inch (35-cm) width of the IR (via reduced magnification of the body part) and, most importantly, to ensure that the heart is not technically enlarged for diagnoses of cardiac enlargement.

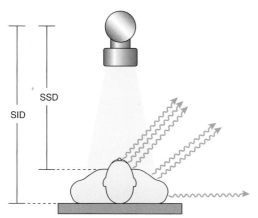

Fig. 1-34 Radiographic tube, patient, and table illustrate SID and SSD.

SOURCE-TO-IMAGE RECEPTOR DISTANCE IN THIS ATLAS

When a specific SID is necessary for optimal image quality, it is identified on the specific projection's page. The sample exposure technique charts in each chapter identify the traditional SID of 40 inches (102 cm). The special SID projections vary from 30 inches (76 cm) to 120 inches (305 cm) for general projections.

SOURCE-TO-SKIN DISTANCE

The distance between the radiography tube and the skin of the patient is termed the *source-to-skin distance* (SSD) (see Fig. 1-34). This distance affects the dose to the patient and is regulated by the National Council on Radiation Protection (NCRP). The current NCRP regulations state that the SSD *shall not* be less than 12 inches (<30 cm) and *should not* be less than 15 inches (<38 cm).[1]

---

[1]National Council on Radiation Protection: *NCRP Report 102*, Bethesda, MD, 1989, The Council.

Collimation of X-ray Beam

The beam of radiation must be narrow enough to irradiate only the area under examination. This restriction of the x-ray beam serves two purposes. First, it minimizes the amount of radiation to the patient and reduces the amount of scatter radiation that can reach the IR. Second, it produces radiographs that show excellent recorded detail and increased radiographic contrast by reducing scatter radiation, producing a shorter scale of contrast, and preventing secondary radiation from unnecessarily exposing surrounding tissues, with resultant image fogging (Fig. 1-35). Many experts regard collimation as the most important aspect of producing an optimal image. Collimation is equally important when using digital systems.

The area of the beam of radiation is reduced to the required size by using an automatic collimator or a specifically shaped diaphragm constructed of lead or other metal with high radiation absorption capability. Because of beam restriction, the peripheral radiation strikes and is absorbed by the collimator metal, and only x-rays in the exit aperture are transmitted to the exposure field.

DIGITAL RADIOGRAPHY

With the introduction of DR imaging systems, there are no film cassettes or imaging plates used as the IR. The table or upright unit contains a 17- × 17-inch (43- × 43-cm) flat panel detector (see Fig. 1-31, *D*). When using cassettes or plates, the collimator automatically adjusts to the size of the IR, or the radiographer could manually reduce collimation when necessary. Collimating to large was seldom a problem. Without cassettes or plates in DR, the collimator has to be manually adjusted by the radiographer to the correct field size. This environment has prompted numerous technical problems in recent years because radiographers have collimated larger than the anatomic area in an effort to avoid clipping anatomy, or they simply try to make their jobs easier.

It is a violation of the Code of Ethics to collimate larger than the required field size. When collimating larger than the required area, the patient receives unnecessary radiation to areas not needed on the image (Fig. 1-36, *A*). In addition, the in-

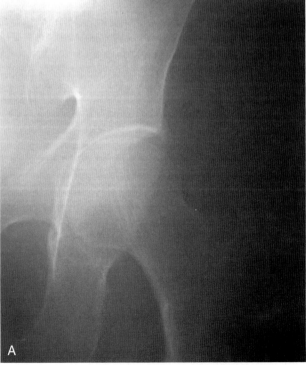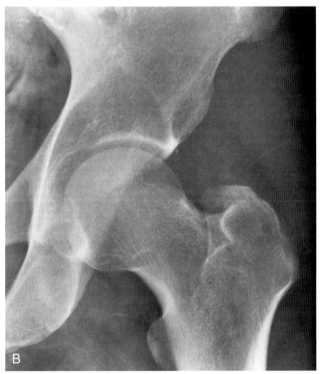

Fig. 1-35 Radiographs of the hip joint and acetabulum. **A,** Collimator inadvertently opened to size 14 × 17 inches (35 × 43 cm). Scatter and secondary radiation have reduced radiographic contrast and a poor-quality image results. **B,** Collimator set correctly to 8 × 10 inches (18 × 24 cm), improving radiographic contrast and visibility of detail.

creased scatter radiation decreases the contrast and recorded detail in the image, reducing the ability to ensure an accurate diagnosis. When using DR systems, the collimator should be adjusted to the same anatomic area size or smaller that would be used for a cassette or plate (Fig. 1-36, *B*). This adjustment has to be manually done on the collimator for each projection performed.

The software included in the computers of DR systems allows for shuttering. Shuttering is used in DR to provide a black background around the original collimation edges. This black background eliminates the distracting clear areas and the associated brightness that comes through to the eyes. Many radiographers open the collimator larger than is necessary and use the shuttering software to "crop-in" or mask unwanted peripheral image information and create the appearance of proper collimation. This technique

irradiates patients unnecessarily, increases scatter radiation, decreases contrast, and increases the radiation dose. Shuttering is an image aesthetic only and should not be a substitute for proper and accurate collimation of the body part. Each projection in this atlas describes exactly the size of the collimation that should be used with DR systems.

Gonad Shielding

The patient's gonads may be irradiated when radiographic examinations of the abdomen, pelvis, and hip areas are performed. When practical, gonad shielding should always be used to protect the patient. Contact, shadow, and large part area shields are used for radiography examinations (Figs. 1-37 through 1-39). The Center for Devices of Radiological Health has developed guidelines recommending gonad shielding in the following instances[1]:

- If the gonads lie within or close to (about 5 cm from) the primary x-ray field despite proper beam limitation
- If the clinical objective of the examination is not compromised
- If the patient has a reasonable reproductive potential

Gonad shielding is often appropriate when limbs are radiographed with the patient seated at the end of the radiographic table (see Fig. 1-11). To ensure that shielding is used appropriately, many departments have a policy that states that the gonads be shielded on every patient and for every projection in which the lead shield would not interfere with the image. Finally, gonad shielding must be considered and used when requested by the patient unless it is contraindicated. Gonad shielding is included in selected illustrations in this atlas.

[1]Bureau of Radiological Health: *Gonad shielding in diagnostic radiology,* Pub No. (FDA) 75-8024, Rockville, MD, 1975, The Bureau.

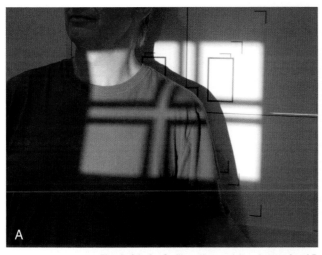
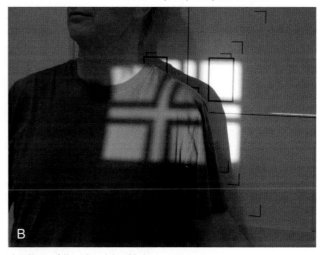

Fig. 1-36 A, Collimation set too large for AP projection of the shoulder. Note unnecessary radiation of thyroid, sternum, and general thoracic tissues. With this large collimation, more than half of the radiation strikes the table directly and results in increased scatter. **B,** Collimation set correctly to 10 × 12 inches (24 × 30 cm). Less tissue receives radiation, and less scatter is produced from the radiation striking table.

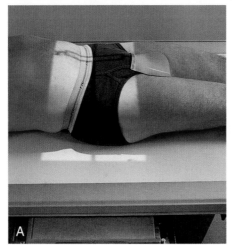
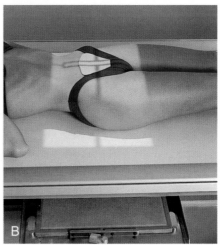

Fig. 1-37 A, Contact shield placed over the gonads of a male patient. **B,** Contact shield placed over the gonads of a female patient.

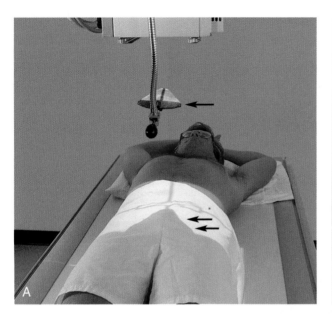

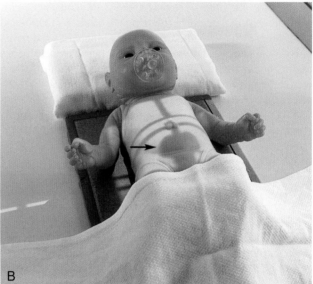

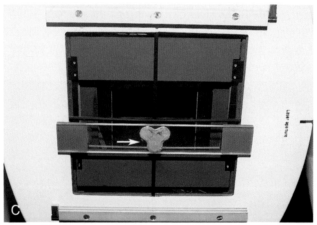

Fig. 1-38 A, Shadow shield used on a male patient. Triangular lead device (*arrow*) is hung from the x-ray tube and positioned so that its shadow falls on the gonads (*double arrows*). **B,** Shadow shield used on female infant. Cloverleaf shield is positioned under the collimator with magnets so that its shadow falls over the gonads (*arrow*). **C,** Cloverleaf-shaped shadow shield (*arrow*) positioned under the collimator with magnets.

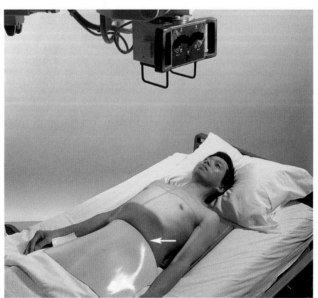

Fig. 1-39 Large piece of flexible lead (*arrow*) is draped over this patient's pelvis to protect the gonads during mobile radiography examination of the chest.

BONE MARROW DOSE

An organ of particular concern is the bone marrow. Bone marrow dose is used to estimate the population *mean marrow dose* (MMD) as an index of the somatic effect of radiation exposure. Table 1-4 relates the MMD associated with various radiographic examinations. Each of these doses results from partial-body exposure and is averaged over the entire body.

GONAD DOSE

Exposure of the gonads to radiation during diagnostic radiology is of concern because of the possible genetic effects of x-radiation. Table 1-5 indicates average gonad doses received during various radiographic examinations. The large difference between males and females results from the shielding of the ovaries by overlying tissue.

TABLE 1-4

Representative bone marrow dose for selected radiographic examinations

Examination	Mean marrow dose (mrad)
Skull	10
Cervical spine	20
Chest	2
Stomach and upper gastrointestinal tract	100
Gallbladder	80
Lumbar spine	60
Intravenous urography	25
Abdomen	30
Pelvis	20
Limb	2

TABLE 1-5

Approximate gonad dose resulting from various radiographic examinations

Examination	Gonad dose (mrad) Male	Female
Skull	<1	<1
Cervical spine	<1	<1
Full-mouth dental	>1	<1
Chest	>1	<1
Stomach and upper gastrointestinal tract	<2	40
Gallbladder	1	20
Lumbar spine	175	400
Intravenous urography	150	300
Abdomen	100	200
Pelvis	300	150
Limb	<1	<1

Digital Imaging

Since the discovery of x-rays in 1895, digital imaging has prompted some of the most technically significant changes in the way radiographs are produced. These systems use computers and digital systems to display the radiographic image. Radiography departments worldwide are slowly converting to digital systems. In the future, all radiographs may eventually be done with digital or some other type of digital technology.

Computed radiography (CR) involves conventional radiographic projection radiography in which the latent image (the unseen image) is produced in digital format using computer technology. The CR system uses a conventional radiography machine and conventional positioning and technical factors. The IR consists of a phosphor material plate that is similar to a conventional intensifying screen, inside a closed cassette rather than on a film in a light-tight cassette. These storage-phosphor IRs are often referred to as "plates" or "imaging plates" (IPs). After exposure the CR cassette is inserted into an image reader device (Fig. 1-40), where it is scanned by a laser beam, and the final image appears on a computer monitor. The radiographer can either adjust the image for appropriate density and contrast and then print it on laser film or store the image in the computer to be read directly from the monitor by the radiologist (Fig. 1-41). A darkroom and film processor are not used with CR systems.

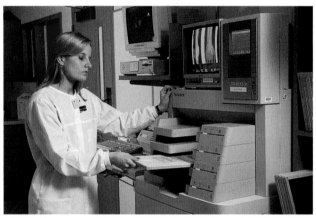

Fig. 1-40 Radiographer inserting IP into an image reader unit on CR system. The unit scans the plate with a laser beam and places the digitized image of the body part in a computer for reading on a monitor or, if necessary, for printing on a laser film.

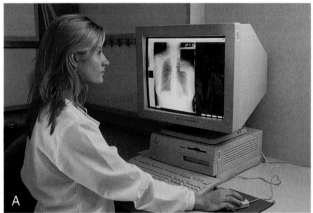 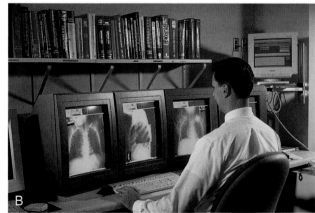

Fig. 1-41 A, Radiographer at the monitor uses the mouse to adjust the CR image of the body part to the proper size, density, and contrast before electronically sending the image for reading. **B,** Radiologist at the monitor is reading several CR images on one patient.

The newest digital x-ray systems are called *digital radiography* (DR) systems. These are similar to CR systems but do not use any type of cassette. The IR, a solid-state flat panel or CCD detector that receives the x-ray image, is built into the x-ray table or wall unit (Fig. 1-42). The built-in IR is 17 × 17 inches (43 × 43 cm) to accommodate lengthwise and crosswise projections (see Fig. 1-31, *D*). An IP reader unit is unnecessary for the solid-state detectors. The image is immediately displayed on the computer monitor after exposure.

Attention to detail is paramount when the radiographer is using CR or DR. The following sections address the technical considerations that are different from those used in conventional radiography.

KILOVOLTAGE

Because of the wider dynamic range of digital systems, a specific kVp setting is not as critical as in conventional radiography. A slightly higher kVp setting may be acceptable for a specific radiography projection. Using a kVp that is too low and does not penetrate the part adequately can create a poor-quality image (Fig. 1-43), however. Slightly overpenetrating the body part is better than underpenetrating it. An optimal kVp range should be posted on the technique chart for all projections using digital systems. In addition, for body parts that have different thicknesses of structures and densities but must be imaged on one projection (e.g., a femur), the thickest part must be well penetrated. Compensating filters should be used for body parts that have extreme differences in tissue density (see Chapter 2).

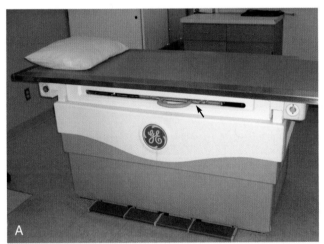
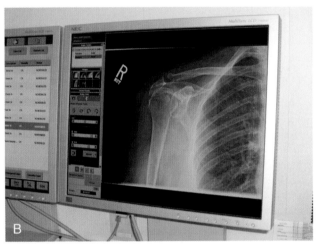

Fig. 1-42 A, DR x-ray table. The flat panel detector system is built into the table (*arrow*). There is no Bucky tray for a cassette. **B,** Image is immediately displayed on the monitor in the x-ray room for viewing.

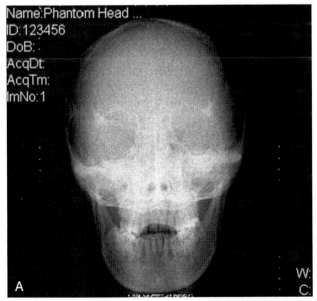
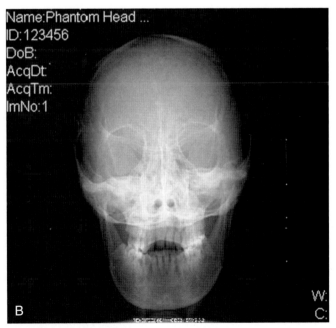

Fig. 1-43 CR images showing effect of underpenetration. **A,** AP projection of the skull underpenetrated at 48 kVp. Computer was unable to create a diagnostic image because not enough x-rays reached IP. **B,** Same projection adequately penetrated at 85 kVp. Determining the correct kVp is critical when using digital systems.

(Courtesy Beth L. Veale, MEd, RT(R), and Christi Carter, MSRS, RT(R).)

PART CENTERING

The body part that is being radiographed must always be placed in or near the center area of the CR plate or DR detector. If the central ray is directed to a body part that is positioned at the periphery of the IR (e.g., a finger placed near the edge), the computer may be unable to form the image properly; this also depends on whether the computer is in the autoprocessing or manual-processing mode. CR imaging plates can be split in half and used for two separate exposures because the image reader notes the two areas of exposure. This practice is not encouraged by the digital manufacturers, however.

SPLIT CASSETTES

If a CR plate is divided in half and used for two separate exposures, the side not receiving the exposure must always be covered with a lead shield. Storage phosphors in the CR plate are hypersensitive to small levels of exposure and may show on the image if not properly shielded. Covering the unused half prevents scatter radiation from reaching the unexposed side of the CR plate. Although this technique is practiced in conventional radiography, it is more critical with CR. Depending on the specific technical factors used, the images may not appear at all, may contain artifacts, or may display other image-processing failures. In addition, technical factors and body part thickness for the two exposures must be relatively close to each other.

COLLIMATION

As with conventional radiology, the body part being radiographed must be collimated cautiously. In addition to the usual image-quality issues associated with excessive scattered or off-focus radiation, poor collimation practices with digital systems can result in digital processing errors. These errors are frequently related to inability of the system to identify and separate image information from primary beam exposure at the collimated edges of the image field, resulting in images with inappropriate brightness or contrast. The body part and collimated field should always be centered to the IR when possible. At the very least, the collimated field should be placed so that all four margins are on the IR. When producing multiple exposures on a CR image receptor, the collimated fields should be spaced and oriented to prevent overlap of adjacent collimated edges.

GRIDS

The IRs used in digital radiography systems are much more sensitive to scatter radiation. Some projections may require a grid if the kVp is above a certain level. One manufacturer requires that a grid be used for any exposure greater than 90 kVp. This consideration is particularly important in mobile radiography, for which many projections are done without a grid. With digital systems, examination routines may need to be reevaluated to determine the need for a grid.

DIGITAL IMAGING IN THIS ATLAS

For most radiographic examinations, radiographic positioning does not markedly change with CR or DR. For some projections, the part centering, central ray, collimation, and other technical factors may be slightly different. When this occurs, a comment is made and indicated under the following icon:

DIGITAL IMAGING

Foundation Exposure Techniques and Charts

An exposure technique chart should be placed in each radiographic room and on mobile machines including machines that use automatic exposure control (AEC) and digital systems.[1-3] A foundation technique chart is one made for all normal-size adults. A well-designed chart also includes suggested adjustments for pediatric, emaciated, and obese patients. The chart should be organized to display all the radiographic projections performed in the room. The specific exposure factors for each projection should also be indicated (Fig. 1-44). A measuring caliper should be used to ascertain the part thickness for accurate technique selection (Fig. 1-45).

Each chapter contains a sample exposure technique chart of the essential projections described in the chapter. This chart is a *sample only,* and the exposure techniques listed should not be used unless all the technical parameters are exactly the same in the user's department. The chart can be used, however, to show typical manual and automatic exposure techniques and the difference between exposures for various body parts and to serve as a baseline for developing accurate charts for a radiology department. The kVp values for each projection are approximate for the three-phase generator used for the charts and can be used for the body part as indicated.

[1]Eastman TR: Digital systems require x-ray charts too, *Radiol Technol* 67:354, 1996.
[2]Gray JE et al: *Quality control in diagnostic imaging,* Rockville, MD, 1983, Aspen.
[3]Eastman TR: Get back to the basics of radiography, *Radiol Technol* 68:285, 1997.

BONY THORAX

Part	cm	kVp*	tm	mA	mAs	AEC	SID	IR	Dose† (mrad)
Sternum—*PA Oblique*‡	20	65	0.22	200s	45		30"	10 × 12 inches	306
Sternum—*Lateral*‡	29	70	0.4	200s	80		72"	10 × 12 inches	710
SC Articulations—*PA*‡	17	65		200s		⚬⚬●	40"	8 × 10 inches	195
SC Articulations—*PA Oblique*‡	18	65	0.15	200s	30		40"	8 × 10 inches	208
Upper Anterior Ribs—*PA*‡	21	70	0.16	200s	32		40"	14 × 17 inches	60
Posterior Ribs—*AP Upper*‡	21	70	0.16	200s	32		40"	14 × 17 inches	60
Posterior Ribs—*AP Lower*‡	21	70		200s		●● ⚬	40"	14 × 17 inches	159
Ribs—Axillary—*AP Oblique*‡	23	70	0.16	200s	32		40"	14 × 17 inches	82
Ribs—Axillary—*PA Oblique*‡	23	70	0.16	200s	32		40"	14 × 17 inches	82

s, Small focal spot.
*kVp values are for a three-phase, 12-pulse generator or high frequency.
†Relative doses for comparison use. All doses are skin entrance for average adult at cm indicated.
‡Bucky, 16:1 grid. Screen/film speed 300 or equivalent CR.

Fig. 1-44 Radiographic exposure technique chart showing manual and AEC technical factors for the examinations identified.

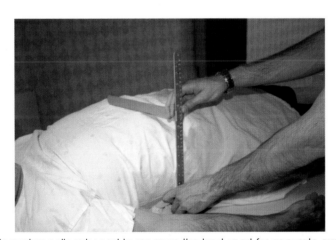

Fig. 1-45 Measuring caliper is used to measure the body part for accurate exposure technique selection.

A satisfactory technique chart can be established only by the radiographer's familiarity with the characteristics of the particular equipment and accessories used and the radiologist's preference in image quality. The following primary factors must be taken into account when the correct foundation technique is being established for each unit:

• Milliamperage (mA)
• Kilovolt (peak) (kVp)
• Exposure time (seconds)
• Automatic exposure controls (AECs)
• Source–to–image receptor distance (SID)
• Grid
• Film and screen speed number
• Electrical supply

With this information available, the exposure factors can be selected for each region of the body and balanced so that the best possible radiographic quality is obtained.

Modern x-ray generators have anatomic programmers that can store a wide range of radiographic exposure techniques for most body parts (Fig. 1-46). The radiographer simply selects the body part, and the technique is automatically set.

Adaptation of Exposure Technique to Patients

The radiographer's responsibility is to select the combination of exposure factors that produces the desired quality of radiographs for each region of the body and to standardize this quality. When the radiographer establishes this standard quality, deviation from the exposure factors should be minimal. These foundation factors should be adjusted for every patient's size to maintain uniform quality. The same definition on all subjects cannot be achieved, however, because of congenital and developmental factors and age and pathologic changes. Some patients have fine, distinct bony trabecular markings, whereas others do not. Individual differences must be considered when the quality of the radiograph is judged.

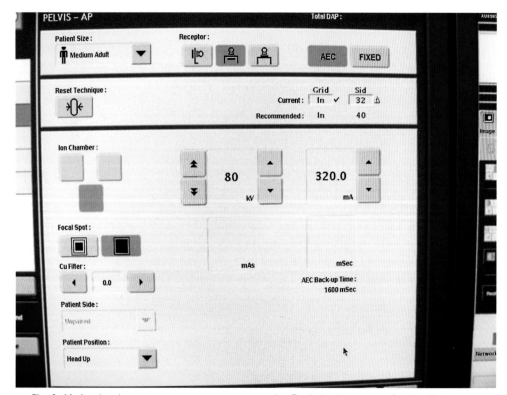

Fig. 1-46 Anatomic programmer on x-ray generator. Technical exposure factors for most body parts are preprogrammed into computer. The factors on this display are for AP projection of the pelvis.

Certain conditions require the radiographer to compensate when establishing an exposure technique (Fig. 1-47). Conditions that require a decrease in technical factors include the following:
- Old age
- Pneumothorax
- Emphysema
- Emaciation
- Degenerative arthritis
- Atrophy

Some conditions require an increase in technical factors to penetrate the part to be examined. These include the following:
- Pneumonia
- Pleural effusion
- Hydrocephalus
- Enlarged heart
- Edema
- Ascites

Preexposure Instructions

The radiographer should instruct the patient in breathing and have the patient practice until the necessary actions are clearly understood. After the patient is in position but before the radiographer leaves to make the exposure, the radiographer should have the patient practice breathing once more. This step requires a few minutes, but it saves much time and the need for repeat radiographs.

Inspiration (inhalation) depresses the diaphragm and abdominal viscera, lengthens and expands the lung fields, elevates the sternum and pushes it anteriorly, and elevates the ribs and reduces their angle near the spine. *Expiration* (exhalation) elevates the diaphragm and abdominal viscera, shortens the lung fields, depresses the sternum, and lowers the ribs and increases their angle near the spine.

During trunk examinations, the patient's phase of breathing is important. When exposures are to be made during shallow breathing, the patient should practice slow, even breathing, so that only the structures above the one being examined move. When lung motion and not rib motion is desired, the patient should practice slow, deep breathing after a compression band has been applied across the chest. (The correct *respiration phase* is printed in the positioning instructions for each projection in the text.)

The eyes of the radiographer should always be on the patient when the exposure is made to ensure that an exposure is not made if the patient moves or breathes. This is particularly important when radiographing pediatric, trauma, unconscious, and some geriatric patients.

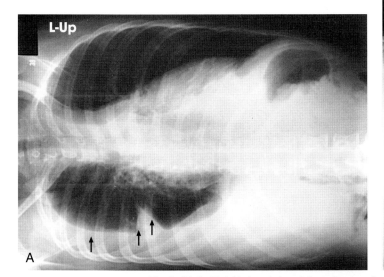 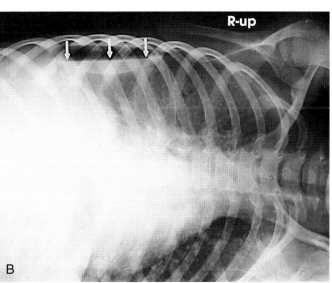

Fig. 1-47 A, Right lateral decubitus chest radiograph showing fluid level (*arrows*). The radiographic exposure technique had to be increased from the standard technique to show the fluid level. **B,** Left lateral decubitus chest radiograph showing air-fluid level (*arrows*). The radiographic exposure technique had to be decreased from the standard technique to show the free air.

Technical Factors

The variation in power delivered by the x-ray tube permits the radiographer to control several prime technical factors: *milliamperage* (mA), *kilovolt peak* (kVp), and *exposure time* (seconds). The radiographer selects the specific factors required to produce a quality radiograph using the generator's control panel after consulting a technique chart. Manual and AEC systems are used to set the factors (Fig. 1-48).

Detailed aspects of each technical factor are presented in physics and imaging courses. Because of the variety of exposure factors and equipment used in clinical practice, exact technical factors are not presented in this atlas. The companion *Merrill's Pocket Guide to Radiography* is designed to allow students and radiographers to organize and write in the technical factors used in respective departments with the different equipment available (Fig. 1-49). Each chapter's technique chart shows an approximate kVp and AEC detector setting as described later. These two parameters do not vary from department to department. The factors mA, exposure time, SID, screens, grids, CR and DR factors are highly variable, however, and not listed.

KILOVOLTAGE IN THIS ATLAS

The kVp setting is a crucial factor that controls the energy and penetrating ability of the x-ray beam. Various kVp settings are used depending on the type of x-ray generators used, the type of grid used, and the contrast of the finished radiograph. A 70-kVp technique with a three-phase generator requires 80 kVp with a single-phase generator to maintain the same contrast level.[1] An approximate kVp value is shown for each essential projection for three-phase generators. These are the kVp values that ensure an adequate penetration of the body part and appropriate dose control.

[1]Cullinan AM, Cullinan JE: *Producing quality radiography,* Philadelphia, 1994, JB Lippincott.

AUTOMATIC EXPOSURE CONTROL IN THIS ATLAS

X-ray generators contain complex AEC systems that require several settings for each exposure—kVp, mA, backup timer, density control, screen setting, and sensor selection. Numerous factors, including the type of examination, tabletop or Bucky technique, patient cooperation, and cassette size, determine which settings are used. For projections that are performed using AEC, an approximate detector selection is shown in the text for each essential projection. The other AEC variables are not shown because of the wide range of settings used in radiology departments (see Fig. 1-49).

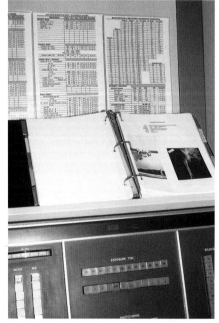

Fig. 1-48 X-ray generator control panel where exposure factors are set. Also note exposure technique chart on the wall. Radiographer uses the chart to set the techniques for each projection performed.

Knee
AP

Patient Position
- Position patient supine with leg extended.
- Adjust patient's body so that pelvis is not rotated.

Part Position
- Center knee to IR at level ½ inch (1.3 cm) below patellar apex.
- Adjust leg so that femoral condyles are parallel with IR.

Central Ray
- Enters point ½ inch (1.3 cm) inferior to patellar apex
- Depending on ASIS to tabletop measurement, direct central ray as follows:

<19 cm	3 to 5 degrees *caudad* (thin pelvis)
19 to 24 cm	0 degrees
>24 cm	3 to 5 degrees *cephalad* (large pelvis)

Collimation:
Adjust to 10 × 12 inches (24 × 30 cm).

kVp: 65   *Reference: 12th edition ATLAS p. 1:296.*

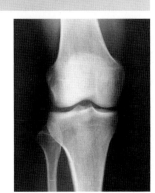

Manual Factors

Part Thickness (cm)	mA	kVp	Time	mAs	SID	IR Size	IR Speed	Grid	HF, 1 or 3Ø

ACE Factors

Part Thickness (cm)	mA	kVp	AEC Detector	mAs	Density Comp.	IR Size	Screen Comp.	Grid	HF, 1 or 3Ø

Notes: _____   Competency: ___/___/___

_____   Instructor: _____

103

Lower Limb

Fig. 1-49 Exposure technique page from *Merrill's Pocket Guide to Radiography* showing how a specific department's manual techniques and AEC techniques can be written in for reference in setting optimal techniques. Note also patient photograph and radiograph. Quick reference can be made to the exact position of the patient, and the radiograph shows how the final image should appear.

Working Effectively with Obese Patients

Radiology departments are having a difficult time acquiring and interpreting images of obese patients. A study found the number of radiology studies that were difficult to interpret because of obesity has doubled over the last 15 years.[1] According to the CDC, approximately 64% of Americans are overweight, obese, or morbidly obese.[2] More than 72 million adults are obese, and more than 6 million are morbidly obese (Fig. 1-50). The prevalence of obesity in children has been steadily increasing. Over the past 25 years, the number of obese children has nearly tripled. Approximately 15% of children 6 to 9 years old are obese.[3] Obesity has an impact on the quality of the radiographic image, and

it affects the radiographer's ability to transfer and position the patient. Obese patients have an effect on the functionality of the imaging equipment, and many obese patients cannot be placed onto radiographic or computed tomographic (CT) tables. Meanwhile, the popularity of bariatric surgery has increased the demand for radiographic procedures in obese patients.

Obesity is defined as an increase in body weight by excessive accumulation of fat. More specifically, obesity is quantified by the body mass index (BMI).[1] A BMI of 30 to 39.9 is classified as obese. A BMI greater than 40 is classified as morbidly obese, or approximately 100 lb overweight. The BMI is not of primary importance when performing radiographic examinations; the patient's *body diameter*

and *weight* are the two important considerations. One or both of these factors determine whether or not a radiographic examination can be performed.

EQUIPMENT

Manufacturers of imaging equipment have defined weight limits. The structural integrity and function of equipment and motors are typically insured by manufacturers up to the stated weight only. Radiographic table weight limits cannot be exceeded without voiding the warranty. Fluoroscopy towers have a maximum diameter, and many obese patients cannot fit under the tower. CT and magnetic resonance imaging (MRI) scanners have gantry and bore diameters that cannot accom-

[1]Trenker SW: Imaging of morbid obesity procedures and their complications, *Abdominal Imaging* 34:335, 2008.

[2]Department of Health and Human Services, Centers for Disease Control and Prevention: *Overweight and obesity: obesity trends: 1991-2001 prevalence of obesity among U.S. adults by state-behavioral risk factor surveillance system 2001,* Available at: www.cdc.gov/nccdphp/dnpa/obesity/trend/prev_reg.htm.

[3]Choudhary AK et al: Diseases associated with childhood obesity, *AJR Am J Roentgenol* 188:1118, 2007.

[1]Uppot RN et al: Impact of obesity on medical imaging and image-guided intervention, *AJR Am J Roentgenol* 188:433, 2007.

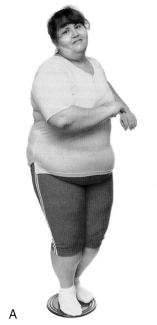
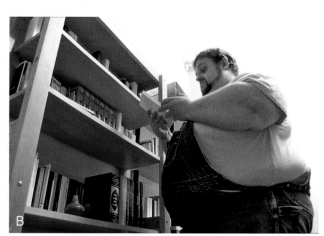

Fig. 1-50 A, Obese patient. **B,** Morbidly obese patient.

(**A,** Used with permission from Fotosearch; **B,** Copyright Phototake, Inc.)

modate some obese patients. Table 1-6 lists the current industry standard weight limits and maximum aperture diameters. For CT and MRI, the aperture diameter is accurate in the horizontal plane. The vertical plane must take into consideration the table thickness entering the gantry or bore. The table takes up 15 to 18 cm of the stated vertical diameter; this limits many patients from having CT or MRI examinations. Most radiology departments do not perform examinations on patients who weigh more than 350 to 450 lb. Radiographers must be aware of the weight and aperture limits of the radiographic equipment in their departments. The radiology department should have a protocol for working with obese patients, and all equipment should be marked with the limits.

To accommodate obese patients, most radiography equipment manufacturers are redesigning their equipment and increasing table weights and aperture dimensions. Table 1-7 shows the limits of the current equipment that has been modified for obese patients. Radiographic and fluoroscopic table weight limits have doubled to 700 lb. CT and MRI table weights and aperture openings have also increased.

TRANSPORTATION

Transportation of obese patients is another way in which obesity affects the delivery of health care to these individuals. Obese patients require larger wheelchairs and larger transport beds or stretchers. Some hospitals have installed larger doorways to accommodate the larger transportation equipment. The availability of these special chairs and beds may be limited and may affect the scheduling of these patients. One manufacturer[1] has designed a special cart that can hold patients weighing 750 lb; this cart has a 34-inch pad width. Many obese patients, unless they are hospitalized, are able to walk around and access clinics and imaging centers. Their weight becomes an issue, however, when they have to get on the radiographic equipment.

A major factor involved in the transportation and transfer of obese patients is the

[1]Pedigo, Vancouver, WA, Available at: www.pedigo.com. Accessed April 1, 2010.

potential risk of injury to the radiographer and other health care workers during movement and positioning of patients. Radiographic examinations of obese patients who are hospitalized must be coordinated carefully between the radiology department and the patient's nursing section. Appropriate measurements must be made in the patient's room in advance by trained radiology personnel. An obese patient should not be transported to the radiology department and find on arrival that he or she cannot be accommodated.

An appropriate number of staff must be available to ensure that there is appropriate moving assistance. Transfer of a patient from the cart to the radiographic table may require 8 to 10 individuals. Obese patients are not lifted; they are moved by sliding. Hydraulic lifts cannot be used because of weight limit restrictions, and most obese patients are too large or wide for plastic moving devices and sliders. It is imperative that proper body mechanics be used by all personnel moving these patients.

TABLE 1-6

Industry standard weight limit and maximum aperture diameter by imaging technique

Imaging technique	Weight limit	Maximum aperture diameter (cm)
Fluoroscopy	350 lb (159 kg)	45
4- to 16-multidetector CT	450 lb (205 kg)	70*
Cylindric bore MRI, 1.5-3.0 T	350 lb (159 kg)	60*
Vertical field MRI, 0.3-1.0 T	550 lb (250 kg)	55*

*Aperture is accurate in horizontal plane only. For vertical plane, about 15 to 18 cm must be subtracted from diameter to account for table thickness.

TABLE 1-7

Advances in weight limit and maximum aperture diameter by imaging technique

Imaging technique	Weight limit	Maximum aperture diameter (cm)
Fluoroscopy	700 lb (318 kg)	60
16-multidetector CT	680 lb (308 kg)	90*
Cylindric bore MRI, 1.5 T	550 lb (250 kg)	70*
Vertical field MRI, 0.3-1.0 T	550 lb (250 kg)	55*

*Aperture is accurate in horizontal plane only. For vertical plane, about 15 to 18 cm must be subtracted from diameter to account for table thickness.

COMMUNICATION

Communication with obese patients may require personnel to be more aware of the issues of obesity. The radiographer must be able to assess the difficulties created by the limitations of equipment in handling an obese patient and be able to communicate with the patient without offending him or her. The dignity of the patient must be kept in mind. Sensitivity training should be provided by the hospital or clinic. For the most part, communications are no different than with a nonobese patient. Reference to the patient's weight should never be made. The radiographer should be sensitive and display compassion. This can be accomplished by clearly explaining the procedure to gain the patient's confidence and trust. After the patient's trust and cooperation have been obtained, it is easier to communicate effectively if any problems or concerns with the examination arise.

There should never be any discussion about the patient in the radiographic room and no discussion within hearing distance of the patient about the poor image quality or the difficulty in obtaining images. If the radiologist and the patient's physician together determine that the patient's weight allows radiographic images to be made, the examination should proceed in the same manner as with any other patient.

More staff may be needed for transfer purposes; however, communications and performance of the examination should remain the same.

IMAGING CHALLENGES

When the patient is on the table, it is imperative that he or she is centered accurately to the center of the table; this is necessary because it may be impossible to palpate traditional landmarks such as the anterior-superior iliac spine (ASIS) and iliac crest (see Chapter 3 for positioning landmarks). One of the most important considerations in positioning an obese patient is to recognize that the bony skeleton and most organs have not changed in position and the organs are not larger. Most of what is seen physically on these patients is fat. In Fig. 1-51, the skeleton is normal size, and most organs fall with their normal position. The only exception would be in morbidly obese patients, in whom the width of the thoracic cage and ribs may be expanded 2 inches, the stomach may be slightly larger, and the colon may be spread out more across the width of the abdomen. Most positioning landmarks used on obese patients will be reference points in the midsagittal plane of the patient.

Radiographic projections of the skull, cervical spine, and upper limb are obtainable on all obese patients. Projections of the lower limb from the knee distally are obtainable. Shoulder and femur projections may be difficult to position but are usually obtainable. All projections of the thorax including lungs, abdomen, thoracic and lumbar spines, pelvis, and hips are very challenging to position and may be impossible to obtain in morbidly obese patients. The patient's lack of mobility makes lateral hip projections virtually impossible. Fig. 1-52 shows that most fat accumulates around the trunk, particularly around the abdomen, pelvis, and hips. Imaging of organs such as the stomach, small bowel, and colon may be impossible. CT may be the only imaging alternative, if the equipment integrity can support the weight and girth of these patients.

Landmarks

Finding traditional positioning landmarks may be possible in some obese patients and impossible in morbidly obese patients. It is appropriate to enlist the patient's assistance in identifying landmarks if it is possible. This gives the patient a sense of being involved in their examination. The *jugular notch* may be the only landmark available for palpation. Traditional landmarks such as the xiphoid, ASIS, iliac crest, pubic symphysis, and greater trochanter are impossible to palpate. The radiographer should not attempt

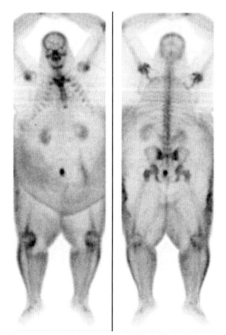

Fig. 1-51 Bone scan on 500-lb patient. Note large physical size of patient, but within the large body are the skeleton and organs of a typical 165-lb body.

(Used with permission from ARRS.)

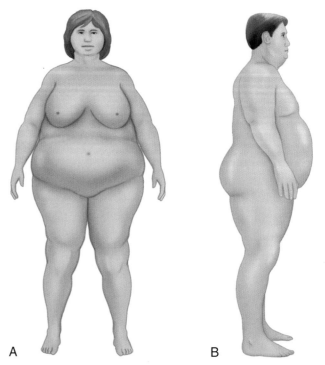

Fig. 1-52 Large amount of body fat that surrounds the abdomen, pelvis, hips, and upper femora on obese patients. Dimensions shown are from actual patient measurements.

to push and prod to find these. Fig. 1-53 shows a morbidly obese patient and how he would appear on the radiographic table. The traditional landmarks would be impossible to find because of excess body fat. If the patient's chin is raised, however, the jugular notch can be palpated.

The importance of the jugular notch cannot be underestimated because most projections of the thorax, abdomen, and pelvis can be obtained by simply finding this landmark. Two items should be available in the radiographic room—tongue depressors and a tape measure. When the jugular notch is found, a tongue depressor should be placed on the notch. With the tape, the radiographer measures straight down the midsagittal plane, from the jugular notch point to the pubic symphysis (Fig. 1-54). The symphysis is found at the following distances from the jugular notch:

Patient height: <5 ft: 21 inches
5 to 6 ft: 22 inches
> 6 ft: 24 inches

At the point of the pubic symphysis, the second tongue depressor is placed. The two depressors presents a visual indication of the trunk of the body. Note the symphysis will not be palpated due to the pendiculum (the fat skirt that hangs down over the symphysis). The indicators above will determine its location. When the radiographer knows where these two anatomic points are, nearly all projections of the trunk can be obtained with moderate accuracy. The bottom edge of a 14- × 17-inch (35- × 43-cm) IR placed lengthwise at the pubic symphysis shows the abdomen and lumbar spine. If the bottom edge of the IR is placed crosswise, it shows the pelvis and hips. The first thoracic vertebra (T1) is located approximately 2 inches (5 cm) above the jugular notch. An understanding of the landmarks related to body structures described in Chapter 3 enables the radiographer to position for nearly all projections of the trunk.

Some variations in obese patients occur. Many of these patients have a very large abdomen only (Fig. 1-55). Although

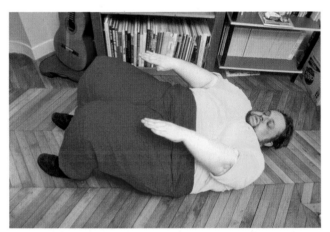

Fig. 1-53 Morbidly obese patient. Traditional landmarks would be impossible to palpate. With the chin raised, the jugular notch can be palpated.

(Copyright Phototake, Inc.)

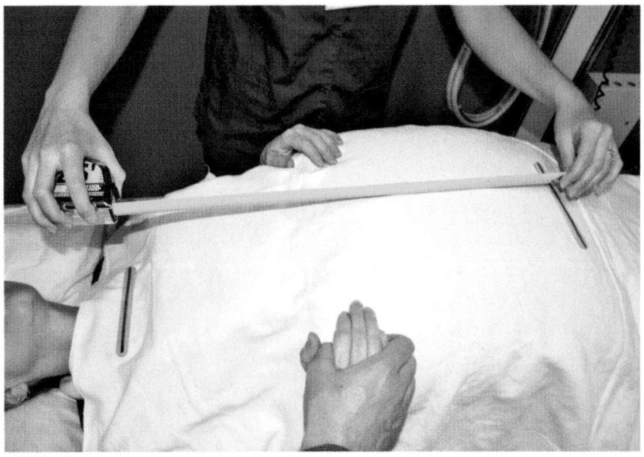

Fig. 1-54 Radiographer measuring jugular notch to pubic symphysis plane.

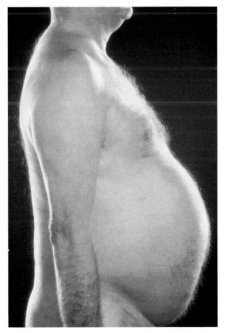

Fig. 1-55 Large abdomen only. Note most body areas other than abdomen are normal size.

(Copyright Phototake, Inc.)

their other body areas are not large, the largeness of the abdomen prevents any type of landmark palpation for lumbar spine, abdomen, and pelvis images. In other obese patients, the abdominal fat is very soft and movable and is layered in "folds" (Fig. 1-56). For these patients, the radiographer can gently move or push the folds of skin out of the way to palpate the ASIS or iliac crest. The patient should be informed of what the radiographer is doing every step of the way.

Oblique and lateral projections

Caution should be used when turning patients on their side for oblique and lateral projections. Turning should always be done with the assistance of the patient and at least three other health care workers. Positioning aids or equipment should be used to prevent injury to the patient and personnel. Before turning the patient, measurements should be taken of the body part width to determine if the exposure technique can be made. Oblique and lateral projections of the hips, lumbar spine, lumbosacral area, sacrum, coccyx and, in some patients, thoracic spine may be prohibited because of x-ray tube limits (Fig. 1-57). The patient should not be turned unless the exposure can be made. Oblique and lateral projections are typically impossible to obtain on a morbidly obese patient. "Cross-table" projections also may be impossible because of the patient's size and the very large amount of scatter radiation produced. Lower grid ratios ingrid holders are typically used for these exposures, and these do not aid in improving the image quality. There may be limited instances when two exposures can be made. The patient must be able to cooperate, however, and this works only on bone projections.

Image receptor sizes and collimation

At first, it may seem that larger size IRs are needed to image obese patients. In most instances, this is not the case. If care is taken to find landmarks, in particular, the jugular notch and pubic symphysis, relatively accurate positioning can be accomplished. Collimation is one of the most important considerations when imaging obese patients. Setting the collimator to the smallest dimensions possible reduces scatter radiation. The reduced scatter increases contrast, which enables improved visibility of the structures (Fig. 1-58). The use of standard size IRs and standard collimation settings for DR keeps scatter radiation to low levels, and scatter radiation fog on the image is reduced. *The collimator should never be set larger than the size of the IR.*

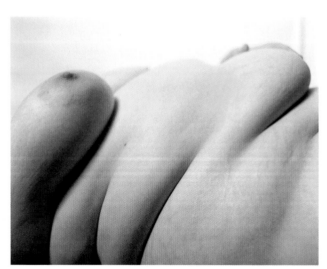

Fig. 1-56 Obese patient with abdominal folds. Skin and fat folds are soft and movable. Landmarks such as ASIS or iliac crest may be found.

(Used with permission from Fotosearch.)

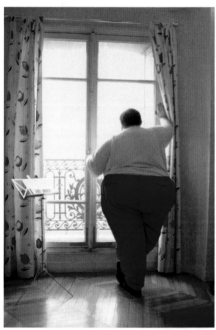

Fig. 1-57 Obese patient with large lateral measurement of lumbar spine area. Lateral projections of this area and possibly thoracic area may be unobtainable.

(Copyright Phototake, Inc.)

Digital radiography

With DR and the availability of the 17- ×17-inch (43- × 43-cm) flat-panel detector built in the table (see Fig. 1-31, *D*), there may be a temptation to use the maximum size of this field on the large patients. *This temptation should be avoided.* This very large collimator setting produces more scatter, increases fog on the radiograph, and reduces contrast. Collimating larger than the traditional 14 × 17 inches (35 × 43 cm) for the body parts that require this dimension images only more fat. Recall from Fig. 1-51 that within the large body is a standard size skeletal frame and organs. A significantly improved diagnostic image is obtained on obese patients when smaller IRs and collimation settings are used. For colon and other abdominal images, it may be necessary to take multiple images on quadrants of the body[1] using smaller collimation settings. When using DR to image obese patients, radiographers should use the collimation settings for the various projections as indicated in this atlas.

[1]Uppot RN et al: Impact of obesity on medical imaging and image-guided intervention, *AJR Am J Roentgenol* 188:433, 2007.

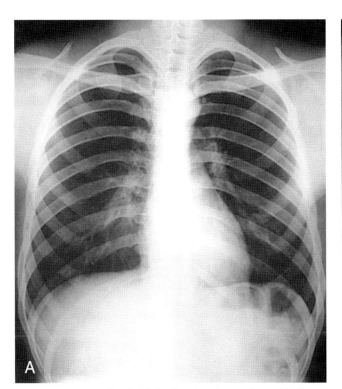
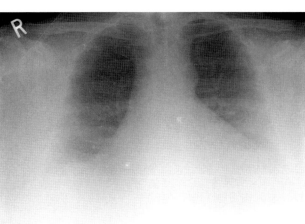

Fig. 1-58 A, Chest radiograph on 160-lb patient. Note very good contrast and visibility of structures. **B,** Chest radiograph on 500-lb patient. Note reduced contrast and fogging on image. A reasonable image was obtained, however.

(**B,** Used with permission from ARRS.)

Field light size

When the collimator size is set automatically for IRs in the Bucky or manually on the collimator for DR equipment, the field light is visible on a nonobese patient's body relatively close to the actual dimensions of the IR (Fig. 1-59, *A*). This light gives the radiographer an accurate visual indication of where the radiation field falls. On obese patients, in whom the vertical dimension of the thorax and abdomen is very large (see Fig. 1-50, *B*), the field light visible on top of the patient appears much smaller than the IR size because the abdomen is closer to the collimator bulb, and less light divergence occurs (Fig. 1-59, *B*). There may be a natural tendency to open the collimator when this small field is seen. *The collimator should not be opened larger than the size of the IR or the stated collimator dimensions for DR.* The radiographer must understand that although the field size visually appears small on top of the patient, the radiation field diverges to expose the entire IR size.

EXPOSURE FACTORS

Modified x-ray exposure techniques need to be used on obese patients. The main factors have to be increased, including the mA, kVp, and exposure time. The major limitation in obtaining images of obese patients is inadequate penetration of the body part. This situation results in increased quantum mottle (noise) and very low image contrast. The increased exposure time required in these patients can also contribute to motion artifacts in the image. The most important adjustment that should be made is an increase in the kVp. Increasing the kVp increases the penetration of the x-ray beam. The mA and exposure time (mAs) have to be increased; however, caution should be used in increasing the mA. Greater exposures can be obtained safely by using low mA settings and longer exposure times. (See tube rating charts in a physics text.)

Motion is not a major problem in imaging obese patients because the weight of the patient prevents most body parts from moving, and mA settings of about 320 can be used. This setting may increase the exposure time; however, with an explanation of the importance of holding the breath, most obese patients can do so. With repeated use of high exposure factors, the x-ray tube can become very hot. Radiographers should ensure that adequate cooling of the anode and tube as a whole occurs; this can be accomplished by simply taking more time in between exposures.

Focal spot

The focal spot in the x-ray tube is controlled by the mA that is selected. The mA for obese patient radiographs may be higher than 250 to 320 mA, which will automatically engage the large focus. Use of the small focal spot, which enables greater recorded detail, may be restricted to the distal limbs because of the higher exposure techniques. Radiographers must have a full understanding of the focal spot limits for the machines they use. These should be posted for use with obese patient projections.

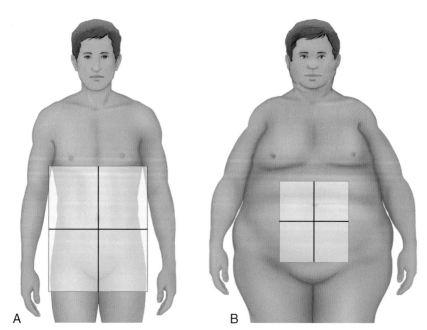

Fig. 1-59 A, Illustration of how collimator light for 14- × 17-inch (43- × 43-cm) IR appears on normal-size patient with 21-cm abdomen measurement. The light is very close in dimension to IR size. **B,** Collimator light shown for same size IR on obese patient with 45-cm vertical abdomen measurement. Although collimator is set to same dimensions, light field appears small on top of the patient.

Bucky and grid

The use of a Bucky grid or a mobile grid can minimize scatter radiation significantly. The grid is automatically used when obtaining standard projections on the x-ray table and for some cross-table lateral images of limbs. Although a grid is never used for elbow, ankle, and leg projections on nonobese patients, it can significantly improve image quality on obese patients and in particular morbidly obese patients. Radiology departments should have a high-ratio mobile grid available for use with obese patients.

Automatic exposure control and anatomically programmed radiography systems

AEC and anatomically programmed radiography (APR) systems are widely used in radiology departments to control technical factors "automatically." Machine-set exposure factors will frequently be inappropriate for obese patients so the kVp, mA, exposure time, AEC detectors, and focal spot should be *manually adjusted*. With AEC, the radiographer should ensure that a high kVp and a moderate mA are used. The radiology department should maintain a special exposure technique chart for obese patients similar to using a special chart for pediatric patients. When possible, all three AEC detectors should be activated.

Mobile radiography

Mobile radiography machines may be used for imaging obese patients; however, their use is very limited. Because the x-ray tubes on these machines have limited ratings, exposure techniques high enough to penetrate these patients cannot be obtained. Depending on the size of the patient, mobile projections are restricted to chest and limbs only. The mobile machine should have a special technique chart outlining the technical factors used for this group of patients.

Radiation dose

Radiographers must use caution in all aspects of working with obese patients, including keeping repeat exposures to a minimum. A study of radiation doses to obese patients having bariatric surgery showed a "fourfold" dose increase compared with nonobese patients having the same examinations.[1] Doses to these patients reached 4500 mrem (45 mSv). Precautions must be taken to minimize patient dose. The radiologist should be involved in evaluating the justification of any radiologic procedure on an obese patient. Radiographers should be especially cautious when holding a limb or an IR

---

[1]Rampado O et al: Radiation dose evaluations during radiological contrast studies in patients with morbid obesity, *Radiol Med* 113:1229, 2008.

during an x-ray exposure on an obese patient. The increased exposure techniques prompt increased scatter, which reaches the person holding the patient. If someone has to hold an obese patient, when possible, the person should stand at a right angle (90 degrees) to the central ray for maximum scatter protection. (See Mobile Chapter 28 for further information.)

Special technical considerations must be followed when working with obese and morbidly obese patients. Box 1-4 summarizes the principal technical factors that should be observed.

BOX 1-4

Technical considerations for working effectively with obese patients

- Warm up x-ray tube before making any exposures.
- Use lower mA settings (<320).
- Use higher kVp settings.
- Do not make repeated exposures near x-ray tube loading limit.
- Use the large focal spot for all but distal limbs.
- Do not use APR systems to determine exposure technique.
- When using AEC systems, ensure kVp is high enough and mA is moderate.
- Collimate to the size of IR or smaller.
- With DR, collimate to suggested field size for the projection.
- Never collimate to the maximum 17- × 17-inch (43- × 43-cm) size of the flat panel DR detector.
- Maintain special exposure technique chart for obese patient projections.
- Stand at right angles (90 degrees) to the central ray when holding an obese patient.

ABBREVIATIONS USED IN CHAPTER 1

AEC	automatic exposure control
AP	anteroposterior
ASRT	American Society of Radiologic Technologists
CAMRT	Canadian Association of Medical Radiation Technologists
CCD	charge-coupled device
CDC	Centers for Disease Control and Prevention
cm	centimeter
CR*	central ray
CR*	computed radiography
DR	digital radiography
IP	image plate
IR	image receptor
kVp	kilovolt peak
L	left
LAO	left anterior oblique
mA	milliamperage
mAs	milliampere second
MMD	mean marrow dose
NCRP	National Council on Radiation Protection
OD	optical density
OID	object-to-image receptor distance
OR	operating room
PA	posteroanterior
R	right
RA	radiologist assistant
RPA	radiology practitioner assistant
RPO	right posterior oblique
SID	source-to-image receptor distance
SSD	source-to-skin distance

See Addendum A for a summary of all abbreviations in Volume 1.
*Note that there are two different abbreviations for CR.

2

COMPENSATING FILTERS

PETER J. BARGER

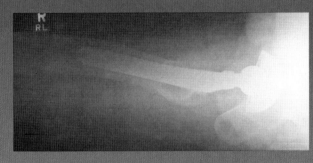

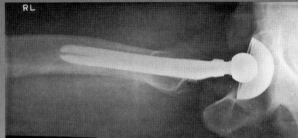

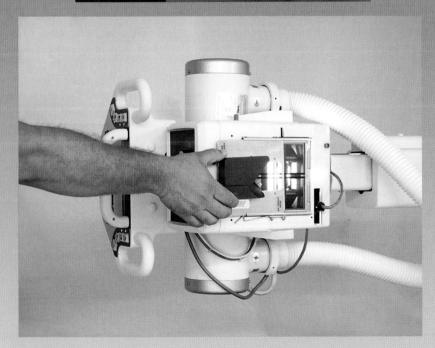

Introduction

In most cases, radiography is accomplished using a single exposure technique for a given body structure. Some structures contain areas of significantly varied tissue thickness and density that must be shown on one image, however. These structures present special challenges in showing the anatomic structures with an acceptable range of densities. Often, two exposures must be made on these body structures, doubling the radiation exposure to the patient.

Typically, if one exposure is used, a technique is selected to penetrate adequately the densest area of anatomy. In this case, the radiologist highlights the dark anatomic area on the image with a "hot-light." These images often have to be viewed by other physicians without having such a light available. With digital radiography systems, the image can be adjusted with the computer to lighten the dark area of anatomy; however, the large difference in transmitted x-rays often exceeds the dynamic range of the software.

Images that appear low in contrast, contain high noise, or show processing artifacts can result. Clinical experience shows that compensating filters improve digital images.

Examples of x-ray projections that have to show significantly varied tissue density include the anteroposterior (AP) projection of the thoracic spine, the axiolateral projection (Danelius-Miller method) of the hip, and the lateral cervicothoracic region (swimmer's technique) (Fig. 2-1). Exposure of these structures with a uni-

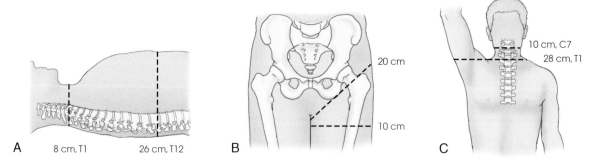

Fig. 2-1 A-C, Body structures with significantly varied tissue thickness and density include thoracic spine (AP) (**A**), hip (lateral) (**B**), and cervicothoracic region (lateral) (**C**). Note different thicknesses in these areas. Use of compensating filters allows these structures to be shown with one exposure.

formly intense x-ray beam results in the production of an image with areas of underexposed or overexposed anatomy. To compensate for these variations in tissue density, specially designed attenuating devices called *compensating filters* can be placed between the radiographic tube and the image receptor (IR). The resulting attenuated beam more appropriately exposes the various tissue densities of the anatomy and reveals more anatomic detail. Equally important, the filter reduces the entrance skin exposure and the dose to some of the organs in the body (Fig. 2-2).

The technique of compensatory filtration was first applied in 1905 by Pfahler,[1] not long after x-rays were first discovered. Pfahler used wet shoe leather as the filter by wrapping it around a patient's arm. Compensating filters of one type or another have been in use since that time. Some of the most common filters in use today are shown in Fig. 2-3. These filters can be used with screen-film and digital

[1]Pfahler GE: A roentgen filter and a universal diaphragm and protecting screen, *Transcripts of the American Roentgen Ray Society* 217, 1906.

imaging systems to improve the image quality of various anatomic areas. With most digital systems, filters are necessary to obtain a diagnostic image of a body part with extreme differences in density. In addition, radiation exposure to the patient is reduced through elimination of extra exposures needed to show all of the anatomy and through the beam-hardening effect of the attenuating filter. The increasing thickness of the filter over the thinner body part also acts to reduce exposure.

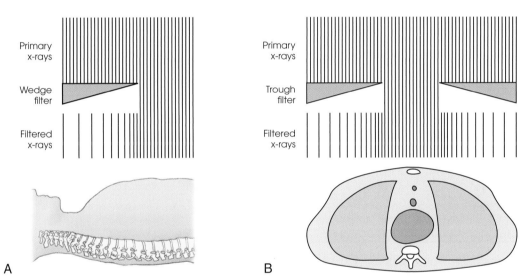

Fig. 2-2 A, Wedge filter in position for AP projection of thoracic spine. Note how thick portion of wedge partially attenuates x-ray beam over upper thoracic area while nonfilter area receives full exposure to penetrate thick portion of spine. An even image density results. **B,** Trough filter in position for AP projection of chest. Note how two side wedges partially attenuate x-ray beam over lung areas while mediastinum receives full exposure. A better-quality image of chest and mediastinal structures results.

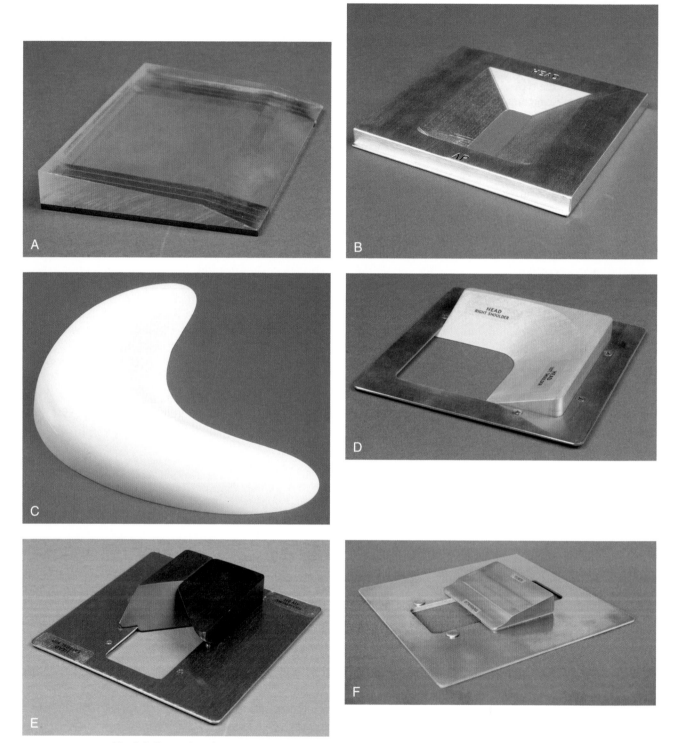

Fig. 2-3 Examples of compensating filters in use today. **A,** Supertech wedge, collimator-mounted Clear Pb filter used for AP projection of hips, knees, and ankles on long (51-inch) film. **B,** Trough, collimator-mounted aluminum filter with double wedge used for AP projections of thoracic spine. **C,** Boomerang contact filter used for AP projections of shoulder and facial bones. **D,** Ferlic collimator-mounted filter used for AP and PA oblique (scapular Y) projections of shoulder. **E,** Ferlic collimator-mounted filter used for lateral projections of cervicothoracic region (swimmer's technique) and axiolateral projections (Danelius-Miller method) of hip. **F,** Ferlic collimator-mounted filter for AP axial projections of foot.

The appropriate use of radiographic compensating filters is an important addition to the radiographer's skill set. The radiographer determines whether or not to use a filter based on an assessment of the patient and determines the type and exact position of the filter. This determination is made while positioning the patient. Radiographic projections of the lateral hip and the lateral C7-T1 cervicothoracic region in most instances require a filter to show all the anatomy on one image. Projections such as the AP shoulder and AP thoracic spine may not need a filter on hyposthenic patients; however, on hypersthenic patients and patients who are "barrel-chested" or obese, a filter is necessary. Pediatric patients seldom require a filter except when posteroanterior (PA) and lateral projections of the full spine are done in cases of spinal curvatures such as scoliosis. Compensating filters for full-spine radiography not only allow the entire spine to be imaged with one exposure, but they also significantly reduce the radiation exposure to the young patients who require these images.[1-3]

Physical Principles

Compensating filters are manufactured in various shapes and are composed of several materials. The shape or material chosen is based on the particular body part to be imaged. The exact placement of the filter also varies, with most being placed between the x-ray tube and the skin surface, although some are placed under the patient. Filters placed under the patient often produce distinct outlines of the filter, which can be objectionable to the radiologist.

SHAPE

The *wedge* is the simplest and most common of the compensating filter shapes. It is used to improve the image quality of a wide variety of body parts. Various filters with more complex shapes have been developed for technically challenging anatomic areas, including the *trough, scoliosis, Ferlic,*[1] and *Boomerang.*[2]

Some filters have multiple uses. A filter that is shaped for one area of the body can also be adapted for other body structures. Filters such as the Ferlic cervicothoracic lateral projection (swimmer's technique) filter can be adapted for the axiolateral projection (Danelius-Miller technique) of the hip with excellent results.

COMPOSITION

Compensating filters are composed of a substance of sufficiently high atomic number to attenuate the x-ray beam. The most common filter materials are aluminum and high-density plastics. These are manufactured with different thickness of the material and generally distributed in a smoothly graduated way that corresponds with the distribution of the different tissue densities of the anatomy (see Fig. 2-2). Aluminum is an efficient attenuator and a common filter material.

Some manufacturers offer compensating filters made from clear leaded plastic, known as *Clear Pb,*[1] which allows the field light to shine through to the patient but still attenuates the x-ray beam (Fig. 2-3, *A*). This leaded plastic is inappropriate for all filter uses, however, such as in the extremely dense area of the shoulder during lateral spine radiography because the thickness required to attenuate the beam sufficiently would result in a prohibitively heavy device. In these cases, aluminum is generally used. The Boomerang (see Fig. 2-3, *C*) filter is composed of an attenuating silicon rubber compound, and some models of this filter have an embedded metal bead chain to mark the filter edge.

[1]ClearPb; Nuclear Associates, Hicksville, NY.

[1]Gray JE, Stears JG, Frank ED: Shaped, lead-loaded acrylic filters for patient exposure reduction and image quality improvement, *Radiology* 146:825, 1983.
[2]Frank ED et al: Use of the posterior-anterior projection as a method of reducing x-ray exposure to specific radiosensitive organs, *Radiol Technol* 54:343, 1983.
[3]Nash CL Jr et al: Risks of exposure to x-rays in patients undergoing long-term treatment for scoliosis, *J Bone Joint Surg Am* 61:371, 1979.

[1]Ferlic; Ferlic Filter Company LLC, White Bear Lake, MN.
[2]Boomerang; Octostop, Inc., Laval, Canada.

PLACEMENT

Compensating filters are most often placed in the x-ray beam between the x-ray tube and patient. Broadly, filters fall into two categories based on their location during use: *collimator-mounted* filters and *contact* filters. Collimator-mounted filters are mounted on the collimator, using either rails installed on both sides of the window on the collimator housing (Fig. 2-4, *A*) or magnets. Contact compensating filters are placed either directly on the patient or between the anatomy and the IR (Fig. 2-4, *B*).

Collimator mounted filters made of aluminum block the field light, which makes positioning of the patient and the central ray more challenging. Many aluminum filters have a 100% x-ray transmission zone (see Fig. 2-3, *B, D, E,* and *F*), and positioning is made slightly easier. Radiographers who use aluminum filters must complete the positioning of the patient and alignment of the central ray first before mounting the filter to the collimator (Fig. 2-5).

Generally, filters placed between the primary beam and the body have the added benefit of a reduction in radiation exposure to the patient because of the beam-hardening effect of the filter, whereas filters placed between anatomy and the IR have no effect on patient exposure. Measurements provided with Ferlic filters show radiation exposure reductions of 50% to 80%, depending on the kilovoltage peak (kVp), in the anatomic area covered by the filter. Measurements by Frank et al.[1] show exposure reductions of 20% to 69% to the thyroid, sternum, and breasts. Both types have the same effect on the finished image, which is a more uniform radiographic density even though the tissue density varied greatly. Filters can be improvised as well, with radiographers creating their own version of attenuation control devices, such as filled bags of saline solution. Bags of solution increase scattered radiation, however. Use of improvised filters is not recommended because there is potential for creating unknown artifacts in the image.

[1]Frank ED et al: Use of the posterior-anterior projection as a method of reducing x-ray exposure to specific radiosensitive organs, *Radiol Technol* 54:343, 1983.

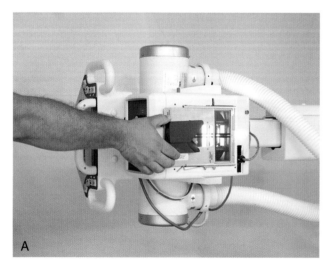
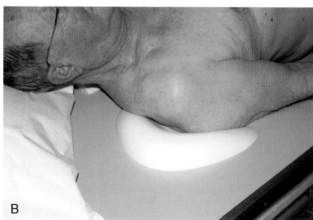

Fig. 2-4 A, Ferlic collimator-mounted filter positioned on collimator for AP projection of shoulder. **B,** Boomerang contact filter in position for AP projection of shoulder.

(**A,** Courtesy Scott Slinkard, College of Nursing and Health Sciences, Cape Girardeau, MO.)

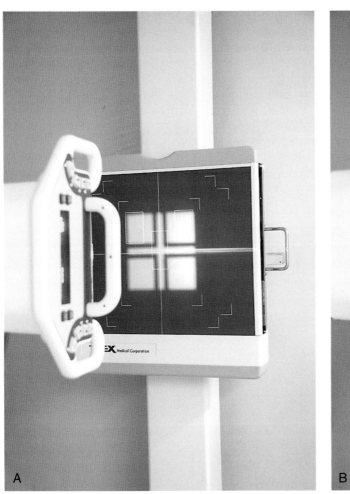
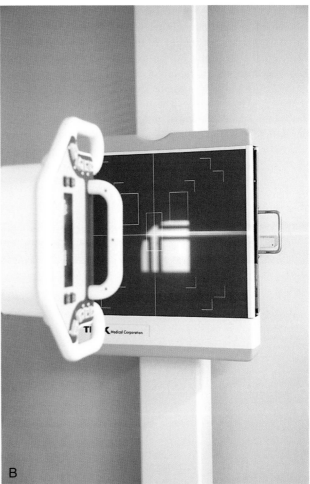

A

B

Fig. 2-5 A, Collimator light adjusted for AP projection of right shoulder. **B,** Ferlic shoulder filter in place showing 100% transmission area (light) and remaining area blocked by aluminum of filter.

(Courtesy Scott Slinkard, College of Nursing and Health Sciences, Cape Girardeau, MO.)

Specific Applications

The choice of compensating filter to be used depends on the distribution of tissue densities of the anatomy to be radiographed. As illustrated in Table 2-1, most of these imaging challenges can be solved with only a few filter shapes. The following are examples of the most common compensating filter applications.

- The *wedge filter* is used for areas of the body where tissue density varies gradually from one end to the other along the long axis of the body. The wedge filter can be used to improve image quality of AP projections of the thoracic spine (Fig. 2-6).
- The *trough filter* is best used for areas of the body where the subject density in

the center is much greater than at the edges. This filter has been successfully applied to improving PA projections of the chest (Fig. 2-7).
- The *Ferlic swimmer's filter* is a collimator-mounted filter created to improve imaging of the lateral projection of the cervicothoracic region (swimmer's technique) (Fig. 2-8), but it is also used for the axiolateral projection of the hip

TABLE 2-1

Common x-ray projections for which filters improve image quality*

Anatomy/Projection	Filter	Type	Thick portion oriented to	Improved demonstration of
Mandible/Axiolateral oblique	Ferlic[†] swimmer's	Collimator	Anterior of mandible	Mandibular symphysis
Nasal bones/Lateral	Wedge	Collimator	Anterior	Nasal bones/ cartilage
Facial bones/Lateral	Boomerang[‡]	Contact	Anterior	Anterior facial structures
Cervicothoracic/Lateral	Ferlic[†] swimmer's	Collimator	Upper cervical	C6-T2
Thoracic spine/AP	Wedge	Collimator	Upper thoracic	Upper thoracic
Shoulder/AP	Boomerang[‡] Ferlic[†] shoulder	Contact and collimator	AC joint AC joint	AC joint AC joint
Shoulder/Axial	Ferlic[†] swimmer's	Collimator	Humerus	Humerus
Shoulder/Oblique	Boomerang[‡] Ferlic[†] shoulder	Contact and collimator	Humeral head Humeral head	Glenoid fossa Glenoid fossa
Chest/AP	Supertech[§]/trough	Collimator	Sides of chest	Mediastinum
Abdomen/AP upright	Wedge	Collimator	Upper abdomen	Diaphragm
Abdomen/AP decubitus	Wedge	Collimator	Side furthest from table	Abdomen side up
Lateral hip/Axiolateral	Ferlic[†] swimmer's	Collimator	Distal femur	Proximal femur
Hip/AP (emaciated patient)	Wedge	Collimator	Greater trochanter	Femoral head
Foot/AP	Wedge/gentle slope	Contact and collimator	Toes	Forefoot
Calcaneus/Axial	Ferlic[†] swimmer's	Collimator	Calcaneus	Posterior calcaneus
Hip-knee-ankle 51 inches/AP	Supertech[§]/ full-length leg Ferlic[†] swimmer's	Collimator	Tibia/fibula	Distal tibia-fibula

*This table is not all-inclusive. Other body structures can be imaged, and other filters are available on the market.
[†]Ferlic; Ferlic Filter Company, LLC, White Bear Lake, MN.
[‡]Boomerang; Octostop, Inc., Laval, Canada.
[§]Supertech, Elkhart, IN.
AC, acromioclavicular joint.

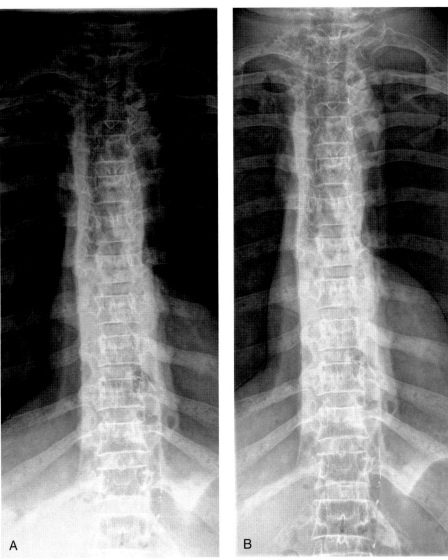

Fig. 2-6 A, AP projection of thoracic spine without compensating filter. **B,** Same projection with Ferlic wedge filter. Note more even density of spine, and all vertebrae are shown.

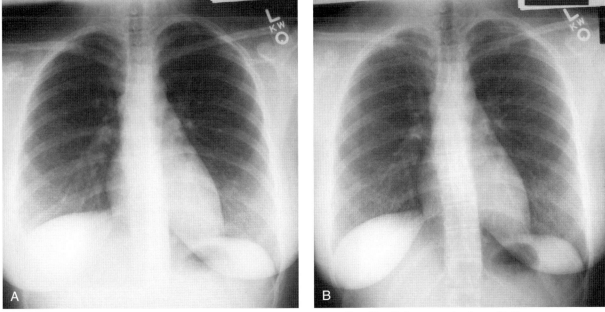

Fig. 2-7 A, AP projection of chest without compensating filter. **B,** Same projection with Supertech trough filter. Lower lung fields and mediastinum are better shown.

61

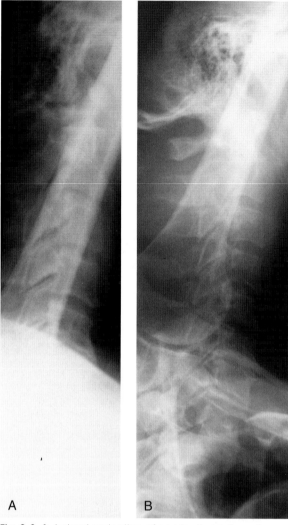

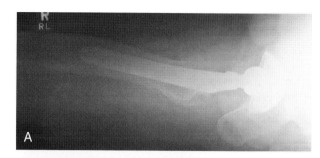

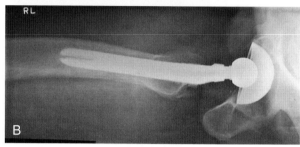

Fig. 2-9 A, Axiolateral projection of hip (Danelius-Miller method) without compensating filter. **B,** Same projection with Ferlic swimmer's filter. Note how acetabulum and end of metal shaft are seen on one image.

Fig. 2-8 A, Lateral projection of cervicothoracic region (swimmer's technique) without compensating filter. **B,** Same projection with Ferlic swimmer's filter. Note how C7-T1 area is penetrated and shown.

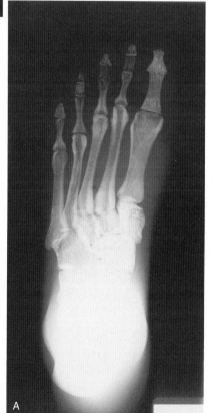

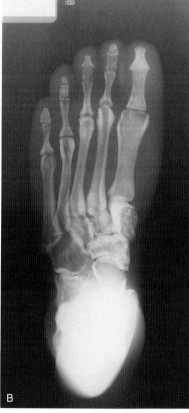

Fig. 2-10 A, AP axial projection of foot. Note dark toe area and light tarsal area without filter. **B,** Same projection with use of Ferlic AP foot filter showing improved visualization of toes and tarsals.

(Danelius-Miller method) (Fig. 2-9). The Ferlic shoulder filter, also a collimator-mounted filter, is designed specifically to image the shoulder in both the supine and upright positions.

• Specialized *wedge* filters are designed for specific uses. Fig. 2-10 shows the results of using the Ferlic foot filter to provide a significantly improved image of the foot with one exposure.

• The *Boomerang filter* was designed to conform to the shape of the shoulder and create images of more uniform radiographic density at the superior margins (Fig. 2-11). This is a contact filter placed between the anatomy and the IR (see Fig. 2-4, *B*). It can also be used effectively for lateral facial bone images. Although effective in compensating for differences in anatomic density, this filter does not reduce radiation exposure because it is located behind the patient. The Ferlic *shoulder filter* is a collimator-mounted filter also designed

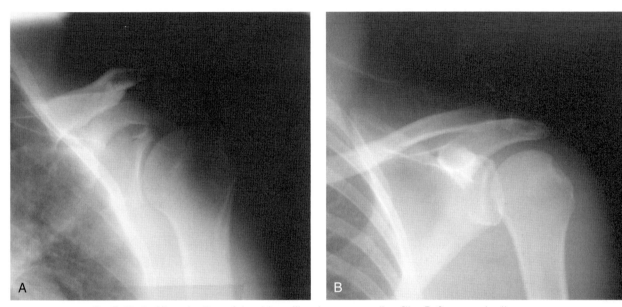

Fig. 2-11 A, AP projection of shoulder without compensating filter. **B,** Same projection using Boomerang contact filter.

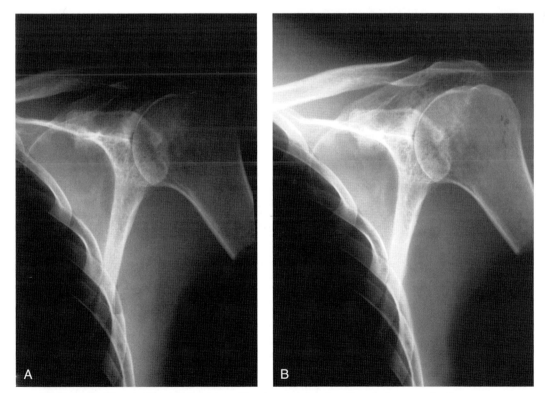

Fig. 2-12 A, AP projection of shoulder without compensating filter. **B,** Same projection using Ferlic shoulder collimator mounted filter. Note greater visualization of acromion, acromioclavicular joint, and humeral head.

specifically to image the shoulder (Fig. 2-12). Because this filter is placed in the primary x-ray beam, it also acts to reduce radiation exposure to the patient.

• The *scoliosis filters* are used with two of the most challenging projections to obtain: the PA (Frank et al. method) and lateral full-spine projections for evaluation of spinal curvatures. These projections are challenging because the cervical, thoracic, and lumbosacral spines have to be shown on one image. One exposure technique has to be set for what normally would be three separate exposures. With the use of compensating filters, the PA projection can be made with a wedge filter positioned over the cervical and thoracic spines (Fig. 2-13, *A*). For the lateral projection, two double-wedge filters are positioned over the mid-thoracic area and the cervical spine (Fig. 2-13, *B*). The exposure technique for the PA and lateral projections is set to penetrate the most dense area—the lumbar spine. The filters attenuate enough of the exposure over the cervical and thoracic areas to show the thoracic and cervical spines adequately.

Highly specialized compensating filters are also used in other areas of the radiology department. During digital fluoroscopy, convex and concave conical-shaped filters are used to compensate for the round image intensifier. In computed tomography (CT), "bow-tie"–shaped filters are used to compensate for the rounded shape of the head.

Radiographers must use caution when mounting and removing compensating filters on the collimator while the x-ray tube is over the patient. There have been instances when filters did not attach properly, did not get positioned into the filter track, or were forgotten and fell onto the patient when the tube was moved. All compensating filters, especially aluminum ones, are moderately heavy with sharp edges; they can cause injury to the patient if dropped. When positioning the filter to the underside of the collimator and when removing it, two hands must be used (Fig. 2-14). One hand should attach the filter while the other is positioned to catch the filter if it does not attach properly.

Compensating Filters in This Atlas

Body structures whose radiographic images can be improved through the use of compensating filters are identified throughout the atlas directly on the projection page. The special icon ◥ identifies the use of a filter.

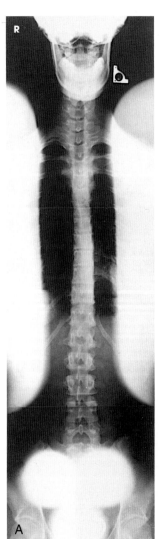
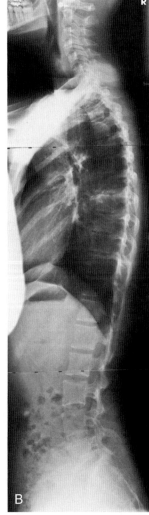

Fig. 2-13 A, PA projection (Frank et al. method) of cervical, thoracic, and lumbar spine using wedge filter. **B,** Lateral projection of cervical, thoracic, and lumbar spine using two bilateral wedge filters. The entire spine can be imaged on both projections with use of compensating filter.

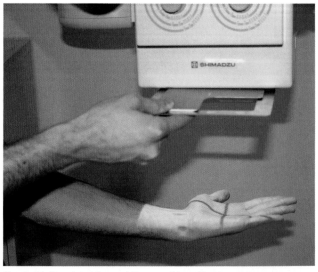

Fig. 2-14 Two hands must be used to attach and remove collimator-mounted filters. One hand is used to catch the filter in case it is dropped.

3

GENERAL ANATOMY AND RADIOGRAPHIC POSITIONING TERMINOLOGY

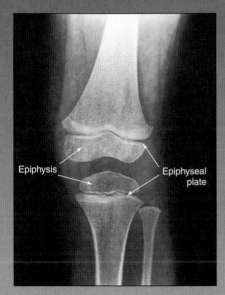

Epiphysis

Epiphyseal
plate

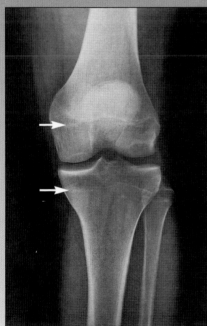

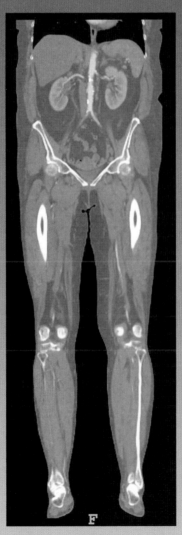

F

General Anatomy

Radiographers must possess a thorough knowledge of anatomy, physiology, and osteology to obtain radiographs that show the desired body part. *Anatomy* is the term applied to the science of the structure of the body. *Physiology* is the study of the function of the body organs. *Osteology* is the detailed study of the body of knowledge relating to the bones of the body.

Radiographers also must have a general understanding of all body systems and their functions. Particular attention must be given to gaining a thorough understanding of the skeletal system and the surface landmarks used to locate different body parts. The radiographer must be able to visualize mentally the internal structures that are to be radiographed. By using external landmarks, the radiographer should properly position body parts to obtain the best diagnostic radiographs possible.

BODY PLANES

The full dimension of the human body as viewed in the *anatomic position* (see Chapter 1) can be effectively subdivided through the use of imaginary body planes. These planes slice through the body at designated levels from all directions. The following four fundamental body planes referred to regularly in radiography are illustrated in Fig. 3-1, *A*:

- Sagittal
- Coronal
- Horizontal
- Oblique

Sagittal plane

A sagittal plane divides the entire body or a body part into right and left segments. The plane passes vertically through the body from front to back (see Fig. 3-1, *A* and *B*). The *midsagittal plane* is a specific sagittal plane that passes through the midline of the body and divides it into equal right and left halves (Fig. 3-1, *C*).

Coronal plane

A coronal plane divides the entire body or a body part into anterior and posterior segments. The plane passes through the body vertically from one side to the other (see Fig. 3-1, *A* and *B*). The *midcoronal plane* is a specific coronal plane that passes through the midline of the body, dividing it into equal anterior and posterior halves (see Fig. 3-1, *C*). This plane is sometimes referred to as the *midaxillary plane*.

Horizontal plane

A *horizontal plane* passes crosswise through the body or a body part at right angles to the longitudinal axis. It is positioned at a right angle to the sagittal and coronal planes. This plane divides the body into superior and inferior portions. Often it is referred to as a *transverse, axial,* or *cross-sectional plane* (see Fig. 3-1, *A*).

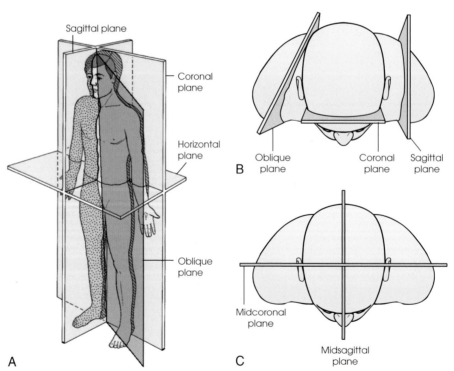

Fig. 3-1 Planes of the body. **A,** A patient in anatomic position with four planes identified. **B,** Top-down perspective of patient's body showing sagittal plane through left shoulder, coronal plane through anterior head, and oblique plane through right shoulder. **C,** Midsagittal plane dividing body equally into right and left halves and midcoronal plane dividing body equally into anterior and posterior halves. Sagittal, coronal, and horizontal planes are always at right angles to one another.

Oblique plane

An oblique plane can pass through a body part at any angle among the three previously described planes (see Fig. 3-1, *A* and *B*). Planes are used in radiographic positioning to center a body part to the image receptor (IR) or central ray and to ensure that the body part is properly oriented and aligned with the IR. The mid-sagittal plane may be centered and perpendicular to the IR with the long axis of the IR parallel to the same plane. Planes can also be used to guide projections of the central ray. The central ray for an anteroposterior (AP) projection passes through the body part parallel to the sagittal plane and perpendicular to the coronal plane. Quality imaging requires attention to all relationships among body planes, the IR, and the central ray.

Body planes are used in computed tomography (CT), magnetic resonance imaging (MRI), and ultrasound (US) to identify the orientation of anatomic cuts or slices shown in the procedure (Fig. 3-2). Imaging in several planes is often used to show large sections of anatomy (Fig. 3-3).

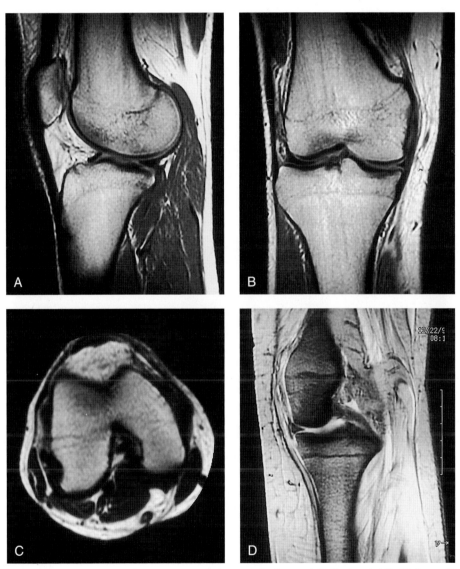

Fig. 3-2 MRI of the knee in four planes. **A,** Sagittal. **B,** Coronal. **C,** Horizontal. **D,** Oblique, 45 degrees.

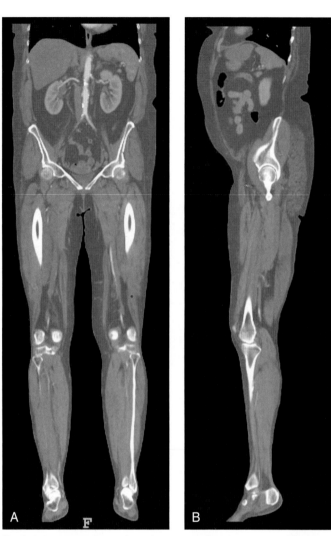

Fig. 3-3 Large sections of anatomy are often imaged in different planes. **A,** Coronal plane of abdomen and lower limb. **B,** Sagittal plane of abdomen and lower limb at level of left kidney, left acetabulum, and left knee.

SPECIAL PLANES

Two special planes are used in radiographic positioning. These planes are localized to a specific area of the body only.

Interiliac plane

The interiliac plane transects the pelvis at the top of the iliac crests at the level of the fourth lumbar spinous process (Fig. 3-4, *A*). It is used in positioning the lumbar spine, sacrum, and coccyx.

Occlusal plane

The occlusal plane is formed by the biting surfaces of the upper and lower teeth with the jaws closed (Fig. 3-4, *B*). It is used in positioning of the odontoid process and some head projections.

BODY CAVITIES

The two great cavities of the torso are the *thoracic* and *abdominal cavities* (Fig. 3-5). The thoracic cavity is subdivided into a pericardial segment and two pleural portions. Although the abdominal cavity has no intervening partition, the lower portion is called the *pelvic cavity*. Some anatomists combine the abdominal and pelvic cavities and refer to them as the *abdominopelvic cavity*. The principal structures located in the cavities are listed on the following page.

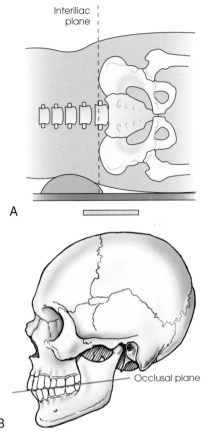

A

B

Fig. 3-4 Special planes. **A,** Interiliac plane transecting trunk at tops of iliac crests. **B,** Occlusal plane formed by biting surfaces of teeth.

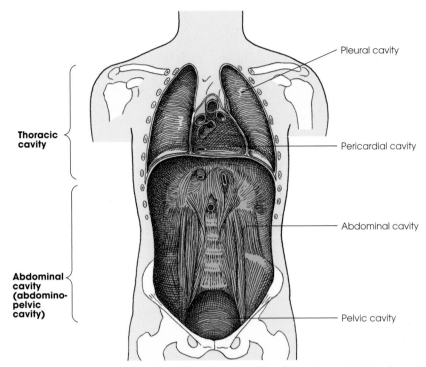

Fig. 3-5 Anterior view of torso showing two great cavities: thoracic and abdominopelvic.

Thoracic cavity

- Pleural membranes
- Lungs
- Trachea
- Esophagus
- Pericardium
- Heart and great vessels

Abdominal cavity

- Peritoneum
- Liver
- Gallbladder
- Pancreas
- Spleen
- Stomach
- Intestines
- Kidneys
- Ureters
- Major blood vessels
- **Pelvic portion**—rectum, urinary bladder, and parts of the reproductive system

DIVISIONS OF THE ABDOMEN

The abdomen is the portion of the trunk that is bordered superiorly by the diaphragm and inferiorly by the superior pelvic aperture (pelvic inlet). The location of organs or an anatomic area can be described by dividing the abdomen according to one of two methods: four quadrants or nine regions.

Quadrants

The abdomen is often divided into four clinical divisions called *quadrants* (Fig. 3-6). The midsagittal plane and a horizontal plane intersect at the umbilicus and create the boundaries. The quadrants are named as follows:

- Right upper quadrant (RUQ)
- Right lower quadrant (RLQ)
- Left upper quadrant (LUQ)
- Left lower quadrant (LLQ)

Dividing the abdomen into four quadrants is useful for describing the location of the various abdominal organs. For example, the spleen can be described as being located in the left upper quadrant.

Regions

Some anatomists divide the abdomen into nine regions by using four planes (Fig. 3-7). These anatomic divisions are not used as often as quadrants in clinical practice. The nine regions of the body, divided into three groups, are named as follows:

Superior

- Right hypochondrium
- Epigastrium
- Left hypochondrium

Middle

- Right lateral
- Umbilical
- Left lateral

Inferior

- Right inguinal
- Hypogastrium
- Left inguinal

In the clinical setting, a patient could be described as having "epigastric" pain. A patient with discomfort in the right lower abdomen could be described as having "RLQ" pain. Sometimes a quadrant term is used, and other times a region term is used.

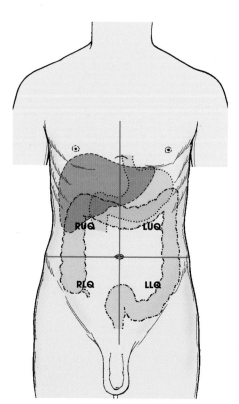

Fig. 3-6 Four quadrants of abdomen.

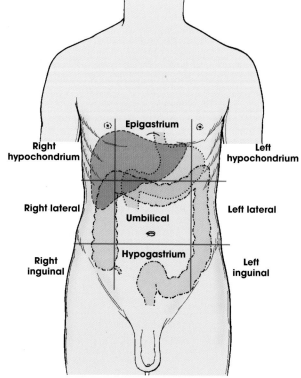

Fig. 3-7 Nine regions of abdomen.

SURFACE LANDMARKS

Most anatomic structures cannot be visualized directly; the radiographer must use various protuberances, tuberosities, and other external indicators to position the patient accurately. These surface landmarks enable the radiographer to obtain radiographs of optimal quality consistently for a wide variety of body types. If surface landmarks are not used for radiographic positioning or if they are used incorrectly, the chance of having to repeat the radiograph greatly increases.

Many commonly used landmarks are listed in Table 3-1 and diagrammed in Fig. 3-8. These landmarks are accepted averages for most patients and should be used only as guidelines. Variations in anatomic build or pathologic conditions may warrant positioning compensation on an individual basis. The ability to compensate is gained through experience.

TABLE 3-1

External landmarks related to body structures at the same level

Body structures	External landmarks
Cervical area (see Fig. 3-6)	
C1	Mastoid tip
C2, C3	Gonion (angle of mandible)
C3, C4	Hyoid bone
C5	Thyroid cartilage
C7, T1	Vertebra prominens
Thoracic area	
T1	Approximately 2 inches (5 cm) above level of jugular notch
T2, T3	Level of jugular notch
T4, T5	Level of sternal angle
T7	Level of inferior angles of scapulae
T9, T10	Level of xiphoid process
Lumbar area	
L2, L3	Inferior costal margin
L4, L5	Level of superiormost aspect of iliac crests
Sacrum and pelvic area	
S1, S2	Level of anterior superior iliac spine (ASIS)
Coccyx	Level of pubic symphysis and greater trochanters

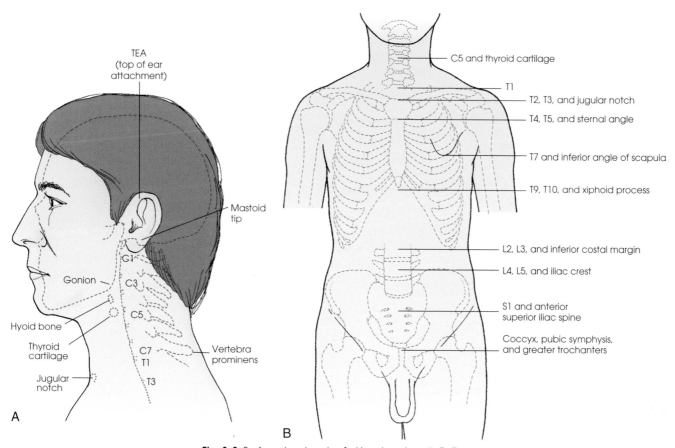

Fig. 3-8 Surface landmarks. **A,** Head and neck. **B,** Torso.

BODY HABITUS

Common variations in the shape of the human body are termed the *body habitus*. Mills[1] determined the primary classifications of body habitus based on his study of 1000 patients. The specific type of body habitus is important in radiography because it determines the size, shape, and position of the organs of the thoracic and abdominal cavities.

Body habitus directly affects the location of the following:
- Heart
- Lungs
- Diaphragm
- Stomach
- Colon
- Gallbladder

An organ such as the gallbladder may vary in position by 8 inches, depending on the body habitus. The stomach may be positioned horizontally, high, and in the center of the abdomen for one type of habitus and positioned vertically, low, and to the side of the midline in another type. Fig. 3-9 shows an example of the placement, shape, and size of the lungs, heart, and diaphragm in patients with four different body habitus types.

Body habitus and the placement of the thoracic and abdominal organs are also important in the determination of technical and exposure factors for the appropriate radiographic density and contrast and the radiation doses. Contrast medium in the gallbladder may affect the automatic exposure control detector. For one type of habitus, the gallbladder may lie directly over the detector (which is undesirable); for another, it may not even be near the detector. The standard placement and size of the IR may have to be changed because of body habitus. The selection of kilovolt (peak) and milliampere-second exposure factors may also be affected by the type of habitus because of wide variations in physical tissue density. These technical considerations are described in greater detail in radiography physics and imaging texts.

[1]Mills WR: The relation of bodily habitus to visceral form, position, tonus, and motility, *AJR* 4:155, 1917.

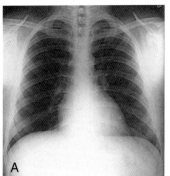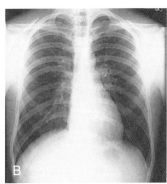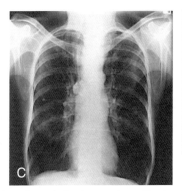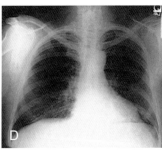

Fig. 3-9 Placement, shape, and size of lungs, heart, and diaphragm in patients with four different body habitus types. **A,** Sthenic. **B,** Hyposthenic. **C,** Asthenic. **D,** Hypersthenic.

Box 3-1 describes specific characteristics of the four types of body habitus and outlines their general shapes and variations. The four major types of body habitus and their approximate frequency in the population are identified as follows:
- Sthenic—50%
- Hyposthenic—35%
- Asthenic—10%
- Hypersthenic—5%

More than 85% of the population has either a *sthenic* or *hyposthenic* body habitus. The sthenic type is considered the dominant type of habitus. The relative shape of patients with a sthenic or hyposthenic body habitus and the position of their organs are referred to in clinical practice as *ordinary* or *average*. All standard radiographic positioning and exposure techniques are based on these two groups. Radiographers must become thoroughly familiar with the characteristics and organ placements of these two body types.

BOX 3-1
Four types of body habitus: prevalence, organ placement, and characteristics

Sthenic, 50%

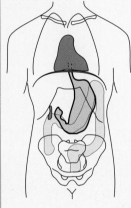

Organs
Heart: Moderately transverse
Lungs: Moderate length
Diaphragm: Moderately high
Stomach: High, upper left
Colon: Spread evenly; slight dip in transverse colon
Gallbladder: Centered on right side, upper abdomen

Characteristics
Build: Moderately heavy
Abdomen: Moderately long
Thorax: Moderately short, broad, and deep
Pelvis: Relatively small

Hyposthenic, 35%

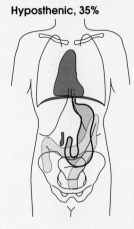

Organs and characteristics for this habitus are intermediate between sthenic and asthenic body habitus types; this habitus is the most difficult to classify

Asthenic, 10%

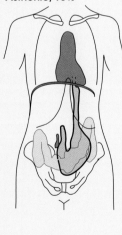

Organs
Heart: Nearly vertical and at midline
Lungs: Long, apices above clavicles, may be broader above base
Diaphragm: Low
Stomach: Low and medial, in the pelvis when standing
Colon: Low, folds on itself
Gallbladder: Low and nearer the midline

Characteristics
Build: Frail
Abdomen: Short
Thorax: Long, shallow
Pelvis: Wide

Hypersthenic, 5%

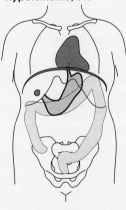

Organs
Heart: Axis nearly transverse
Lungs: Short, apices at or near clavicles
Diaphragm: High
Stomach: High, transverse, and in the middle
Colon: Around periphery of abdomen
Gallbladder: High, outside, lies more parallel

Characteristics
Build: Massive
Abdomen: Long
Thorax: Short, broad, deep
Pelvis: Narrow

Note the significant differences between the two extreme habitus types (i.e., asthenic and hypersthenic). The differences between the sthenic and hyposthenic types are less distinct.

Radiographers must also become familiar with the two extreme habitus types: *asthenic* and *hypersthenic*. In these two small groups (15% of the population), the placement and size of the organs significantly affect positioning and the selection of exposure factors. Consequently, radiography of these patients can be challenging. Experience and professional judgment enable the radiographer to determine the correct body habitus and to judge the specific location of the organs.

Body habitus is not an indication of disease or other abnormality, and it is not determined by the body fat or physical condition of the patient. Habitus is simply a classification of the four general shapes of the *trunk* of the human body. When positioning patients, the radiographer should be conscious that habitus is not associated with height or weight. Four patients of equal height could have four different trunk shapes (Fig. 3-10).

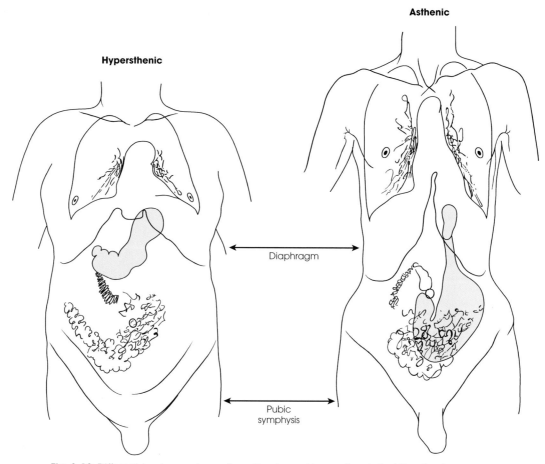

Fig. 3-10 Different trunks are shown for asthenic and hypersthenic habitus, the two extremes. The abdomen is the same length in both patients (diaphragm to pubic symphysis). The abdominal organs are in completely different positions. Note high stomach in hypersthenic habitus (*green color*) and low stomach in asthenic habitus.
(Art is based on actual autopsy findings by R. Walter Mills, MD.)

Osteology

The adult human skeleton is composed of 206 primary bones. Ligaments unite the bones of the skeleton. Bones provide the following:

- Attachment for muscles
- Mechanical basis for movement
- Protection of internal organs
- A frame to support the body
- Storage for calcium, phosphorus, and other salts
- Production of red and white blood cells

The 206 bones of the body are divided into two main groups:

- Axial skeleton
- Appendicular skeleton

The axial skeleton supports and protects the head and trunk with 80 bones (Table 3-2). The appendicular skeleton allows the body to move in various positions and from place to place with its 126 bones (Table 3-3). Fig. 3-11 identifies these two skeletal areas.

TABLE 3-2

Axial skeleton: 80 bones

Area	Bones	No.
Skull	Cranial	8
	Facial	14
	Auditory ossicles*	6
Neck	Hyoid	1
Thorax	Sternum	1
	Ribs	24
Vertebral column	Cervical	7
	Thoracic	12
	Lumbar	5
	Sacrum	1
	Coccyx	1

*Auditory ossicles are small bones in the ears. They are not considered official bones of the axial skeleton but are placed here for convenience.

TABLE 3-3

Appendicular skeleton: 126 bones

Area	Bones	No.
Shoulder girdle	Clavicles	2
	Scapulae	2
Upper limbs	Humeri	2
	Ulnae	2
	Radii	2
	Carpals	16
	Metacarpals	10
	Phalanges	28
Lower limbs	Femora	2
	Tibias	2
	Fibulae	2
	Patellae	2
	Tarsals	14
	Metatarsals	10
	Phalanges	28
Pelvic girdle	Hip bones	2

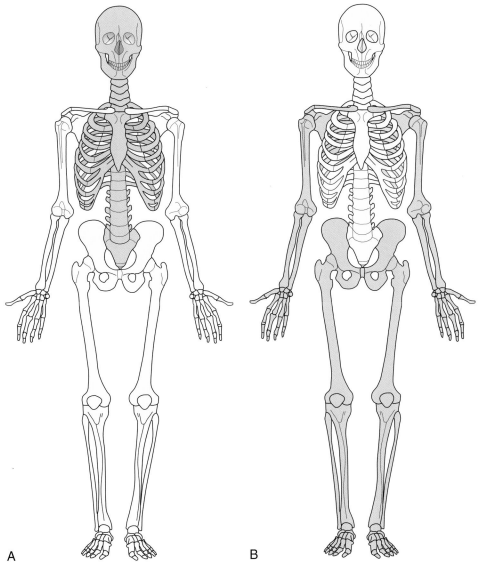

A   B

Fig. 3-11 Two main groups of bones. **A,** Axial skeleton. **B,** Appendicular skeleton.

GENERAL BONE FEATURES

The general features of most bones are shown in Fig. 3-12. All bones are composed of a strong, dense outer layer called the *compact bone* and an inner portion of less dense *spongy bone*. The hard outer compact bone protects the bone and gives it strength for supporting the body. The softer spongy bone contains a spiculated network of interconnecting spaces called the *trabeculae* (Fig. 3-13). The trabeculae are filled with red and yellow marrow. Red marrow produces red and white blood cells, and yellow marrow stores adipose (fat) cells. Long bones have a central cavity called the *medullary cavity,* which contains trabeculae filled with yellow marrow. In long bones, the red marrow is concentrated at the ends of the bone and not in the medullary cavity.

A tough, fibrous connective tissue called the *periosteum* covers all bony surfaces except the articular surfaces, which are covered by the articular cartilage. The tissue lining the medullary cavity of bones is called the *endosteum.* Bones contain various knoblike projections called *tubercles* and *tuberosities,* which are covered by the periosteum. Muscles, tendons, and ligaments attach to the periosteum at these projections. Blood vessels and nerves enter and exit the bone through the periosteum.

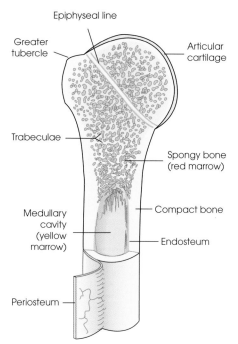

Epiphyseal line

Greater tubercle

Articular cartilage

Trabeculae

Spongy bone (red marrow)

Medullary cavity (yellow marrow)

Compact bone

Endosteum

Periosteum

Fig. 3-12 General bone features and anatomic parts.

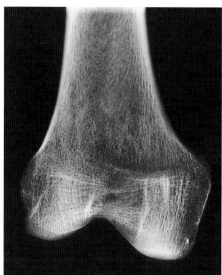

Fig. 3-13 Radiograph of distal femur and condyles showing bony trabeculae within entire bone.

BONE VESSELS AND NERVES

Bones are live organs and must receive a blood supply for nourishment or they die. Bones also contain a supply of nerves. Blood vessels and nerves enter and exit the bone at the same point, through openings called the *foramina*. Near the center of all long bones is an opening in the periosteum called the *nutrient foramen*. The nutrient artery of the bone passes into this opening and supplies the cancellous bone and marrow. The epiphyseal artery separately enters the ends of long bones to supply the area, and periosteal arteries enter at numerous points to supply the compact bone. Veins exiting the bones carry blood cells to the body (Fig. 3-14).

BONE DEVELOPMENT

Ossification is the term given to the development and formation of bones. Bones begin to develop in the 2nd month of embryonic life. Ossification occurs separately by two distinct processes: *intermembranous ossification* and *endochondral ossification*.

Intermembranous ossification

Bones that develop from fibrous membranes in the embryo produce the flat bones—bones of the skull, clavicles, mandible, and sternum. Before birth, these bones are not joined. As flat bones grow after birth, they join and form sutures. Other bones in this category merge and create the various *joints* of the skeleton.

Endochondral ossification

Bones created by endochondral ossification develop from hyaline cartilage in the embryo and produce the short, irregular, and long bones. Endochondral ossification occurs from two distinct centers of development called the *primary* and *secondary centers of ossification*.

Primary ossification

Primary ossification begins before birth and forms the entire bulk of the short and irregular bones. This process forms the long central shaft in long bones. During development only, the long shaft of the bone is called the *diaphysis* (Fig. 3-15, *A*).

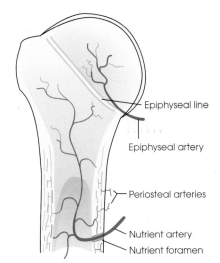

Fig. 3-14 Long bone end showing its rich arterial supply. Arteries, veins, and nerves enter and exit bone at the same point.

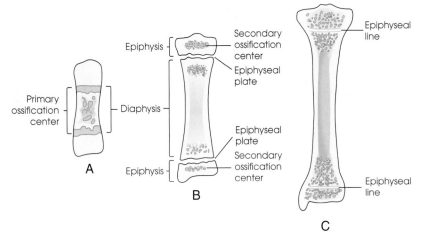

Fig. 3-15 Primary and secondary ossification of bone. **A,** Primary ossification of tibia before birth. **B,** Secondary ossification, which forms two *epiphyses* after birth. **C,** Full growth into single bone, which occurs by age 21 years.

Secondary ossification

Secondary ossification occurs after birth when a separate bone begins to develop at both ends of each long bone. Each end is called the *epiphysis* (Fig. 3-15, *B*). At first, the diaphysis and epiphysis are distinctly separate. As growth occurs, a plate of cartilage called the *epiphyseal plate* develops between the two areas (Fig. 3-15, *C*). This plate is seen on long bone radiographs of all pediatric patients (Fig. 3-16, *A*). The epiphyseal plate is important radiographically because it is a common site of fractures in pediatric patients. Near age 21 years, full ossification occurs, and the two areas become completely joined; only a moderately visible *epiphyseal line* appears on the bone (Fig. 3-16, *B*).

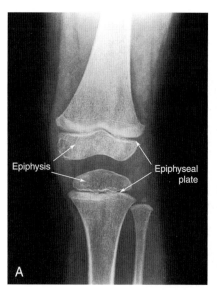
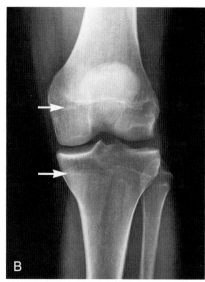
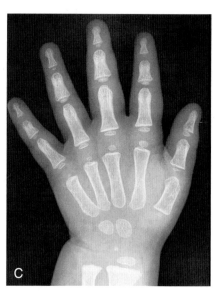

Fig. 3-16 A, Radiograph of a 6-year-old child. Epiphysis and epiphyseal plate shown on knee radiograph (*arrows*). **B,** Radiograph of same area in a 21-year-old adult. Full ossification has occurred, and only subtle epiphyseal lines are seen (*arrows*). **C,** PA radiograph of hand of a 2½-year-old child. Note early stages of ossification in epiphyses at proximal ends of phalanges and first metacarpal, distal ends of other metacarpals, and radius.

(**C,** From Standring S: *Gray's anatomy,* ed 40, New York, 2009, Churchill Livingstone.)

CLASSIFICATION OF BONES

Bones are classified by shape, as follows (Fig. 3-17):

- Long
- Short
- Flat
- Irregular
- Sesamoid

Long bones

Long bones are found only in the limbs. They consist primarily of a long cylindric shaft called the *body* and two enlarged, rounded ends that contain a smooth, slippery articular surface. A layer of articular cartilage covers this surface. The ends of these bones all articulate with other long bones. The femur and humerus are typical long bones. The phalanges of the fingers and toes are also considered long bones. A primary function of long bones is to provide support.

Short bones

Short bones consist mainly of cancellous bone containing red marrow and have a thin outer layer of compact bone. The carpal bones of the wrist and the tarsal bones of the ankles are the only short bones. They are varied in shape and allow minimum flexibility of motion in a short distance.

Flat bones

Flat bones consist largely of two tables of compact bone. The narrow space between the inner and outer tables contains cancellous bone and red marrow, or *diploë,* as it is called in flat bones. The bones of the cranium, sternum, and scapula are examples of flat bones. The flat surfaces of these bones provide protection, and their broad surfaces allow muscle attachment.

Irregular bones

Irregular bones are so termed because their peculiar shapes and variety of forms do not place them in any other category. The vertebrae and the bones in the pelvis and face fall into this category. Similar to other bones, they have compact bone on the exterior and cancellous bone containing red marrow in the interior. Their shape serves many functions, including attachment for muscles, tendons, and ligaments, or they attach to other bones to create joints.

Sesamoid bones

Sesamoid bones are small and oval. They develop inside and beside tendons. Their precise role is not understood. Experts believe that they alter the direction of muscle pull and decrease friction. The largest sesamoid bone is the patella, or the kneecap. Other sesamoids are located beneath the first metatarsophalangeal articulation of the foot and on the palmar aspect of the thumb at the metacarpophalangeal joint of the hand. Two small but prominent sesamoids are located beneath the base of the large toe. Similar to all other bones, they can be fractured.

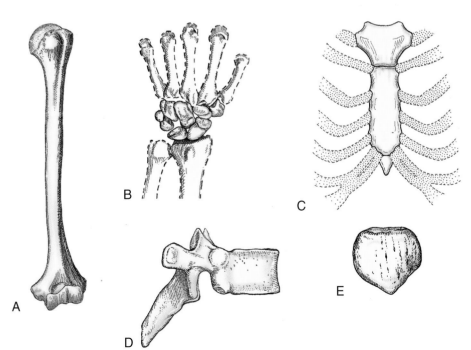

Fig. 3-17 Bones are classified by shape. **A,** Humerus is a long bone. **B,** Carpals of the wrist are short bones. **C,** Sternum is a flat bone. **D,** Vertebra is an irregular bone. **E,** Patella is a sesamoid bone.

TABLE 3-4

Structural classification of joints

Connective tissue	Classification	Movement
Fibrous	1. Syndesmosis	Slightly movable
	2. Suture	Immovable
	3. Gomphosis	Immovable
Cartilaginous	4. Symphysis	Slightly movable
	5. Synchondrosis	Immovable
Synovial	6. Gliding	Freely movable
	7. Hinge	Freely movable
	8. Pivot	Freely movable
	9. Ellipsoid	Freely movable
	10. Saddle	Freely movable
	11. Ball and socket	Freely movable

Arthrology

Arthrology is the study of the joints, or articulations between bones. Joints make it possible for bones to support the body, protect internal organs, and create movement. Various specialized articulations are necessary for these functions to occur.

The two classifications of joints described in anatomy books are *functional* and *structural*. Studying both classifications can be confusing. The most widely used and primary classification is the structural classification, which is used to describe all the joints in this atlas. This is also the classification recognized by *Nomina Anatomica*. For academic interest, a brief description of the functional classification is also provided.

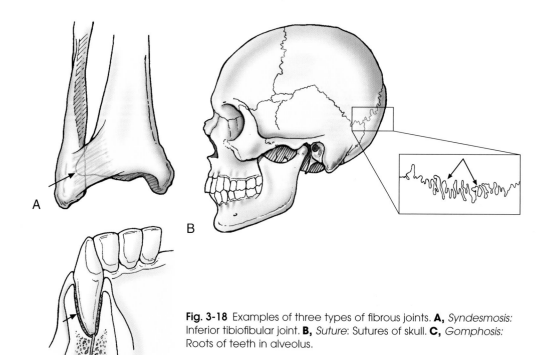

Fig. 3-18 Examples of three types of fibrous joints. **A,** *Syndesmosis:* Inferior tibiofibular joint. **B,** *Suture:* Sutures of skull. **C,** *Gomphosis:* Roots of teeth in alveolus.

FUNCTIONAL CLASSIFICATION

When joints are classified as functional, they are broken down into three classifications. These classifications are based on the mobility of the joint, as follows:
- Synarthroses—immovable joints
- Amphiarthroses—slightly movable
- Diarthroses—freely movable

STRUCTURAL CLASSIFICATION

The structural classification of joints is based on the types of tissues that unite or bind the articulating bones. A thorough study of this classification is easier if radiographers first become familiar with the terminology and breakdown of the structural classification identified in Table 3-4.

Structurally, joints are classified into three distinct groups on the basis of their connective tissues: fibrous, cartilaginous, and synovial. Within these three broad categories are the 11 specific types of joints. They are numbered in the text for easy reference to Table 3-4.

Fibrous joints

Fibrous joints do not have a joint cavity. They are united by various fibrous and connective tissues or ligaments. These are the strongest joints in the body because they are virtually immovable. The three types of fibrous joints are as follows:

1. *Syndesmosis:* An immovable joint or slightly movable joint united by sheets of fibrous tissue. The inferior tibiofibular joint is an example (Fig. 3-18, *A*).
2. *Suture:* An immovable joint occurring only in the skull. In this joint, the interlocking bones are held tightly together by strong connective tissues. The sutures of the skull are an example (Fig. 3-18, *B*).
3. *Gomphosis:* An immovable joint occurring only in the roots of the teeth. The roots of the teeth that lie in the alveolar sockets are held in place by fibrous periodontal ligaments (Fig. 3-18, *C*).

Cartilaginous joints

Cartilaginous joints are similar to fibrous joints in two ways: (1) They do not have a joint cavity, and (2) they are virtually immovable. Hyaline cartilage or fibrocartilage unites these joints. The two types of cartilaginous joints are as follows:

4. *Symphysis:* A slightly movable joint. The bones in this joint are separated by a pad of fibrocartilage. The ends of the bones contain hyaline cartilage. A symphysis joint is designed for strength and shock absorbency. The joint between the two pubic bones (pubic symphysis) is an example of a symphysis joint (Fig. 3-19, *A*). Another example of a symphysis joint is the joint between each vertebral body. These joints all contain a fibrocartilaginous pad or disk.
5. *Synchondrosis:* An immovable joint. This joint contains a rigid cartilage that unites two bones. An example is the epiphyseal plate found between the epiphysis and diaphysis of a growing long bone (Fig. 3-19, *B*). Before adulthood, these joints consist of rigid hyaline cartilage that unites two bones. When growth stops, the cartilage ossifies, making this type of joint a temporary joint.

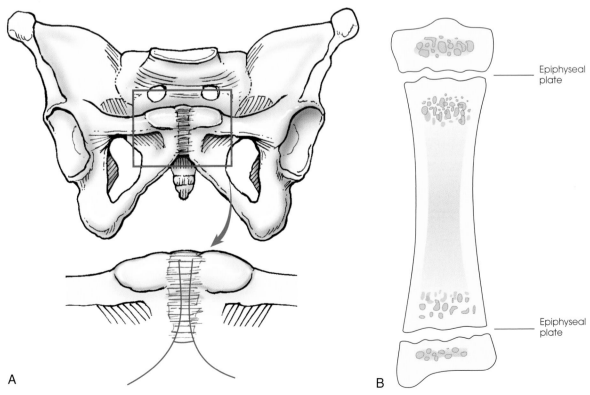

Epiphyseal plate

Epiphyseal plate

A   B

Fig. 3-19 Examples of two types of cartilaginous joints. **A,** *Symphysis:* Pubic symphysis. **B,** *Synchondrosis:* Epiphyseal plate found between epiphysis and diaphysis of growing long bones.

Synovial joints

Synovial joints permit a wide range of motion, and they all are freely movable. These joints are the most complex joints in the body. Fig. 3-20 shows their distinguishing features.

An articular capsule completely surrounds and enfolds all synovial joints to join the separate bones together. The outer layer of the capsule is called the *fibrous capsule,* and its fibrous tissue connects the capsule to the periosteum of the two bones. The *synovial membrane,* which is the inner layer, surrounds the entire joint to create the joint cavity. The membrane produces a thick, yellow, viscous fluid called *synovial fluid.* Synovial fluid lubricates the joint space to reduce friction between the bones. The ends of the adjacent bones are covered with articular cartilage. This smooth and slippery cartilage permits ease of motion. The two cartilages do not actually touch because they are separated by a thin layer of synovial membrane and fluid.

Some synovial joints contain a pad of fibrocartilage called the *meniscus,* which surrounds the joint. Specific menisci intrude into the joint from the capsular wall. They act as shock absorbers by conforming to and filling in the large gaps around the periphery of the bones. Some synovial joints also contain synovial fluid–filled sacs outside the main joint cavity, which are called the *bursae.* Bursae help reduce friction between skin and bones, tendons and bones, and muscles and bones. The menisci, bursae, and other joint structures can be visualized radiographically by injecting iodine-based contrast medium or air directly into the synovial cavity. This procedure, called *arthrography,* is detailed in Chapter 12.

The 6 synovial joints complete the 11 types of joints within the structural classification. They are listed in order of increasing movement. The most common name of each joint is identified, and the less frequently used name is given in parentheses.

6. *Gliding (plane):* Uniaxial movement. This is the simplest synovial joint. Joints of this type permit slight movement. They have flattened or slightly curved surfaces, and most glide slightly in only one axis. The intercarpal and intertarsal joints of the wrist and foot are examples of gliding joints (Fig. 3-21, *A*).
7. *Hinge (ginglymus):* Uniaxial movement. A hinge joint permits only flexion and extension. The motion is similar to that of a door. The elbow, knee, and ankle are examples of this type of joint (Fig. 3-21, *B*).
8. *Pivot (trochoid):* Uniaxial movement. These joints allow only rotation around a single axis. A rounded or pointed surface of one bone articulates within a ring formed partially by the other bone. An example of this joint is the articulation of the atlas and axis of the cervical spine. The atlas rotates around the dens of the axis and allows the head to rotate to either side (Fig. 3-21, *C*).
9. *Ellipsoid (condyloid):* Biaxial movement, primary. An ellipsoid joint permits movement in two directions at right angles to each other. The radiocarpal joint of the wrist is an example. Flexion and extension occur along with abduction and adduction. Circumduction, a combination of both movements, can also occur (Fig. 3-21, *D*).
10. *Saddle (sellar):* biaxial movement. This joint permits movement in two axes, similar to the ellipsoid joint. The joint is so named because the articular surface of one bone is saddle-shaped and the articular surface of the other bone is shaped like a rider sitting in a saddle. The two saddlelike structures fit into each other. The carpometacarpal joint between the trapezium and the first metacarpal is the only saddle joint in the body. The face of each bone end has a concave and a convex aspect. The opposing bones are shaped in a manner that allows side-to-side and up-and-down movement (Fig. 3-21, *E*).
11. *Ball and socket (spheroid):* multiaxial movement. This joint permits movement in many axes, including flexion and extension, abduction and adduction, circumduction, and rotation. In a ball-and-socket joint, the round head of one bone rests within the cup-shaped depression of the other bone. The hip and shoulder are examples (Fig. 3-21, *F*).

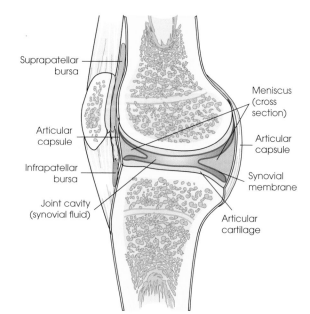

Fig. 3-20 Lateral cutaway view of knee showing distinguishing features of a synovial joint.

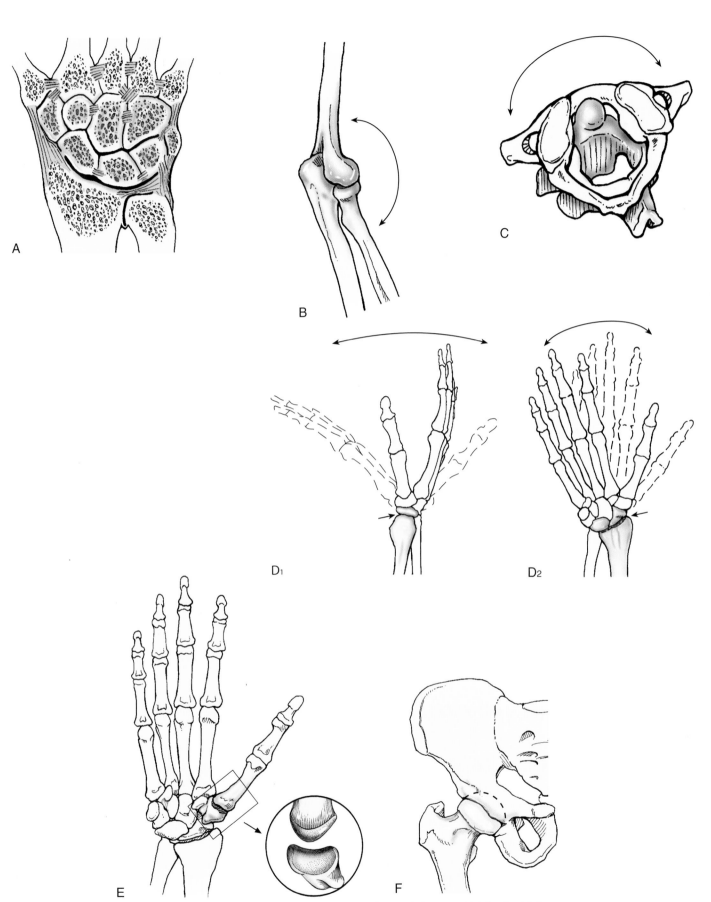

Fig. 3-21 Examples of six types of synovial joints. **A,** *Gliding:* Intercarpal joints of wrist. **B,** *Hinge:* Elbow joint. **C,** *Pivot:* Atlas and axis of cervical spine (viewed from above). **D,** *Ellipsoid:* Radiocarpal joint of wrist. **E,** *Saddle:* Carpometacarpal joint. **F,** *Ball and socket:* Hip joint.

Bone Markings and Features

The following anatomic terms are used to describe either processes or depressions on bones.

PROCESSES OR PROJECTIONS

Processes or projections extend beyond or project out from the main body of a bone and are designated by the following terms:

condyle rounded process at an articular extremity
coracoid or coronoid beaklike or crownlike process
crest ridgelike process
epicondyle projection above a condyle
facet small, smooth-surfaced process for articulation with another structure
hamulus hook-shaped process
head expanded end of a long bone
horn hornlike process on a bone
line less prominent ridge than a crest; a linear elevation
malleolus club-shaped process
protuberance projecting part or prominence
spine sharp process
styloid long, pointed process

trochanter either of two large, rounded, and elevated processes (greater or major and lesser or minor) located at junction of neck and shaft of femur
tubercle small, rounded, and elevated process
tuberosity large, rounded, and elevated process

DEPRESSIONS

Depressions are hollow or depressed areas and are described by the following terms:

fissure cleft or deep groove
foramen hole in a bone for transmission of blood vessels and nerves
fossa pit, fovea, or hollow space
groove shallow linear channel
meatus tubelike passageway running within a bone
notch indentation into border of a bone
sinus recess, groove, cavity, or hollow space, such as (1) recess or groove in bone, as used to designate a channel for venous blood on inner surface of cranium; (2) air cavity in bone or hollow space in other tissue (used to designate a hollow space within a bone, as in paranasal sinuses); or (3) fistula or suppurating channel in soft tissues
sulcus furrow, trench, or fissurelike depression

Fractures

A fracture is a break in the bone. Fractures are classified according to the nature of the break. Several general terms can pertain to them:

closed fracture that does not break through the skin
displaced serious fracture in which bones are not in anatomic alignment
nondisplaced fracture in which bone retains its normal alignment
open serious fracture in which broken bone or bones project through the skin

Common classifications of fractures are listed as follows and identified in Fig. 3-22:
- Compression
- Open or compound
- Simple
- Greenstick
- Transverse
- Spiral or oblique
- Comminuted
- Impacted

Many fractures fall into more than one category. A fracture could be spiral, closed, *and* nondisplaced.

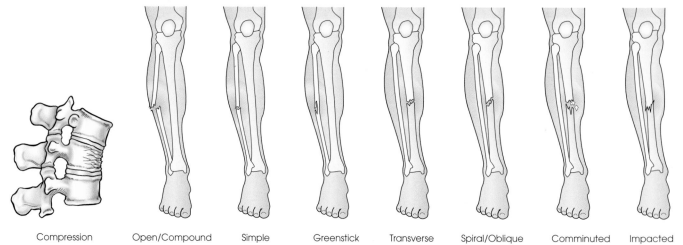

Compression   Open/Compound   Simple   Greenstick   Transverse   Spiral/Oblique   Comminuted   Impacted

Fig. 3-22 Common classifications of fractures.

Anatomic Relationship Terms

Various terms are used to describe the relationship of parts of the body in the anatomic position. Radiographers should be thoroughly familiar with these terms, which are commonly used in clinical practice. Most of the following positioning and anatomic terms are paired as opposites. Fig. 3-23 illustrates two commonly used sets of terms.

anterior (ventral) refers to forward or front part of body or forward part of an organ

posterior (dorsal) refers to back part of body or organ (note, however, that the superior surface of the foot is referred to as the dorsal surface)

caudad refers to parts away from the head of the body

cephalad refers to parts toward the head of the body

inferior refers to nearer the feet or situated below

superior refers to nearer the head or situated above

central refers to middle area or main part of an organ

peripheral refers to parts at or near the surface, edge, or outside of another body part

contralateral refers to part or parts on the opposite side of body

ipsilateral refers to part or parts on the same side of body

lateral refers to parts away from the median plane of body or away from the middle of another body part to the right or left

medial refers to parts toward the median plane of body or toward the middle of another body part

deep refers to parts far from the surface

superficial refers to parts near the skin or surface

distal refers to parts farthest from the point of attachment, point of reference, origin, or beginning; away from center of body

proximal refers to parts nearer the point of attachment, point of reference, origin, or beginning; toward the center of body

external refers to parts outside an organ or on the outside of body

internal refers to parts within or on the inside of an organ

parietal refers to the wall or lining of a body cavity

visceral refers to the covering of an organ

dorsum refers to the top or anterior surface of the foot or to the back or posterior surface of the hand

palmar refers to the palm of the hand

plantar refers to the sole of the foot

Radiographic Positioning Terminology

Radiography is the process of recording an image of a body part using one or more types of IRs (cassette/film, cassette/phosphor plate, or fluoroscopic screen/TV). The terminology used to position the patient and to obtain the radiograph was developed through convention. Attempts to analyze the usage often lead to confusion because the manner in which the terms are used does not follow one specific rule. During the preparation of this chapter, contact was maintained with the American Registry of Radiologic Technologists (ARRT) and the Canadian Association of Medical Radiation Technologists (CAMRT). The ARRT first distributed the "Standard Terminology for Positioning and Projection" in 1978[1]; it has not been substantially revised since initial distribution.[2] Despite its title, the ARRT document did not actually define selected positioning terms.[3] Terms not defined by the ARRT are defined in this atlas.

Approval of Canadian positioning terminology is the responsibility of the CAMRT Radiography Council on Education. This council provided information for the development of this chapter and clearly identified the terminology differences between the United States and Canada.[4]

---

[1]*ARRT educator's handbook,* ed 3, 1990, ARRT.
[2]*ARRT educator guide,* Spring 2010.
[3]ARRT, personal communication and permission, May 2006.
[4]CAMRT, Radiography Council on Education, personal communication, July 1993.

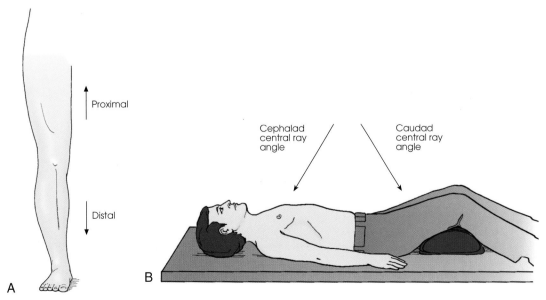

Fig. 3-23 A, Use of common radiology terms *proximal* and *distal.* **B,** Use of common radiology terms *caudad angle* and *cephalad angle.*

BOX 3-2

Primary x-ray projections and body positions

Projections	Positions
Anteroposterior (AP)	General body positions
Posteroanterior (PA)	Upright
Lateral	Seated
AP oblique	Supine
PA oblique	Prone
Axial	Recumbent
AP axial	Fowler
PA axial	Trendelenburg
AP axial oblique	Radiographic body positions
PA axial oblique	Lateral
Axiolateral	Right
Axiolateral oblique	Oblique
Transthoracic	Right posterior oblique (RPO)
Craniocaudal	Left posterior oblique (LPO)
Tangential	Right anterior oblique (RAO)
Inferosuperior	Left anterior oblique (LAO)
Superoinferior	Decubitus
Plantodorsal	Right lateral
Dorsoplantar	Left lateral
Lateromedial	Ventral
Mediolateral	Dorsal
Submentovertical	Lordotic
Acanthoparietal	
Parietoacanthial	
Acanthioparietal	
Orbitoparietal	
Parieto-orbital	

The terminology used by the ARRT and CAMRT is consistent overall with that used in this atlas. The only difference is that the term *view* is commonly used in Canada for some projections and positions.

The following are the four positioning terms most commonly used in radiology:
- Projection
- Position
- View
- Method

PROJECTION

The term *projection* is defined as the path of the central ray as it exits the x-ray tube and goes through the patient to the IR. Most projections are defined by the entrance and exit points in the body and are based on the *anatomic position*. When the central ray enters anywhere in the front (anterior) surface of the body and exits the back (posterior), an *anteroposterior (AP) projection* is obtained. Regardless of which body position the patient is in (e.g., supine, prone, upright), if the central ray enters the anterior body surface and exits the posterior body surface, the projection is termed an *AP projection* (Fig. 3-24).

Projections can also be defined by the relationship formed between the central ray and the body as the central ray passes through the entire body or body part. Examples include the *axial* and *tangential projections*.

All radiographic examinations described in this atlas are standardized and titled by their x-ray projection. The x-ray projection accurately and concisely defines each image produced in radiography. A complete list of the projection terms used in radiology is provided in Box 3-2. The essential radiographic projections follow.

Anteroposterior projection

In Fig. 3-25, a perpendicular central ray enters the anterior body surface and exits the posterior body surface. This is an *AP projection*. The patient is shown in the supine or dorsal recumbent body position. AP projections can also be achieved with upright, seated, or lateral decubitus positions.

Posteroanterior projection

In Fig. 3-26, a perpendicular central ray is shown entering the posterior body surface and exiting the anterior body surface. This illustrates a *posteroanterior (PA) projection* with the patient in the upright body position. PA projections can also be achieved with seated, prone (ventral recumbent), and lateral decubitus positions.

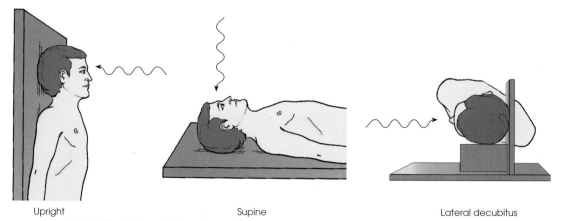

Upright   Supine   Lateral decubitus

Fig. 3-24 Patient's head placed in upright, supine, and lateral decubitus positions for a radiograph. All three body positions produce AP projection of skull.

Axial projection

In an axial projection (Fig. 3-27), there is *longitudinal angulation* of the central ray with the long axis of the body or a specific body part. This angulation is based on the anatomic position and is most often produced by angling the central ray cephalad or caudad. The longitudinal angulation in some examinations is achieved by angling the entire body or body part while maintaining the central ray perpendicular to the IR.

The term *axial,* as used in this atlas, refers to all projections in which the longitudinal angulation between the central ray and the long axis of the body part is *10 degrees or more.* When a range of central ray angles (e.g., 5 to 15 degrees) is recommended for a given projection, the term *axial* is used because the angulation could exceed 10 degrees. Axial projections are used in a wide variety of examinations and can be obtained with the patient in virtually any body position.

Tangential projection

Occasionally the central ray is directed toward the outer margin of a curved body surface to profile a body part just under the surface and project it free of superimposition. This is called a *tangential projection* because of the tangential relationship formed between the central ray and the entire body or body part (Fig. 3-28).

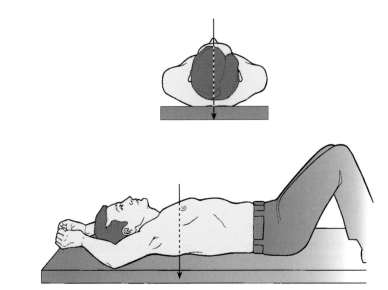

Fig. 3-25 AP projection of chest. Central ray enters anterior aspect and exits posterior aspect.

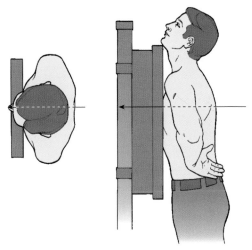

Fig. 3-26 PA projection of chest. Central ray enters posterior aspect and exits anterior aspect. Patient is in upright position.

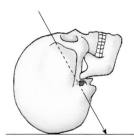

Fig. 3-27 AP axial projection of skull. Central ray enters anterior aspect at an angle and exits posterior aspect.

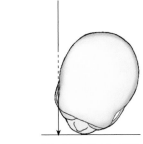

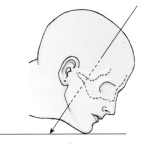

Fig. 3-28 Tangential projection of zygomatic arch. Central ray skims surface of the skull.

Lateral projection

For a lateral projection, a perpendicular central ray enters one side of the body or body part, passes transversely along the coronal plane, and exits on the opposite side. Lateral projections can enter from either side of the body or body part as needed for the examination. This can be determined by the patient's condition or ordered by the physician. When a lateral projection is used for head, chest, or abdominal radiography, the direction of the central ray is described with reference to the associated radiographic position. A left lateral position or right lateral position specifies the *side of the body closest to the IR* and corresponds with the side exited by the central ray (Fig. 3-29). For a right lateral position, the central ray enters the left side of the body and exits the right side (see Fig. 3-29). Lateral projections of the limbs are clarified further by the terms *lateromedial* or *mediolateral* to indicate the sides entered and exited by the central ray (Fig. 3-30). The *transthoracic projection* is a unique lateral projection used for shoulder radiography and is described in Chapter 5.

Oblique projection

During an oblique projection, the central ray enters the body or body part from a side angle following an oblique plane. Oblique projections may enter from either side of the body and from anterior or posterior surfaces. If the central ray enters the anterior surface and exits the opposite posterior surface, it is an *AP oblique projection;* if it enters the posterior surface and exits anteriorly, it is a *PA oblique projection* (Fig. 3-31).

Most oblique projections are achieved by rotating the patient with the central ray perpendicular to the IR. As in the lateral projection, the direction of the central ray for oblique projections is described with reference to the associated radiographic position. A right posterior oblique position (RPO) places the right posterior surface of the body closest to the IR and corresponds with an AP oblique projection exiting through the same side. This relationship is discussed later. Oblique projections can also be achieved for some examinations by angling the central ray diagonally along the horizontal plane rather than rotating the patient.

Complex projections

For additional clarity, projections may be defined by entrance and exit points and by the central ray relationship to the body at the same time. In the PA axial projection, the central ray enters the posterior body surface and exits the anterior body surface following an axial or angled trajectory relative to the entire body or body part. Axiolateral projections also use angulations of the central ray, but the ray enters and exits through lateral surfaces of the entire body or body part.

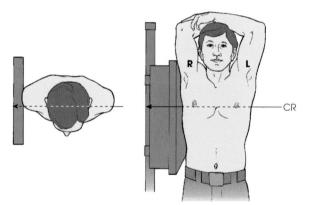

Fig. 3-29 Lateral projection of chest. The patient is placed in right lateral position. Right side of the chest is touching IR. Central ray (*CR*) enters left or opposite side of body.

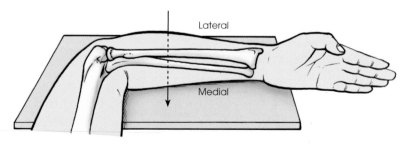

Fig. 3-30 Lateromedial projection of forearm. Central ray enters lateral aspect of forearm and exits medial aspect.

True projections

The term *true* (*true AP, true PA,* and *true lateral*)[1] is often used in clinical practice. *True* is used specifically to indicate that the body part must be placed exactly in the anatomic position.

A true AP or PA projection is obtained when the central ray is perpendicular to the coronal plane and parallel to the sagittal plane. A true lateral projection is obtained when the central ray is parallel to the normal plane and perpendicular to the sagittal plane. When a body part is rotated for an AP or PA oblique projection, a true AP or PA projection cannot be obtained. In this atlas, the term *true* is used only when the body part is placed in the anatomic position.

In-profile

In-profile is an outlined or silhouette view of an anatomic structure that has a distinctive shape. The distinctive aspect is not superimposed. The view is frequently seen from the side.

[1]Bontrager KL: *Textbook of radiographic positioning,* ed 7, St Louis, 2009, Mosby.

POSITION

The term *position* is used in two ways in radiology. One way identifies the overall posture of the patient or the general body position. The patient may be described as upright, seated, or supine. The second use of *position* refers to the specific placement of the body part in relation to the radiographic table or IR during imaging. This is the radiographic position and may be a right lateral, left anterior oblique, or other position depending on the examination and anatomy of interest. A list of all general body positions and radiographic positions is provided in Box 3-2.

During radiography, general body positions are combined with radiographic positions to produce the appropriate image. For clarification of the positioning for an examination, it is often necessary to include references to both because a particular radiographic position, such as right lateral, can be achieved in several general body positions (e.g., upright, supine, lateral recumbent) with differing image outcomes. Specific descriptions of general body positions and radiographic positions follow.

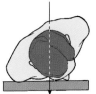

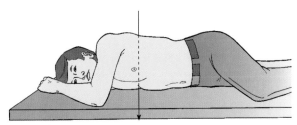

Fig. 3-31 PA oblique projection of chest. Central ray enters posterior aspect of body (even though it is rotated) and exits anterior aspect.

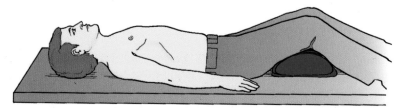

Fig. 3-32 Supine position of body, also termed *dorsal recumbent position*. The patient's knees are flexed for comfort.

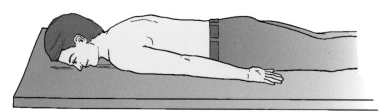

Fig. 3-33 Prone position of body, also termed *ventral recumbent position*.

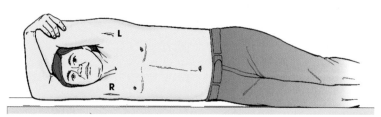

Fig. 3-34 Recumbent position of body, specifically *right lateral recumbent position*.

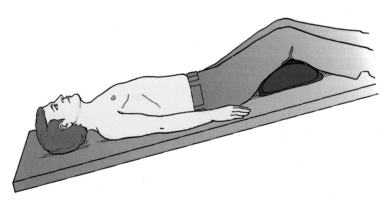

Fig. 3-35 Trendelenburg position of body. Feet are higher than the head.

General body positions

The following list describes the general body positions. All are commonly used in radiography practice.

upright erect or marked by a vertical position (see Fig. 3-26)

seated upright position in which the patient is sitting on a chair or stool

recumbent general term referring to lying down in any position, such as dorsal recumbent (Fig. 3-32), ventral recumbent (Fig. 3-33), or lateral recumbent (Fig. 3-34)

supine lying on the back (see Fig. 3-32)

prone lying face down (see Fig. 3-33)

Trendelenburg position supine position with head tilted downward (Fig. 3-35)

Fowler position supine position with head higher than the feet (Fig. 3-36)

Sims position recumbent position with the patient lying on the left anterior side (semi-prone) with left leg extended and right knee and thigh partially flexed (Fig. 3-37)

lithotomy position supine position with knees and hip flexed and thighs abducted and rotated externally, supported by ankle or knee supports (Fig. 3-38)

Lateral position

Lateral radiographic positions are always named according to the side of the patient that is placed closest to the IR (Figs. 3-39 and 3-40). In this atlas, the right or left lateral positions are indicated as subheadings for all lateral x-ray projections of the head, chest, and abdomen in which either the left or the right side of the patient is placed adjacent to the IR. The specific side selected depends on the condition of the patient, the anatomic structure of clinical interest, and the purpose of the examination. In Figs. 3-39 and 3-40, the x-ray projection for the positions indicated is lateral projection.

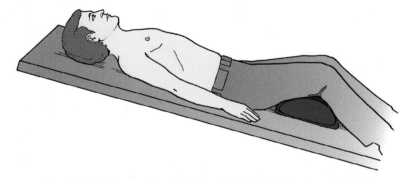

Fig. 3-36 Fowler position of the body. Head is higher than the feet.

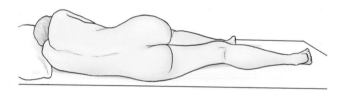

Fig. 3-37 Sims position of body. The patient is on the left side in recumbent oblique position.

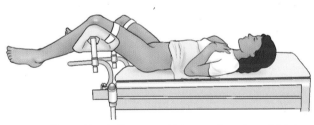

Fig. 3-38 Lithotomy position of body. Knees and hips are flexed, and thighs are abducted and rotated laterally.

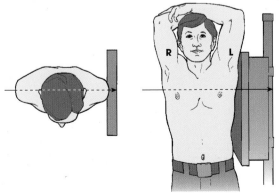

Fig. 3-39 Left lateral radiographic position of chest results in lateral projection.

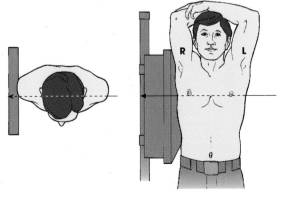

Fig. 3-40 Right lateral radiographic position of chest results in lateral projection.

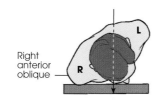

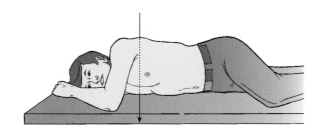

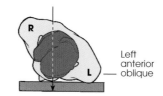

Fig. 3-41 RAO radiographic position of chest results in PA oblique projection.

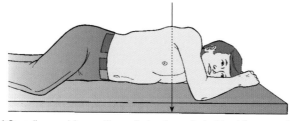

Fig. 3-42 LAO radiographic position of chest results in PA oblique projection.

Oblique position

An oblique radiographic position is achieved when the entire body or body part is rotated so that the coronal plane is not parallel with the radiographic table or IR. The angle of oblique rotation varies with the examination and structures to be shown. In this atlas, an angle is specified for each oblique position (e.g., rotated 45 degrees from the prone position).

Oblique positions, similar to lateral positions, are always named according to the side of the patient that is placed closest to the IR. In Fig. 3-41, the patient is rotated with the right anterior body surface in contact with the radiographic table. This is a *right anterior oblique (RAO) position* because the right side of the anterior body surface is closest to the IR. Fig. 3-42 shows the patient placed in a *left anterior oblique (LAO) position.*

The relationship between oblique position and oblique projection can be summarized simply. Anterior oblique positions result in PA oblique projections as shown in Figs. 3-41 and 3-42. Similarly, posterior oblique positions result in AP oblique projections as illustrated in Figs. 3-43 and 3-44.

The oblique positioning terminology used in this atlas has been standardized using RAO and LAO or RPO and LPO positions along with the appropriate PA or AP oblique projection. For oblique positions of the limbs, the terms *medial rotation* and *lateral rotation* have been standardized to designate the direction in which the limbs have been turned from the anatomic position (Fig. 3-45).

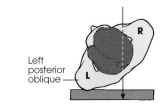

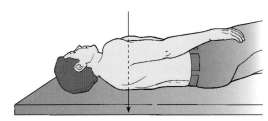

Fig. 3-43 LPO radiographic position of chest results in AP oblique projection.

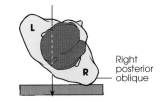

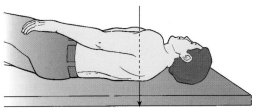

Fig. 3-44 RPO radiographic position of chest results in AP oblique projection.

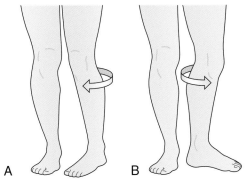

Fig. 3-45 A, Medial rotation of knee. **B,** Lateral rotation of knee.

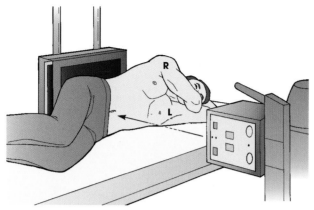

Fig. 3-46 Left lateral decubitus radiographic position of abdomen results in AP projection. Note horizontal orientation of central ray.

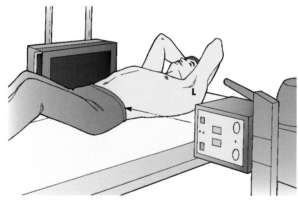

Fig. 3-47 Right dorsal decubitus radiographic position of abdomen results in right lateral projection. Note horizontal orientation of central ray.

Decubitus position

In radiographic positioning terminology, the term *decubitus* indicates that the patient is lying down and that the central ray is horizontal and parallel with the floor. Three primary decubitus positions are named according to the body surface on which the patient is lying: *lateral decubitus (left or right), dorsal decubitus,* and *ventral decubitus.* Of these, the lateral decubitus position is used most often to show the presence of air-fluid levels or free air in the chest and abdomen.

In Fig. 3-46, the patient is placed in the left lateral decubitus radiographic position with the back (posterior surface) closest to the IR. In this position, a horizontal central ray provides an AP projection. Fig. 3-46 is accurately described as an AP projection with the body in the left lateral decubitus position. Alternatively, the patient may be placed with the front of the body (anterior surface) facing the IR, resulting in a PA projection. This would be correctly described as a PA projection of the body in the left lateral decubitus position. Right lateral decubitus positions may be necessary with AP or PA projections, depending on the examination.

In Fig. 3-47, the patient is shown in a dorsal decubitus radiographic position with one side of the body next to the IR. The horizontal central ray provides a lateral projection. This is correctly described as a lateral projection with the patient placed in the dorsal decubitus position. Either side may face the IR, depending on the examination or the patient's condition.

The ventral decubitus radiographic position (Fig. 3-48) also places a side of the body adjacent to the IR, resulting in a lateral projection. Similar to the earlier examples, the accurate terminology is lateral projection with the patient in the ventral decubitus position. Either side may face the IR.

Lordotic position

The lordotic position is achieved by having the patient lean backward while in the upright body position so that only the shoulders are in contact with the IR (Fig. 3-49). An angulation forms between the central ray and the long axis of the upper body, producing an AP axial projection. This position is used for the visualization of pulmonary apices (see Chapter 10) and clavicles (see Chapter 5).

Note to educators, students, and clinicians

In clinical practice, the terms *position* and *projection* are often incorrectly used. These are two distinct terms that should not be interchanged. Incorrect use leads to confusion for the student who is attempting to learn the correct terminology of the profession. Educators and clinicians are encouraged to use the term *projection* generally when describing any examination performed. The word *projection* is the only term that accurately describes how the body part is being examined. The term *position* should be used only when referring to the placement of the patient's body. A correct example is, "We are going to perform a PA projection of the chest with the patient in the upright position."

VIEW

The term *view* is used to describe the body part as seen by the IR. Use of this term is restricted to the general discussion of a finished radiograph or image. *View* and *projection* are exact opposites. For many years, *view* and *projection* were often used interchangeably, which led to confusion. In the United States, *projection* has replaced *view* as the preferred terminology for describing radiographic images. In Canada, *view* remains an acceptable positioning term. For consistency, this atlas refers to all views as *images* or *radiographs*.

METHOD

Some radiographic projections and procedures are named after individuals (e.g., Waters, Towne) in recognition of their development of a method to show a specific anatomic part. *Method*, which was first described in the fifth edition of this atlas, describes the specific radiographic projection that the individual developed. The majority of methods are named after an individual, however a few are for unique projections. The method specifies the x-ray projection and body position, and it may include specific items such as IR, CR, or other unique aspects. In this atlas, standard projection terminology is used first, and a named method is listed secondarily (e.g., PA axial projection; Towne method). The ARRT and CAMRT use the standard anatomic projection terminology and list the originator in parentheses.

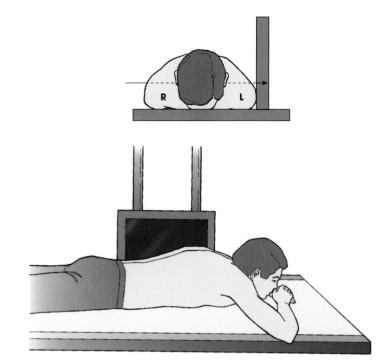

Fig. 3-48 Left ventral decubitus radiographic position of abdomen results in left lateral projection. Note horizontal orientation of central ray.

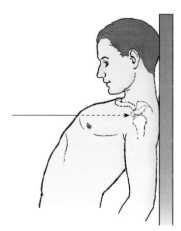

Fig. 3-49 Lordotic radiographic position of chest results in AP axial projection. Central ray is not angled; however, it enters chest axially as a result of body position.

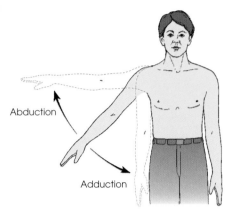

Fig. 3-50 Abduction and adduction of arm.

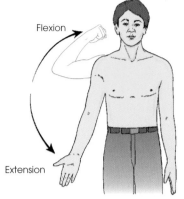

Fig. 3-51 Extension of arm (anatomic position) and flexion (bending).

Body Movement Terminology

The following terms are used to describe movement related to the limbs. These terms are often used in positioning descriptions and in the patient history provided to the radiographer by the referring physician. They must be studied thoroughly.

abduct or abduction movement of a part away from the central axis of the body or body part

adduct or adduction movement of a part toward the central axis of the body or body part (Fig. 3-50)

extension straightening of a joint; when both elements of the joint are in the anatomic position; normal position of a joint (Fig. 3-51)

flexion act of bending a joint; opposite of extension (Fig. 3-52)

hyperextension forced or excessive extension of a limb or joints

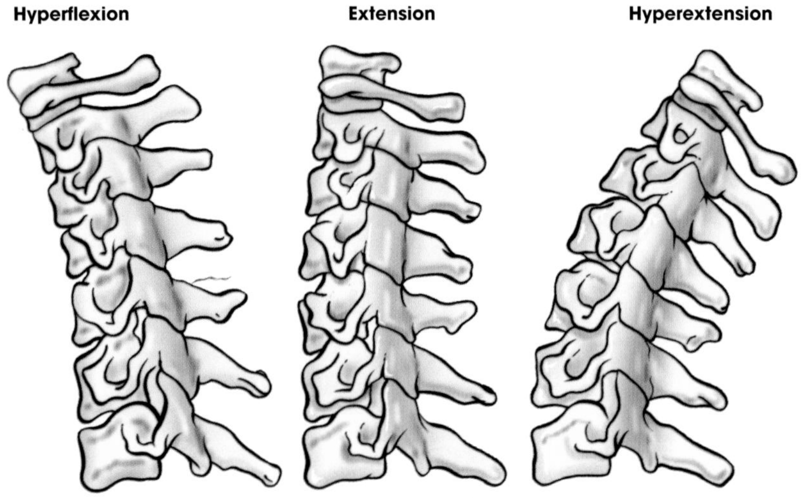

Hyperflexion **Extension** **Hyperextension**

Fig. 3-52 Hyperextension, extension, and hyperflexion of neck.

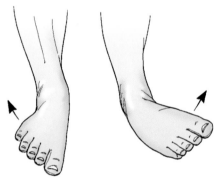

Fig. 3-53 Eversion and inversion of foot at ankle joint.

hyperflexion forced overflexion of a limb or joints (see Fig. 3-52)

evert/eversion outward turning of the foot at the ankle

invert/inversion inward turning of the foot at the ankle (Fig. 3-53)

pronate/pronation rotation of the forearm so that the palm is down

supinate/supination rotation of the forearm so that the palm is up (in the anatomic position) (Fig. 3-54)

rotate/rotation turning or rotating of body or a body part around its axis (Fig. 3-55, *A*); rotation of a limb is either medial (toward the midline of the body from the anatomic position [Fig. 3-55, *B*]) or lateral (away from the midline of the body from the anatomic position [Fig. 3-55, *C*])

circumduction circular movement of a limb (Fig. 3-56)

tilt tipping or slanting a body part slightly; tilt is in relation to the long axis of the body (Fig. 3-57)

deviation turning away from the regular standard or course (Fig. 3-58)

dorsiflexion flexion or bending the foot toward the leg (Fig. 3-59)

plantar flexion flexion or bending the foot downward toward the sole (see Fig. 3-59)

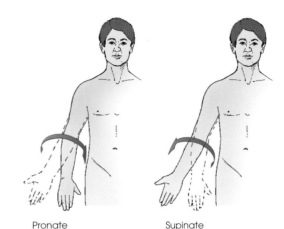

Pronate — Supinate

Fig. 3-54 Pronation and supination of forearm.

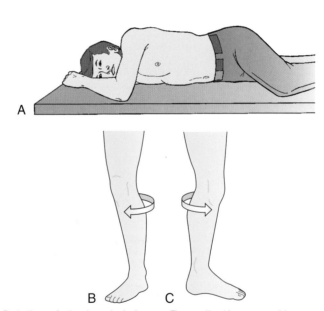

Fig. 3-55 A, Rotation of chest and abdomen. The patient's arm and knee are flexed for comfort. **B,** Medial rotation of left leg. **C,** Lateral rotation of left leg.

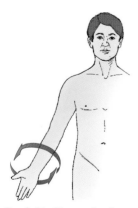

Fig. 3-56 Circumduction of arm.

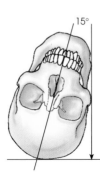

Fig. 3-57 Tilt of skull is 15 degrees from long axis.

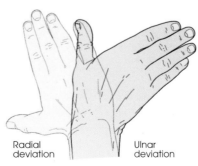

Radial deviation — Ulnar deviation

Fig. 3-58 Radial deviation of hand (turned to radial side) and ulnar deviation (turned to ulnar side).

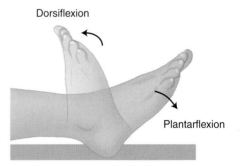

Dorsiflexion — Plantarflexion

Fig. 3-59 Foot in dorsiflexion and plantar flexion. Note movement is at ankle joint.

TABLE 3-5
Greek and Latin nouns: common singular and plural forms

Singular	Plural	Examples: singular—plural
-a	-ae	maxilla—maxillae
-ex	-ces	apex—apices
-is	-es	diagnosis—diagnoses
-ix	-ces	appendix—appendices
-ma	-mata	condyloma—condylomata
-on	-a	ganglion—ganglia
-um	-a	antrum—antra
-us	-i	ramus—rami

TABLE 3-6
Frequently misused single and plural word forms

Singular	Plural	Singular	Plural
adnexus	adnexa	mediastinum	mediastina
alveolus	alveoli	medulla	medullae
areola	areolae	meninx	meninges
bronchus	bronchi	meniscus	menisci
bursa	bursae	metastasis	metastases
calculus	calculi	mucosa	mucosae
coxa	coxae	omentum	omenta
diagnosis	diagnoses	paralysis	paralyses
diverticulum	diverticula	plexus	plexi
fossa	fossae	pleura	pleurae
gingiva	gingivae	pneumothorax	pneumothoraces
haustrum	haustra	ramus	rami
hilum	hila	ruga	rugae
ilium	ilia	sulcus	sulci
labium	labia	thrombus	thrombi
lamina	laminae	vertebra	vertebrae
lumen	lumina	viscus	viscera

Medical Terminology

Single and plural word endings for common Greek and Latin nouns are presented in Table 3-5. Single and plural word forms are often confused. Examples of commonly misused word forms are listed in Table 3-6; the singular form generally is used when the plural form is intended.

ABBREVIATIONS USED IN CHAPTER 3	
ARRT	American Registry of Radiologic Technologists
ASIS	Anterior superior iliac spine
CT	Computed tomography
LAO	Left anterior oblique
LLQ	Left lower quadrant
LPO	Left posterior oblique
LUQ	Left upper quadrant
MRI	Magnetic resonance imaging
RAO	Right anterior oblique
RLQ	Right lower quadrant
RPO	Right posterior oblique
RUQ	Right upper quadrant
US	Ultrasound

⸱ See Addendum A for a summary of all abbreviations used in Volume 1.

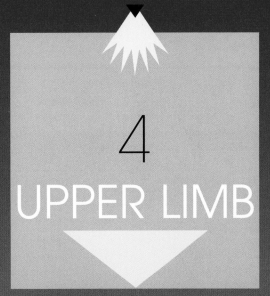

4

UPPER LIMB

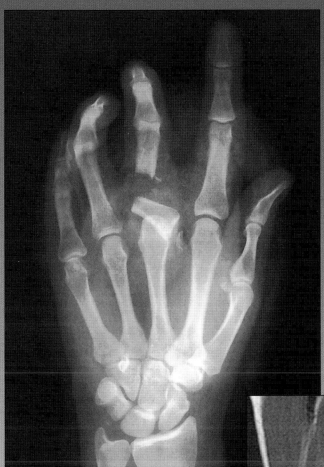

SUMMARY OF PROJECTIONS

PROJECTIONS, POSITIONS, AND METHODS

Page	Essential	Anatomy	Projection	Position	Method
110	🌲	Digits (second through fifth)	PA		
112	🌲	Digits (second through fifth)	Lateral	Lateromedial, mediolateral	
114	🌲	Digits (second through fifth)	PA oblique	Lateral rotation	
116	🌲	First digit (thumb)	AP		
116		First digit (thumb)	PA		
116	🌲	First digit (thumb)	Lateral		
117	🌲	First digit (thumb)	PA oblique		
118		First digit (thumb): *First carpometacarpal joint*	AP		ROBERT
120		First digit (thumb): *First carpometacarpal joint*	AP		BURMAN
122		First digit (thumb): *First metacarpophalangeal joint*	PA		FOLIO
124	🌲	Hand	PA		
126	🌲	Hand	PA oblique	Lateral rotation	
128	🌲	Hand	Lateral	Extension and fan lateral	
130		Hand	Lateral	Flexion	
130		Hand	AP oblique	Medial rotation	NORGAARD
132	🌲	Wrist	PA		
133		Wrist	AP		
134	🌲	Wrist	Lateral		
136	🌲	Wrist	PA oblique	Lateral rotation	
137		Wrist	AP oblique	Medial rotation	
138	🌲	Wrist	PA	Ulnar deviation	
139		Wrist	PA	Radial deviation	
140	🌲	Wrist: *Scaphoid*	PA axial		STECHER
142		Wrist: *Scaphoid series*	PA, PA axial	Ulnar deviation	RAFERT-LONG
144		Wrist: *Trapezium*	PA axial oblique		CLEMENTS-NAKAYAMA
145		Carpal bridge	Tangential		
146	🌲	Carpal canal	Tangential		GAYNOR-HART
148	🌲	Forearm	AP		
150	🌲	Forearm	Lateral		
151	🌲	Elbow	AP		
152	🌲	Elbow	Lateral		
154	🌲	Elbow	AP oblique	Medial rotation	
155	🌲	Elbow	AP oblique	Lateral rotation	
156	🌲	Elbow: *Distal humerus*	AP	Partial flexion	
157	🌲	Elbow: *Proximal forearm*	AP	Partial flexion	
158		Elbow: *Distal humerus*	AP	Acute flexion	
159		Elbow: *Proximal forearm*	PA	Acute flexion	
160		Elbow: *Radial head*	Lateral		
162	🌲	Elbow: *Radial head, coronoid process*	Axiolateral	Lateral	COYLE
165		Distal humerus	PA axial		
166		Olecranon process	PA axial		
167	🌲	Humerus	AP	Upright	
168	🌲	Humerus	Lateral	Upright	
169	🌲	Humerus	AP	Recumbent	
170	🌲	Humerus	Lateral	Recumbent	
171	🌲	Humerus	Lateral	Recumbent, lateral recumbent	

The icons in the Essential column indicate projections frequently performed in the United States and Canada. Students should demonstrate competence in these projections.

Anatomists divide the bones of the upper limbs, or extremities, into the following main groups:
• Hand
• Forearm
• Arm
• Shoulder girdle

The proximal arm and shoulder girdle are discussed in Chapter 5.

Hand

The *hand* consists of 27 bones, which are subdivided into the following groups:
• *Phalanges*: Bones of the digits (fingers and thumb)
• *Metacarpals*: Bones of the palm
• *Carpals*: Bones of the wrist (Fig. 4-1)

DIGITS

The five *digits* are described by numbers and names; however, description by number is the more correct practice. Beginning at the lateral, or thumb, side of the hand, the numbers and names are as follows:
• First digit (thumb)
• Second digit (index finger)
• Third digit (middle finger)
• Fourth digit (ring finger)
• Fifth digit (small finger)

The digits contain 14 *phalanges* (*phalanx,* singular), which are long bones that consist of a cylindric body and articular ends. Nine phalanges have two articular ends. The first digit has two phalanges—the *proximal* and *distal.* The other digits have three phalanges—the *proximal, middle,* and *distal.* The proximal phalanges are the closest to the palm, and the distal phalanges are the farthest from the palm. The distal phalanges are small and flattened, with a roughened rim around their distal anterior end; this gives them a spatulalike appearance. Each phalanx has a *head, body,* and *base.*

METACARPALS

Five *metacarpals,* which are cylindric in shape and slightly concave anteriorly, form the palm of the hand (see Fig. 4-1). They are long bones consisting of a *body* and two articular ends—the *head* distally and the *base* proximally. The area below the head is the *neck* where fractures often occur. The first metacarpal contains two small *sesamoid* bones on its palmar aspect below the neck (see Fig. 4-1). A single

sesamoid is often seen at this same level on the second metacarpal. The metacarpal heads, commonly known as the *knuckles,* are visible on the dorsal hand in flexion. The metacarpals are also numbered 1 to 5, beginning from the lateral side of the hand.

CARPAL TERMINOLOGY CONVERSION	
Preferred	**Synonyms**
Proximal row	
Scaphoid	Navicular
Lunate	Semilunar
Triquetrum	Triquetral, cuneiform, or triangular
Pisiform	(none)
Distal row	
Trapezium	Greater multangular
Trapezoid	Lesser multangular
Capitate	Os magnum
Hamate	Unciform

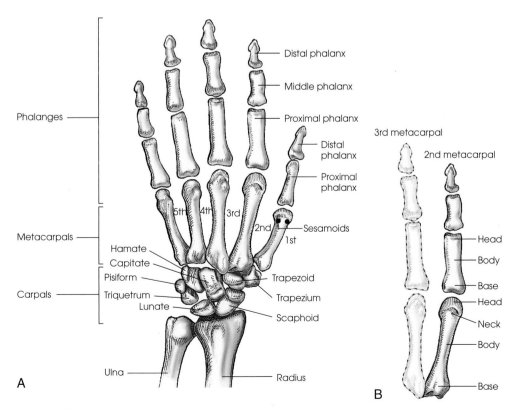

Fig. 4-1 **A,** Anterior aspect of right hand and wrist. **B,** Second metacarpal and phalanges showing head, neck, body, and base on second digit.

WRIST

The *wrist* has eight *carpal* bones, which are fitted closely together and arranged in two horizontal rows (see Fig. 4-1). The carpals are classified as short bones and are composed largely of cancellous tissue with an outer layer of compact bony tissue. These bones, with one exception, have two or three names; this atlas uses the preferred terms (see box). The proximal row of carpals, which is nearest the forearm, contains the scaphoid, lunate, triquetrum, and pisiform. The distal row includes the trapezium, trapezoid, capitate, and hamate.

Each carpal contains identifying characteristics. Beginning at the proximal row of carpals on the lateral side, the *scaphoid,* the largest bone in the proximal carpal row, has a tubercle on the anterior and lateral aspect for muscle attachment and is palpable near the base of the thumb. The *lunate* articulates with the radius proximally and is easy to recognize because of its crescent shape. The *triquetrum* is roughly pyramidal and articulates anteriorly with the hamate. The *pisiform* is a pea-shaped bone situated anterior to the triquetrum and is easily palpated.

Beginning at the distal row of carpals on the lateral side, the *trapezium* has a tubercle and groove on the anterior surface. The tubercles of the trapezium and scaphoid constitute the lateral margin of the carpal groove. The *trapezoid* has a smaller surface anteriorly than posteriorly. The *capitate* articulates with the base of the third metacarpal and is the largest and most centrally located carpal. The wedge-shaped *hamate* exhibits the prominent *hook of hamate,* which is located on the anterior surface. The hamate and the pisiform form the medial margin of the carpal groove.

A triangular depression is located on the posterior surface of the wrist and is visible when the thumb is abducted and extended. This depression, known as the *anatomic snuffbox,* is formed by the tendons of the two major muscles of the thumb. The anatomic snuffbox overlies the scaphoid bone and the radial artery, which carries blood to the dorsum of the hand. Tenderness in the snuffbox area is a clinical sign suggesting fracture of the scaphoid—the most commonly fractured carpal bone.

CARPAL SULCUS

The anterior or palmar surface of the wrist is concave from side to side and forms the *carpal sulcus* (Figs. 4-2 and 4-3). The *flexor retinaculum,* a strong fibrous band, attaches medially to the pisiform and hook of hamate and laterally to the tubercles of the scaphoid and trapezium. The *carpal tunnel* is the passageway created between the carpal sulcus and flexor retinaculum. The *median nerve* and the *flexor tendons* pass through the carpal canal. Carpal tunnel syndrome results from compression of the median nerve inside the carpal tunnel.

Forearm

The *forearm* contains two bones that lie parallel to each other—the *radius* and *ulna.* Similar to other long bones, they have a body and two articular extremities. The radius is located on the lateral side of the forearm, and the ulna is located on the medial side (Figs. 4-4 and 4-5).

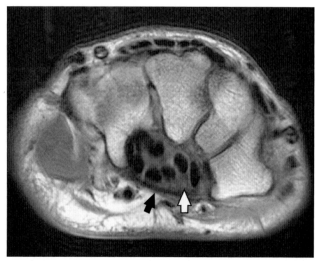

Fig. 4-2 Axial MRI of wrist. Bones in same position as in Fig. 4-3. Note arched position of carpal bones and carpal sulcus protecting tendons of fingers (*black circles* within sulcus) and median nerve (*white arrow*). Flexor retinaculum (*black arrow*) is also seen.

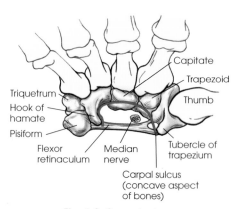

Fig. 4-3 Carpal sulcus.

ULNA

The *body* of the ulna is long and slender and tapers inferiorly. The upper portion of the ulna is large and presents two beaklike processes and concave depressions (Fig. 4-6). The proximal process, or *olecranon process,* concaves anteriorly and slightly inferiorly and forms the proximal portion of the *trochlear notch.* The more distal *coronoid process* projects anteriorly from the anterior surface of the body and curves slightly superiorly. The process is triangular and forms the lower portion of the trochlear notch. A depression called the *radial notch* is located on the lateral aspect of the coronoid process.

The distal end of the ulna includes a rounded process on its lateral side called the *head* and a narrower conic projection on the posteromedial side called the *ulnar styloid process.* An articular disk separates the head of the ulna from the wrist joint.

RADIUS

The proximal end of the radius is small and presents a flat disklike *head* above a constricted area called the *neck.* Just inferior to the neck on the medial side of the *body* of the radius is a roughened process called the *radial tuberosity.* The distal end of the radius is broad and flattened and has a conic projection on its lateral surface called the *radial styloid process.*

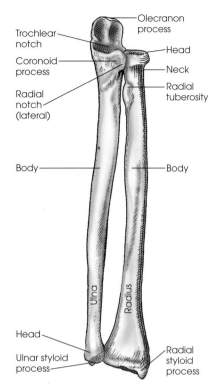

Fig. 4-4 Anterior aspect of left radius and ulna.

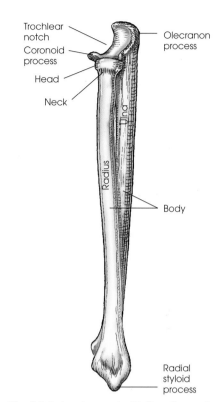

Fig. 4-5 Lateral aspect of left radius and ulna.

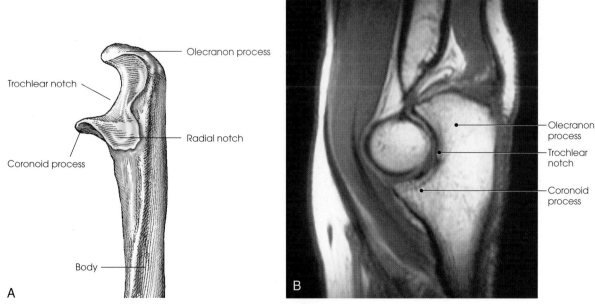

Fig. 4-6 A, Radial aspect of left proximal ulna. **B,** Sagittal MRI of elbow joint showing trochlear notch surrounding trochlea of humerus.

(**B,** Modified from Kelley LL, Petersen CM: *Sectional anatomy for imaging professionals,* ed 2, St Louis, 2007, Mosby.)

Forearm

Arm

The arm has one bone called the *humerus,* which consists of a *body* and two articular ends (Fig. 4-7, *A* and *B*). The proximal part of the humerus articulates with the shoulder girdle and is described further in Chapter 5. The distal humerus is broad and flattened and presents numerous processes and depressions.

The entire distal end of the humerus is called the *humeral condyle* and includes two smooth elevations for articulation with the bones of the forearm—the *trochlea* on the medial side and the *capitulum* on the lateral side. The *medial* and *lateral epicondyles* are superior to the condyle and easily palpated. On the anterior surface superior to the trochlea, a shallow depression called the *coronoid fossa* receives the coronoid process when the elbow is flexed. The relatively small *radial fossa,* which receives the radial head when the elbow is flexed, is located lateral to the coronoid fossa and proximal to the capitulum. The *olecranon fossa* is a deep depression found immediately behind the coronoid fossa on the posterior surface and accommodates the olecranon process when the elbow is extended (Fig. 4-7, *C*).

The proximal end of the humerus contains the *head,* which is large, smooth, and rounded and lies in an oblique plane on the superomedial side. Just below the head, lying in the same oblique plane, is

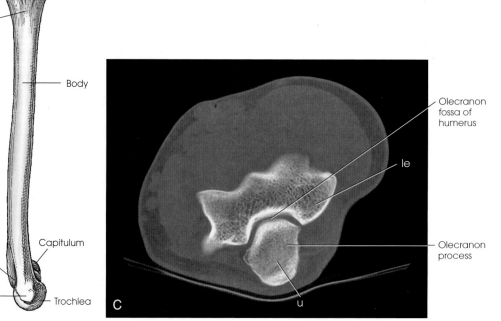

Fig. 4-7 **A,** Anterior aspect of left humerus. **B,** Medial aspect of left humerus. **C,** Axial CT scan of elbow. *le,* lateral epicondyle; *u,* ulna.

the narrow, constricted *anatomic neck*. The constriction of the body just below the tubercles is called the *surgical neck*, which is the site of many fractures.

The *lesser tubercle* is situated on the anterior surface of the bone immediately below the anatomic neck. The tendon of the subscapularis muscle inserts at the lesser tubercle. The *greater tubercle* is located on the lateral surface of the bone just below the anatomic neck and is separated from the lesser tubercle by a deep depression called the *intertubercular groove*.

Upper Limb Articulations

Table 4-1 contains a summary of the joints of the upper limb. A detailed description of the upper limb articulations follows.

The *interphalangeal* (IP) articulations between the phalanges are *synovial hinge* type and allow only flexion and extension (Fig. 4-8). The IP joints are named by location and are differentiated as either *proximal interphalangeal* (PIP) or *distal interphalangeal* (DIP), by the digit number, and by right or left hand (e.g., the PIP articulation of the fourth digit of the left hand) (Fig. 4-9, *A* and *B*). Because the first digit has only two phalanges, the joint between the two phalanges is simply called the IP joint.

The metacarpals articulate with the phalanges at their distal ends and the carpals at their proximal ends. The *metacarpophalangeal* (MCP) articulations are *synovial ellipsoidal* joints and have the movements of flexion, extension, abduction, adduction, and circumduction. Because of the less convex and wider surface of the MCP joint of the thumb, only limited abduction and adduction are possible.

TABLE 4-1

Joints of the upper limb

Joint	Structural classification		Movement
	Tissue	**Type**	**Movement**
Interphalangeal	Synovial	Hinge	Freely movable
Metacarpophalangeal	Synovial	Ellipsoidal	Freely movable
Carpometacarpal			
First digit	Synovial	Saddle	Freely movable
Second to fifth digits	Synovial	Gliding	Freely movable
Intercarpal	Synovial	Gliding	Freely movable
Radiocarpal	Synovial	Ellipsoidal	Freely movable
Radioulnar			
Proximal	Synovial	Pivot	Freely movable
Distal	Synovial	Pivot	Freely movable
Humeroulnar	Synovial	Hinge	Freely movable
Humeroradial	Synovial	Hinge	Freely movable

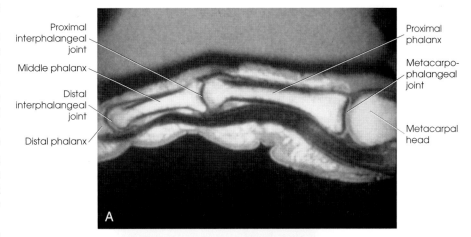

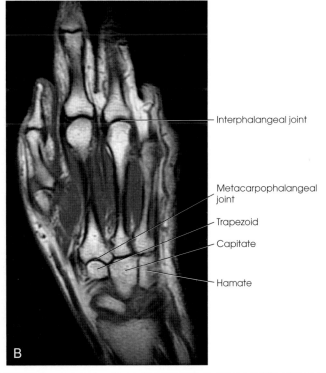

Fig. 4-8 A, Sagittal MRI of finger showing IP and MCP joints. **B,** Coronal MRI of hand and wrist showing same joints.

The carpals articulate with each other, the metacarpals, and the radius of the forearm. In the *carpometacarpal* (CMC) articulations, the first metacarpal and trapezium form a *synovial saddle* joint, which permits the thumb to oppose the fingers (touch the fingertips). The articulations between the second, third, fourth, and fifth metacarpals and the trapezoid, capitate, and hamate form *synovial glid-* ing joints. The *intercarpal* articulations are also *synovial gliding* joints. The articulations between the lunate and scaphoid form a gliding joint. The *radiocarpal* articulation is a *synovial ellipsoidal* type. This joint is formed by the articulation of the scaphoid, lunate, and triquetrum, with the radius and the articular disk just distal to the ulna (Fig. 4-9, *C*).

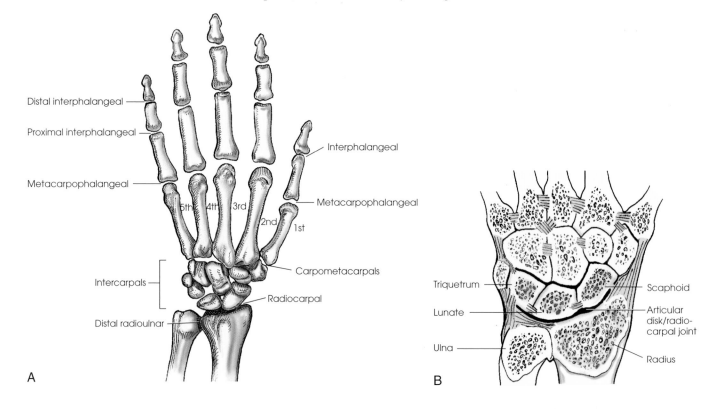

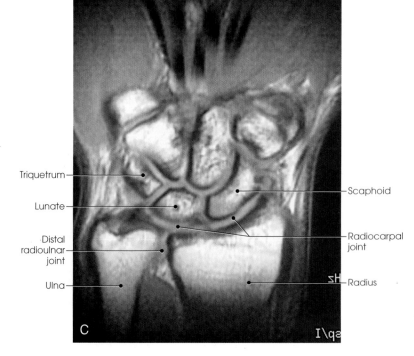

Fig. 4-9 A, Articulations of hand and wrist. **B,** Radiocarpal articulation formed by scaphoid, lunate, and triquetrum with radius. **C,** Coronal MRI of wrist showing bones and joints of wrist.

The *distal* and *proximal radioulnar* articulations are synovial pivot joints. The distal ulna articulates with the ulnar notch of the distal radius. The proximal head of the radius articulates with the radial notch of the ulna at the medial side. The movements of supination and pronation of the forearm and hand largely result from the combined rotary action of these two joints. In pronation, the radius turns medially and crosses over the ulna at its upper third, and the ulna makes a slight counter-rotation that rotates the humerus medially.

The elbow joint proper includes the proximal radioulnar articulation and the articulations between the humerus and the radius and ulna. The three joints are enclosed in a common capsule. The trochlea of the humerus articulates with the ulna at the trochlear notch. The capitulum of the humerus articulates with the flattened head of the radius. The *humeroulnar* and *humeroradial* articulations form a *synovial hinge* joint and allow only flexion and extension movement (Figs. 4-10 and 4-11, *A*). The proximal humerus and its articulations are described with the shoulder girdle in Chapter 5.

Fat Pads

The three areas of fat[1,2] associated with the elbow joint can be visualized only in the lateral projection (Fig. 4-11, *B* and *C*). The *posterior fat pad* covers the largest area and lies within the olecranon fossa of the posterior humerus. The superimposed coronoid and radial fat pads, which lie in the coronoid and radial fossae of the anterior humerus, form the *anterior fat pad*. The *supinator fat pad* is positioned anterior to and parallel with the anterior aspect of the proximal radius.

When the elbow is flexed 90 degrees for the lateral projection, only the anterior and supinator fat pads are visible, and the posterior fat pad is depressed within the olecranon fossa. The anterior fat pad resembles a teardrop, and the supinator fat pad appears as shown in Fig. 4-11, *B*. The fat pads become significant radiographically when an elbow injury causes effusion and displaces the fat pads or alters their shape. Visualization of the posterior fat pad is a reliable indicator of elbow pathology. Exposure factors designed to show soft tissues are extremely important on lateral elbow radiographs because visualization of the fat pads may be the only evidence of injury.

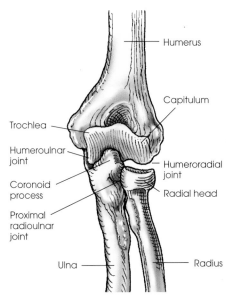

Fig. 4-10 Anterior aspect of left elbow joint.

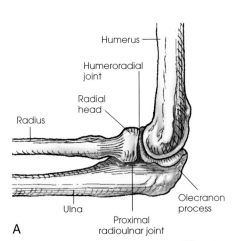

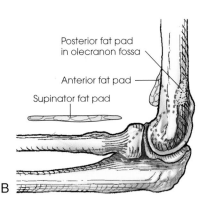

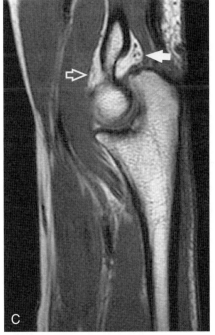

Fig. 4-11 A, Lateral aspect of elbow. **B,** Fat pads of elbow joint. **C,** Sagittal MRI of elbow joint showing posterior fat pad (*solid arrow*) and anterior fat pad (*open arrow*).

SUMMARY OF ANATOMY

Hand
Phalanges (bones of digits)
Digits
  Head
  Body
  Base
Metacarpals
Carpals

Metacarpals
First to fifth metacarpals
  Head
  Neck
  Body
  Base
Sesamoids

Wrist
Scaphoid
Lunate
Triquetrum
Pisiform

Trapezium
Trapezoid
Capitate
Hamate
Hook of hamate
Anatomic snuffbox

Carpal sulcus
Carpal tunnel
Flexor retinaculum
Median nerve
Flexor tendons

Forearm
Ulna
Radius

Ulna
Olecranon process
Trochlear notch
Coronoid process
Radial notch
Body

Head
Ulnar styloid process

Radius
Head
Neck
Radial tuberosity
Body
Radial styloid process

Arm
Humerus

Humerus
Humeral condyle
Trochlea
Capitulum
Medial epicondyle
Lateral epicondyle
Coronoid fossa
Radial fossa
Olecranon fossa
Body

Surgical neck
Lesser tubercle
Greater tubercle
Intertubercular groove
Anatomic neck
Head

Articulations
Interphalangeal
Metacarpophalangeal
Carpometacarpal
Intercarpal
Radiocarpal
Radioulnar
Humeroulnar
Humeroradial

Fat pads
Anterior fat pads
Posterior fat pad
Supinator fat pad

EXPOSURE TECHNIQUE CHART ESSENTIAL PROJECTIONS

UPPER LIMB

Part	cm	kVp*	tm	mA	mAs	AEC	SID	IR	Dose (mrad)†
Digits‡	Ave	54	.01	200s	2		40″	8 × 10 in-2	5
Hand—*PA*‡	Ave	54	.01	200s	2		40″	24 × 30 cm-2	5
Hand—*Oblique*‡	Ave	57	.01	200s	2		40″	24 × 30 cm-2	7
Hand—*Lateral*‡	Ave	60	.01	200s	2		40″	24 × 30 cm-2	11
Wrist—*PA, AP*‡	Ave	54	.01	200s	2		40″	24 × 30 cm-2	5
Wrist—*Lateral*‡	Ave	60	.01	200s	2		40″	24 × 30 cm-2	11
Carpal canal‡	Ave	65	.01	200s	2		40″	8 × 10 in	18
Forearm—*AP, lateral*‡	7	60	.02	200s	4		40″	18 × 43 cm	24
Elbow—*AP, lateral*§	8	60	.01	200s	2		40″	24 × 30 cm-2	4
Elbow—*Distal humerus*§	9	65	.01	200s	2		40″	8 × 10 in	4
Elbow—*Proximal forearm*§	9	65	.01	200s	2		40″	8 × 10 in	4
Humerus—*AP, lateral*ǁ	12	70	.06	200s	2		40″	35 × 43 cm	28
Humerus—*Lateral recumbent*§	12	70	.01	200s	2		40″	30 × 35 cm	5
Cast—*Fiberglass*	Increase mAs 25% *or* 4 kVp								
Cast—*Plaster medium*	Increase mAs 50% *or* 7 kVp								
Cast—*Plaster large*	Increase mAs 100% *or* 10 kVp¶								

*kVp values are for a three-phase, 12-pulse or high-frequency generator.
†Relative doses for comparison use. All doses are skin entrance for average adult at cm indicated.
‡Tabletop, extremity IR. Screen-film speed 100.
§Tabletop, standard IR. Screen-film speed 300.
ǁBucky, 16:1 grid. Screen-film speed 300 or equivalent CR.

¶Gratale P, Turner GW, Burns CB: Using the same exposure factors for wet and dry casts, *Radiol Technol* 57:328, 1986.
s, small focal spot.

SUMMARY OF PATHOLOGY

Condition	Definition
Bone cyst	Fluid-filled cyst with wall of fibrous tissue
Bursitis	Inflammation of bursa
Dislocation	Displacement of bone from joint space
Fracture	Disruption in continuity of bone
Bennett	Fracture at base of first metacarpal
Boxer's	Fracture of metacarpal neck
Colles	Fracture of distal radius with posterior (dorsal) displacement
Smith	Fracture of distal radius with anterior (palmar) displacement
Torus or buckle	Impacted fracture with bulging of periosteum
Gout	Hereditary form of arthritis in which uric acid is deposited in joints
Joint effusion	Accumulation of fluid in joint associated with underlying condition
Metastases	Transfer of cancerous lesion from one area to another
Osteoarthritis or degenerative joint disease	Form of arthritis marked by progressive cartilage deterioration in synovial joints and vertebrae
Osteomyelitis	Inflammation of bone owing to pyogenic infection
Osteopetrosis	Increased density of atypically soft bone
Osteoporosis	Loss of bone density
Rheumatoid arthritis	Chronic, systemic, inflammatory collagen disease
Tumor	New tissue growth where cell proliferation is uncontrolled
Chondrosarcoma	Malignant tumor arising from cartilage cells
Enchondroma	Benign tumor consisting of cartilage
Ewing sarcoma	Malignant tumor of bone arising in medullary tissue
Osteosarcoma	Malignant, primary tumor of bone with bone or cartilage formation

Rob Hughes, MS, RT(R), contributed the new pathology terms and definitions for each chapter of this edition of the atlas.

ABBREVIATIONS USED IN CHAPTER 4

CMC	Carpometacarpal
DIP	Distal interphalangeal
IP*	Interphalangeal
MC	Metacarpal
MCP	Metacarpophalangeal
PIP	Proximal interphalangeal

See Addendum A for a summary of all abbreviations used in Volume 1.
*Note that IP has two different meanings; it is used in Chapter 1 to mean "image plate."

General Procedures

When the upper limb is radiographed, the following steps should be initiated:

- Remove rings, watches, and other radiopaque objects, and place them in secure storage during the procedure.
- Seat the patient at the side or end of the table to avoid a strained or uncomfortable position.
- Place the IR at a location and angle that allows the patient to be in the most comfortable position. Because the degree of immobilization (particularly of the hand and digits) is limited, the patient must be comfortable to promote relaxation and cooperation in maintaining the desired position.
- Unless otherwise specified, direct the central ray at a right angle to the midpoint of the IR. Because the joint spaces of the limbs are narrow, accurate centering is essential to avoid obscuring the joint spaces.
- Radiograph each side *separately* when performing a bilateral examination of the hands or wrists; this prevents distortion, particularly of the joint spaces.
- *Shield gonads* from scattered radiation with a sheet of lead-impregnated rubber or a lead apron placed over the patient's pelvis (Fig. 4-12).
- Use close collimation. This technique is recommended for all upper limb radiographs.
- Placing multiple exposures on one IR is a common practice. The side of the unexposed IR should always be covered with lead, especially when the new computed radiography IRs are used.
- Use right or left markers and all other vital identification markers when appropriate.

Digits (Second Through Fifth)

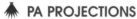 PA PROJECTIONS

Image receptor: 8 × 10 inch (18 × 24 cm) lengthwise or crosswise for two or more images on one IR

Position of patient

- Seat the patient at the end of the radiographic table.

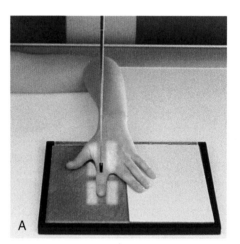 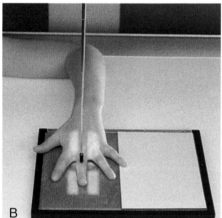

Fig. 4-13 **A,** PA second digit. **B,** PA third digit.

Position of part

When radiographing individual digits (except the first), take the following steps:

- Place the extended digit with the palmar surface down on the unmasked portion of the IR.
- Separate the digits slightly, and center the digit under examination to the midline portion of the IR.
- Center the PIP joint to the IR (Figs. 4-13 to 4-15).
- *Shield gonads.*

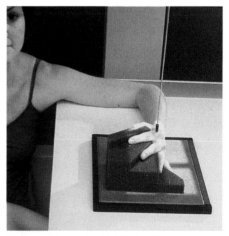

Fig. 4-12 Properly shielded patient.

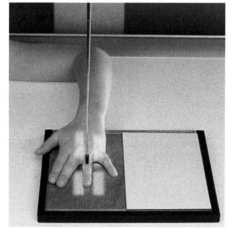

Fig. 4-14 PA fourth digit.

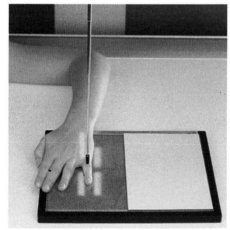

Fig. 4-15 PA fifth digit.

Digits (Second through Fifth)

Central ray
- Perpendicular to the PIP joint of the affected digit

Collimation
- 1 inch (2.5 cm) on all sides of the digit, including 1 inch (2.5 cm) proximal to the MCP joint

 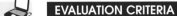

The digit for all projections must be centered to the plate or plate section with four collimator margins or with no margins at all. Two images can be projected on one plate; however, there should be four collimator margins for each projection. A lead blocker must cover the unexposed side when two images are made on one IR.

Structures shown
A PA projection of the appropriate digit is visualized (Figs. 4-16 through 4-19).

EVALUATION CRITERIA

The following should be clearly shown:
- Evidence of proper collimation
- No rotation of the digit
- Concavity of the phalangeal shafts and an equal amount of soft tissue on both sides of the phalanges
- Fingernail, if visualized and normal, centered over the distal phalanx
- Entire digit from fingertip to distal portion of the adjoining metacarpal
- No soft tissue overlap from adjacent digits
- Open IP and MCP joint spaces without overlap of bones
- Soft tissue and bony trabeculation

NOTE: Digits that cannot be extended can be examined in small sections. When joint injury is suspected, an AP projection is recommended instead of a PA projection.

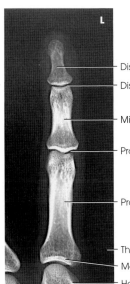

Distal phalanx
Distal interphalangeal joint
Middle phalanx
Proximal interphalangeal joint
Proximal phalanx
Thumb
Metacarpophalangeal joint
Head of metacarpal

Fig. 4-16 PA second digit.

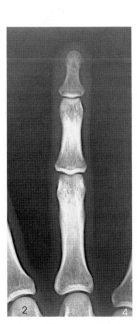

Fig. 4-17 PA third digit.

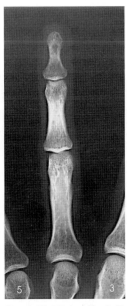

Fig. 4-18 PA fourth digit.

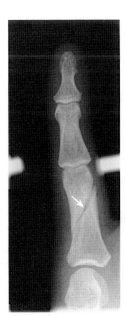

Fig. 4-19 Fractured fifth digit (*arrow*).

Digits (Second through Fifth)

♠ LATERAL PROJECTION
Lateromedial or mediolateral

Image receptor: 8 × 10 inch (18 × 24 cm) lengthwise or crosswise for two or more images on one IR

Position of patient
- Seat the patient at the end of the radiographic table.

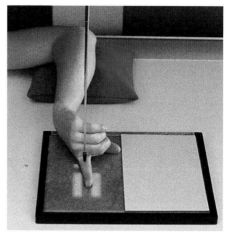

Fig. 4-20 Lateral second digit.

Position of part
- Because lateral digit positions are difficult to hold, tell the patient how the digit is adjusted on the IR and demonstrate with your own finger. Let the patient assume the most comfortable arm position.
- Ask the patient to extend the digit to be examined. Close the rest of the digits into a fist and hold them in complete flexion with the thumb.
- Support the elbow on sandbags or provide other suitable support when the elbow must be elevated to bring the digit into position.
- With the digit under examination extended and other digits folded into a fist, have the patient's hand rest on the lateral, or radial, surface for the second or third digit (Figs. 4-20 and 4-21) or on the medial, or ulnar, surface for the fourth or fifth digit (Figs. 4-22 and 4-23).

- Before making the final adjustment of the digit position, place the IR so that the midline of its unmasked portion is parallel with the long axis of the digit. Center the IR to the PIP joint.
- Rest the second and fifth digits directly on the IR, but for an accurate image of the bones and joints, elevate the third and fourth digits and place their long axes parallel with the plane of the IR. A radiolucent sponge may be used to support the digits.
- Immobilize the extended digit by placing a strip of adhesive tape, a tongue depressor, or other support against its palmar surface. The patient can hold the support with the opposite hand.
- Adjust the anterior or posterior rotation of the hand to obtain a true lateral position of the digit.
- *Shield gonads.*

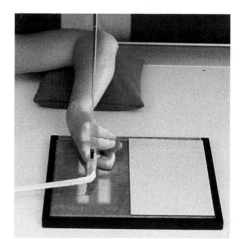

Fig. 4-21 Lateral third digit (*adhesive tape*).

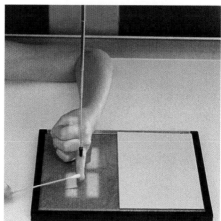

Fig. 4-22 Lateral fourth digit (*cotton swab*).

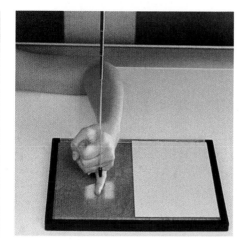

Fig. 4-23 Lateral fifth digit.

Upper Limb

Central ray
- Perpendicular to the PIP joint of the affected digit

Collimation
- 1 inch (2.5 cm) on all sides of the digit, including 1 inch (2.5 cm) proximal to the MCP joint

Structures shown
A lateral projection of the affected digit is shown (Figs. 4-24 through 4-27).

EVALUATION CRITERIA

The following should be clearly shown:
- Evidence of proper collimation
- Entire digit in a true lateral position
  - Fingernail in profile, if visualized and normal
  - Concave, anterior surfaces of the phalanges
  - No rotation of the phalanges
- No obstruction of the proximal phalanx or MCP joint by adjacent digits
- Open IP joint spaces
- Soft tissue and bony trabeculation

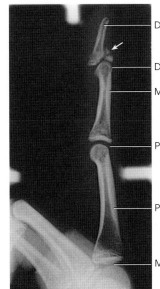

Distal phalanx

Distal interphalangeal joint

Middle phalanx

Proximal interphalangeal joint

Proximal phalanx

Metacarpophalangeal joint

Fig. 4-24 Lateral digit showing chip fracture (*arrow*) and dislocation involving DIP joint of second digit (*arrow*).

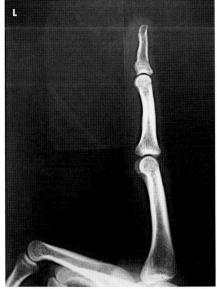

Fig. 4-25 Lateral third digit.

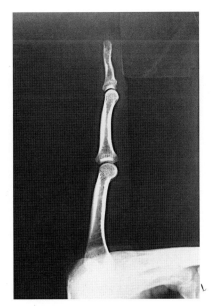

Fig. 4-26 Lateral fourth digit.

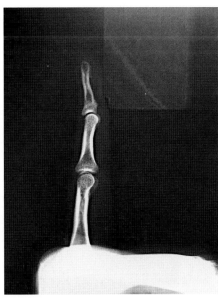

Fig. 4-27 Lateral fifth digit.

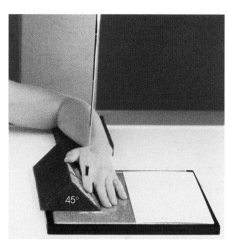

Fig. 4-28 PA oblique second digit.

☀ PA OBLIQUE PROJECTION
Lateral rotation

Image receptor: 8 × 10 inch (18 × 24 cm) lengthwise or crosswise for two or more images on one IR

Position of patient
- Seat the patient at the end of the radiographic table.

Position of part
- Place the patient's forearm on the table with the hand pronated and the palm resting on the IR.
- Center the IR at the level of the PIP joint.
- Rotate the hand laterally until the digits are separated and supported on a 45-degree foam wedge. The wedge supports the digits in a position parallel with the IR plane (Figs. 4-28 through 4-31) so that the IP joint spaces are open.
- *Shield gonads.*

Central ray
- Perpendicular to the PIP joint of the affected digit

Collimation
- 1 inch (2.5 cm) on all sides of the digit, including 1 inch (2.5 cm) proximal to the MCP joint

Structures shown
The resultant image shows a PA oblique projection of the bones and soft tissue of the affected digit (Figs. 4-32 through 4-35).

EVALUATION CRITERIA
The following should be clearly shown:
- Evidence of proper collimation
- Entire digit rotated at a 45-degree angle, including the distal portion of the adjoining metacarpal
- No superimposition of the adjacent digits over the proximal phalanx or MCP joint
- Open IP and MCP joint spaces
- Soft tissue and bony trabeculation

OPTION: Some radiographers rotate the second digit medially from the prone position (Fig. 4-36). The advantage of medially rotating the digit is that the part is closer to the IR for improved recorded detail and increased visibility of certain fractures.[1]

[1]Street JM: Radiographs of phalangeal fractures: importance of the internally rotated oblique projection for diagnosis, *AJR Am J Roentgenol* 160:575, 1993.

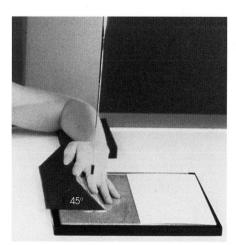

Fig. 4-29 PA oblique third digit.

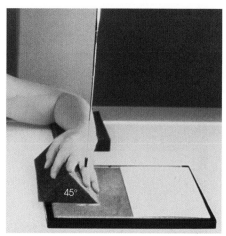

Fig. 4-30 PA oblique fourth digit.

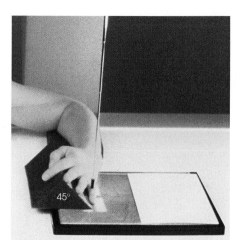

Fig. 4-31 PA oblique fifth digit.

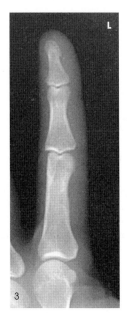

Fig. 4-32 PA oblique second digit.

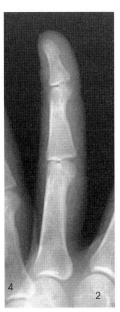

Fig. 4-33 PA oblique third digit.

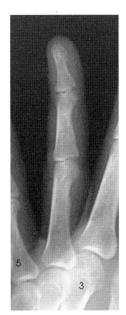

Fig. 4-34 PA oblique fourth digit.

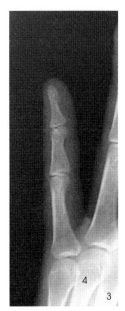

Fig. 4-35 PA oblique fifth digit.

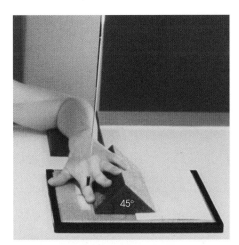

Fig. 4-36 PA oblique second digit (alternative method, medial rotation).

First Digit (Thumb)

AP, PA, LATERAL, AND PA OBLIQUE PROJECTIONS

Image receptor: 8 × 10 inch (18 × 24 cm) lengthwise or crosswise for two or more images on one IR

▲ AP PROJECTION

Position of patient

- Seat the patient at the end of the radiographic table with the arm internally rotated.

Position of part

- Demonstrate how to avoid motion or rotation with the hand. By adjusting the body position on the chair, the patient can place the hand in the correct position with the least amount of strain on the arm.
- Put the patient's hand in a position of extreme medial rotation. Have the patient hold the extended digits back with tape or the opposite hand. Rest the thumb on the IR. If the elbow is elevated, place a support under it and have the patient rest the opposite forearm against the table for support (Fig. 4-37).
- Center the long axis of the thumb parallel with the long axis of the IR. Adjust the position of the hand to ensure a true AP projection of the thumb. Place the fifth metacarpal back far enough to avoid superimposition.
- Lewis[1] suggested directing the central ray 10 to 15 degrees along the long axis of the thumb toward the wrist to show the first metacarpal free of the soft tissue of the palm.
- *Shield gonads.*

---

[1]Lewis S: New angles on the radiographic examination of the hand—II, *Radiogr Today* 54:29, 1988.

PA PROJECTION

Position of patient

- Seat the patient at the end of the radiographic table with the hand resting on its medial surface.

Position of part

- If a PA projection of the first CMC joint and first digit is to be performed, place the hand in the lateral position. Rest the elevated and abducted thumb on a radiographic support, or hold it up with a radiolucent stick. Adjust the hand to place the dorsal surface of the digit parallel with the IR. This position magnifies the part (Fig. 4-38).
- Center the MCP joint to the center of the IR.
- *Shield gonads.*

▲ LATERAL PROJECTION

Position of patient

- Seat the patient at the end of the radiographic table with the relaxed hand placed on the IR.

Position of part

- Place the hand in its natural arched position with the palmar surface down and fingers flexed or resting on a sponge.
- Place the midline of the IR parallel with the long axis of the digit. Center the IR to the MCP joint.
- Adjust the arching of the hand until a true lateral position of the thumb is obtained (Fig. 4-39).

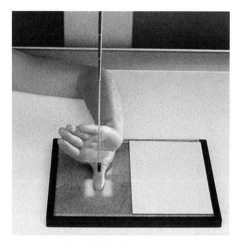

Fig. 4-37 AP first digit.

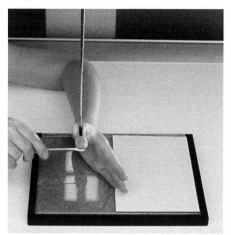

Fig. 4-38 PA first digit (*cotton swab*).

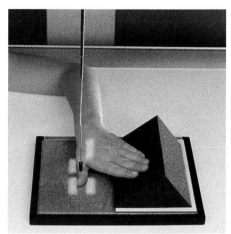

Fig. 4-39 Lateral first digit.

🔥 PA OBLIQUE PROJECTION

Position of patient

- Seat the patient at the end of the radiographic table with the palm of the hand resting on the IR.

Position of part

- With the thumb abducted, place the palmar surface of the hand in contact with the IR. Ulnar deviate the hand slightly. This relatively normal placement positions the thumb in the oblique position.
- Align the longitudinal axis of the thumb with the long axis of the IR. Center the IR to the MCP joint (Fig. 4-40).
- *Shield gonads.*

Central ray

- Perpendicular to the MCP joint for AP, PA, lateral, and oblique projections

Collimation

- 1 inch (2.5 cm) on all sides of the digit, including 1 inch (2.5 cm) proximal to the CMC joint

Structures shown

AP, PA, lateral, and PA oblique projections of the thumb are shown (Figs. 4-41 through 4-44).

EVALUATION CRITERIA

AP and PA thumb

The following should be clearly shown:
- Evidence of proper collimation
- No rotation
    - □ Concavity of the phalangeal and metacarpal shafts
    - □ Equal amount of soft tissue on both sides of the phalanges
    - □ Thumbnail, if visualized, in the center of the distal thumb
- Area from the distal tip of the thumb to the trapezium
- Open IP and MCP joint spaces without overlap of bones
- Overlap of soft tissue profile of the palm over the mid-shaft of the first metacarpal
- Soft tissue and bony trabeculation
- PA thumb projection magnified compared with AP projection

Lateral thumb

The following should be clearly shown:
- First digit in a true lateral projection
    - □ Thumbnail, if visualized and normal, in profile
    - □ Concave, anterior surface of the proximal phalanx
    - □ No rotation of the phalanges
- Area from the distal tip of the thumb to the trapezium
- Open IP and MCP joint spaces
- Soft tissue and bony trabeculation

Oblique thumb

The following should be clearly shown:
- Proper rotation of phalanges, soft tissue, and first metacarpal
- Area from the distal tip of the thumb to the trapezium
- Open IP and MCP joint spaces
- Soft tissue and bony trabeculation

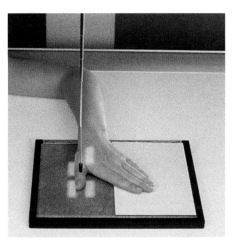

Fig. 4-40 PA oblique first digit.

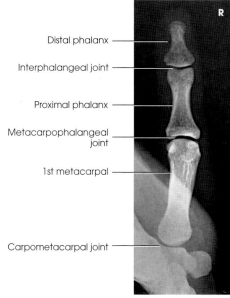

Distal phalanx
Interphalangeal joint
Proximal phalanx
Metacarpophalangeal joint
1st metacarpal
Carpometacarpal joint

Fig. 4-41 AP first digit.

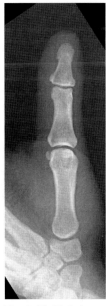

Fig. 4-42 PA first digit.

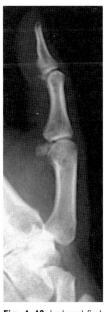

Fig. 4-43 Lateral first digit.

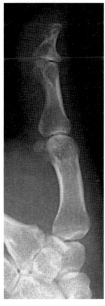

Fig. 4-44 PA oblique first digit.

First Carpometacarpal Joint

AP PROJECTION

ROBERT METHOD

Robert[1] first described the radiographic projection of the first CMC joint in 1936. Lewis[2] modified the central ray for this projection in 1988, and Long and Rafert[3] further modified the central ray in 1995. This projection is commonly performed to show arthritic changes, fractures, displacement of the first CMC joint, and Bennett fracture. The Robert method does not replace the initial AP or PA thumb projection.

Image receptor: 8 × 10 inch (18 × 24 cm) lengthwise

---

[1]Robert M: X-ray of trapezo-metacarpal articulation: the arthroses of this joint, *Bulletins et memories de la Societe de Radiologie Medicale de France* 24:687, 1936.
[2]Lewis S: New angles on the radiographic examination of the hand—II, *Radiogr Today* 54:29, 1988.
[3]Long B, Rafert J: *Orthopaedic radiography,* Philadelphia, 1995, Saunders.

Position of patient

• Seat the patient sideways at the end of the radiographic table. The patient should be positioned low enough to place the shoulder, elbow, and wrist on the same plane. The entire limb *must* be on the same plane to prevent elevation of the carpal bones and closing of the first CMC joint (Fig. 4-45, *A*).

Position of part

• Extend the limb straight out on the radiographic table.
• Rotate the arm internally to place the posterior aspect of the thumb on the IR with the thumbnail down (Fig. 4-45, *B*).

• Place the thumb in the center of the IR.
• Hyperextend the hand so that the soft tissue over the ulnar aspect does not obscure the first CMC joint (Fig. 4-46). Ensure that the thumb is not oblique.
• Long and Rafert[1] stated that the patient may hold the fingers back with the other hand.
• Steady the hand on a sponge if necessary.
• *Shield gonads.*

---

[1]Long B, Rafert J: *Orthopaedic radiography,* Philadelphia, 1995, Saunders.

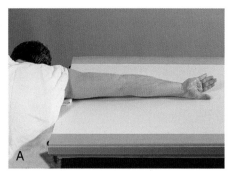
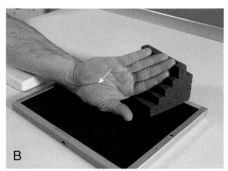

Fig. 4-45 A, Patient in position for AP thumb to show first CMC joint: Robert method. The patient leans forward to place entire arm on same plane and for ease of maximum internal arm rotation. **B,** Thumb, hand, and wrist in correct position for AP of first CMC joint. Note specific area of wrist where joint is located (*arrow*).

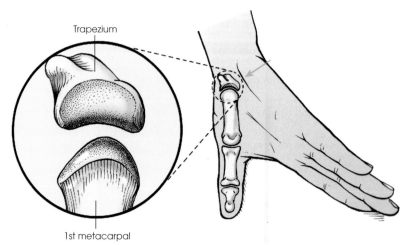

Trapezium

1st metacarpal

Fig. 4-46 Hyperextended hand and thumb position for AP projection of first CMC joint: Robert method. Soft tissue of palm (*arrow*) is positioned out of the way so that joint is clearly shown. *Inset:* First CMC joint is a saddle joint; articular surfaces are shown.

First Digit (Thumb)

Central ray (Fig. 4-47)
Robert method
- Perpendicular entering at the first CMC joint

Long and Rafert modification
- Angled 15 degrees proximally along the long axis of the thumb and entering the first CMC joint
- Collimation to include the entire thumb

Lewis modification
- Angled 10 to 15 degrees proximally along the long axis of the thumb and entering the first MCP joint

NOTE: Angulation of the central ray serves two purposes: (1) It may help project the soft tissue of the hand away from the first CMC joint, and (2) it can help open the joint space when the space is not shown with a perpendicular central ray.

Structures shown
This projection shows the first CMC joint free of superimposition of the soft tissues of the hand (Fig. 4-48).

EVALUATION CRITERIA
The following should be clearly shown:
- First CMC joint free of superimposition of the hand or other bony elements
- First metacarpal with the base in convex profile
- Trapezium

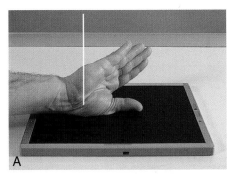 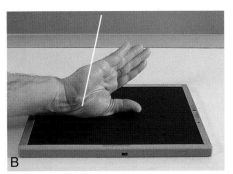 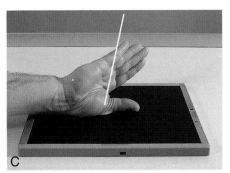

Fig. 4-47 Central ray angulation choices to show first CMC joint. **A,** Robert method, 0 degrees to CMC joint. **B,** Long-Rafert modification, 15 degrees proximal to CMC joint. **C,** Lewis modification, 10 to 15 degrees proximal to MCP joint.

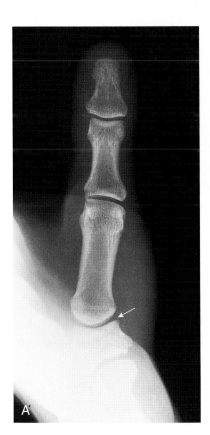 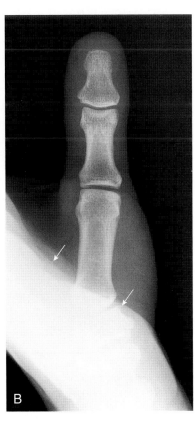

Fig. 4-48 A, Optimal radiograph of AP first CMC joint (*arrow*): Robert method. **B,** Example of typical repeat radiograph. Soft tissue of palm (*arrows*) obscured first CMC joint. Long-Rafert or Lewis modification of central ray would help show the joint on this patient.

119

First Carpometacarpal Joint

AP PROJECTION

BURMAN METHOD

When hyperextension of the wrist is not contraindicated, Burman[1] stated that this projection provides a clearer image of the first CMC joint than the standard AP projection.

Image receptor: 8 × 10 inch (18 × 24 cm) lengthwise

SID: The recommended distance is 18 inches; this produces a magnified image that creates a greater field of view of the concavoconvex aspect of this joint.

---

[1]Burman M: Anteroposterior projection of the carpometacarpal joint of the thumb by radial shift of the carpal tunnel view, *J Bone Joint Surg Am* 40:1156, 1958.

Position of patient

- Seat the patient at the end of the radiographic table so that the forearm can be adjusted to lie approximately parallel with the long axis of the IR.

Position of part

- Place the IR under the wrist, and center the first CMC joint to the center of the IR.
- Hyperextend the hand, and have the patient hold the position with the opposite hand or with a bandage looped around the digits.
- Rotate the hand internally, and abduct the thumb so that it is flat on the IR (Fig. 4-49).
- *Shield gonads.*

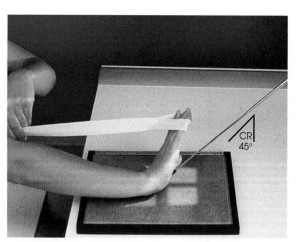

Fig. 4-49 Hyperextended hand and abducted thumb position for AP of first CMC joint: Burman method.

First Digit (Thumb)

Central ray
- Through the first CMC joint at a 45-degree angle toward the elbow

Structures shown
This image shows a magnified concavo-convex outline of the first CMC joint (Fig. 4-50).

The following should be clearly shown:
- First metacarpal
- Trapezium in concave profile
- Base of the first metacarpal in convex profile
- First CMC joint, unobscured by adjacent carpals

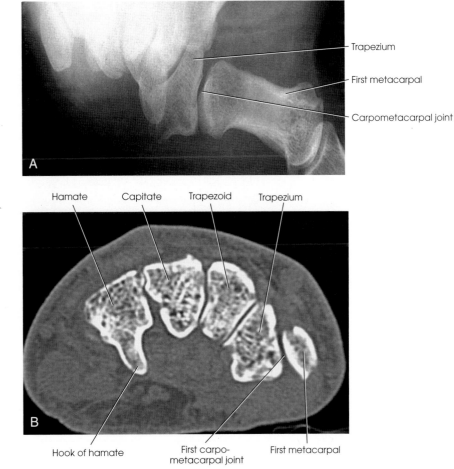

Fig. 4-50 **A,** AP thumb to demonstrate show the first CMC joint: Burman method. **B,** Axial CT scan through distal carpals. Note CMC joint is well visualized.

(**A,** Courtesy Michael Burman.)

First Metacarpophalangeal Joint

PA PROJECTION
FOLIO METHOD

This projection is useful for the diagnosis of ulnar collateral ligament (UCL) rupture in the MCP joint of the thumb, also known as "skier's thumb."[1]

Image receptor: 8 × 10 inch (18 × 24 cm) crosswise

---

[1]Folio L: Patient-controlled stress radiography of the thumb, *Radiol Technol* 70:465, 1999.

Position of patient
- Seat the patient at the end of the radiographic table.

Position of part
- Place the patient's hands on the cassette, resting them on their medial aspects.
- Tightly wrap a rubber band around the distal portion of both thumbs and place a roll of medical tape between the bodies of the first metacarpals.
- Ensure the thumbs remain in the PA plane by keeping the thumbnails parallel to the cassette (Fig. 4-51).
- Before exposure, instruct the patient to pull the thumbs apart and hold.
- *Shield gonads.*

Central ray
- Perpendicular to a point midway between both hands at the level of the MCP joints

NOTE: To avoid motion, have the correct technical factors set on the generator and be ready to make the exposure before instructing the patient to pull the thumbs apart.

Structures shown
This projection shows the MCP joints and MCP angles bilaterally (Fig. 4-52).

EVALUATION CRITERIA

The following should be clearly shown:
- No rotation of the thumbs
- First metacarpals
- Diagnostic image of the first MCP joint
- Rubber band and medical tape in correct position
- Thumbs centered to the center of the image

RESEARCH: Catherine E. Hearty, MS, RT(R), performed the research and provided this new projection for the atlas.

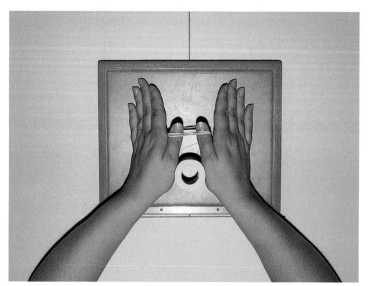

Fig. 4-51 Hands and thumbs in position for PA first MCP joints: Folio method. Note roll of tape between thumbs.

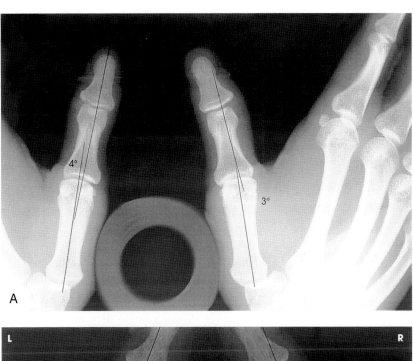

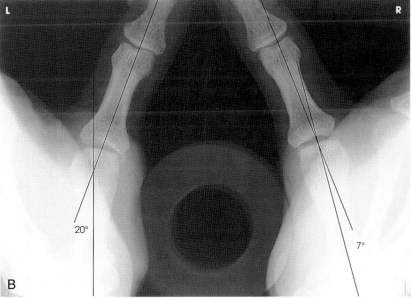

Fig. 4-52 First MCP joint, Folio method. **A,** Normal thumbs with acceptable MCP joints bilaterally. Roll of tape between metacarpals and rubber band holding distal aspects of thumbs are visible. **B,** Increased angulation of left MCP joint with 13-degree difference compared with right MCP joint. Partially torn left UCL measures 20 degrees between long axis of first metacarpal and proximal phalanx, whereas uninjured side measures 7 degrees.

🦅 PA PROJECTION

Image receptor: 8 × 10 inch (18 × 24 cm) for hand of average size or 10 × 12 inch (24 × 30 cm) crosswise for two images

Position of patient

- Seat the patient at the end of the radiographic table.
- Adjust the patient's height so that the forearm is resting on the table (Fig. 4-53, *A*).

Position of part

- Rest the patient's forearm on the table, and place the hand with the palmar surface down on the IR.
- Center the IR to the MCP joints, and adjust the long axis of the IR parallel with the long axis of the hand and forearm.
- Spread the fingers slightly (Fig. 4-53, *B*).
- Ask the patient to relax the hand to avoid motion. Prevent involuntary movement with the use of adhesive tape or positioning sponges. A sandbag may be placed over the distal forearm.
- *Shield gonads.*

Central ray

- Perpendicular to the third MCP joint

Collimation

- 1 inch (2.5 cm) on all sides of the hand, including 1 inch (2.5 cm) proximal to the ulnar styloid

COMPUTED RADIOGRAPHY

The hand must be centered to the plate or plate section with four collimator margins or with no margins at all. Two images can be projected on one plate; however, because the hand takes up most of the plate half, collimate to the margins of the plate. A lead blocker must cover the opposite side when two images are made on one IR.

Structures shown

PA projections of the carpals, metacarpals, phalanges (except the thumb), interarticulations of the hand, and distal radius and ulna are shown in Fig. 4-54. This image also shows a PA oblique projection of the first digit.

EVALUATION CRITERIA

The following should be clearly shown:
- Evidence of proper collimation
- No rotation of the hand
  - ☐ Equal concavity of the metacarpal and phalangeal shafts on both sides
  - ☐ Equal amount of soft tissue on both sides of the phalanges
  - ☐ Fingernails, if visualized, in the center of each distal phalanx
  - ☐ Equal distance between the metacarpal heads
- Open MCP and IP joints, indicating that the hand is placed flat on the IR
- Slightly separate digits with no soft tissue overlap
- All anatomy distal to the radius and ulna
- Soft tissue and bony trabeculation

NOTE: When the MCP joints are under examination and the patient cannot extend the hand enough to place its palmar surface in contact with the IR, the position of the hand can be reversed for an AP projection. This position is also used for the metacarpals when the hand cannot be extended because of an injury, a pathologic condition, or the use of dressings.

SPECIAL TECHNIQUES: Clements and Nakayama[1] described a special exposure technique for imaging early rheumatoid arthritis. Lewis[2] described a positioning variation to place the second through fifth metacarpals parallel to the IR, resulting in a true PA projection.

[1]Clements RW, Nakayama HK: Technique for detecting early rheumatoid arthritis, *Radiol Technol* 62:443, 1991.
[2]Lewis S: New angles on the radiographic examination of the hand—I, *Radiogr Today* 54:44-45, 1988.

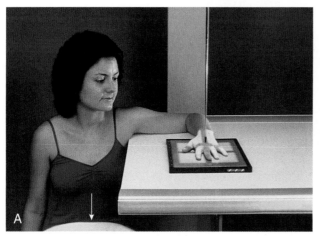
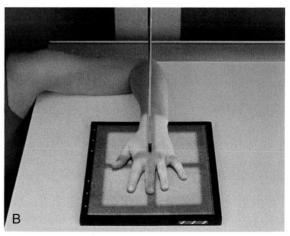

Fig. 4-53 A, Properly shielded patient in position for PA hand. **B,** PA hand.

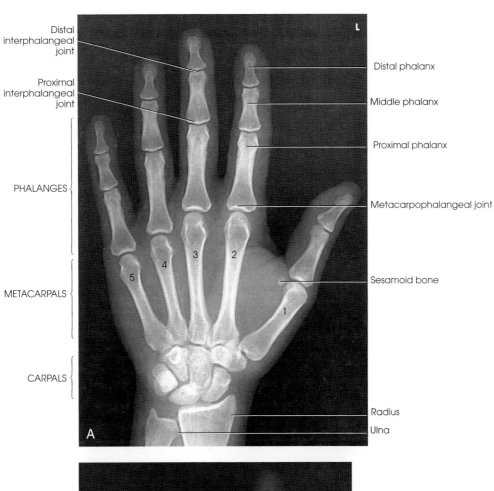

Distal interphalangeal joint

Proximal interphalangeal joint

PHALANGES

METACARPALS

CARPALS

Distal phalanx

Middle phalanx

Proximal phalanx

Metacarpophalangeal joint

Sesamoid bone

Radius

Ulna

A

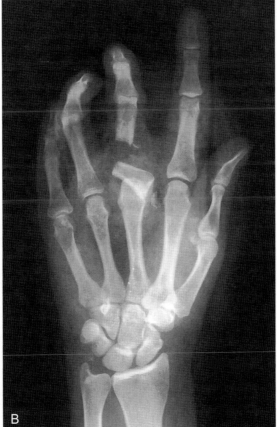

B

Fig. 4-54 A, PA hand. **B,** PA hand showing closed, displaced, transverse fracture of third proximal phalanx with dislocation of MCP joint. Overall hand was placed in correct position despite trauma. This gives physician accurate information about displacement of bone.

⚘ PA OBLIQUE PROJECTION
Lateral rotation

Image receptor: 8 × 10 inch (18 × 24 cm) lengthwise or 10 × 12 inch (24 × 30 cm) crosswise for two images

Position of patient
- Seat the patient at the end of the radiographic table.
- Adjust the patient's height to rest the forearm on the table.

Position of part
- Rest the patient's forearm on the table with the hand pronated and the palm resting on the IR.
- Adjust the obliquity of the hand so that the MCP joints form an angle of approximately 45 degrees with the IR plane.
- Use a 45-degree foam wedge to support the fingers in the extended position to show the IP joints (Figs. 4-55 and 4-56).

- When examining the metacarpals, obtain a PA oblique projection of the hand by rotating the patient's hand laterally (externally) from the pronated position until the fingertips touch the IR (Fig. 4-57).
- If it is impossible to obtain the correct position with all fingertips resting on the IR, elevate the index finger and thumb on a suitable radiolucent material (see Fig. 4-56). Elevation opens the joint spaces and reduces the degree of foreshortening of the phalanges.
- For either approach, center the IR to the MCP joints and adjust the midline to be parallel with the long axis of the hand and forearm.
- *Shield gonads.*

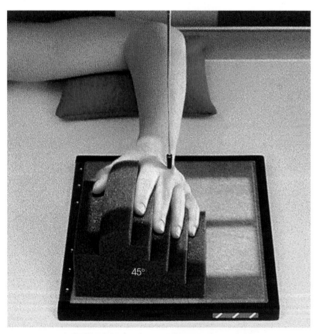

Fig. 4-55 PA oblique hand to show joint spaces.

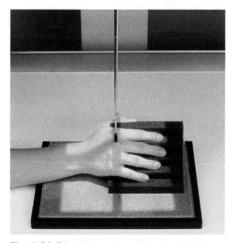

Fig. 4-56 PA oblique hand to show joint spaces.

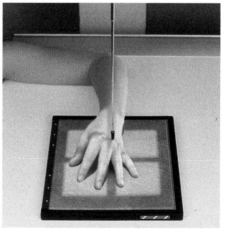

Fig. 4-57 PA oblique hand to show metacarpals.

Central ray
- Perpendicular to the third MCP joint

Collimation
- 1 inch (2.5 cm) on all sides of the hand, including 1 inch (2.5 cm) proximal to the ulnar styloid

Structures shown
The resulting image shows a PA oblique projection of the bones and soft tissues of the hand (Fig. 4-58). This supplemental position is used for investigating fractures and pathologic conditions.

EVALUATION CRITERIA
The following should be clearly shown:
- Evidence of proper collimation
- Minimal overlap of the third-fourth and fourth-fifth metacarpal shafts
- Slight overlap of the metacarpal bases and heads
- Separation of the second and third metacarpals
- Open IP and MCP joints
- Digits separated slightly with no overlap of their soft tissues
- All anatomy distal to the distal radius and ulna
- Soft tissue and bony trabeculation

NOTE: Lane et al.[1] recommended the inclusion of a reverse oblique projection to show severe metacarpal deformities or fractures better. This projection is accomplished by having the patient rotate the hand 45 degrees medially (internally) from the palm-down position.

Kallen[2] recommended using a tangential oblique projection to show metacarpal head fractures. From the PA hand position, the MCP joints are flexed 75 to 80 degrees with the dorsum of the digits resting on the IR. The hand is rotated 40 to 45 degrees toward the ulnar surface. Then the hand is rotated 40 to 45 degrees forward until the affected MCP joint is projected beyond its proximal phalanx. The perpendicular central ray is directed tangentially to enter the MCP joint of interest. Variations of rotation are described to show the second metacarpal head free of superimposition.

[1]Lane CS, Kennedy JF, Kuschner SH: The reverse oblique x-ray film: metacarpal fractures revealed, *J Hand Surg Am* 17:504, 1992.
[2]Kallen MJ: Kallen projection reveals metacarpal head fractures, *Radiol Technol* 65:229, 1994.

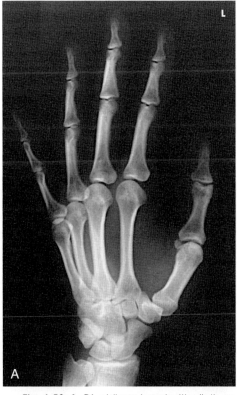
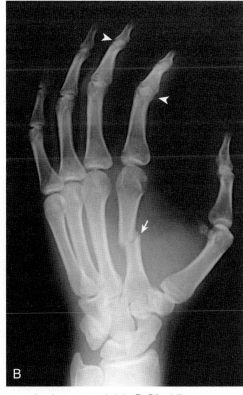

Fig. 4-58 A, PA oblique hand with digits on sponge to show open joints. **B,** PA oblique hand without support sponge, showing fracture (*arrow*). IP joints (*arrowheads*) are not entirely open, and phalanges are foreshortened.

LATERAL PROJECTION
Mediolateral or lateromedial
Extension and fan lateral

Image receptor: 8 × 10 inch (18 × 24 cm) lengthwise for hand of average size or 10 × 12 inch (24 × 30 cm) crosswise for two images

Position of patient
- Seat the patient at the end of the radiographic table with the forearm in contact with the table and the hand in the lateral position with the ulnar aspect down (Fig. 4-59).

- Alternatively, place the radial side of the wrist against the IR (Fig. 4-60). This position is more difficult for the patient to assume.
- If the elbow is elevated, support it with sandbags.

Position of part
- Extend the patient's digits and adjust the first digit at a right angle to the palm.
- Place the palmar surface perpendicular to the IR.

- Center the IR to the MCP joints, and adjust the midline to be parallel with the long axis of the hand and forearm. If the hand is resting on the ulnar surface, immobilization of the thumb may be necessary.
- The two extended digit positions result in superimposition of the phalanges. A modification of the lateral hand is the *fan lateral position,* which eliminates superimposition of all but the proximal phalanges. For the fan lateral position, place the digits on a sponge wedge. Abduct the thumb and place it on the radiolucent sponge for support (Fig. 4-61).
- *Shield gonads.*

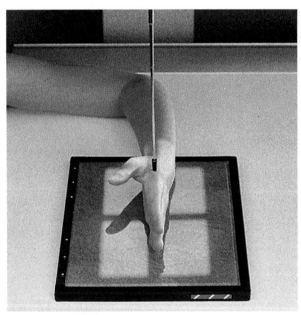

Fig. 4-59 Lateral hand with ulnar surface to IR: lateromedial.

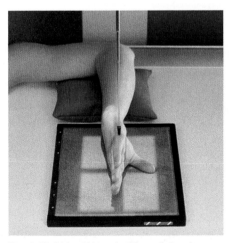

Fig. 4-60 Lateral hand with radial surface to IR: mediolateral.

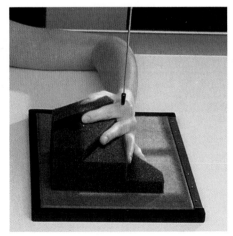

Fig. 4-61 Fan lateral hand.

Central ray

- Perpendicular to the *second digit* MCP joint

Collimation

- 1 inch (2.5 cm) on all sides of the shadow of the hand and thumb, including 1 inch (2.5 cm) proximal to the ulnar styloid

Structures shown

This image, which shows a lateral projection of the hand in extension (Fig. 4-62), is the customary position for localizing foreign bodies and metacarpal fracture displacement. The exposure technique depends on the foreign body.

The fan lateral superimposes the metacarpals but shows almost all of the individual phalanges. The most proximal portions of the proximal phalanges remain superimposed (Fig. 4-63).

EVALUATION CRITERIA

The following should be clearly shown:
- Evidence of proper collimation
- Hand is in a true lateral position if the following are seen:
  - ☐ Superimposed phalanges (individually shown on fan lateral)
  - ☐ Superimposed metacarpals
  - ☐ Superimposed distal radius and ulna
- Extended digits
- Thumb free of motion and superimposition
- Each bone outlined through the superimposed shadows of the other metacarpals

NOTE: To show fractures of the fifth metacarpal better, Lewis[1] recommended rotating the hand 5 degrees posteriorly from the true lateral position. This positioning removes the superimposition of the second through fourth metacarpals. The thumb is extended as much as possible, and the hand is allowed to become hollow by relaxation. The central ray is angled so that it passes parallel to the extended thumb and enters the midshaft of the fifth metacarpal.

[1]Lewis S: New angles on the radiographic examination of the hand—II, *Radiogr Today* 54:29, 1988.

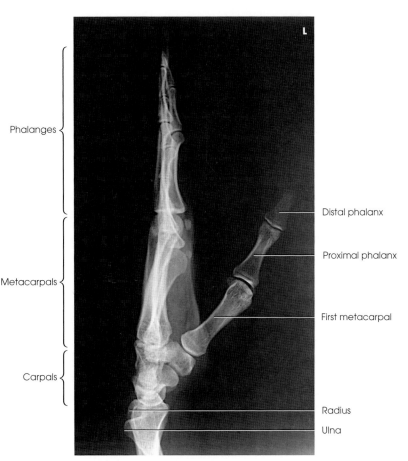

Fig. 4-62 Lateral hand.

Phalanges

Metacarpals

Carpals

Distal phalanx

Proximal phalanx

First metacarpal

Radius

Ulna

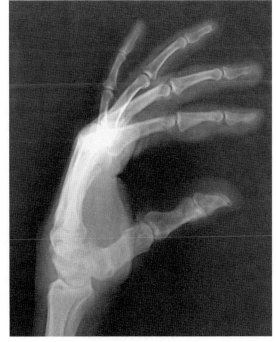

Fig. 4-63 Fan lateral hand.

LATERAL PROJECTION
Lateromedial in flexion

This projection is useful when a hand injury prevents the patient from extending the fingers.

Image receptor: 8 × 10 inch (18 × 24 cm) lengthwise

Position of patient

- Seat the patient at the end of the radiographic table.
- Ask the patient to rest the forearm on the table, and place the hand on the IR with the ulnar aspect down.

Position of part

- Center the IR to the MCP joints, and adjust it so that its midline is parallel with the long axis of the hand and forearm.
- With the patient relaxing the digits to maintain the natural arch of the hand, arrange the digits so that they are perfectly superimposed (Fig. 4-64).
- Have the patient hold the thumb parallel with the IR, or, if necessary, immobilize the thumb with tape or a sponge.
- *Shield gonads.*

Central ray

- Perpendicular to the MCP joints, entering MCP joint of the second digit

Structures shown

This projection produces a lateral image of the bony structures and soft tissues of the hand in their normally flexed position (Fig. 4-65). It also shows anterior or posterior displacement in fractures of the metacarpals.

EVALUATION CRITERIA

The following should be clearly shown:
- Superimposed phalanges and metacarpals
- Superimposed distal radius and ulna
- Flexed digits
- No motion or superimposition of the first digit
- Radiographic density similar to frontal and oblique hand images, which requires increased exposure factors to compensate for greater hand thickness
- Clear outline of each bone through the superimposed shadows of the other metacarpals

AP OBLIQUE PROJECTION
NORGAARD METHOD
Medial rotation

The Norgaard method,[1-3] sometimes referred to as the *ball-catcher's position,* assists in detecting early radiologic changes in the dorsoradial aspects of the second through fifth proximal phalangeal bases, needed to diagnose rheumatoid arthritis. Norgaard reported that it is often possible to make an early diagnosis of rheumatoid arthritis by using this position before laboratory tests are positive.[3] He also stated that extremely fine-grain intensifying screens should be used to show high resolution. Low kVp (60 to 65 kVp) is recommended to obtain necessary contrast.

In a more recent article, Stapczynski[3] recommended this projection to show fractures of the base of the fifth metacarpal.

Image receptor: 10 × 12 inch (24 × 30 cm) crosswise

Position of patient

- Seat the patient at the end of the radiographic table. Norgaard recommended that both hands be radiographed in the half-supinated position for comparison.

Position of part

- Have the patient place the palms of both hands together. Center the MCP joints on the medial aspect of both hands to the IR. Both hands should be in the lateral position.
- Place two 45-degree radiolucent sponges against the posterior aspect of each hand.
- Rotate the patient's hands to a half-supinated position until the dorsal surface of each hand rests against each 45-degree sponge support (Fig. 4-66).
- Extend the patient's fingers, and abduct the thumbs slightly to avoid superimposing them over the second MCP joint.

[1]Norgaard F: Earliest roentgenological changes in polyarthritis of the rheumatoid type: rheumatoid arthritis, *Radiology* 85:325, 1965.
[2]Norgaard F: Early roentgen changes in polyarthritis of the rheumatoid type, *Radiology* 92:299, 1969.
[3]Stapczynski JS: Fracture of the base of the little finger metacarpal: importance of the "ball-catcher" radiographic view, *J Emerg Med* 9:145, 1991.

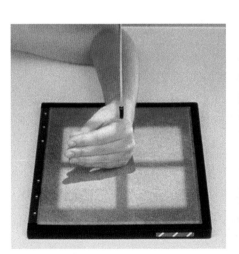

Fig. 4-64 Lateral hand in flexion.

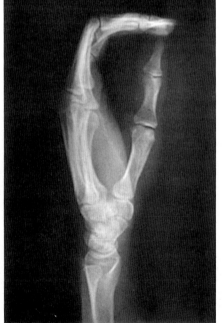

Fig. 4-65 Lateral hand in flexion.

- The original method of positioning the hands is often modified. The patient is positioned similar to the method described except that the fingers are not extended. Instead the fingers are cupped as though the patient were going to catch a ball (Fig. 4-67). Comparable diagnostic information is provided using either position.
- *Shield gonads.*

Central ray

- Perpendicular to a point midway between both hands at the level of the MCP joints for either of the two patient positions

Structures shown

The resulting image shows an AP 45-degree oblique projection of both hands (Fig. 4-68). The early radiologic change significant in making the diagnosis of rheumatoid arthritis is a symmetric, very slight, indistinct outline of the bone corresponding to the insertion of the joint capsule dorsoradial on the proximal end of the first phalanx of the four fingers. In addition, associated demineralization of the bone structure is always present in the area directly below the contour defect.

EVALUATION CRITERIA

The following should be clearly shown:
- Both hands from the carpal area to the tips of the digits
- Metacarpal heads and proximal phalangeal bases free of superimposition
- Useful level of density over the heads of the metacarpals

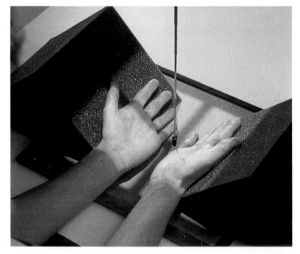

Fig. 4-66 AP oblique hands, semisupinated position.

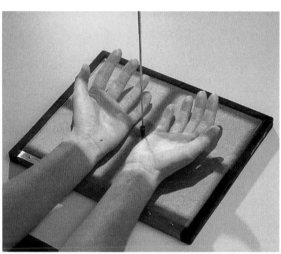

Fig. 4-67 Ball-catcher's position.

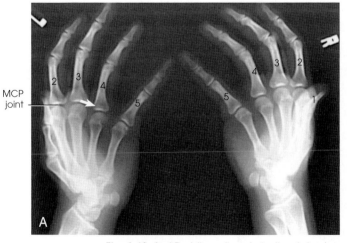
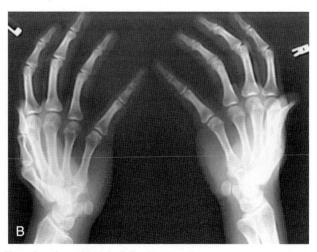

Fig. 4-68 A, AP oblique hands, ball-catcher's position, showing where indistinct area occurs at dorsoradial aspect of proximal phalangeal base (*arrow*). **B,** Ball-catcher's position.

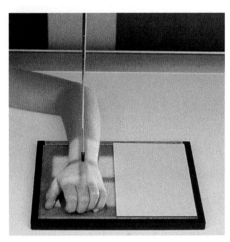

Fig. 4-69 PA wrist.

✦ PA PROJECTION

Image receptor: 8 × 10 inch (18 × 24 cm) lengthwise or crosswise for two or more images on one IR

Position of patient

- Seat the patient low enough to place the axilla in contact with the table, or elevate the limb to shoulder level on a suitable support. This position places the shoulder, elbow, and wrist joints in the same plane to permit right-angle rotation of the ulna and radius for the lateral position.

Position of part

- Have the patient rest the forearm on the table, and center the wrist joint to the IR area. The wrist (radiocarpal) joint is at a level just distal to the ulnar styloid.
- When it is difficult to determine the exact location of the radiocarpal joint because of a swollen wrist, ask the patient to flex the wrist slightly, and center the IR to the point of flexion. When the wrist is in a cast or splint, the exact point of centering can be determined by comparison with the opposite side.

- Adjust the hand and forearm to lie parallel with the long axis of the IR.
- Slightly arch the hand at the MCP joints by flexing the digits to place the wrist in close contact with the IR (Fig. 4-69).
- When necessary, place a support under the digits to immobilize them.
- *Shield gonads.*

Central ray

- Perpendicular to the midcarpal area

Collimation

- 2.5 inches (6 cm) proximal and distal to the wrist joint and 1 inch (2.5 cm) on the sides

COMPUTED RADIOGRAPHY

The wrist must be centered to the plate or plate section with four collimator margins or with no margins at all. Two images can be projected on one plate; however, there must be four collimator margins for each projection. A lead blocker must cover the opposite side when two images are made on one IR.

Structures shown

A PA projection of the carpals, distal radius and ulna, and proximal metacarpals is shown (Fig. 4-70). The projection gives a slightly oblique rotation to the ulna. When the ulna is under examination, an AP projection should be taken.

EVALUATION CRITERIA

The following should be clearly shown:
- Evidence of proper collimation
- Distal radius and ulna, carpals, and proximal half of metacarpals
- No rotation in carpals, metacarpals, or radius
- Open radioulnar joint space
- Soft tissue and bony trabeculation
- No excessive flexion to overlap and obscure metacarpals with digits

NOTE: To show the scaphoid and capitate better, Daffner et al.[1] recommended angling the central ray when the patient is positioned for a PA radiograph. A central ray angle of 30 degrees toward the elbow elongates the scaphoid and capitate, whereas an angle of 30 degrees toward the fingertips elongates only the capitate.

[1]Daffner RH, Emmerling EW, Buterbaugh GA: Proximal and distal oblique radiography of the wrist: value in occult injuries, *J Hand Surg Am* 17:499, 1992.

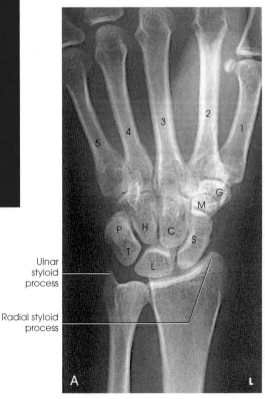

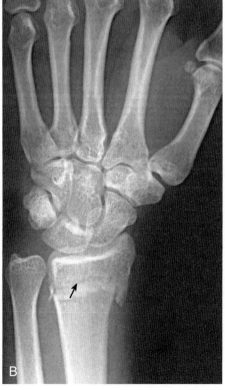

Ulnar styloid process

Radial styloid process

Fig. 4-70 A, PA wrist. *C,* capitate; *G,* trapezium; *H,* hamate; *L,* lunate; *M,* trapezoid; *P,* pisiform; *S,* scaphoid; *T,* triquetrum. **B,** PA wrist showing Smith fracture of distal radius (*arrow*).

AP PROJECTION

Image receptor: 8 × 10 inch (18 × 24 cm) lengthwise or crosswise for two or more images on one IR

Position of patient
• Seat the patient at the end of the radiographic table.

Position of part
• Have the patient rest the forearm on the table, with the arm and hand supinated.
• Place the IR under the wrist, and center it to the carpals.
• Elevate the digits on a suitable support to place the wrist in close contact with the IR.
• Have the patient lean laterally to prevent rotation of the wrist (Fig. 4-71).
• *Shield gonads.*

Central ray
• Perpendicular to the midcarpal area

Structures shown
The *carpal interspaces* are better shown in the AP image than the PA image. Because of the oblique direction of the interspaces, they are more closely parallel with the divergence of the x-ray beam (Fig. 4-72).

EVALUATION CRITERIA
The following should be clearly shown:
■ Distal radius and ulna, carpals, and proximal half of the metacarpals
■ No rotation of the carpals, metacarpals, radius, and ulna
■ Well-shown soft tissue and bony trabeculation
■ No overlapping or obscuring of the metacarpals as a result of excessive flexion

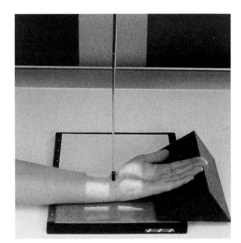

Fig. 4-71 AP wrist.

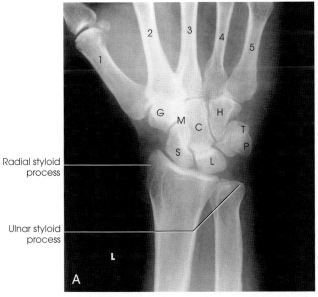

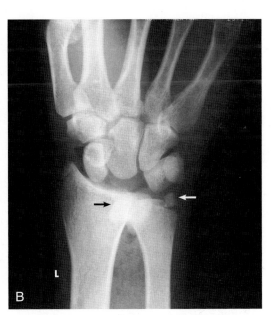

Fig. 4-72 A, AP wrist. *C,* capitate; *G,* trapezium; *H,* hamate; *L,* lunate; *M,* trapezoid; *P,* pisiform; *S,* scaphoid; *T,* triquetrum. **B,** AP wrist showing complete dislocation of lunate (*black arrow*) and fracture of ulnar styloid process (*white arrow*).

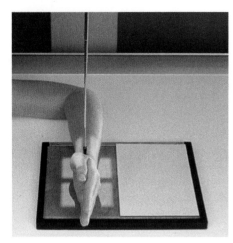

Fig. 4-73 Lateral wrist with ulnar surface to IR.

🌾 LATERAL PROJECTION
Lateromedial

Image receptor: 8 × 10 inch (18 × 24 cm) lengthwise or crosswise for two images

Position of patient
- Seat the patient at the end of the radiographic table.
- Have the patient rest the arm and forearm on the table to ensure that the wrist is in a lateral position.

Position of part
- Have the patient flex the elbow 90 degrees to rotate the ulna to the lateral position.
- Center the IR to the wrist (radiocarpal) joint, and adjust the forearm and hand so that the wrist is in a true lateral position (Fig. 4-73).
- *Shield gonads.*

Central ray
- Perpendicular to the wrist joint

Collimation
- 2.5 inches (6 cm) proximal and distal to the wrist joint and 1 inch (2.5 cm) on the palmar and dorsal surfaces

Structures shown
This image shows a lateral projection of the proximal metacarpals, carpals, and distal radius and ulna (Fig. 4-74). An image obtained with the radial surface against the IR (Fig. 4-75) is shown for comparison. This position can also be used to show anterior or posterior displacement in fractures.

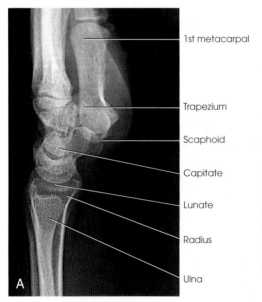

1st metacarpal

Trapezium

Scaphoid

Capitate

Lunate

Radius

Ulna

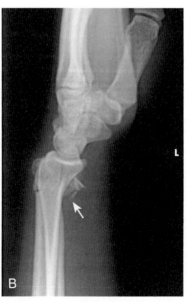

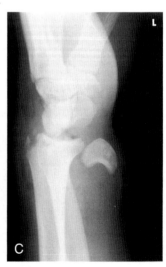

Fig. 4-74 A, Lateral wrist with ulnar surface to IR. **B,** Lateral with Smith fracture (*arrow*). This is the same patient as in Fig. 4-70, *B*. **C,** Lateral wrist showing obvious complete anterior dislocation of lunate bone. This is the same patient as in Fig. 4-72, *A*. A lighter exposure was used to show soft tissue.

EVALUATION CRITERIA

The following should be clearly shown:
- Evidence of proper collimation
- Distal radius and ulna, carpals, and proximal half of metacarpals
- Superimposed distal radius and ulna
- Superimposed metacarpals
- Radiographic density similar to PA or AP and oblique radiographs, which requires increased exposure factors to compensate for greater part thickness

NOTE: Burman et al.[1] suggested that the lateral position of the scaphoid should be obtained with the wrist in palmar flexion because this action rotates the bone anteriorly into a dorsovolar position (Fig. 4-76). This position is valuable, however, only when sufficient flexion is permitted.

Fiolle[2,3] was the first to describe a small bony growth occurring on the dorsal surface of the third CMC joint. He termed the condition *carpe bossu* (carpal boss) and found that it is shown best in a lateral position with the wrist in palmar flexion (see Fig. 4-76).

[1]Burman MS et al: Fractures of the radial and ulnar axes, *AJR Am J Roentgenol* 51:455, 1944.
[2]Fiolle J: Le "carpe bossu," *Bull Soc Chir Paris* 57:1687, 1931.
[3]Fiolle J et al: Nouvelle observation de "carpe bossu," *Bull Soc Chir Paris* 58:187, 1932.

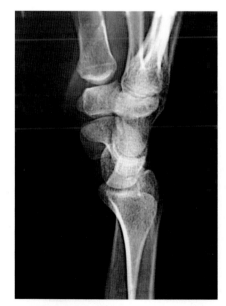

Fig. 4-75 Lateral wrist with radial surface to IR.

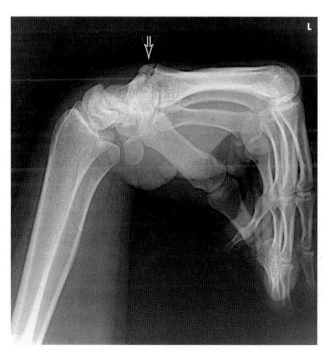

Fig. 4-76 Lateral wrist with palmar flexion of wrist, showing carpal boss (*arrow*).

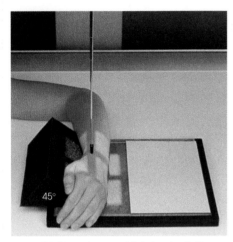

Fig. 4-77 PA oblique wrist: lateral rotation.

⚘ PA OBLIQUE PROJECTION
Lateral rotation

Image receptor: 8 × 10 inch (18 × 24 cm) lengthwise or crosswise for two images on one IR

Position of patient

- Seat the patient at the end of the radiographic table, placing the axilla in contact with the table.

Position of part

- Rest the palmar surface of the wrist on the IR.
- Adjust the IR so that its center point is under the scaphoid when the wrist is rotated from the pronated position.
- From the pronated position, rotate the wrist laterally (externally) until it forms an angle of approximately 45 degrees with the plane of the IR. For exact positioning and to ensure duplication in follow-up examinations, place a 45-degree foam wedge under the elevated side of the wrist.
- Extend the wrist slightly, and if the digits do not touch the table, support them in place (Fig. 4-77).
- When the scaphoid is under examination, adjust the wrist in ulnar deviation. Place a sandbag across the forearm.
- *Shield gonads.*

Central ray

- Perpendicular to the midcarpal area; it enters just distal to the radius

Collimation

- 2.5 inches (6 cm) proximal and distal to the wrist joint and 1 inch (2.5 cm) on the sides

Structures shown

This projection shows the carpals on the lateral side of the wrist, particularly the trapezium and the scaphoid. The scaphoid is superimposed on itself in the direct PA projection (Figs. 4-78 and 4-79).

EVALUATION CRITERIA

The following should be clearly shown:

- Evidence of proper collimation
- A well-shown trapezium and the distal half of the scaphoid
- Distal radius and ulna, carpals, and proximal half of metacarpals
- Open trapeziotrapezoid and scaphotrapezial joint space
- Usually, adequate amount of obliquity in the following circumstances
  - Slight interosseus space between the third-fourth and fourth-fifth metacarpal shafts
  - Slight overlap of the distal radius and ulna
- Soft tissue and bony trabeculation

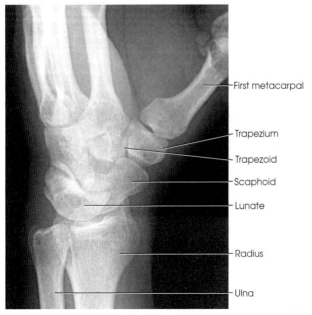

Fig. 4-78 PA oblique wrist.

First metacarpal

Trapezium

Trapezoid

Scaphoid

Lunate

Radius

Ulna

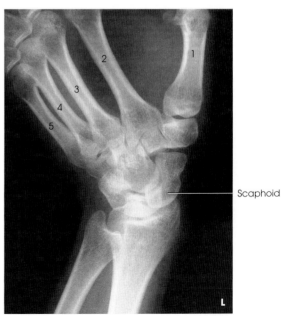

Fig. 4-79 PA oblique wrist with ulnar deviation.

Scaphoid

AP OBLIQUE PROJECTION[1]
Medial rotation

Image receptor: 8 × 10 inch (18 × 24 cm) lengthwise or crosswise for two images on one IR

Position of patient
- Seat the patient at the end of the radiographic table.
- Have the patient rest the forearm on the table in the supine position.

Position of part
- Place the IR under the wrist and center it at the dorsal surface of the wrist.
- Rotate the wrist medially (internally) until it forms a semisupinated position of approximately 45 degrees to the IR (Fig. 4-80).
- *Shield gonads.*

Central ray
- Perpendicular to the midcarpal area; it enters the anterior surface of the wrist midway between its medial and lateral borders

Structures shown
This position separates the pisiform from the adjacent carpal bones. It also provides a more distinct radiograph of the triquetrum and hamate (compare Figs. 4-81 and 4-82).

EVALUATION CRITERIA
The following should be clearly shown:
- Carpals on medial side of wrist
- Triquetrum, hook of hamate, and pisiform free of superimposition and in profile
- Distal radius and ulna, carpals, and proximal half of metacarpals
- Radiographic-quality soft tissue and bony trabeculation

---

[1]McBride E: Wrist joint injuries, a plea for greater accuracy in treatment, *J Okla Med Assoc* 19:67, 1926.

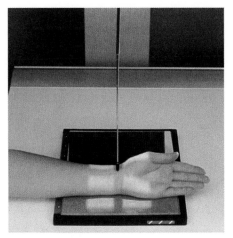

Fig. 4-80 AP oblique wrist: medial rotation.

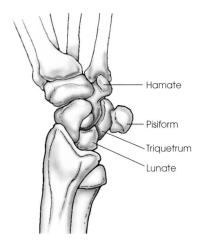

Hamate
Pisiform
Triquetrum
Lunate

Fig. 4-81 AP oblique wrist.

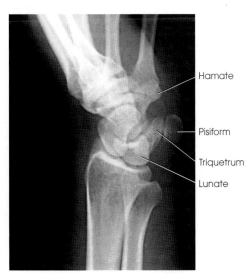
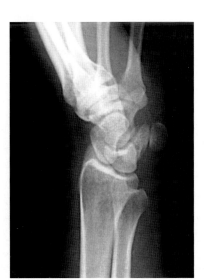

Hamate
Pisiform
Triquetrum
Lunate

Fig. 4-82 AP oblique wrist.

Upper Limb

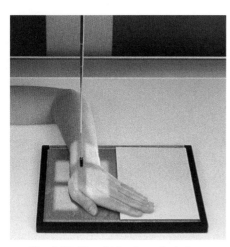

Fig. 4-83 PA wrist in ulnar deviation.

PA PROJECTION
Ulnar deviation[1]

Image receptor: 8 × 10 inch (18 × 24 cm) lengthwise or crosswise for two images

Position of patient
- Seat the patient at the end of the radiographic table with the arm and forearm resting on the table. The elbow should be at a 90° angle.

Position of part
- Position the wrist on the IR for a PA projection.
- Without moving the forearm, turn the hand outward until the wrist is in extreme ulnar deviation (Fig. 4-83).
- *Shield gonads.*

---

[1]Frank ED et al: Two terms, one meaning, *Radiol Technol* 69:517, 1998.

Central ray
- Perpendicular to the scaphoid
- Central ray angulation of 10 to 15 degrees proximally or distally sometimes required for clear delineation

Collimation
- 2.5 inches (6 cm) proximal and distal to the wrist joint and 1 inch (2.5 cm) on the sides

Structures shown
This position corrects foreshortening of the scaphoid, which occurs with a perpendicular central ray. It also opens the spaces between the adjacent carpals (Fig. 4-84).

EVALUATION CRITERIA

The following should be clearly shown:
- Evidence of proper collimation
- Scaphoid with adjacent articulations open
- No rotation of wrist
- Extreme ulnar deviation, as revealed by the angle formed between longitudinal axes of the forearm compared with the longitudinal axes of the metacarpals
- Soft tissue and bony trabeculation

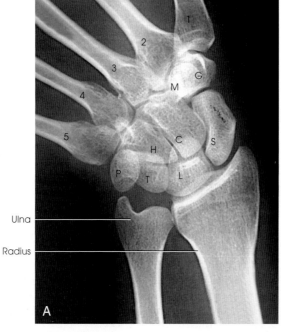
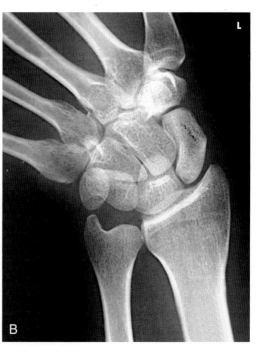

Fig. 4-84 A, PA wrist in ulnar deviation. *C,* capitate; *G,* trapezium; *H,* hamate; *L,* lunate; *M,* trapezoid; *P,* pisiform; *S,* scaphoid; *T,* triquetrum. **B,** Wrist in ulnar deviation.

PA PROJECTION
Radial deviation[1]

Image receptor: 8 × 10 inch (18 × 24 cm) lengthwise or crosswise for two images

Position of patient

- Seat the patient at the end of the radiographic table with the arm and forearm resting on the table.

Position of part

- Position the wrist on the IR for a PA projection.
- Without moving the forearm, turn the hand medially until the wrist is in extreme radial deviation (Fig. 4-85).
- *Shield gonads.*

---

[1]Frank ED et al: Two terms, one meaning, *Radiol Technol* 69:517, 1998.

Central ray

- Perpendicular to midcarpal area

Structures shown

Radial deviation opens the interspaces between the carpals on the medial side of the wrist (Fig. 4-86).

EVALUATION CRITERIA

The following should be clearly shown:

- Carpals and their articulations on the medial side of the wrist
- No rotation of wrist
- Extreme radial deviation, as revealed by the angle formed between longitudinal axes of forearm compared with the longitudinal axes of the metacarpals
- Soft tissue and bony trabeculation

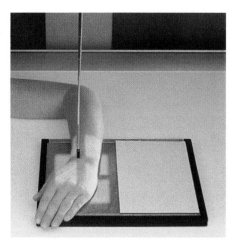

Fig. 4-85 PA wrist in radial deviation.

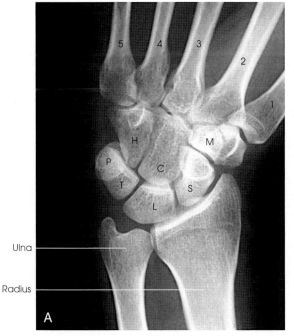
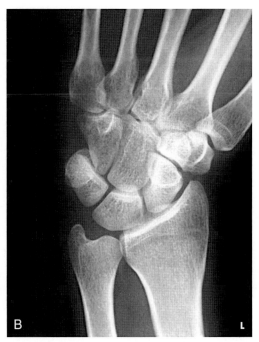

Fig. 4-86 A, PA wrist in radial deviation. *C,* capitate; *G,* trapezium; *H,* hamate; *L,* lunate; *M,* trapezoid; *P,* pisiform; *S,* scaphoid; *T,* triquetrum. **B,** Wrist in radial deviation.

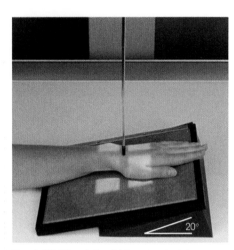

Fig. 4-87 PA axial wrist for scaphoid: Stecher method with IR angled 20 degrees.

Scaphoid

⚜ PA AXIAL PROJECTION
STECHER METHOD[1]

Image receptor: 8 × 10 inch (18 × 24 cm) lengthwise

Position of patient

- Seat the patient at the end of the radiographic table with the arm and axilla in contact with the table.
- Rest the forearm on the table.

Position of part

- Place one end of the IR on a support, and adjust the IR so that the finger end of the IR is elevated 20 degrees (Fig. 4-87).
- Adjust the wrist on the IR for a PA projection, and center the wrist to the IR.
- Bridgman[2] suggested positioning the wrist in ulnar deviation for this radiograph.
- *Shield gonads.*

[1]Stecher WR: Roentgenography of the carpal navicular bone, *AJR Am J Roentgenol* 37:704, 1937.
[2]Bridgman CF: Radiography of the carpal navicular bone, *Med Radiogr Photogr* 25:104, 1949.

Central ray

- Perpendicular to the table and directed to enter the scaphoid

Collimation

- 2.5 inches (6 cm) proximal and distal to the wrist joint and 1 inch (2.5 cm) on the sides

Structures shown

The 20-degree angulation of the wrist places the scaphoid at right angles to the central ray so that it is projected without self-superimposition (Figs. 4-88 and 4-89).

EVALUATION CRITERIA

The following should be clearly shown:
- Evidence of proper collimation
- Scaphoid
- No rotation of carpals, metacarpals, radius, or ulna
- Distal radius and ulna, carpals, and proximal half of the metacarpals
- Soft tissue and bony trabeculation

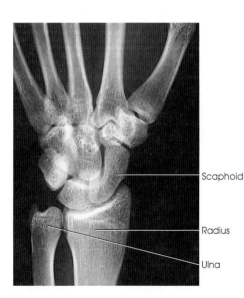

Fig. 4-88 PA axial wrist for scaphoid: Stecher method.

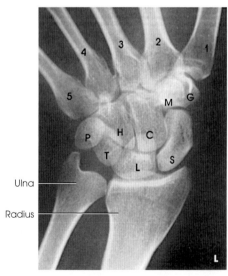

Fig. 4-89 PA axial wrist for scaphoid: Bridgman method, ulnar deviation. *C,* capitate; *G,* trapezium; *H,* hamate; *L,* lunate; *M,* trapezoid; *P,* pisiform; *S,* scaphoid; *T,* triquetrum.

Variations

Stecher[1] recommended the previous method as preferable; however, a similar position can be obtained by placing the IR and wrist horizontally and directing the central ray 20 degrees toward the elbow (Fig. 4-90).

To show a fracture line that angles superoinferiorly, these positions may be reversed. In other words, the wrist may be angled inferiorly, or from the horizontal position the central ray may be angled toward the digits.

A third method recommended by Stecher is to have the patient clench the fist. This elevates the distal end of the scaphoid so that it lies parallel with the IR; it also widens the fracture line. The wrist is positioned as for the PA projection, and no central ray angulation is used.

[1]Stecher WR: Roentgenography of the carpal navicular bone, *AJR Am J Roentgenol* 37:704, 1937.

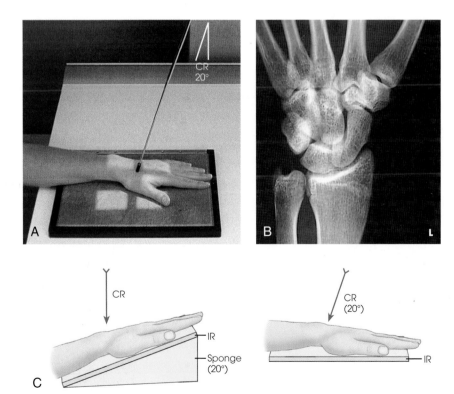

Fig. 4-90 A, PA axial wrist for scaphoid: Stecher method with 20-degree angulation of central ray. **B,** PA axial wrist: Stecher method. **C,** Angled IR and angled central ray (*CR*) methods achieve same projection.

Scaphoid Series

PA AND PA AXIAL PROJECTIONS
RAFERT-LONG METHOD

Ulnar deviation

Scaphoid fractures account for 60% of all carpal bone injuries. In 1991, Rafert and Long[1] described this method of diagnosing scaphoid fractures using a four-image, multiple-angle central ray series. The series is performed after routine wrist radiographs do not identify a fracture.

Image receptor: 8 × 10 inch (18 × 24 cm) crosswise for two images

[1]Rafert JA, Long BW: Technique for diagnosis of scaphoid fractures, *Radiol Technol* 63:16, 1991.

Position of patient
- Seat the patient at the end of the radiographic table with the arm and forearm resting on the table.

Position of part
- Position the wrist on the IR for a PA projection.
- Without moving the forearm, turn the hand outward until the wrist is in extreme ulnar deviation (Fig. 4-91).
- *Shield gonads.*

Central ray
- Perpendicular and with multiple cephalad angles; with the hand and wrist in the same position for each projection, four separate exposures made at 0, 10, 20, and 30 degrees cephalad
- The central ray should directly enter the scaphoid bone.
- Collimation should be close to improve image quality.

Structures shown
The scaphoid is shown with minimal superimposition (Fig. 4-92).

The following should be clearly shown:
- No rotation of the wrist
- Scaphoid with adjacent articular areas open
- Extreme ulnar deviation

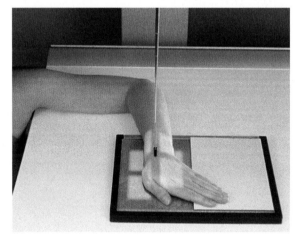

Fig. 4-91 PA wrist in ulnar deviation.

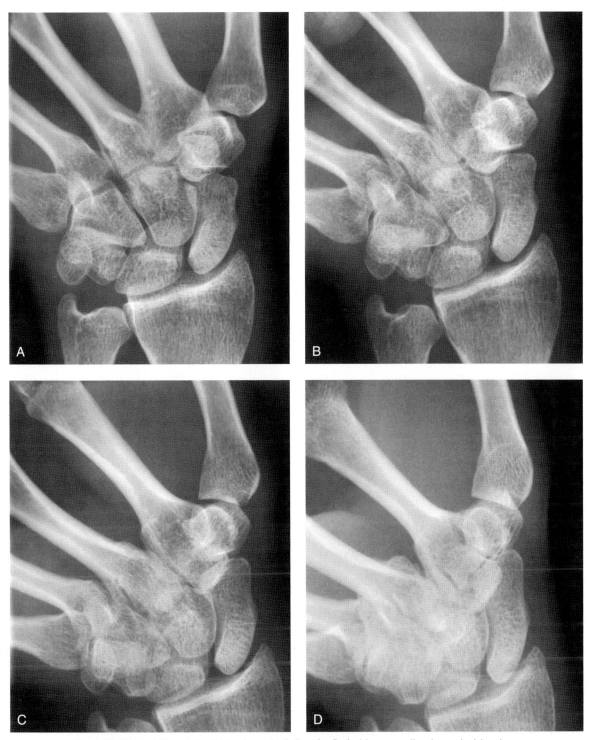

Fig. 4-92 PA and PA axial wrist in ulnar deviation for Rafert-Long method scaphoid series. Radiographs are all from the same patient. **A,** PA wrist with 0-degree central ray angle. **B,** PA axial wrist with 10-degree cephalad angle. **C,** PA axial wrist with 20-degree cephalad angle. **D,** PA axial wrist with 30-degree cephalad angle.

(From Rafert JA, Long BW: Technique for diagnosis of scaphoid fractures. *Radiol Technol* 63:16, 1991.)

Trapezium

PA AXIAL OBLIQUE PROJECTION

CLEMENTS-NAKAYAMA METHOD

Fractures of the trapezium are rare; however, if undiagnosed, these fractures can lead to functional difficulties. In certain cases, the articular surfaces of the trapezium should be evaluated to treat patients with osteoarthritis.[1]

Image receptor: 8 × 10 inch (18 × 24 cm) lengthwise

Position of patient

- With the patient seated at the end of the radiographic table, place the hand on the IR in the lateral position.

[1]Clements R, Nakayama H: Radiography of the polyarthritic hands and wrists, *Radiol Technol* 53:203, 1981.

Position of part

- Place the wrist in the lateral position, resting on the ulnar surface over the center of the IR.
- Place a 45-degree sponge wedge against the anterior surface, and rotate the hand to come in contact with the sponge.
- If the patient is able to achieve ulnar deviation, adjust the IR so that the long axis of the IR and the forearm align with the central ray (Fig. 4-93).
- If the patient is unable to achieve ulnar deviation comfortably, align the straight wrist to the IR, and rotate the elbow end of the IR and arm 20 degrees away from the central ray (Fig. 4-94).
- *Shield gonads.*

Central ray

- Angled 45 degrees distally to enter the anatomic snuffbox of the wrist and pass through the trapezium

Structures shown

The image clearly shows the trapezium and its articulations with the adjacent carpal bones (Fig. 4-95). The articulation of the trapezium and scaphoid is not shown on this image.

EVALUATION CRITERIA

The following should be clearly shown:

- Trapezium projected free of the other carpal bones with the exception of the articulation with the scaphoid

NOTE: Holly[1] recommended a variation of this method with the hand in ulnar deviation on a 37-degree sponge wedge. The central ray is directed vertically, entering just proximal to the first metacarpal base.

[1]Holly EW: Radiography of the greater multangular bone, *Med Radiogr Photogr* 24:79, 1948.

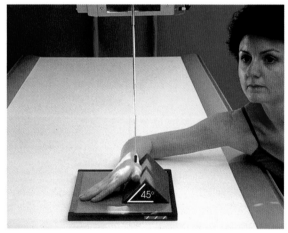

Fig. 4-93 PA axial oblique wrist for trapezium: Clements-Nakayama method; alignment with ulnar deviation.

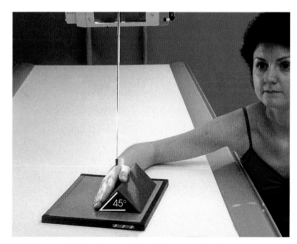

Fig. 4-94 PA axial oblique wrist for trapezium: Clements-Nakayama method; alignment without ulnar deviation.

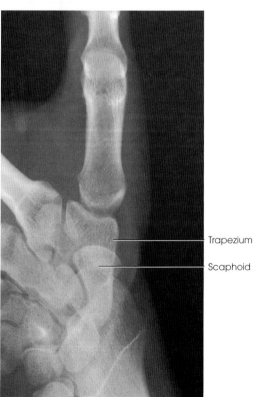

Trapezium

Scaphoid

Fig. 4-95 PA axial oblique wrist for trapezium: Clements-Nakayama method.

Carpal Bridge

TANGENTIAL PROJECTION

Image receptor: 8 × 10 inch (18 × 24 cm) lengthwise

Position of patient

- Seat or stand the patient at the side of the radiographic table to permit the required manipulation of the arm or x-ray tube.

Position of part

- The originators[1] of this projection recommended that the hand lie palm upward on the IR with the hand at right angle to the forearm (Fig. 4-96).

[1]Lentino W et al: The carpal bridge view, *J Bone Joint Surg Am* 39:88, 1957.

- When the wrist is too painful to be adjusted in the position just described, a similar image can be obtained by elevating the forearm on sandbags or other suitable support. Then with the wrist flexed in right-angle position, place the IR in the vertical position (Fig. 4-97).
- *Shield gonads.*

Central ray

- Directed to a point about 1½ inches (3.8 cm) proximal to the wrist joint at a caudal angle of 45 degrees

Structures shown

The carpal bridge is shown on the image in Figs. 4-98 and 4-99. The originators recommended this procedure to show fractures of the scaphoid, lunate dislocations, calcifications and foreign bodies in the dorsum of the wrist, and chip fractures of the dorsal aspect of the carpal bones.

EVALUATION CRITERIA

The following should be clearly shown:
- Dorsal aspect of the wrist
- Carpals
- Dorsal surface of the carpals free of superimposition by the metacarpal bases

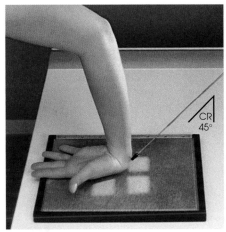

Fig. 4-96 Tangential carpal bridge, original method.

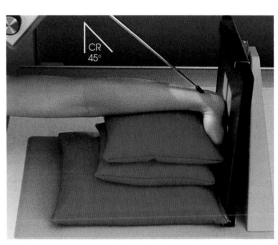

Fig. 4-97 Tangential carpal bridge, modified method.

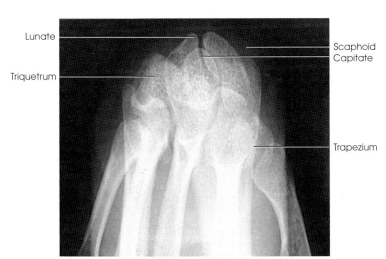

Lunate
Triquetrum
Scaphoid
Capitate
Trapezium

Fig. 4-98 Tangential carpal bridge, original method.

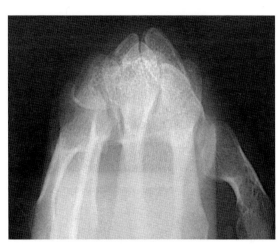

Fig. 4-99 Tangential carpal bridge, modified method.

⚜ TANGENTIAL PROJECTIONS
GAYNOR-HART METHOD[1]

The carpal canal contains the tendons of the flexors of the fingers and the median nerve. Compression of the median nerve results in pain. Radiography is performed to identify abnormality of the bones or soft tissue of the canal.

Fractures of the hook of hamate, pisiform, and trapezium are increasingly seen in athletes. The tangential projection is helpful in identifying fractures of these carpal bones. This projection was added as an essential projection based on the 1997 survey performed by Bontrager.[2]

Image receptor: 8 × 10 inch (18 × 24 cm) lengthwise

---

[1]Hart VL, Gaynor V: Roentgenographic study of the carpal canal, *J Bone Joint Surg* 23:382, 1941.
[2]Bontrager KL: *Textbook of radiographic positioning and related anatomy,* ed 7, St Louis, 2009, Mosby.

Inferosuperior
Position of patient

- Seat the patient at the end of the radiographic table so that the forearm can be adjusted to lie parallel with the long axis of the table.

Position of part

- Hyperextend the wrist, and center the IR to the joint at the level of the radial styloid process.
- For support, place a radiolucent pad approximately ¾ inch (1.9 cm) thick under the lower forearm.
- Adjust the position of the hand to make its long axis as vertical as possible.
- To prevent superimposition of the shadows of the hamate and pisiform bones, rotate the hand slightly toward the radial side.
- Have the patient grasp the digits with the opposite hand, or use a suitable device to hold the wrist in the extended position (Fig. 4-100).
- *Shield gonads.*

Central ray

- Directed to the palm of the hand at a point approximately 1 inch (2.5 cm) distal to the base of the third metacarpal and at an angle of 25 to 30 degrees to the long axis of the hand
- When the wrist cannot be extended to within 15 degrees of vertical, McQuillen Martensen[1] suggested that the central ray first be aligned parallel to the palmar surface, then angled an additional 15 degrees toward the palm.

Collimation

- 1 inch (2.5 cm) on the three sides of the shadow of the wrist

Structures shown

This image of the carpal canal (carpal tunnel) shows the palmar aspect of the trapezium; the tubercle of the trapezium; and the scaphoid, capitate, hook of hamate, triquetrum, and entire pisiform (Fig. 4-101).

---

[1]McQuillen Martensen K: *Radiographic image analysis,* ed 3, St Louis, 2010, Saunders.

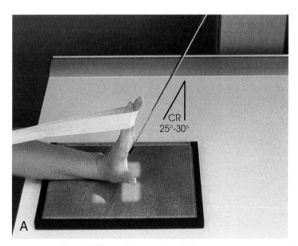
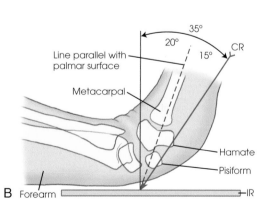

Fig. 4-100 A, Tangential (inferosuperior) carpal canal: Gaynor-Hart method. **B,** Suggested central ray (*CR*) alignment when wrist cannot be extended within 15 degrees of vertical. CR is angled 15 degrees more than angle of metacarpals.

(Modified from McQuillen Martensen K: *Radiographic image analysis,* ed 3, St Louis, 2010, Saunders.)

Superoinferior

Position of patient

- When the patient cannot assume or maintain the previously described wrist position, a similar image may be obtained.
- Have the patient dorsiflex the wrist as much as is tolerable and lean forward to place the carpal canal tangent to the IR (Fig. 4-102). The canal is easily palpable on the palmar aspect of the wrist as the concavity between the trapezium laterally and hook of hamate and pisiform medially.

Position of part

- When dorsiflexion of the wrist is limited, Marshall[1] suggested placing a 45-degree angle sponge under the palmar surface of the hand. The sponge slightly elevates the wrist to place the carpal canal tangent to the central ray. A slight degree of magnification exists because of the increased object-to-IR distance (OID) (Fig. 4-103).

Central ray

- Tangential to the carpal canal at the level of the midpoint of the wrist
- Angled toward the hand approximately 20 to 35 degrees from the long axis of the forearm

Collimation

- Include palmar aspect of wrist, proximal one third of metacarpals, and 1 inch (2.5 cm) on the sides

EVALUATION CRITERIA

With either approach, the following should be clearly shown:
- Evidence of proper collimation
- Carpals in an arch arrangement
- Pisiform in profile and free of superimposition
- Hamulus of hamate
- All carpals

[1]Marshall J: Imaging the carpal tunnel, *Radiogr Today* 56:11, 1990.

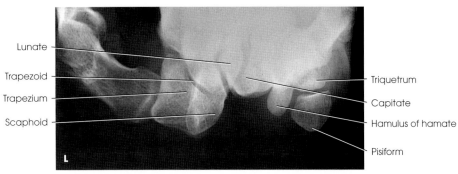

Fig. 4-101 Tangential (inferosuperior) carpal canal: Gaynor-Hart method.

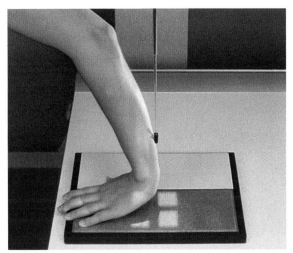

Fig. 4-102 Tangential (superoinferior) carpal canal.

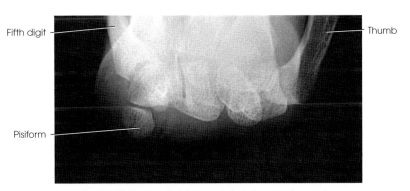

Fig. 4-103 Tangential (superoinferior) carpal canal.

♠ AP PROJECTION

The IR should be long enough to include the entire forearm from the olecranon process of the ulna to the styloid process of the radius and the wrist and elbow joints. Both images of the forearm may be taken on one IR by alternately covering one half of the IR with a lead mask. Space should be allowed for the patient identification marker so that no part of the radiographic image is cut off.

Image receptor: Lengthwise—7 × 17 inch (18 × 43 cm) single; 14 × 17 inch (35 × 43 cm) divided

Position of patient

- Seat the patient close to the radiographic table and low enough to place the entire limb in the same plane.

Position of part

- Supinate the hand, extend the elbow, and center the unmasked half of the IR to the forearm. Ensure that the joint of interest is included.
- Adjust the IR so that the long axis is parallel with the forearm.
- Have the patient lean laterally until the forearm is in a true supinated position (Fig. 4-104).
- Because the proximal forearm is commonly rotated in this position, palpate and adjust the humeral epicondyles to be equidistant from the IR.
- Ensure that the hand is supinated (Fig. 4-105). Pronation of the hand crosses the radius over the ulna at its proximal third and rotates the humerus medially, resulting in an oblique projection of the forearm (Fig. 4-106).
- *Shield gonads.*

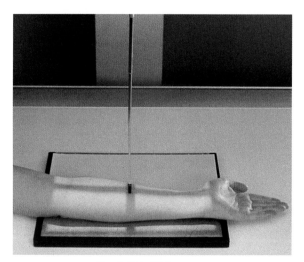

Fig. 4-104 AP forearm.

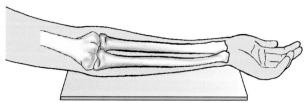

Fig. 4-105 AP forearm with hand supinated.

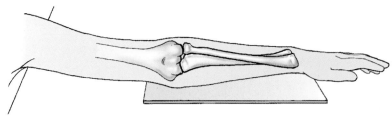

Fig. 4-106 AP forearm with hand pronated—incorrect.

Forearm

Central ray

- Perpendicular to the midpoint of the forearm

Collimation

- 2 inches (5 cm) distal to the wrist joint and proximal to the elbow joint and 1 inch (2.5 cm) on the sides

COMPUTED RADIOGRAPHY

The forearm must be centered to the plate or plate section with four collimator margins or with no margins at all. Two images can be projected on one plate; however, because the arm takes up most of the plate half, collimate to the margins of the plate. A lead blocker must cover the opposite side when two images are made on one IR.

Structures shown

An AP projection of the forearm shows the elbow joint, the radius and ulna, and the proximal row of slightly distorted carpal bones (Fig. 4-107).

EVALUATION CRITERIA

The following should be clearly shown:

- Evidence of proper collimation
- Wrist and distal humerus
- Slight superimposition of the radial head, neck, and tuberosity over the proximal ulna
- No elongation or foreshortening of the humeral epicondyles
- Partially open elbow joint if the shoulder was placed in the same plane as the forearm
- Open radioulnar space
- Similar radiographic densities of the proximal and distal forearm

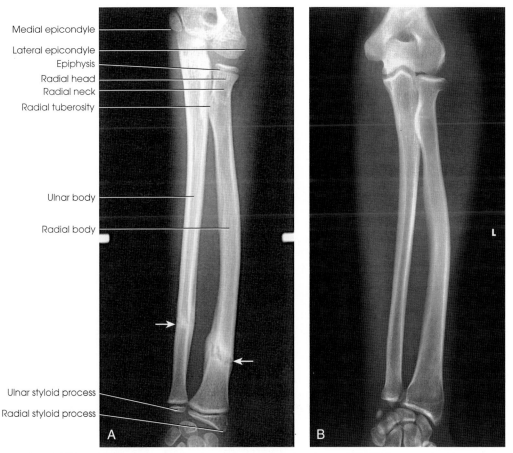

Fig. 4-107 **A,** AP forearm with fractured radius and ulna (*arrows*). **B,** AP forearm showing both joints.

✤ LATERAL PROJECTION
Lateromedial

Image receptor: Lengthwise—7 × 17 inch (18 × 43 cm) single; 14 × 17 inch (35 × 43 cm) divided

Position of patient
- Seat the patient close to the radiographic table and low enough that the humerus, shoulder joint, and elbow lie in the same plane.

Position of part
- Flex the elbow 90 degrees, and center the forearm over the unmasked half of the IR and parallel with the long axis of the forearm.
- Ensure that the entire joint of interest is included.
- Adjust the limb in a true lateral position. The thumb side of the hand must be up (Fig. 4-108).
- *Shield gonads.*

Central ray
- Perpendicular to the midpoint of the forearm

Collimation
- 2 inches (5 cm) distal to the wrist joint and proximal to the elbow joint, and 1 inch (2.5 cm) on the sides

Structures shown
The lateral projection shows the bones of the forearm, the elbow joint, and the proximal row of carpal bones (Fig. 4-109).

EVALUATION CRITERIA
The following should be clearly shown:
- Evidence of proper collimation
- Wrist and distal humerus
- Superimposition of the radius and ulna at their distal end
- Superimposition by the radial head over the coronoid process
- Radial tuberosity facing anteriorly
- Superimposed humeral epicondyles
- Elbow flexed 90 degrees
- Soft tissue and bony trabeculation along the entire length of the radial and ulnar shafts

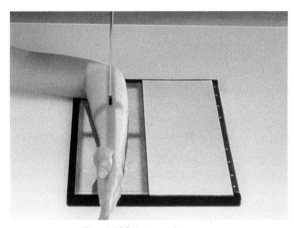

Fig. 4-108 Lateral forearm.

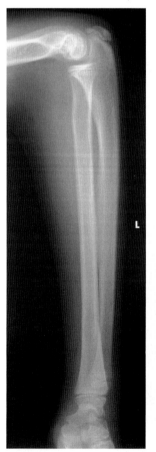
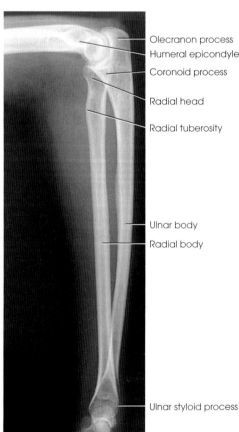

Olecranon process
Humeral epicondyle
Coronoid process

Radial head

Radial tuberosity

Ulnar body

Radial body

Ulnar styloid process

Fig. 4-109 Lateral forearm.

✿ AP PROJECTION

Image receptor: 8 × 10 inch (18 × 24 cm) single or 10 × 12 inch (24 × 30 cm) divided

Position of patient

- Seat the patient near the radiographic table and low enough to place the shoulder joint, humerus, and elbow joint in the same plane.

Position of part

- Extend the elbow, supinate the hand, and center the IR to the elbow joint.
- Adjust the IR to make it parallel with the long axis of the part (Fig. 4-110).
- Have the patient lean laterally until the humeral epicondyles and anterior surface of the elbow are parallel with the plane of the IR.
- Supinate the hand to prevent rotation of the bones of the forearm.
- *Shield gonads.*

Central ray

- Perpendicular to the elbow joint

Collimation

- 3 inches (8 cm) proximal and distal to the elbow joint and 1 inch (2.5 cm) on the sides

COMPUTED RADIOGRAPHY

The elbow must be centered to the plate or plate section with four collimator margins or with no margins at all. Two images can be projected on one plate; however, because the elbow projection takes up most of the plate half, collimate to the margins of the plate. A lead blocker must cover the opposite side when two images are made on one IR.

Structures shown

An AP projection of the elbow joint, distal arm, and proximal forearm is presented (Fig. 4-111).

EVALUATION CRITERIA

The following should be clearly shown:
- Evidence of proper collimation
- Radial head, neck, and tuberosity slightly superimposed over the proximal ulna
- Elbow joint open and centered to the central ray
- No rotation of humeral epicondyles (coronoid and olecranon fossae approximately equidistant to epicondyles)
- Soft tissue and bony trabeculation

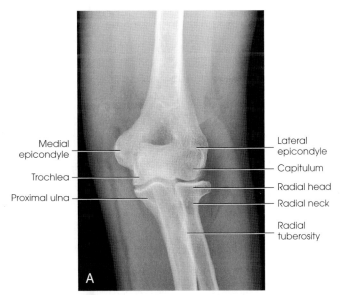

Fig. 4-110 AP elbow.

Medial epicondyle
Trochlea
Proximal ulna

Lateral epicondyle
Capitulum
Radial head
Radial neck
Radial tuberosity

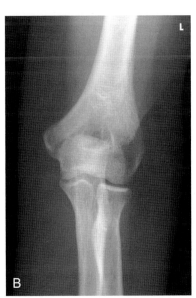

Fig. 4-111 A, AP elbow with wide latitude exposure technique for soft tissue detail. **B,** AP elbow with normal exposure technique.

Upper Limb

⚜ LATERAL PROJECTION
Lateromedial

Griswold[1] gave two reasons for the importance of flexing the elbow 90 degrees: (1) The olecranon process can be seen in profile, and (2) the elbow fat pads are the least compressed. In partial or complete extension, the olecranon process elevates the posterior elbow fat pad and simulates joint pathology.

Image receptor: 8 × 10 inch (18 × 24 cm) single or 10 × 12 inch (24 × 30 cm) divided

---

[1]Griswold R: Elbow fat pads: a radiography perspective, *Radiol Technol* 53:303, 1982.

Position of patient
- Seat the patient at the end of the radiographic table low enough to place the humerus and elbow joint in the same plane.

Position of part
- From the supine position, flex the elbow 90 degrees, and place the humerus and forearm in contact with the table.
- Center the IR to the elbow joint. Adjust the elbow joint so that its long axis is parallel with the long axis of the forearm (Figs. 4-112 and 4-113). On patients with muscular forearms, elevate the wrist to place the forearm parallel with the IR.

- Adjust the IR diagonally to include more of the arm and forearm (Fig. 4-114).
- To obtain a lateral projection of the elbow, adjust the hand in the lateral position and ensure that the humeral epicondyles are perpendicular to the plane of the IR.
- *Shield gonads.*

Central ray
- Perpendicular to the elbow joint, regardless of its location on the IR

Collimation
- 3 inches (8 cm) proximal and distal to the elbow joint

Structures shown
The lateral projection shows the elbow joint, distal arm, and proximal forearm (see Figs. 4-113 and 4-114).

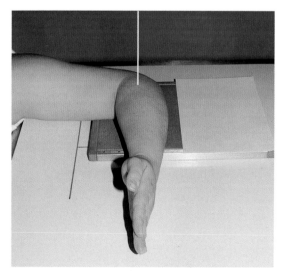

Fig. 4-112 Lateral elbow.

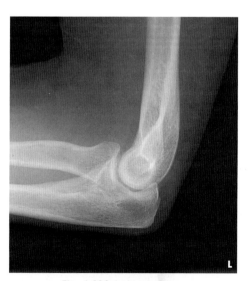

Fig. 4-113 Lateral elbow.

EVALUATION CRITERIA

The following should be clearly shown:
- Evidence of proper collimation
- Open elbow joint centered to the central ray
- Elbow flexed 90 degrees
- Superimposed humeral epicondyles
- Radial tuberosity facing anteriorly
- Radial head partially superimposing the coronoid process
- Olecranon process seen in profile
- Bony trabeculation and any elevated fat pads in the soft tissue at the anterior and posterior distal humerus and the anterior proximal forearm

NOTE: When injury to the soft tissue around the elbow is suspected, the joint should be flexed only 30 or 35 degrees (Fig. 4-115). This partial flexion does not compress or stretch the soft structures as does the full 90-degree lateral flexion. The posterior fat pad may become visible in this position.

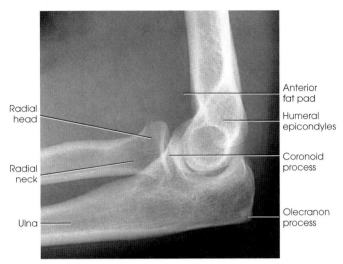

Fig. 4-114 Lateral elbow.

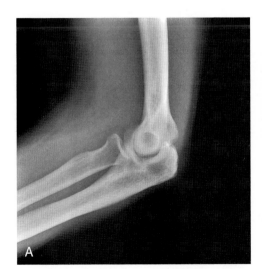
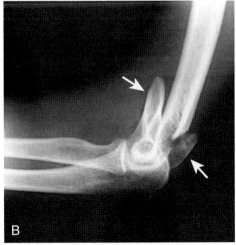

Fig. 4-115 A, Lateral elbow in partial flexion position for soft tissue image. **B,** Lateral elbow of patient who fell from a tree, resulting in impaction fracture (*arrows*) of distal humerus.

Upper Limb

♠ AP OBLIQUE PROJECTION
Medial rotation

Image receptor: 8 × 10 inch (18 × 24 cm) single or 10 × 12 inch (24 × 30 cm) divided

Position of patient
- Seat the patient at the end of the radiographic table with the arm extended and in contact with the table.

Position of part
- Extend the limb in position for an AP projection, and center the midpoint of the IR to the elbow joint (Fig. 4-116).
- Medially (internally) rotate or pronate the hand, and adjust the elbow to place its anterior surface at an angle of 45 degrees. This degree of obliquity usually clears the coronoid process of the radial head.
- *Shield gonads.*

Central ray
- Perpendicular to the elbow joint

Collimation
- 3 inches (8 cm) proximal and distal to the elbow joint and 1 inch (2.5 cm) on the sides

Structures shown
The image shows an oblique projection of the elbow with the coronoid process projected free of superimposition (Fig. 4-117).

EVALUATION CRITERIA
The following should be clearly shown:
- Evidence of proper collimation
- Coronoid process in profile
- Trochlea
- Elongated medial humeral epicondyle
- Ulna superimposed by the radial head and neck
- Olecranon process within the olecranon fossa
- Soft tissue and bony trabeculation

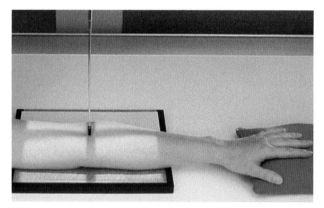

Fig. 4-116 AP oblique elbow: medial rotation.

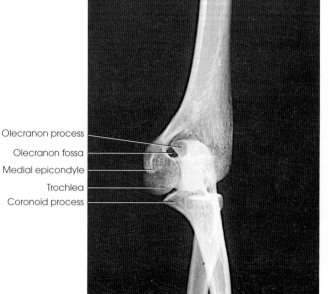
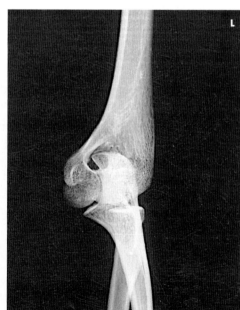

Olecranon process
Olecranon fossa
Medial epicondyle
Trochlea
Coronoid process

Fig. 4-117 AP oblique elbow.

♠ AP OBLIQUE PROJECTION
Lateral rotation

Image receptor: 8 × 10 inch (18 × 24 cm) single or 10 × 12 inch (24 × 30 cm) divided

Position of patient

- Seat the patient at the end of the radiographic table with the arm extended and in contact with the table.

Position of part

- Extend the patient's arm in position for an AP projection, and center the midpoint of the IR to the elbow joint.
- Rotate the hand laterally (externally) to place the posterior surface of the elbow at a 45-degree angle (Fig. 4-118). When proper lateral rotation is achieved, the patient's first and second digits should touch the table.
- *Shield gonads.*

Central ray

- Perpendicular to the elbow joint

Collimation

- 3 inches (8 cm) proximal and distal to the elbow joint and 1 inch (2.5 cm) on the sides

Structures shown

The image shows an oblique projection of the elbow with the radial head and neck projected free of superimposition of the ulna (Fig. 4-119).

EVALUATION CRITERIA

The following should be clearly shown:
- Evidence of proper collimation
- Radial head, neck, and tuberosity projected free of the ulna
- Capitulum
- Open elbow joint
- Soft tissue and bony trabeculation

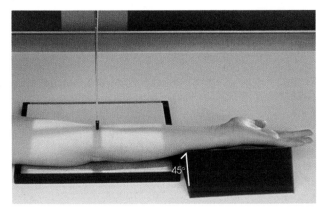

Fig. 4-118 AP oblique elbow: lateral rotation.

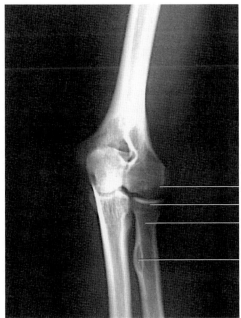
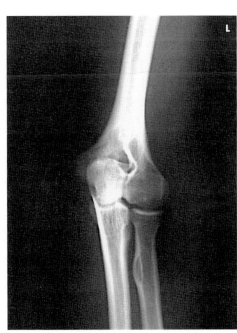

Capitulum
Radial head
Radial neck
Radial tuberosity

Fig. 4-119 AP oblique elbow.

Distal Humerus
♠ AP PROJECTION
Partial flexion

When the patient cannot completely extend the elbow, the lateral position is easily performed; however, two AP projections must be obtained to avoid distortion. Separate AP projections of the distal humerus and proximal forearm are required.

Image receptor: Both exposures can be made on one 8 × 10 inch (18 × 24 cm) IR or on one IR placed crosswise by alternately covering one half of the IR with a lead mask.

Position of patient
• Seat the patient low enough to place the entire humerus in the same plane. Support the elevated forearm.

Position of part
• If possible, supinate the hand. Place the IR under the elbow, and center it to the condyloid area of the humerus (Fig. 4-120).
• *Shield gonads.*

Central ray
• Perpendicular to the humerus, traversing the elbow joint
• Depending on the degree of flexion, angle the central ray distally into the joint.

Collimation
• 3 inches (8 cm) proximal and distal to the elbow joint and 1 inch (2.5 cm) on the sides

Structures shown
This projection shows the distal humerus when the elbow cannot be fully extended (Figs. 4-121 and 4-122).

EVALUATION CRITERIA
The following should be clearly shown:
■ Evidence of proper collimation
■ Distal humerus without rotation or distortion
■ Proximal radius superimposed over the ulna
■ Closed elbow joint
■ Greatly foreshortened proximal forearm
■ Trabecular detail on the distal humerus

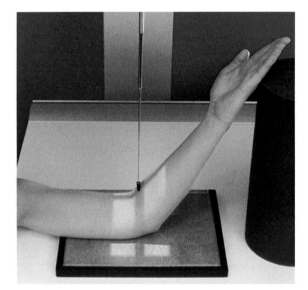

Fig. 4-120 AP elbow, partially flexed.

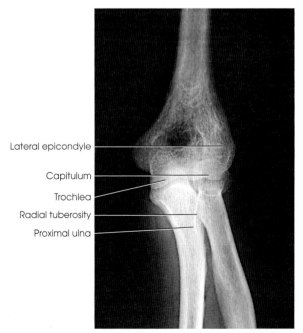

Lateral epicondyle
Capitulum
Trochlea
Radial tuberosity
Proximal ulna

Fig. 4-121 AP elbow, partially flexed, showing distal humerus.

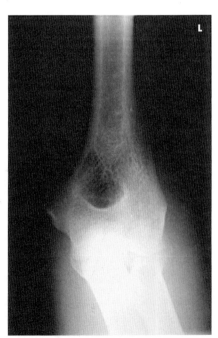

Fig. 4-122 AP elbow, partially flexed, showing distal humerus. White proximal radius and ulna result from overlap of anterior dislocated elbow (see Fig. 4-125).

Proximal Forearm

⚹ AP PROJECTION
Partial flexion

Image receptor: 8 × 10 inch (18 × 24 cm)

Position of patient
- Seat the patient at the end of the radiographic table with the hand supinated.

Position of part
- Seat the patient high enough to permit the dorsal surface of the forearm to rest on the table (Fig. 4-123). If this position is impossible, elevate the limb on a support, adjust the limb in the lateral position, place the IR in the vertical position behind the upper end of the forearm, and direct the central ray horizontally.
- *Shield gonads.*

Central ray
- Perpendicular to the elbow joint and long axis of the forearm
- Adjust the IR so that the central ray passes to its midpoint.

Collimation
- 3 inches (8 cm) proximal and distal to the elbow joint and 1 inch (2.5 cm) on the sides

Structures shown
This projection shows the proximal forearm when the elbow cannot be fully extended (Figs. 4-124 and 4-125).

EVALUATION CRITERIA
The following should be clearly shown:
- Evidence of proper collimation
- Proximal radius and ulna without rotation or distortion
- Radial head, neck, and tuberosity slightly superimposed over the proximal ulna
- Partially open elbow joint
- Foreshortened distal humerus
- Trabecular detail on the proximal forearm

NOTE: Holly[1] described a method of obtaining the AP projection of the radial head. The patient is positioned as described for the distal humerus. The elbow is extended as much as possible, and the forearm is supported. The forearm should be supinated enough to place the horizontal plane of the wrist at an angle of 30 degrees from horizontal.

[1]Holly EW: Radiography of the radial head, *Med Radiogr Photogr* 32:13, 1956.

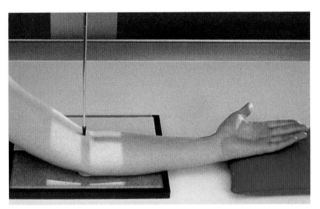

Fig. 4-123 AP elbow, partially flexed.

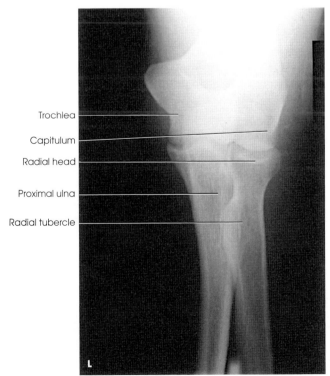

Trochlea
Capitulum
Radial head
Proximal ulna
Radial tubercle

Fig. 4-124 AP elbow, partially flexed, showing proximal forearm. This is a view of the dislocated elbow of the patient shown in Fig. 4-125. White distal humerus is due to dislocated humerus overlapping proximal radius and ulna.

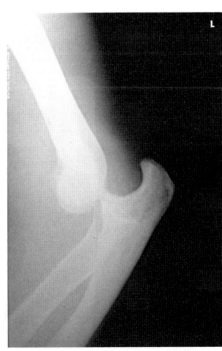

Fig. 4-125 Lateral elbow showing dislocation on same patient as shown in Figs. 4-122 and 4-124.

Distal Humerus

AP PROJECTION

Acute flexion

When fractures around the elbow are being treated using the Jones orthopedic technique (complete flexion), the lateral position offers little difficulty, but the frontal projection must be made through the superimposed bones of the AP arm and PA forearm. This projection is sometimes known as the *Jones method,* although no "Jones" reference has been found.

Image receptor: 8 × 10 inch (18 × 24 cm); may be divided for two images on one IR

Position of patient

- Seat the patient at the end of the radiographic table with the elbow fully flexed (unless contraindicated).

Position of part

- Center the IR proximal to the epicondylar area of the humerus. The long axis of the arm and forearm should be parallel with the long axis of the IR (Figs. 4-126 and 4-127).
- Adjust the arm or the radiographic tube and IR to prevent rotation.
- *Shield gonads.*

Central ray

- Perpendicular to the humerus, approximately 2 inches (5 cm) superior to the olecranon process

Structures shown

This position superimposes the bones of the forearm and arm. The olecranon process should be clearly shown (Fig. 4-128).

EVALUATION CRITERIA

The following should be clearly shown:
- Forearm and humerus superimposed
- No rotation
- Olecranon process and distal humerus
- Soft tissue outside the olecranon process

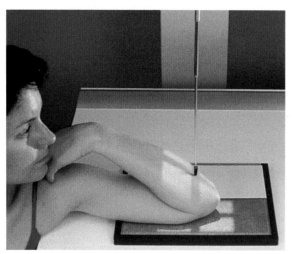

Fig. 4-126 AP distal humerus: acute flexion of elbow.

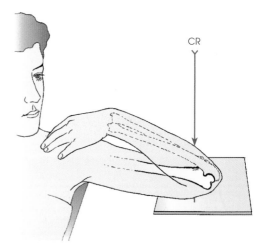

Fig. 4-127 AP distal humerus: acute flexion of elbow.

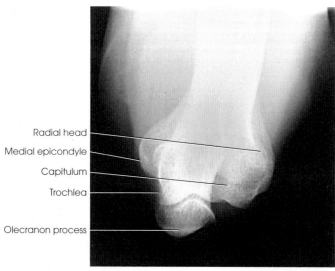

Radial head
Medial epicondyle
Capitulum
Trochlea
Olecranon process

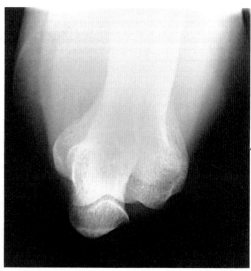

Fig. 4-128 AP distal humerus: acute flexion of elbow.

Proximal Forearm

PA PROJECTION
Acute flexion

Image receptor: 8 × 10 inch (18 × 24 cm)

Position of patient

- Seat the patient at the end of the radiographic table with the elbow fully flexed.

Position of part

- Center the flexed elbow joint to the center of the IR. The long axis of the superimposed forearm and arm should be parallel with the long axis of the IR (Figs. 4-129 and 4-130).
- Move the IR toward the shoulder so that the central ray passes to the midpoint.
- *Shield gonads.*

Central ray

- Perpendicular to the flexed forearm, entering approximately 2 inches (5 cm) distal to the olecranon process

Structures shown

The superimposed bones of the arm and forearm are outlined (Fig. 4-131). The elbow joint should be more open than for projections of the distal humerus.

EVALUATION CRITERIA

The following should be clearly shown:
- Forearm and humerus superimposed
- No rotation
- Proximal radius and ulna

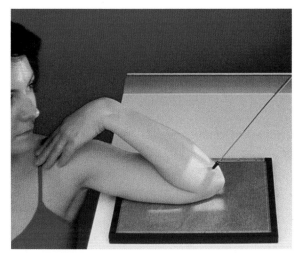

Fig. 4-129 PA proximal forearm: full flexion of elbow.

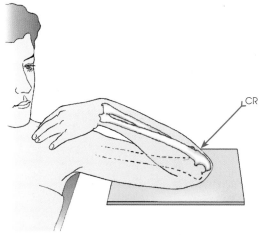

Fig. 4-130 PA proximal forearm: full flexion of elbow.

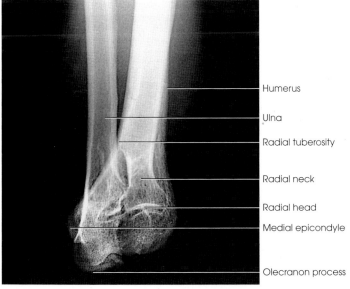

Humerus
Ulna
Radial tuberosity
Radial neck
Radial head
Medial epicondyle
Olecranon process

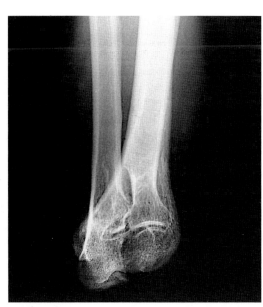

Fig. 4-131 PA proximal forearm: full flexion of elbow.

Radial Head

LATERAL PROJECTION
Lateromedial

Four-position series

Place the IR in position, and cover the unused section with a sheet of lead. To show the entire circumference of the radial head free of superimposition, four projections with varying positions of the hand are performed.

Image receptor: 8 × 10 inch (18 × 24 cm) single or 10 × 12 inch (24 × 30 cm) divided

Position of patient

- Seat the patient low enough to place the entire arm in the same horizontal plane.

Position of part

- Flex the elbow 90 degrees, center the joint to the unmasked IR, and place the joint in the lateral position.
- Make the first exposure with the hand supinated as much as is possible (Fig. 4-132).

- Shift the IR and make the second exposure with the hand in the lateral position, that is, with the thumb surface up (Fig. 4-133).
- Shift the IR, then make the third exposure with the hand pronated (Fig. 4-134).
- Shift the IR, and make the fourth exposure with the hand in extreme internal rotation, that is, resting on the thumb surface (Fig. 4-135).
- *Shield gonads.*

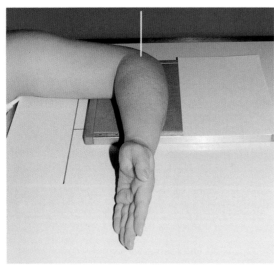

Fig. 4-132 Lateral elbow, radius with hand supinated as much as possible.

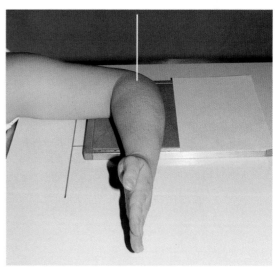

Fig. 4-133 Lateral elbow, radius with hand lateral.

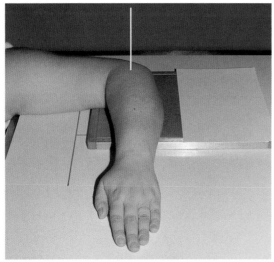

Fig. 4-134 Lateral elbow, radius with hand pronated.

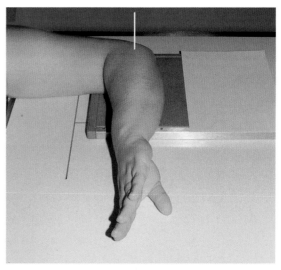

Fig. 4-135 Lateral elbow, radius with hand internally rotated.

Central ray

• Perpendicular to the elbow joint

Structures shown

The radial head is projected in varying degrees of rotation (Figs. 4-136 through 4-139).

The following should be clearly shown:

■ Radial tuberosity facing anteriorly for the first and second images and posteriorly for the third and fourth images (see Figs. 4-136 to 4-139)
■ Elbow flexed 90 degrees
■ Radial head partially superimposing the coronoid process but seen in all images

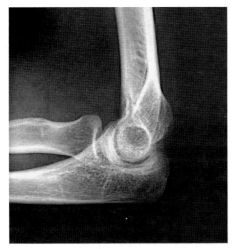

Fig. 4-136 Lateral elbow, radius with hand supinated.

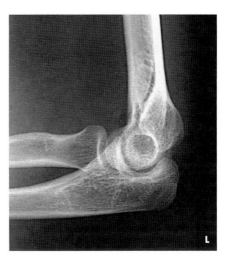

Fig. 4-137 Lateral elbow, radius with hand lateral.

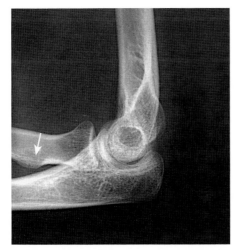

Fig. 4-138 Lateral elbow, radius with hand pronated (radial tuberosity, *arrow*).

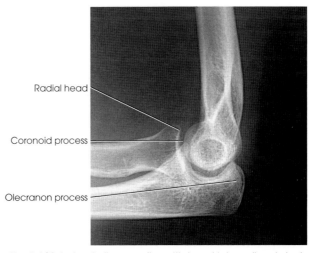

Fig. 4-139 Lateral elbow, radius with hand internally rotated.

Upper Limb

Radial Head and Coronoid Process

♠ AXIOLATERAL PROJECTION
COYLE METHOD
Lateral

NOTE: This projection was devised for obtaining images of the radial head and coronoid process on patients who cannot fully extend the elbow for medial and lateral oblique projections.[1] It is particularly useful in imaging a traumatized elbow.

[1]Coyle GF: *Radiographing immobile trauma patients, Unit 7, Special angled views of joints—elbow, knee, ankle,* Denver, 1980, Multi-Media Publishing.

Image receptor: 8 × 10 inch (18 × 24 cm)

Position of patient
- Seat the patient at the end of the radiographic table.
- Position the patient supine for imaging a traumatized elbow.

Position of part
Seated position
- Seat the patient at the end of the radiographic table low enough to place the humerus, elbow, and wrist joints on the same plane.
- Pronate the hand and flex the elbow 90 degrees to show the radial head or 80 degrees to show the coronoid process.
- Center the IR to the elbow joint. For patients with muscular forearms, elevate the wrist to place forearm parallel with IR (Fig. 4-140).

Supine position for trauma

- In most instances of trauma, the patient is lying in the supine position on a cart. The projection is easily performed in this position.
- Elevate the distal humerus on a radiolucent sponge.
- Place the IR in vertical position centered to the elbow joint.
- Epicondyles should be approximately perpendicular to the IR.
- Slowly flex the elbow 90 degrees to show the radial head or 80 degrees for the coronoid process. Turn the hand so that the palmar aspect is facing medially. An assistant may need to hold the hand depending on the severity of trauma (Fig. 4-141).
- *Shield gonads.*

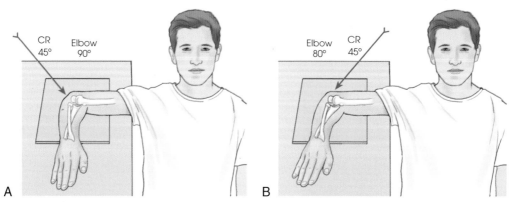

Fig. 4-140 A, Axiolateral projection of elbow (Coyle method) to show radial head and capitulum. Forearm is 90 degrees, and central ray (*CR*) is directed 45 degrees toward shoulder. **B,** To show coronoid process and trochlea, forearm is positioned at 80 degrees, and CR is directed 45 degrees away from shoulder.

Central ray

Seated position
Radial head
- Directed *toward* the shoulder at an angle of 45 degrees to the radial head; central ray enters the joint at mid-elbow (see Fig. 4-140, *A*)

Coronoid process
- Directed *away* from the shoulder at an angle of 45 degrees to the coronoid process; central ray enters the joint at mid-elbow (see Fig. 4-140, *B*)

Supine position for trauma
Radial head
- The horizontal central ray is directed *cephalad* at an angle of 45 degrees to the radial head, entering the joint at mid-elbow (see Fig. 4-141, *A*).

Coronoid process
- The horizontal central ray is directed *caudad* at an angle of 45 degrees to the coronoid process, entering the joint at mid-elbow (see Fig. 4-141, *B*).

Collimation
- 3 inches (8 cm) proximal and distal to the elbow joint

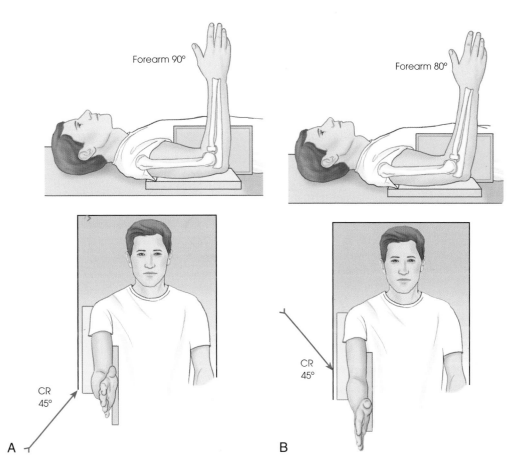

Fig. 4-141 Axiolateral projection of elbow (Coyle method) in trauma. **A,** Patient is supine with humerus on a block, arm is 90 degrees, and central ray (*CR*) is directed cephalad for radial head and capitulum. **B,** Arm is 80 degrees, and CR is directed caudad to show coronoid process and trochlea.

Upper Limb

Structures shown

The resulting projections show an open elbow joint between the radial head and capitulum (Fig. 4-142) or the coronoid process and trochlea (Fig. 4-143) with the area of interest in profile. These projections are used to show pathologic processes or trauma in the area of the radial head and coronoid process. The value of the projections is evident in the trauma images shown in Fig. 4-144.[1]

---

[1]Greenspan A, Norman A, Rosen H: Radial head capitulum view in elbow trauma: clinical applications and anatomic correlation, *AJR Am J Roentgenol* 143:355, 1984.

The following should be clearly shown:

Radial head

- Evidence of proper collimation
- Open joint space between radial head and capitulum
- Radial head, neck, and tuberosity in profile and free from superimposition with the exception of a small portion of the coronoid process
- Humeral epicondyles distorted owing to central ray angulation
- Radial tuberosity facing posteriorly
- Elbow flexed 90 degrees
- Soft tissue and bony trabeculation

Coronoid process

- Open joint space between coronoid process and trochlea
- Coronoid process in profile and elongated
- Radial head and neck superimposed by ulna
- Elbow flexed 80 degrees
- Soft tissue and bony trabeculation

RESEARCH: This projection was researched and standardized for the atlas by Tammy Curtis, MS, RT(R).

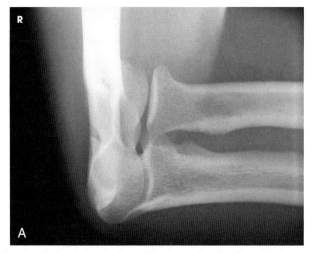

Fig. 4-142 Axiolateral elbow (Coyle method) with radial head and capitulum shown.

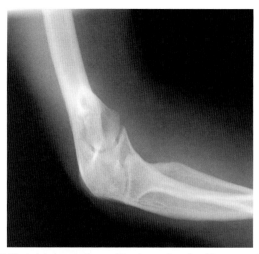

Fig. 4-143 Axiolateral elbow (Coyle method) with coronoid process and trochlea shown.

(From Bontrager KL, Lampignano JP: *Textbook of radiographic positioning and related anatomy*, ed 7, St Louis, 2009, Mosby.)

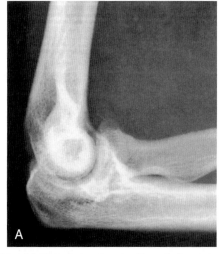
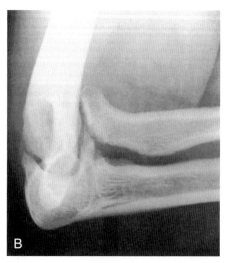

Fig. 4-144 A, Lateral projection of elbow shows fracture of radial head, but bony overlap prevents exact evaluation of extent of fracture line. **B,** Axiolateral projection (Coyle method) clearly shows displaced articular fracture involving posterior third of radial head.

(Used with permission from Greenspan A, Norman A, Rosen H: Radial head capitulum view in elbow trauma: clinical applications and anatomic correlation, *AJR Am J Roentgenol* 143:355, 1984.)

Distal Humerus

PA AXIAL PROJECTION

Image receptor: 8 × 10 inch (18 × 24 cm) for one or two images on one IR

Position of patient

- Seat the patient high enough to enable the forearm to rest on the radiographic table with the arm in the vertical position. The patient must be seated so that the forearm can be adjusted parallel with the long axis of the table.

Position of part

- Ask the patient to rest the forearm on the table, and then adjust the forearm so that its long axis is parallel with the table.
- Center a point midway between the epicondyles and the center of the IR.

- Flex the patient's elbow to place the arm in a nearly vertical position so that the humerus forms an angle of approximately 75 degrees from the forearm (approximately 15 degrees between the central ray and the long axis of the humerus).
- Confirm that the patient is not leaning anteriorly or posteriorly.
- Supinate the hand to prevent rotation of the humerus and ulna, and have the patient immobilize it with the opposite hand (Fig. 4-145).
- *Shield gonads.*

Central ray

- Perpendicular to the ulnar sulcus, entering at a point just medial to the olecranon process

Structures shown

This projection shows the epicondyles, trochlea, ulnar sulcus (groove between the medial epicondyle and the trochlea), and olecranon fossa (Fig. 4-146). The projection is used in radiohumeral bursitis (tennis elbow) to detect otherwise obscured calcifications located in the ulnar sulcus.

NOTE: Long and Rafert[1] describe an AP oblique distal humerus projection that specifically shows the ulnar sulcus.

EVALUATION CRITERIA

The following should be clearly shown:
- Outline of the ulnar sulcus (groove)
- Soft tissue outside the distal humerus
- Forearm and humerus superimposed
- No rotation

[1]Long BW, Rafert JA: The elbow. In: *Orthopedic radiography,* Philadelphia, 1995, Saunders.

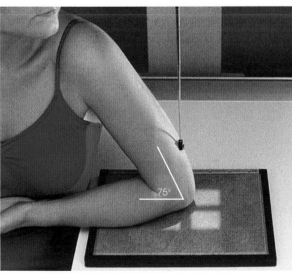

Fig. 4-145 PA axial distal humerus.

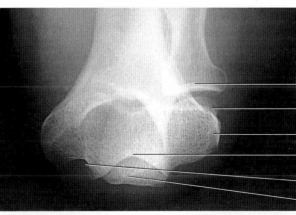
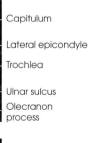

Radial head

Capitulum

Lateral epicondyle

Trochlea

Ulnar sulcus

Olecranon process

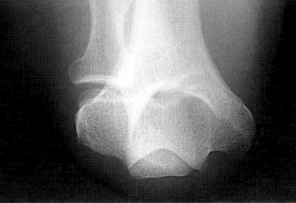

Fig. 4-146 PA axial distal humerus.

Olecranon Process

PA AXIAL PROJECTION

Image receptor: 8 × 10 inch (18 × 24 cm)

Position of patient

- Seat the patient at the end of the radiographic table, high enough that the forearm can rest flat on the IR.

Position of part

- Adjust the arm at an angle of 45 to 50 degrees from the vertical position, and ensure that the patient is not leaning anteriorly or posteriorly.
- Supinate the hand and have the patient immobilize it with the opposite hand.
- Center a point midway between the epicondyles and the center of the IR.
- *Shield gonads.*

Central ray

- Perpendicular to the olecranon process to show the dorsum of the olecranon process and at a 20-degree angle toward the wrist to show the curved extremity and articular margin of the olecranon process (Fig. 4-147)

Structures shown

The projection shows the olecranon process and the articular margin of the olecranon and humerus (Figs. 4-148 through 4-150).

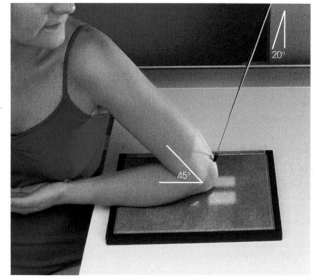

Fig. 4-147 PA axial olecranon process with central ray angled 20 degrees.

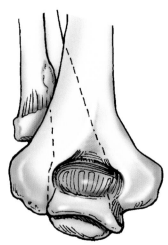

Fig. 4-148 PA axial olecranon process.

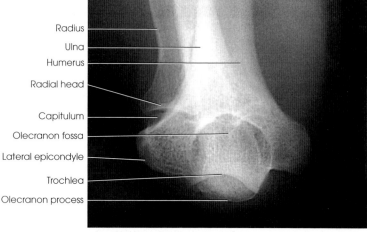

Radius
Ulna
Humerus
Radial head
Capitulum
Olecranon fossa
Lateral epicondyle
Trochlea
Olecranon process

Fig. 4-149 PA axial olecranon process with central ray angulation of 0 degrees.

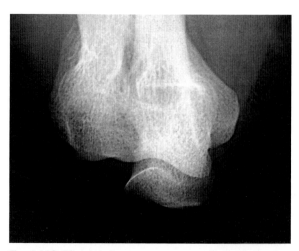

Fig. 4-150 PA axial olecranon process with central ray angulation of 20 degrees.

Upper Limb

✲ AP PROJECTION
Upright

Shoulder and arm abnormalities, whether traumatic or pathologic in origin, are extremely painful. For this reason, an upright position, either standing or seated, should be used whenever possible. With rotation of the patient's body as required, the arm can be positioned quickly and accurately with minimal discomfort to the patient.

Image receptor: Lengthwise—7 × 17 inch (18 × 43 cm); 14 × 17 inch (35 × 43 cm)

Position of patient
- Place the patient in a seated-upright or standing position facing the x-ray tube.
- Fig. 4-151 illustrates the body position used for an AP projection of a freely movable arm. The body position, whether oblique or facing toward or away from the IR, is unimportant as long as a true frontal radiograph of the arm is obtained.

Position of part
- Adjust the height of the IR to place its upper margin about 1½ inches (3.8 cm) above the head of the humerus.
- Abduct the arm slightly, and supinate the hand.
- A coronal plane passing through the epicondyles should be parallel with the IR plane for the AP (or PA) projection (see Fig. 4-151).
- *Shield gonads.*
- *Respiration:* Suspend.

Central ray
- Perpendicular to the mid-portion of the humerus and the center of the IR

Collimation
- 2 inches (5 cm) distal to the elbow joint and superior to the shoulder and 1 inch (2.5 cm) on the sides

Structures shown
The AP projection shows the entire length of the humerus. The accuracy of the position is shown by the epicondyles (Fig. 4-152).

The following should be clearly shown:
- Evidence of proper collimation
- Elbow and shoulder joints
- Maximal visibility of epicondyles without rotation
- Humeral head and greater tubercle in profile
- Outline of the lesser tubercle, located between the humeral head and the greater tubercle
- Beam divergence possibly partially closing the elbow joint
- No great variation in radiographic densities of the proximal and distal humerus

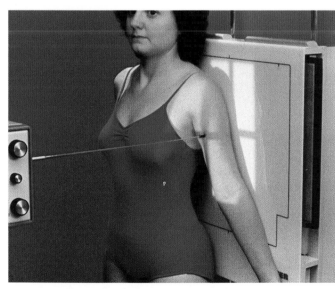

Fig. 4-151 Upright position for AP humerus.

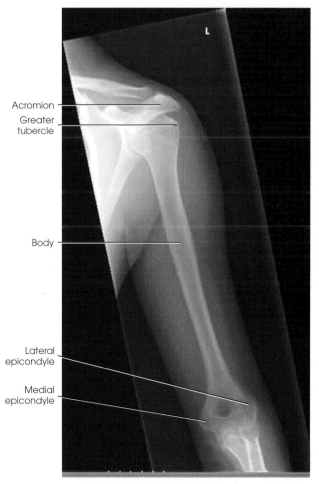

Acromion
Greater tubercle
Body
Lateral epicondyle
Medial epicondyle

Fig. 4-152 Upright AP humerus.

♠ LATERAL PROJECTION
Lateromedial, mediolateral
Upright

Image receptor: 7 × 17 inch (18 × 43 cm); 14 × 17 inch (35 × 43 cm)

Position of patient
- Place the patient in a seated-upright or standing position facing the x-ray tube. The body position, whether oblique or facing toward or away from the IR, is not critical as long as a true projection of the lateral arm is obtained.

Position of part
- Place the top margin of the IR approximately 1½ inches (3.8 cm) above the level of the head of the humerus.

- Unless contraindicated by possible fracture, internally rotate the arm, flex the elbow approximately 90 degrees, and place the patient's anterior hand on the hip. This places the humerus in lateral position. A coronal plane passing through the epicondyles should be perpendicular with the IR plane (Fig. 4-153).
- A patient with a broken humerus may be easier to position by performing a *mediolateral* projection as shown in Fig. 4-154. Face the sitting or standing patient toward the IR and incline the thorax as necessary to align the humerus for the mediolateral projection. If the patient is not already holding the hand of the broken arm, have the patient do so.
- *Shield gonads.*
- *Respiration:* Suspend.

Central ray
- Perpendicular to the mid-portion of the humerus and the center of the IR

Collimation
- 2 inches (5 cm) distal to the elbow joint and superior to the shoulder and 1 inch (2.5 cm) on the sides

Structures shown
The lateral projection shows the entire length of the humerus. A true lateral image is confirmed by superimposed epicondyles (Fig. 4-155).

EVALUATION CRITERIA

The following should be clearly shown:
- Evidence of proper collimation
- Elbow and shoulder joints
- Superimposed epicondyles
- Lesser tubercle in profile
- Greater tubercle superimposed over the humeral head
- Beam divergence possibly partially closing the elbow joint
- No great variation in radiographic densities of the proximal and distal humerus

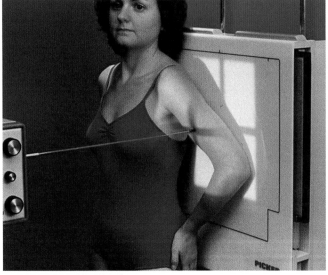

Fig. 4-153 Upright position for lateral humerus. Note hand placement on hip.

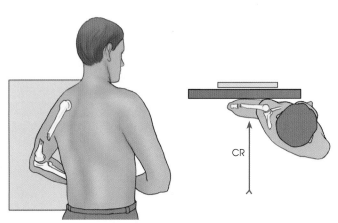

Fig. 4-154 A patient with broken humerus may be easier to position for *mediolateral* projection as shown.

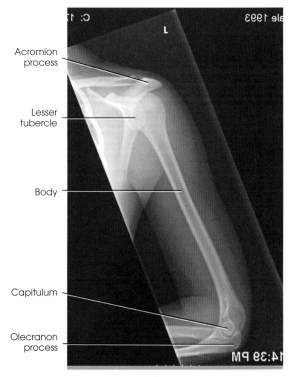

Acromion process
Lesser tubercle
Body
Capitulum
Olecranon process

Fig. 4-155 Upright lateral humerus.

AP PROJECTION
Recumbent

The IR size selected should be long enough to include the entire humerus.

Image receptor: Lengthwise—7 × 17 inch (18 × 43 cm); 14 × 17 (35 × 43 cm)

Position of patient

• With the patient in the supine position, adjust the IR to include the entire length of the humerus.

Position of part

• Place the upper margin of the IR approximately 1½ inches (3.8 cm) above the humeral head.
• Elevate the opposite shoulder on a sandbag to place the affected arm in contact with the IR, or elevate the arm and IR on sandbags.

• Unless contraindicated, supinate the hand and adjust the limb to place the epicondyles parallel with the plane of the IR (Fig. 4-156).
• *Shield gonads.*
• *Respiration:* Suspend.

Central ray

• Perpendicular to the mid-portion of the humerus and the center of the IR

Collimation

• 2 inches (5 cm) distal to the elbow joint and superior to the shoulder and 1 inch (2.5 cm) on the sides

Structures shown

The AP projection shows the entire length of the humerus. The accuracy of the position is shown by the epicondyles (see Fig. 4-156).

The following should be clearly shown:
■ Evidence of proper collimation
■ Elbow and shoulder joints
■ Maximal visibility of epicondyles without rotation
■ Humeral head and greater tubercle in profile
■ Outline of the lesser tubercle, located between the humeral head and the greater tubercle
■ Beam divergence possibly partially closing the elbow joint
■ No great variation in radiographic densities of the proximal and distal humerus

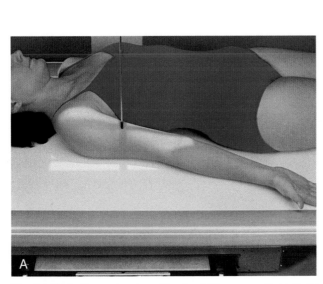

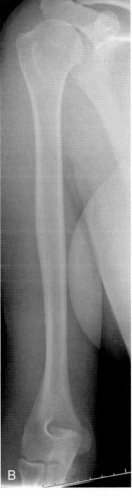

Fig. 4-156 A, Recumbent position for AP humerus. Note that hand is supinated. **B,** AP humerus in correct position.

⚜ LATERAL PROJECTION
Lateromedial
Recumbent

Position of patient
- Place the patient in the supine position with the humerus centered to the IR, or use a Bucky tray.

Position of part
- Adjust the top of the IR to be approximately 1½ inches (3.8 cm) above the level of the head of the humerus.
- Unless contraindicated by possible fracture, abduct the arm and center the IR under it.
- Rotate the forearm medially to place the epicondyles perpendicular to the plane of the IR, and rest the *posterior aspect* of the hand against the patient's side. This movement turns the epicondyles in the lateral position without flexing the elbow (see Fig. 4-153). (The elbow may be flexed slightly for comfort.)

- Adjust the position of the IR to include the entire length of the humerus (Fig. 4-157).
- *Shield gonads.*
- *Respiration:* Suspend.

Central ray
- Perpendicular to the mid-portion of the humerus and the center of the IR

Collimation
- 2 inches (5 cm) distal to the elbow joint and superior to the shoulder and 1 inch (2.5 cm) on the sides

Structures shown
The lateral projection shows the entire length of the humerus. A true lateral image is confirmed by superimposed epicondyles (see Fig. 4-157).

EVALUATION CRITERIA
The following should be clearly shown:
- Evidence of proper collimation
- Elbow and shoulder joints
- Superimposed epicondyles
- Lesser tubercle in profile
- Greater tubercle superimposed over the humeral head
- Beam divergence possibly partially closing the elbow joint
- No great variation in radiographic densities of the proximal and distal humerus

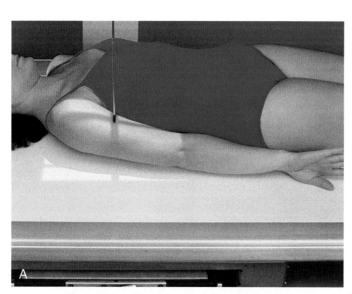

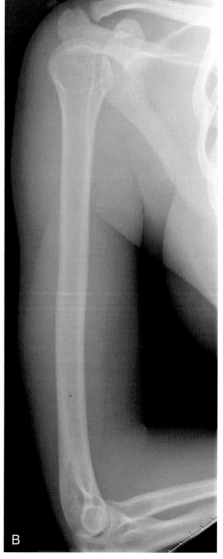

Fig. 4-157 A, Recumbent position for lateral humerus. Note posterior aspect of the patient's hand against thigh. **B,** Lateral humerus, supine position. Note epicondyles are perpendicular to IR. Distal aspect of forearm could not be included because of patient's condition, separate lateral elbow was performed.

⚛ LATERAL PROJECTION
Lateromedial
Recumbent or lateral recumbent

Position of patient
- When a known or suspected fracture exists, position the patient in the recumbent or lateral recumbent position, place the IR close to the axilla, and center the humerus to the midline of the IR.
- Unless contraindicated, flex the elbow, turn the thumb surface of the hand up, and rest the humerus on a suitable support (Fig. 4-158).
- Adjust the position of the body to place the lateral surface of the humerus perpendicular to the central ray.
- *Shield gonads.*
- *Respiration:* Suspend.

Central ray
Recumbent
- Horizontal and perpendicular to the mid-portion of the humerus and the center of the IR
Lateral recumbent
- Directed to the center of the IR, which exposes only the distal humerus (see Fig. 4-158)

Collimation
- 2 inches (5 cm) distal to the elbow joint and 1 inch (2.5 cm) on the sides; top collimator margin should extend no further than edge of the IR

Structures shown
The lateral projection shows the distal humerus (Fig. 4-159).

EVALUATION CRITERIA
The following should be clearly shown:
- Evidence of proper collimation
- Distal humerus
- Superimposed epicondyles

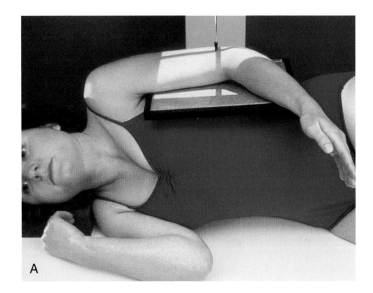

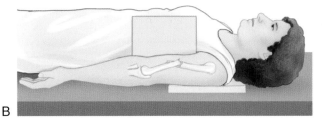

Fig. 4-158 A, Lateral recumbent body position to show distal lateral humerus. **B,** Patient and IR positioned for trauma cross-table lateral projection of humerus.

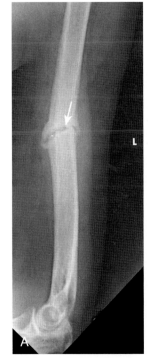
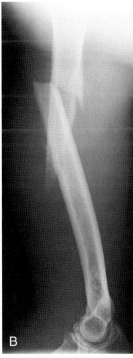

Fig. 4-159 A, Lateral recumbent humerus, showing healing fracture (*arrow*). **B,** Lateral recumbent humerus showing comminuted fracture. Radiograph had to be obtained using lateral recumbent position owing to the patient's pain.

5

SHOULDER GIRDLE

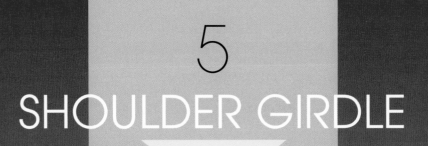

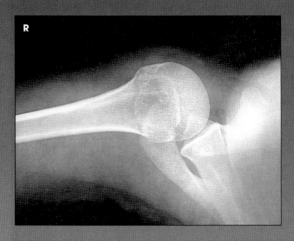

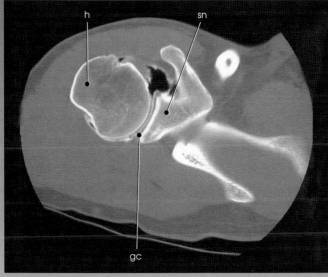

PROJECTIONS, POSITIONS, AND METHODS

Page	Essential	Anatomy	Projection	Position	Method
183	🪶	Shoulder	AP	External, neutral, internal, rotation humerus	
188	🪶	Shoulder joint: *glenoid cavity*	AP oblique	RPO or LPO	GRASHEY
190		Shoulder joint: *glenoid cavity*	AP oblique	RPO or LPO	APPLE
192	🪶	Shoulder	Transthoracic lateral	R or L	LAWRENCE
194	🪶	Shoulder joint	Inferosuperior axial		LAWRENCE
194		Shoulder joint	Inferosuperior axial		RAFERT ET AL. MODIFICATION
196		Shoulder joint	Inferosuperior axial		WEST POINT
198		Shoulder joint	Superoinferior axial		
199	🪶	Shoulder joint: *scapular Y*	PA oblique	RAO or LAO	
202		Shoulder joint: *supraspinatus "outlet"*	Tangential	RAO or LAO	NEER
203		Shoulder joint	AP axial		
204		Shoulder joint: *proximal humerus*	AP axial		STRYKER "NOTCH"
205		Shoulder joint: *glenoid cavity*	AP axial oblique	RPO or LPO	GARTH
207	🪶	Proximal humerus: *intertubercular groove*	Tangential		FISK MODIFICATION
209	🪶	Acromioclavicular articulations	AP	Bilateral	PEARSON
211		Acromioclavicular articulations	AP axial		ALEXANDER
213	🪶	Clavicle	AP		
214	🪶	Clavicle	AP axial	Lordotic	
215	🪶	Clavicle	PA		
215	🪶	Clavicle	PA axial		
216	🪶	Scapula	AP		
218	🪶	Scapula	Lateral	RAO or LAO	
220		Scapula	AP oblique	RPO or LPO	
222		Scapula: *coracoid process*	AP axial		
224		Scapular spine	Tangential		LAQUERRIÈRE-PIERQUIN

The icons in the Essential column indicate projections frequently performed in the United States and Canada. Students should become competent in these projections.

Shoulder Girdle

The *shoulder girdle* is formed by two bones—the *clavicle* and *scapula*. The function of these bones is to connect the upper limb to the trunk. Although the alignment of these two bones is considered a girdle, it is incomplete in front and in back. The girdle is completed in front by the sternum, which articulates with the medial end of the clavicle. The scapulae are widely separated in the back. The proximal portion of the humerus is part of the upper limb and not the shoulder girdle proper; however, because the proximal humerus is included in the shoulder joint, its anatomy is considered with that of the shoulder girdle (Figs. 5-1 and 5-2).

Clavicle

The *clavicle,* classified as a long bone, has a body and two articular extremities (see Fig. 5-1). The clavicle lies in a horizontal oblique plane just above the first rib and forms the anterior part of the shoulder girdle. The lateral aspect is termed the *acromial extremity,* and it articulates with the acromion process of the scapula. The *medial* aspect, termed the *sternal extremity,* articulates with the manubrium of the sternum and the first costal cartilage. The clavicle, which serves as a fulcrum for the movements of the arm, is doubly curved for strength. The curvature is more acute in males than in females.

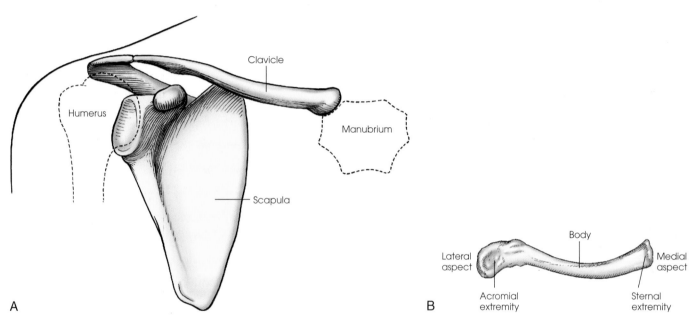

Fig. 5-1 **A,** Anterior aspect of shoulder girdle: clavicle and scapula. Girdle attaches to humerus and manubrium of sternum. **B,** Superior aspect of right clavicle.

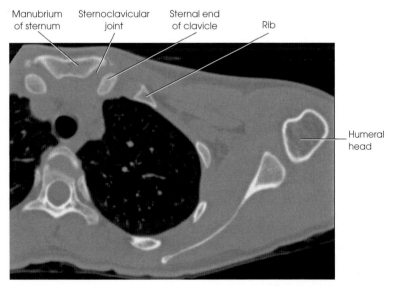

Fig. 5-2 Axial CT scan of shoulder showing relationship of anatomy. Note 45- to 60-degree angle of scapula.

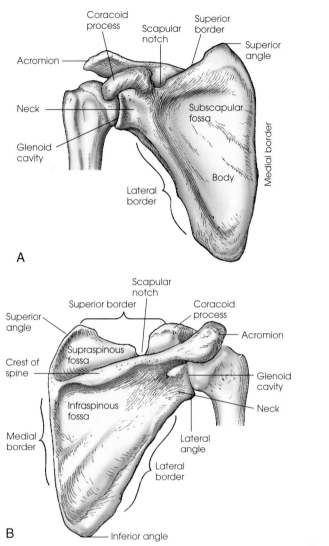

Fig. 5-3 Scapula. **A,** Costal surface (anterior aspect). **B,** Dorsal surface (posterior aspect).

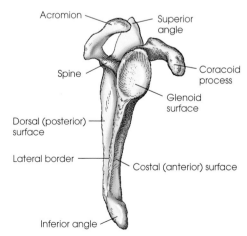

Fig. 5-4 Lateral aspect of scapula.

Scapula

The *scapula,* classified as a flat bone, forms the posterior part of the shoulder girdle (Figs. 5-3 and 5-4). Triangular in shape, the scapula has two surfaces, three borders, and three angles. Lying on the superoposterior thorax between the second and seventh ribs, the *medial border* of the scapula runs parallel with the vertebral column. The body of the bone is arched from top to bottom for greater strength, and its surfaces serve as the attachment sites of numerous muscles. The flat aspect of the bone lies at about a 45- to 60-degree angle in relation to the anatomic position (see Fig. 5-2).

The *costal (anterior) surface* of the scapula is slightly concave and contains the *subscapular fossa.* It is filled almost entirely by the attachment of the subscapularis muscle. The anterior serratus muscle attaches to the medial border of the costal surface from the *superior angle* to the *inferior angle.*

The *dorsal (posterior) surface* is divided into two portions by a prominent spinous process. The *crest of spine* arises at the superior third of the medial border from a smooth, triangular area and runs obliquely superior to end in a flattened, ovoid projection called the *acromion.* The area above the spine is called the *supraspinous fossa* and gives origin to the supraspinatus muscle. The infraspinatus muscle arises from the portion below the spine, which is called the *infraspinous fossa.* The teres minor muscle arises from the superior two thirds of the lateral border of the dorsal surface, and the teres major arises from the distal third and the inferior angle. The dorsal surface of the medial border affords attachment of the levator muscles of the scapulae, greater rhomboid muscle, and lesser rhomboid muscle.

The *superior border* extends from the superior angle to the *coracoid process* and at its lateral end has a deep depression, the *scapular notch.* The *medial border* extends from the superior to the inferior angles. The *lateral border* extends from the *glenoid cavity* to the inferior angle.

The *superior angle* is formed by the junction of the superior and medial borders. The *inferior angle* is formed by the junction of the medial (vertebral) and lateral borders and lies over the seventh rib. The *lateral angle,* the thickest part of the body of the scapula, ends in a shallow, oval depression called the *glenoid cavity.* The constricted region around the glenoid cavity is called the *neck* of the scapula. The coracoid process arises from a thick base that extends from the scapular notch to the superior portion of the neck of the scapula. This process projects first anteriorly and medially and then curves on itself to project laterally. The coracoid process can be palpated just distal and slightly medial to the acromioclavicular articulation.

Humerus

The proximal end of the *humerus* consists of a head, an anatomic neck, two prominent processes called the *greater* and *lesser tubercles,* and the surgical neck (Fig. 5-5). The *head* is large, smooth, and rounded, and it lies in an oblique plane on the superomedial side of the humerus. Just below the head, lying in the same oblique plane, is the narrow, constricted *anatomic neck.* The constriction of the body just below the tubercles is called the *surgical neck,* which is the site of many fractures.

The *lesser tubercle* is situated on the anterior surface of the bone, immediately below the anatomic neck (Figs. 5-6 and 5-7; see Fig. 5-5). The tendon of the sub-scapular muscle inserts at the lesser tubercle. The *greater tubercle* is located on the lateral surface of the bone, just below the anatomic neck, and is separated from the lesser tubercle by a deep depression called the *intertubercular (bicipital) groove.* The superior surface of the greater tubercle slopes posteriorly at an angle of approximately 25 degrees and has three flattened impressions for muscle insertions. The anterior impression is the highest of the three and affords attachment to the tendon of the supraspinatus muscle. The middle impression is the point of insertion of the infraspinatus muscle. The tendon of the upper fibers of the teres minor muscle inserts at the posterior impression (the lower fibers insert into the *body* of the bone immediately below this point).

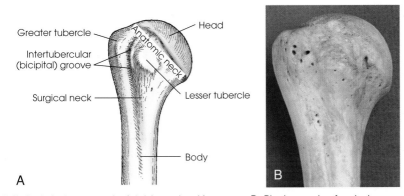

A

Fig. 5-5 **A,** Anterior aspect of right proximal humerus. **B,** Photograph of anterior aspect of proximal humerus.

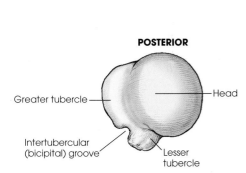

Fig. 5-6 Superior aspect of humerus.

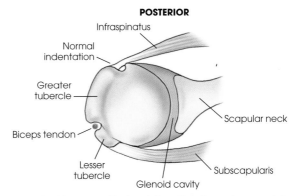

Fig. 5-7 Superior aspect of humerus. Horizontal section through scapulohumeral joint showing normal anatomic relationships.

177

Bursae are small, synovial fluid–filled sacs that relieve pressure and reduce friction in tissue. They are often found between the bones and the skin, and they allow the skin to move easily when the joint is moved. Bursae are found also between bones and ligaments, muscles, or tendons. One of the largest bursae of the shoulder is the *subacromial bursa* (Fig. 5-8). It is located under the acromion process and lies between the deltoid muscle and the shoulder joint capsule. The subacromial bursa does not normally communicate with the joint. Other bursae of the shoulder are found superior to the acromion, between the coracoid process and the joint capsule, and between the capsule and the tendon of the subscapular muscle. Bursae become important radiographically when injury or age causes the deposition of calcium.

Shoulder Girdle Articulations

The three joints of the shoulder girdle are summarized in Table 5-1, and a detailed description follows.

SCAPULOHUMERAL ARTICULATION

The *scapulohumeral articulation* between the glenoid cavity and the head of the humerus forms a *synovial ball-and-socket* joint, allowing movement in all directions (Figs. 5-9 and 5-10). This joint is often referred to as the *glenohumeral* joint. Although many muscles connect with, support, and enter into the function of the shoulder joint, radiographers are chiefly concerned with the insertion points of the short rotator cuff muscles (Fig. 5-11). The insertion points of these muscles—the subscapular, supraspinatus, infraspinatus, and teres minor—have already been described.

TABLE 5-1

Joints of the shoulder girdle

Joint	Structural classification		
	Tissue	Type	Movement
Scapulohumeral	Synovial	Ball and socket	Freely movable
Acromioclavicular	Synovial	Gliding	Freely movable
Sternoclavicular	Synovial	Double gliding	Freely movable

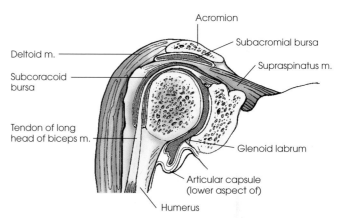

Fig. 5-8 Right shoulder bursae and muscles.

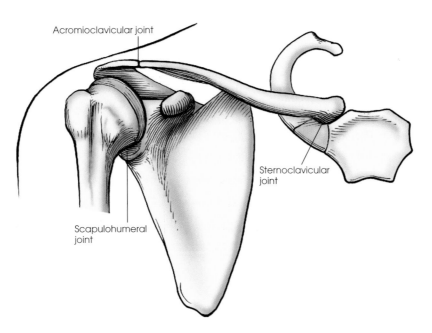

Fig. 5-9 Articulations of scapula and humerus.

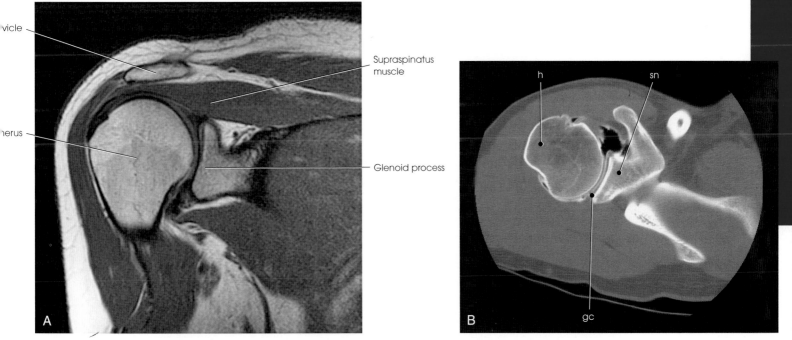

Fig. 5-10 A, Coronal MRI of shoulder. Note articular cartilage around humeral head and muscles closely surrounding bone. **B,** Axial CT of shoulder, mid-joint. Note position of bones relative to each other and articular cartilage in glenoid cavity. *gc,* glenoid cavity; *h,* humerus; *sn,* scapular neck.

(From Kelley LL, Petersen CM: *Sectional anatomy for imaging professionals,* ed 2, St Louis, 2007, Mosby.)

An articular capsule completely encloses the shoulder joint. The tendon of the long head of the biceps brachii muscle, which arises from the superior margin of the glenoid cavity, passes through the capsule of the shoulder joint, goes between its fibrous and synovial layers, arches over the head of the humerus, and descends through the intertubercular (bicipital) groove. The short head of the biceps arises from the coracoid process and, with the long head of the muscle, inserts in the radial tuberosity. Because it crosses with the shoulder and elbow joints, the biceps help synchronize their action.

The interaction of movement among the wrist, elbow, and shoulder joints makes the position of the hand important in radiography of the upper limb. Any rotation of the hand also rotates the joints. The best approach to the study of the mechanics of joint and muscle action is to perform all movements ascribed to each joint and carefully note the reaction in remote parts.

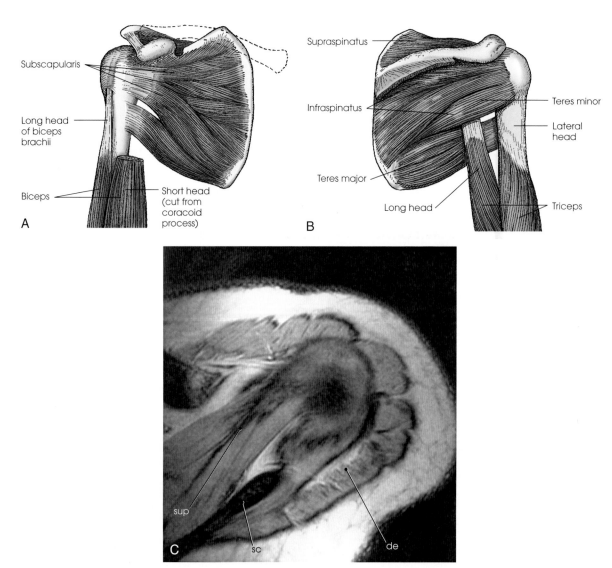

Fig. 5-11 A, Muscles on costal (anterior) surface of scapula and proximal humerus. **B,** Muscles on dorsal (posterior) surface of scapula and proximal humerus. **C,** Axial MRI of shoulder (view from top) showing muscles of shoulder. Supraspinatus (*sup*) and deltoid (*de*) muscles are shown. Note scapular spine (*sc*) for reference.

(From Kelley LL, Petersen CM: *Sectional anatomy for imaging professionals,* ed 2, St Louis, 2007, Mosby.)

ACROMIOCLAVICULAR ARTICULATION

The *acromioclavicular* (AC) articulation between the *acromion* process of the scapula and the acromial extremity of the *clavicle* forms a *synovial gliding joint* (see Fig. 5-12). It permits gliding and rotary (elevation, depression, protraction, and retraction) movement. Because the end of the clavicle rides higher than the adjacent surface of the acromion, the slope of the surfaces tends to favor displacement of the acromion downward and under the clavicle.

STERNOCLAVICULAR ARTICULATION

The *sternoclavicular* (SC) articulation is formed by the sternal extremity of the clavicle with two bones: the manubrium and the first rib cartilage (see Fig. 5-12). The union of the clavicle with the manubrium of the sternum is the only bony union between the upper limb and trunk. This articulation is a *synovial double-gliding* joint. The joint is adapted by a fibrocartilaginous disk, however, to provide movements similar to a ball-and-socket joint: circumduction, elevation, depression, and forward and backward movements. The clavicle carries the scapula with it through any movement.

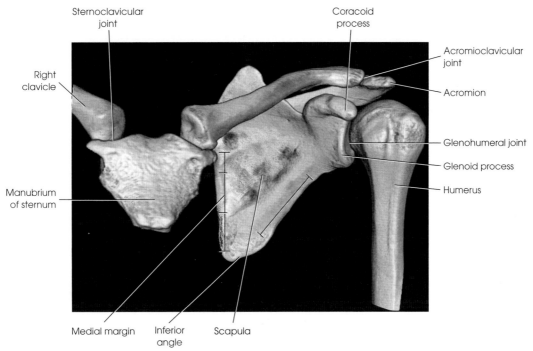

Fig. 5-12 Three-dimensional CT image of shoulder girdle. Note three articulations.

SUMMARY OF ANATOMY

Shoulder girdle	Dorsal surface	**Humerus (proximal aspect)**
Clavicle	Crest of spine	
Scapula	Acromion	Head
	Supraspinous fossa	Anatomic neck
Clavicle	Infraspinous fossa	Surgical neck
Body	Superior border	Intertubercular groove
Acromial extremity	Coracoid process	Greater tubercles
Sternal extremity	Scapular notch	Lesser tubercles
	Lateral border	Body
Scapula	Glenoid cavity	Bursae
Medial border	Lateral angle	Subacromial bursa
Body	Neck	
Costal surface		**Shoulder articulations**
Subscapular fossa		Scapulohumeral
Superior angle		Acromioclavicular
Inferior angle		Sternoclavicular

ABBREVIATIONS USED IN CHAPTER 5

AC	Acromioclavicular
SC	Sternoclavicular

See Addendum A for a summary of all abbreviations used in Volume 1.

SUMMARY OF PATHOLOGY

Condition	Definition
Bursitis	Inflammation of the bursa
Dislocation	Displacement of a bone from the joint space
Fracture	Disruption in the continuity of bone
Hills-Sachs defect	Impacted fracture of posterolateral aspect of the humeral head with dislocation
Metastases	Transfer of a cancerous lesion from one area to another
Osteoarthritis or degen-erative joint disease	Form of arthritis marked by progressive cartilage deterioration in synovial joints and vertebrae
Osteopetrosis	Increased density of atypically soft bone
Osteoporosis	Loss of bone density
Rheumatoid arthritis	Chronic, systemic, inflammatory collagen disease
Tendinitis	Inflammation of the tendon and tendon-muscle attachment
Tumor	New tissue growth where cell proliferation is uncontrolled
Chondrosarcoma	Malignant tumor arising from cartilage cells

EXPOSURE TECHNIQUE CHART ESSENTIAL PROJECTIONS

SHOULDER GIRDLE

Part	cm	kVp*	tm	mA	mAs	AEC	SID	IR	Dose† (mrad)
Shoulder—*AP*‡	18	75		200s		•	40"	24 × 30 cm	41
Shoulder—*Transthoracic lateral*‡	40	80		200s		•	40"	24 × 30 cm	914
Shoulder—*Axillary*§	18	75	.08	200s	16		40"	10 × 12 in	59
Shoulder—*PA Oblique Scapular Y*‡	24	85	.08	200s	16		40"	24 × 30 cm	115
Intertubercular Gr.¶	3	55	.01	200s	2		40"	8 × 10 in	13
AC Articulation—*AP*‡	14	70	.15	200s	30		72"	18 × 43 cm	90
Clavicle—*AP, PA*‡	16	70	.06	200s	12		40"	24 × 30 cm	36
Scapula—*AP*‡	18	75		200s			40"	24 × 30 cm	41
Scapula—*Lateral*‡	24	85	.08	200s	16	•	40"	24 × 30 cm	115

*kVp values are for a three-phase, 12-pulse generator or high frequency.
†Relative doses for comparison use. All doses are skin entrance for average adult at cm indicated.
‡Bucky, 16:1 grid. Screen-film speed 300.
§Tabletop, 8:1 grid. Screen-film speed 300.
¶Tabletop, standard IR. Screen-film speed 300 or equivalent CR.
s, small focal spot.

Radiation Protection

Protection of the patient from unnecessary radiation is a professional responsibility of the radiographer (see Chapters 1 and 2 for specific guidelines). In this chapter, the *Shield gonads* statement at the end of the *Position of part* section indicates that the patient is to be protected from unnecessary radiation by using proper collimation *and* placing lead shielding between the gonads and the radiation source to restrict the radiation beam.

PROJECTIONS REMOVED

The following projections have been removed from the atlas because of the increased use of CT and MRI for imaging the shoulders. The projections may be reviewed in their entirety in the eleventh edition and all previous editions.
Shoulder joint
- Inferosuperior axial, Clements method
Acromioclavicular articulations
- PA axial oblique, Alexander method
Clavicle
- Tangential
Scapula
- PA oblique, Lorenz, Lilienfeld method
- Tangential

Shoulder

AP PROJECTION

External, neutral, internal rotation humerus

NOTE: Do not have the patient rotate the arm if fracture or dislocation is suspected.

Image receptor: 10 × 12 inch (24 × 30 cm) crosswise

Position of patient

- Examine the patient in the upright or supine position, with coronal plane of thorax parallel to IR. Shoulder and arm lesions, whether traumatic or pathologic in origin, are extremely sensitive to movement and pressure. For this reason, the upright position should be used whenever possible.

Position of part

- Center the shoulder joint to the midline of the grid.
- Adjust the position of the IR so that its center is 1 inch (2.5 cm) inferior to the coracoid process.

TABLE 5-2

Hand position and its effect on the proximal humerus

Description	Hand position	Proximal humerus position
Supinating hand and adjusting epicondyles parallel to the plane of the IR positions the humerus in *external rotation*	A	B AP shoulder. External rotation humerus. Greater tubercle (*arrow*).
Palm of the hand placed against hip and epicondyles adjusted at about a 45-degree angle with the plane of the IR positions the humerus in *neutral rotation*	A	B AP shoulder. Neutral rotation humerus. Greater tubercle (*arrows*).
Posterior aspect of hand may be placed against hip and epicondyles adjusted perpendicular to the plane of the IR to position the humerus in *internal rotation*	A	B AP shoulder. Internal rotation humerus. Greater tubercle (*arrows*); lesser tubercle in profile (*arrowhead*).

External rotation humerus:
- Ask the patient to supinate the hand, unless contraindicated (Table 5-2).
- Abduct the arm slightly, and rotate it so that the epicondyles are parallel with the plane of the IR. Externally rotating the entire arm from the neutral position places the shoulder and entire humerus in the true anatomic position (Fig. 5-13).

Neutral rotation humerus:
- Ask the patient to rest the palm of the hand against the thigh (see Table 5-2). This position of the arm rolls the humerus slightly internal into a neutral position, placing the epicondyles at an angle of about 45 degrees with the plane of the IR.

Internal rotation humerus:
- Ask the patient to flex the elbow, rotate the arm internally, and rest the back of the hand on the hip (see Table 5-2).
- Adjust the arm to place the epicondyles perpendicular to the plane of the IR.
- *Shield gonads.*
- *Respiration:* Suspend.

Central ray
- Perpendicular to a point 1 inch (2.5 cm) inferior to the coracoid process

Collimation
- Adjust to 10 × 12 inches (24 × 30 cm) on the collimator.

◣ COMPENSATING FILTER
Use of a specially designed compensating filter for the shoulder improves the quality of the image. These filters are particularly useful when digital imaging (CR or DR) systems are used for this projection.

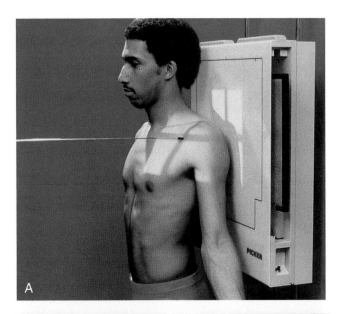

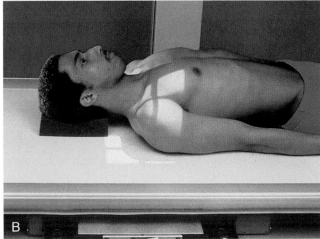

Fig. 5-13 A, AP shoulder, external rotation humerus, standing position. **B,** Same projection in supine position.

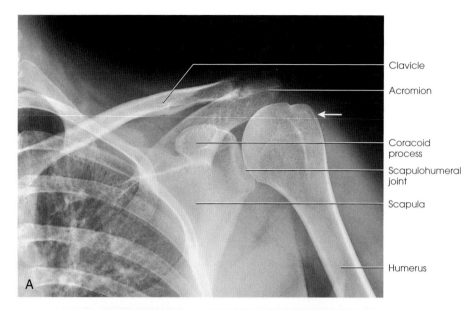

Clavicle

Acromion

Coracoid process

Scapulohumeral joint

Scapula

Humerus

A

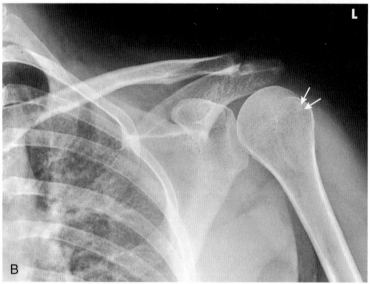

L

B

Fig. 5-14 A, AP shoulder, external rotation humerus: greater tubercle in profile (*arrow*). **B,** AP shoulder, neutral rotation humerus: greater tubercle (*arrow*).

Structures shown

The image shows the bony and soft structures of the shoulder and proximal humerus in the anatomic position (Figs. 5-14 to 5-16). The scapulohumeral joint relationship is seen.

External rotation: The greater tubercle of the humerus and the site of insertion of the supraspinatus tendon are visualized (see Fig. 5-14, *A*).

Neutral rotation: The posterior part of the supraspinatus insertion, which sometimes profiles small calcific deposits not otherwise visualized (see Fig. 5-14, *B*), is seen.

Internal rotation: The proximal humerus is seen in a true lateral position. When the arm can be abducted enough to clear the lesser tubercle of the head of the scapula, a profile image of the site of the insertion of the subscapular tendon is seen (see Fig. 5-15).

EVALUATION CRITERIA

The following should be clearly shown:
- Evidence of proper collimation
- Superior scapula, lateral half of the clavicle, and proximal humerus
- Soft tissue around the shoulder, along with bony trabecular detail
  External rotation:
- Humeral head in profile
- Greater tubercle in profile on lateral aspect of the humerus
- Scapulohumeral joint visualized with slight overlap of humeral head on glenoid cavity
- Outline of lesser tubercle between the humeral head and greater tubercle
  Neutral rotation:
- Greater tubercle partially superimposing the humeral head
- Humeral head in partial profile
- Slight overlap of the humeral head on the glenoid cavity
  Internal rotation:
- Lesser tubercle in profile and pointing medially
- Outline of the greater tubercle superimposing the humeral head
- Greater amount of humeral overlap of the glenoid cavity than in the external and neutral positions

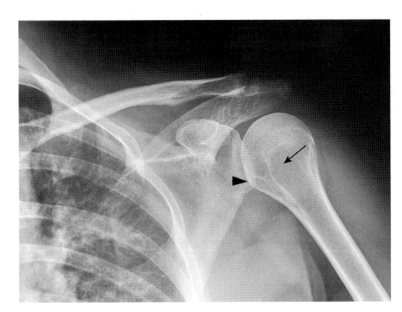

Fig. 5-15 AP shoulder, internal rotation humerus: greater tubercle (*arrow*); lesser tubercle in profile (*arrowhead*).

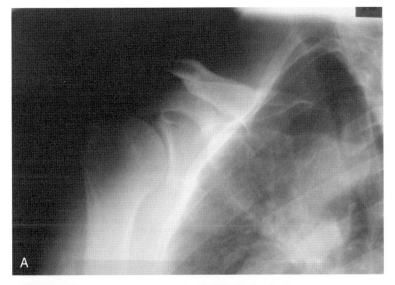

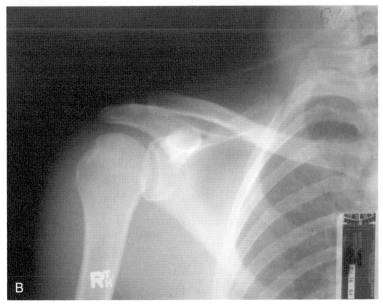

Fig. 5-16 **A,** AP oblique projection of right shoulder without use of compensating filter. **B,** AP projection of same patient with compensating filter. Note improvement of visualization of bony and soft tissue areas with filter.

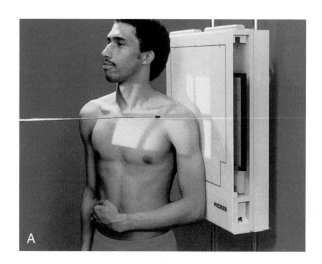

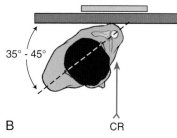

Fig. 5-17 A, Upright AP oblique glenoid cavity: Grashey method. **B,** Note position of shoulder and patient in relationship to IR.

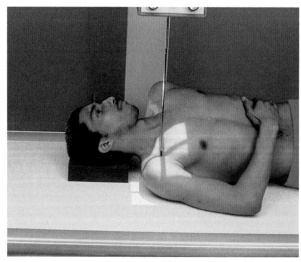

Fig. 5-18 Recumbent AP oblique glenoid cavity: Grashey method.

Glenoid Cavity
♠ AP OBLIQUE PROJECTION
GRASHEY METHOD
RPO or LPO position

Image receptor: 8 × 10 inch (18 × 24 cm) crosswise

Position of patient
- Place the patient in the supine or upright position. The upright position is more comfortable for the patient and assists in accurate adjustment of the part.

Position of part
- Center the IR to the scapulohumeral joint. The joint is 2 inches (5 cm) medial and 2 inches (5 cm) inferior to the superolateral border of the shoulder.
- Rotate the body approximately 35 to 45 degrees toward the affected side (Fig. 5-17).
- Adjust the degree of rotation to place the scapula parallel with the plane of the IR. This is accomplished by orienting the plane through the superior angle of the scapula and acromial tip, parallel to the IR.* The head of the humerus is in contact with the IR.
- If the patient is in the recumbent position, the body may need to be rotated more than 45 degrees (up to 60 degrees) to place the scapula parallel to the IR.
- Support the elevated shoulder and hip on sandbags (Fig. 5-18).
- Abduct the arm slightly in internal rotation, and place palm of the hand on the abdomen.
- *Shield gonads.*
- *Respiration:* Suspend.

*NOTE: These landmarks are recommended by Johnston et al.[1] as useful to identify the plane through the scapular body.

[1]Johnston J et al: Landmarks for lateral scapula and scapular Y positioning, *Radiol Technol* 79:397, 2008.

Central ray

• Perpendicular to the IR; the central ray should be at a point 2 inches (5 cm) medial and 2 inches (5 cm) inferior to the superolateral border of the shoulder

Collimation

• Adjust to 8 × 10 inches (18 × 24 cm) on the collimator.

Structures shown

The joint space between the humeral head and the glenoid cavity (scapulohumeral joint) is shown (Figs. 5-19 and 5-20).

EVALUATION CRITERIA

The following should be clearly shown:
■ Evidence of proper collimation
■ Open joint space between the humeral head and glenoid cavity
■ Glenoid cavity in profile
■ Soft tissue at the scapulohumeral joint along with trabecular detail on the glenoid and humeral head

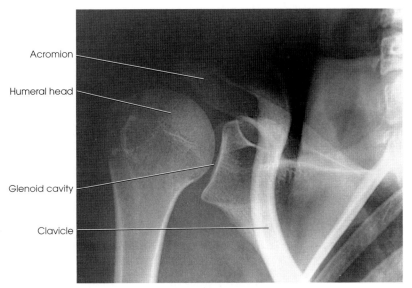

Acromion

Humeral head

Glenoid cavity

Clavicle

Fig. 5-19 AP oblique glenoid cavity: Grashey method.

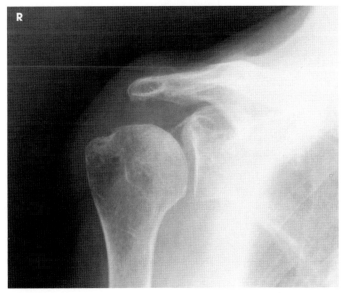

Fig. 5-20 AP oblique glenoid cavity: Grashey method showing moderate deterioration of scapulohumeral joint.

Glenoid Cavity
AP OBLIQUE PROJECTION
APPLE METHOD
RPO or LPO position

The Apple method[1] is similar to the Grashey method but uses weighted abduction to show a loss of articular cartilage in the scapulohumeral joint.

Image receptor: 10 × 12 inch (24 × 30 cm) crosswise

[1]Apple A et al: The weighted abduction Grashey shoulder method, *Radiol Technol* 69:151, 1997.

Position of patient
- Place the patient in a seated or upright position.

Position of part
- Center the IR to the scapulohumeral joint.
- Rotate the body approximately 35 to 45 degrees toward the affected side.
- The posterior surface of affected side is closest to the IR.

- The scapula should be positioned parallel to the plane of the IR (see Grashey method for positioning details).
- The patient should hold a 1-lb weight in the hand on the same side as the affected shoulder in a neutral position.
- While holding the weight, the patient should abduct the arm 90 degrees from the midline of the body (Fig. 5-21).
- *Shield gonads.*
- *Respiration:* Suspend.

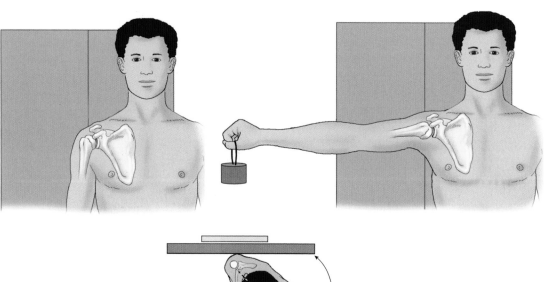

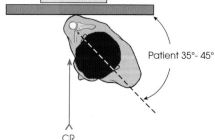

Fig. 5-21 Axial oblique projection: Apple method.

Central ray

- Perpendicular to the IR at the level of the coracoid process

NOTE: To avoid motion, have the correct technical factors set on the generator and be ready to make the exposure before the patient abducts the arm.

Structures shown

The scapulohumeral joint (Fig. 5-22) is seen.

The following should be clearly shown:
- Open joint space between the humeral head and the glenoid cavity
- Glenoid cavity in profile
- Soft tissue at the scapulohumeral joint along with trabecular detail on the glenoid and the humeral head
- The arm in a 90-degree position

RESEARCH: Catherine E. Hearty, MS, RT(R), performed the research and provided this new projection for this edition of the atlas.

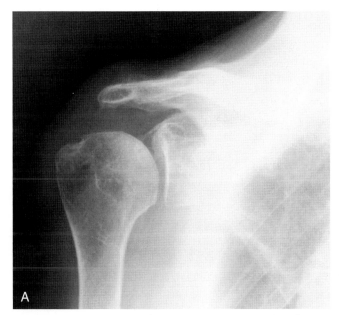 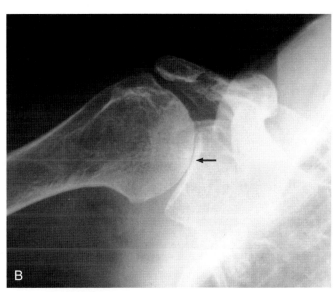

Fig. 5-22 A, AP oblique projection: Grashey method, with shoulder showing normal scapulohumeral joint space. **B,** AP oblique projection: Apple method, with weighted abduction showing loss of articular cartilage (*arrow*).

TRANSTHORACIC LATERAL PROJECTION
LAWRENCE METHOD
R or L position

The Lawrence[1] method is used when trauma exists, and the arm cannot be rotated or abducted because of an injury. This projection shows the proximal humerus in a 90-degree projection from the AP projection and shows its relationship to the scapula and clavicle.

Image receptor: 10 × 12 inch (24 × 30 cm) lengthwise

Position of patient

- Although this projection can be carried out with the patient in the upright or supine position, the upright position is much easier on a trauma patient. It also assists accurate adjustment of the shoulder.

---

[1]Lawrence WS: A method of obtaining an accurate lateral roentgenogram of the shoulder joint, *AJR Am J Roentgenol* 5:193, 1918.

- For upright positioning, seat or stand the patient in the lateral position before a vertical grid device (Fig. 5-23).
- If an upright position is impossible, place the patient in a recumbent position on the table with radiolucent pads elevating the head and shoulders (Fig. 5-24).

Position of part

- Have the patient raise the noninjured arm, rest the forearm on the head, and elevate the shoulder as much as possible (see Fig. 5-23). Elevation of the noninjured shoulder drops the injured side, separating the shoulders to prevent superimposition. Ensure that the midcoronal plane is perpendicular to the IR.
- No attempt should be made to rotate or otherwise to move the injured arm.
- Center the IR to the surgical neck area of the affected humerus.

- *Shield gonads.*
- *Respiration:* Full inspiration. Having the lungs full of air improves the contrast and decreases the exposure necessary to penetrate the body.
- If the patient can be sufficiently immobilized to prevent voluntary motion, a breathing technique can be used. In this case, instruct the patient to practice slow, deep breathing. A minimum exposure time of 3 seconds (4 to 5 seconds is desirable) gives excellent results when a low milliamperage is used.

Central ray

- Perpendicular to the IR, entering the midcoronal plane at the level of the surgical neck
- If the patient cannot elevate the unaffected shoulder, angle the central ray 10 to 15 degrees cephalad to obtain a comparable radiograph.

Collimation

- Adjust to 10 × 12 inches (24 × 30 cm) on the collimator. The field of light on the skin appears smaller than this size because of the distance from the IR. Do not collimate larger than stated size.

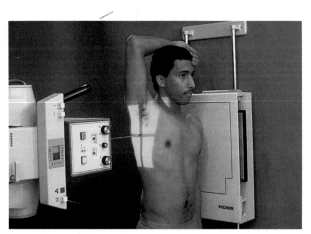

Fig. 5-23 Upright transthoracic lateral shoulder: Lawrence method.

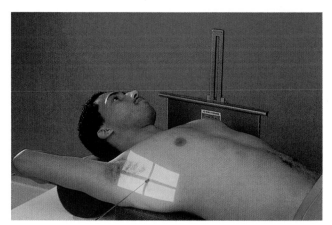

Fig. 5-24 Recumbent transthoracic lateral shoulder: Lawrence method.

Structures shown

A lateral image of the shoulder and proximal humerus is projected through the thorax (Figs. 5-25 and 5-26).

EVALUATION CRITERIA

The following should be clearly shown:
- Evidence of proper collimation
- Proximal humerus
- Scapula, clavicle, and humerus seen through the lung field
- Scapula superimposed over the thoracic spine
- Unaffected clavicle and humerus projected above the shoulder closest to the IR

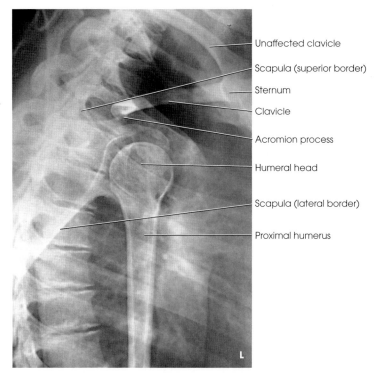

Unaffected clavicle
Scapula (superior border)
Sternum
Clavicle
Acromion process
Humeral head
Scapula (lateral border)
Proximal humerus

Fig. 5-25 Transthoracic lateral shoulder: Lawrence method.

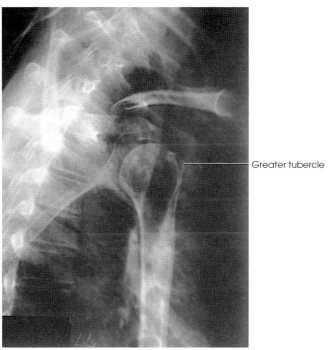

Greater tubercle

Fig. 5-26 Transthoracic lateral shoulder (patient breathing): Lawrence method.

♠ INFEROSUPERIOR AXIAL PROJECTION
LAWRENCE METHOD[1]

INFEROSUPERIOR AXIAL PROJECTION
RAFERT ET AL.[2] MODIFICATION

Image receptor: 10 × 12 inch (24 × 30 cm) grid crosswise, placed in the vertical position in contact with the superior surface of the shoulder

Position of patient
• With the patient in the supine position, elevate the head, shoulders, and elbow about 3 inches (7.6 cm).

Position of part
Lawrence method
• As much as possible, abduct the arm of the affected side at right angles to the long axis of the body.
• Keep the humerus in *external rotation,* and adjust the forearm and hand in a comfortable position, grasping a vertical support or extended on sandbags or a firm pillow. Support may be necessary under the forearm and hand. Provide the patient with an extension board for the arm.
• Have the patient turn the head away from the side being examined so that the IR can be placed against the neck.
• Place the IR on edge against the shoulder and as close as possible to the neck.

• Support the IR in position with sandbags, or use a vertical IR holder (Fig. 5-27).
Rafert modification
• Anterior dislocation of the humeral head can result in a wedge-shaped compression fracture of the articular surface of the humeral head, called the *Hill-Sachs defect.*[1] The fracture is located on the posterolateral humeral head. An *exaggerated external rotation* of the arm may be required to see the defect.
• With the patient in position exactly as for the Lawrence method, externally rotate the extended arm until the hand forms a 45-degree oblique angle. The thumb is pointing downward (Fig. 5-28).
• Assist the patient in rotating the arm to avoid overstressing the shoulder joint.
• *Shield gonads.*
• *Respiration:* Suspend.

Central ray
Lawrence method
• Horizontally through the axilla to the region of the AC articulation. The degree of medial angulation of the central ray depends on the degree of abduction of the arm. The degree of medial angulation is often between 15 degrees and 30 degrees. The greater the abduction, the greater the angle.
Rafert modification
• Horizontal and angled approximately 15 degrees medially, entering the axilla and passing through the AC joint.

Collimation
• Adjust to 12 inches (30 cm) in length and 1 inch (2.5 cm) above the anterior shadow of the shoulder.

Structures shown
An inferosuperior axial image shows the proximal humerus, the scapulohumeral joint, the lateral portion of the coracoid process, and the AC articulation. The insertion site of the subscapular tendon on the lesser tubercle of the humerus and the point of insertion of the teres minor tendon on the greater tubercle of the humerus are also shown. A Hill-Sachs compression fracture on the posterolateral humeral head may be seen using the Rafert modification (Figs. 5-29 and 5-30).

The following should be clearly shown:
■ Evidence of proper collimation
■ Scapulohumeral joint with slight overlap
■ Coracoid process, pointing anteriorly
■ Lesser tubercle in profile and directed anteriorly
■ AC joint, acromion, and acromial end of clavicle projected through the humeral head
■ Soft tissue in the axilla with bony trabecular detail

[1]Lawrence WS: New position in radiographing the shoulder joint, *AJR Am J Roentgenol* 2:728, 1915.
[2]Rafert JA et al: Axillary shoulder with exaggerated rotation: the Hill-Sachs defect, *Radiol Technol* 62:18, 1990.

[1]Hill H, Sachs M: The grooved defect of the humeral head: a frequently unrecognized complication of dislocations of the shoulder joint, *Radiology* 35:690, 1940.

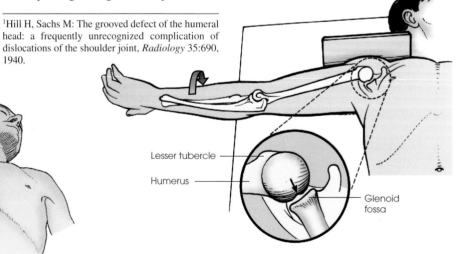

Lesser tubercle
Humerus
Glenoid fossa

Fig. 5-28 Inferosuperior axial shoulder joint: Rafert modification. Note exaggerated external rotation of arm and thumb pointing downward. If present, a Hill-Sachs defect would show as a wedge-shaped depression on posterior aspect of articulating surface of humeral head (*arrow*).

(From Rafert JA et al: Axillary shoulder with exaggerated rotation: the Hill-Sachs defect, *Radiol Technol* 62:18, 1990.)

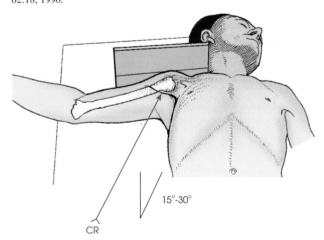

15°-30°

CR

Fig. 5-27 Inferosuperior axial shoulder joint: Lawrence method.

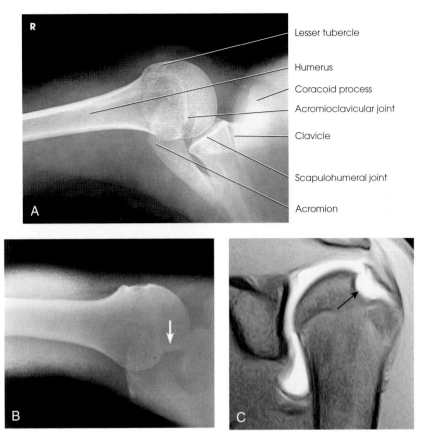

Lesser tubercle

Humerus

Coracoid process

Acromioclavicular joint

Clavicle

Scapulohumeral joint

Acromion

Fig. 5-29 A, Inferosuperior axial shoulder joint: Lawrence method. **B,** Inferosuperior axial shoulder joint: Rafert modification showing Hill-Sachs defect (*arrow*). **C,** Coronal MRI of shoulder joint showing Hill-Sachs defect (*arrow*) after recurring shoulder dislocation.

(**A** and **B,** From Rafert JA et al: Axillary shoulder with exaggerated rotation: the Hill-Sachs defect, *Radiol Technol* 62:18, 1990. **C,** From Jackson SA, Thomas RM: *Cross-sectional imaging made easy,* New York, 2004, Churchill Livingstone.)

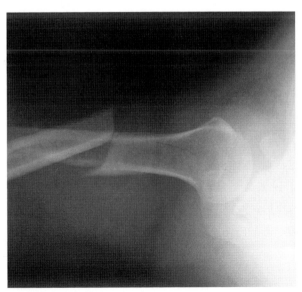

Fig. 5-30 Inferosuperior axial shoulder joint: Lawrence method showing comminuted fracture of humerus. The patient came into emergency department with arm extended out.

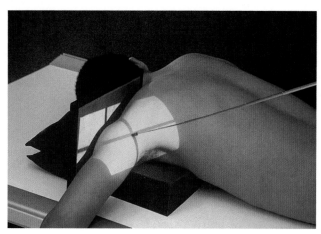

Fig. 5-31 Inferosuperior axial shoulder joint: West Point method.

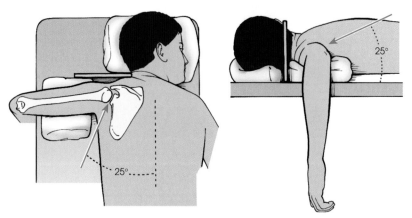

Fig. 5-32 West Point method with anterior and medial central ray angulation.

INFEROSUPERIOR AXIAL PROJECTION

WEST POINT METHOD

The West Point[1] method is used when chronic instability of the shoulder is suspected and to show bony abnormalities of the anterior inferior glenoid rim. Associated Hill-Sachs defect of the posterior lateral aspect of the humeral head is also shown.

Image receptor: 8 × 10 inch (18 × 24 cm) crosswise placed in the vertical position in contact with the superior surface of the shoulder

Position of patient

- Adjust the patient in the prone position with approximately a 3-inch (7.6-cm) pad under the shoulder being examined.
- Turn the patient's head away from the side being examined.

Position of part

- Abduct the arm of the affected side *90 degrees,* and rotate so that the forearm rests over the edge of the table or a Bucky tray, which may be used for support (Figs. 5-31 and 5-32).
- Place a vertically supported IR against the superior aspect of the shoulder with the edge of the IR in contact with the neck.
- Support the IR with sandbags or a vertical IR holder.
- *Shield gonads.*
- *Respiration:* Suspend.

---

[1]Rokous JR et al: Modified axillary roentgenogram, *Clin Orthop Relat Res* 82:84, 1972.

Central ray

- Directed at a dual angle of 25 degrees *anteriorly* from the horizontal and 25 degrees *medially*. The central ray enters approximately 5 inches (13 cm) inferior and 1½ inch (3.8 cm) medial to the acromial edge and exits the glenoid cavity.

Structures shown

The resulting image shows bony abnormalities of the anterior inferior rim of the glenoid and Hill-Sachs defects of the posterolateral humeral head in patients with chronic instability of the shoulder (Fig. 5-33).

EVALUATION CRITERIA

The following should be clearly shown:
- Humeral head projected free of the coracoid process
- Articulation between the head of the humerus and the glenoid cavity
- Acromion superimposed over the posterior portion of the humeral head
- Shoulder joint

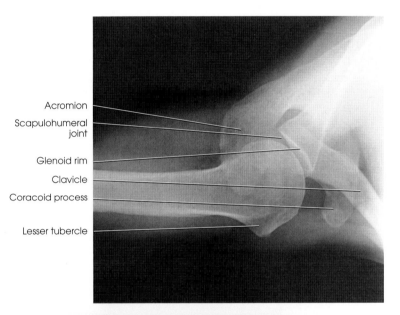

Acromion
Scapulohumeral joint
Glenoid rim
Clavicle
Coracoid process
Lesser tubercle

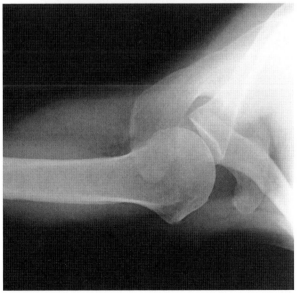

Fig. 5-33 Inferosuperior axial shoulder joint: West Point method.

Shoulder Joint

SUPEROINFERIOR AXIAL PROJECTION

Image receptor: 8 × 10 inch (18 × 24 cm) placed lengthwise for accurate centering to shoulder joint

Position of patient

- Seat the patient at the end of the table on a stool or chair high enough to enable extension of the shoulder under examination well over the IR.

Position of part

- Place the IR near the end of the table and parallel with its long axis.
- Have the patient lean laterally over the IR until the shoulder joint is over the midpoint of the IR.
- Bring the elbow to rest on the table.
- Flex the patient's elbow 90 degrees, and place the hand in the prone position (Fig. 5-34).
- Have the patient tilt the head toward the unaffected shoulder.
- To obtain direct lateral positioning of the head of the humerus, adjust any anterior or posterior leaning of the body to place the humeral epicondyles in the vertical position.
- *Shield gonads.*
- *Respiration:* Suspend.

Central ray

- Angled 5 to 15 degrees through the shoulder joint and toward the elbow; a greater angle is required when the patient cannot extend the shoulder over the IR.

Structures shown

A superoinferior axial image shows the joint relationship of the proximal end of the humerus and the glenoid cavity (Fig. 5-35). The AC articulation, the outer portion of the coracoid process, and the points of insertion of the subscapularis muscle (at body of scapula) and teres minor muscle (at inferior axillary border) are shown.

The following should be clearly shown:
- Scapulohumeral joint (not open on patients with limited flexibility)
- Coracoid process projected above the clavicle
- Lesser tubercle in profile
- AC joint through the humeral head

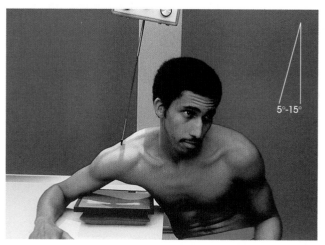

Fig. 5-34 Superoinferior axial shoulder joint: standard IR.

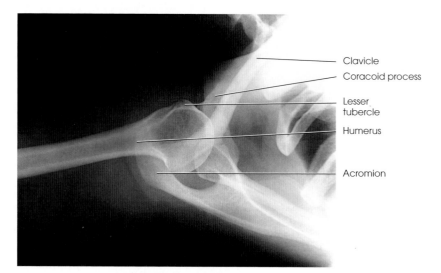

Clavicle
Coracoid process
Lesser tubercle
Humerus
Acromion

Fig. 5-35 Superoinferior axial shoulder joint.

Scapular Y

⚘ PA OBLIQUE PROJECTION

RAO or LAO position

This projection, described by Rubin et al.,[1] obtained its name as a result of the appearance of the scapula. The body of the scapula forms the vertical component of the Y, and the acromion and coracoid processes form the upper limbs. This projection is useful in the evaluation of suspected shoulder dislocations.

Image receptor: 10 × 12 inch (24 × 30 cm) lengthwise

[1]Rubin SA et al: The scapular Y: a diagnostic aid in shoulder trauma, *Radiology* 110:725, 1974.

Position of patient

- Radiograph the patient in the upright or recumbent body position; the upright position is preferred.
- When the patient is severely injured, modify the anterior oblique position by placing the patient in the posterior oblique position.

Position of part

- Position the anterior surface of the shoulder being examined against the upright table.
- Rotate the patient so that the midcoronal plane forms an angle of 45 to 60 degrees to the IR. The position of the arm is not critical because it does not alter the relationship of the humeral head to the glenoid cavity (Fig. 5-36). Palpate the scapula, and place its flat surface perpendicular to the IR. According to Johnson et al.,[1] this is accomplished by orienting the plane through the superior angle of the scapula and acromial tip, perpendicular to the IR.

- Position the center of the IR at the level of the scapulohumeral joint.
- *Shield gonads.*
- *Respiration:* Suspend.

▼ COMPENSATING FILTER

Use of a specially designed compensating filter for the shoulder improves the quality of the image because of the large amount of primary beam radiation striking the IR. These filters are particularly useful when digital imaging (CR or DR) systems are used with this projection.

[1]Johnston J et al: Landmarks for lateral scapula and scapular Y positioning, *Radiol Technol* 79:397, 2008.

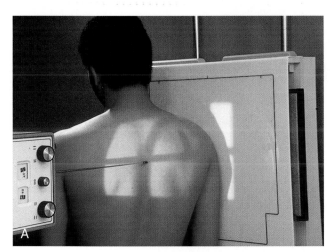
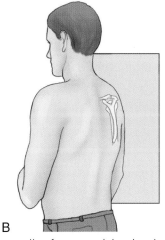
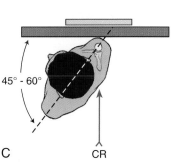

45° - 60°

CR

Fig. 5-36 A, PA oblique shoulder joint. **B,** Perspective from x-ray tube showing scapula centered in true lateral position. **C,** Top-down view showing positioning landmarks used for proper orientation of scapular body.

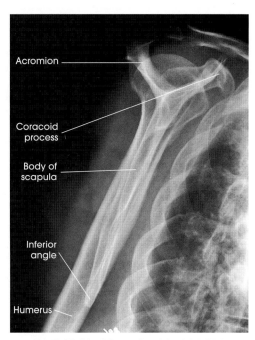
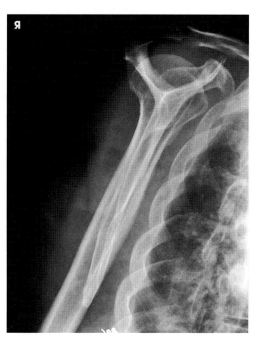

Acromion

Coracoid process

Body of scapula

Inferior angle

Humerus

Fig. 5-37 PA oblique shoulder joint. Note scapular Y components—body, acromion, and coracoid.

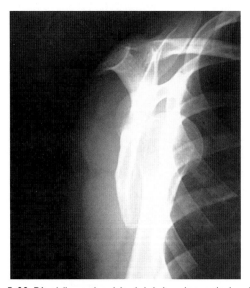

Fig. 5-38 PA oblique shoulder joint showing anterior dislocation (humeral head projected beneath coracoid process).

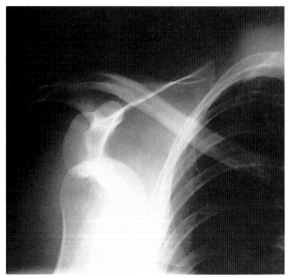

Fig. 5-39 AP shoulder (same patient as in Fig. 5-38).

Shoulder Joint

Central ray
- Perpendicular to the scapulohumeral joint (Table 5-3)

Collimation
- Adjust to 12 inches (30 cm) in length and 1 inch (2.5 cm) from the lateral shadow.

Structures shown
The scapular Y is shown on an oblique image of the shoulder. In the normal shoulder, the humeral head is directly superimposed over the junction of the Y (Fig. 5-37). In anterior (subcoracoid) dislocations, the humeral head is beneath the coracoid process (Fig. 5-38); in posterior (subacromial) dislocations, it is projected beneath the acromion process. An AP shoulder projection is shown for comparison (Fig. 5-39).

Shoulder Joint

TABLE 5-3
Similar shoulder projections

Name	Body rotation (degrees)	Scapula relationship to IR	Central ray angle*	Central ray entrance point*	Arm position*
Shoulder joint: Neer method	45-60	Perpendicular	10-15 degrees border caudad	Superior humeral	At side
Shoulder joint: scapular Y	45-60	Perpendicular	0 degrees	Scapulohumeral joint	At side
Scapula lateral	45-60	Perpendicular	0 degrees	Center of medial border of scapula	Variable

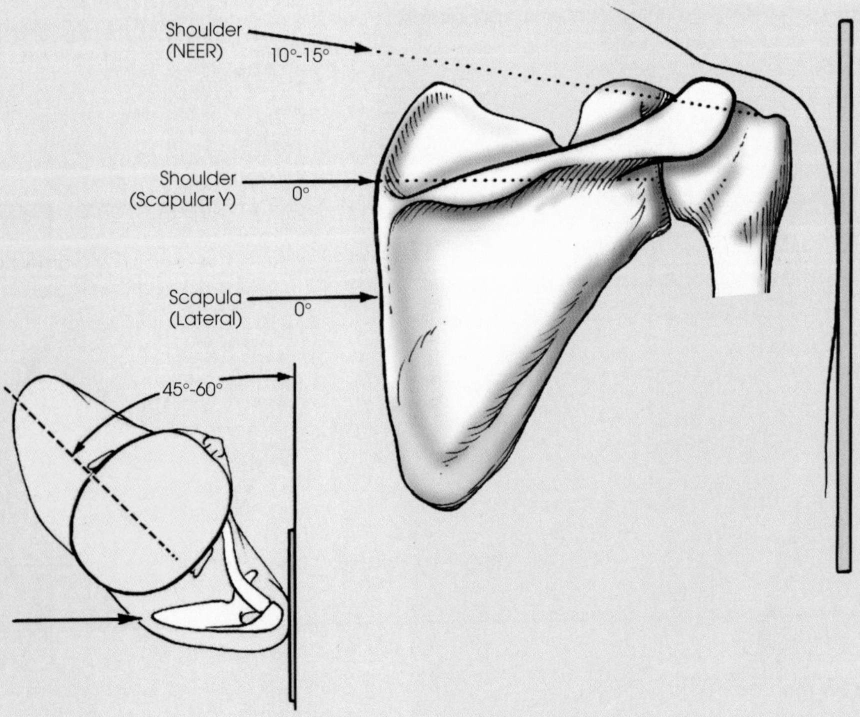

*Central ray angles and entrance points and arm positions are the only differences among these three projections.

Supraspinatus "Outlet"
TANGENTIAL PROJECTION
NEER METHOD

RAO or LAO position

This radiographic projection is useful to show tangentially the coracoacromial arch or outlet to diagnose shoulder impingement.[1,2] The tangential image is obtained

[1]Neer CS II: Supraspinatus outlet, *Orthop Trans* 11:234, 1987.
[2]Neer CS II: *Shoulder reconstruction,* Philadelphia, 1990, Saunders, pp 14-24.

by projecting the x-ray beam under the acromion and AC joint, which defines the superior border of the coracoacromial outlet.

Image receptor: 8 × 10 inch (18 × 24 cm) lengthwise

Position of patient

- Place the patient in a seated or standing position facing the vertical grid device.

Position of part

- With the patient's affected shoulder centered and in contact with the IR, rotate the patient's unaffected side away from the IR. Palpate the flat aspect of the affected scapula and place it perpendicular to the IR. The degree of patient obliquity varies from patient to patient. The average degree of patient rotation varies from 45 to 60 degrees from the plane of the IR (Fig. 5-40).
- Place the patient's arm at the patient's side.
- *Shield gonads.*
- *Respiration:* Suspend.

Central ray

- Angled 10 to 15 degrees caudad, entering the superior aspect of the humeral head (see Table 5-3)

Structures shown

The tangential outlet image shows the posterior surface of the acromion and the AC joint identified as the superior border of the coracoacromial outlet (Figs. 5-41 and 5-42).

EVALUATION CRITERIA

The following should be clearly shown:
- Humeral head projected below the AC joint
- Humeral head and AC joint with bony detail
- Humerus and scapular body, generally parallel

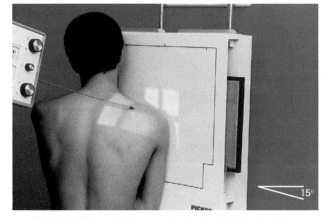

Fig. 5-40 Tangential supraspinatus "outlet" projection.

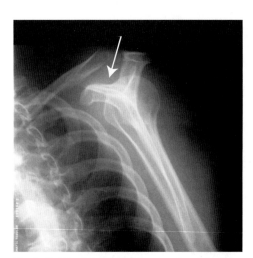

Fig. 5-41 Shoulder joint: Neer method. Supraspinatus outlet (*arrow*).

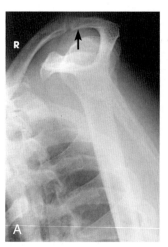 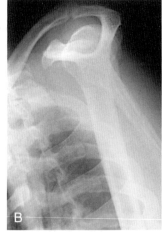

Fig. 5-42 A, Tangential supraspinatus outlet projection showing impingement of shoulder outlet by subacromial spur (*arrow*). **B,** Radiograph of same patient as in Fig. 5-41 after surgical removal of posterolateral surface of clavicle.

Shoulder Girdle

Shoulder Joint

AP AXIAL PROJECTION

Image receptor: 8 × 10 inch (18 × 24 cm) crosswise

Position of patient
- Position the patient in the upright or supine position.

Position of part
- Center the scapulohumeral joint of the shoulder being examined to the midline of the grid (Fig. 5-43).
- *Shield gonads.*
- *Respiration:* Suspend.

Central ray
- Directed through the scapulohumeral joint at a cephalic angle of 35 degrees

Structures shown
The axial image shows the relationship of the head of the humerus to the glenoid cavity. This is useful in diagnosing cases of posterior dislocation (Fig. 5-44).

EVALUATION CRITERIA
The following should be clearly shown:
- Scapulohumeral joint
- Proximal humerus
- Clavicle projected above superior angle of scapula

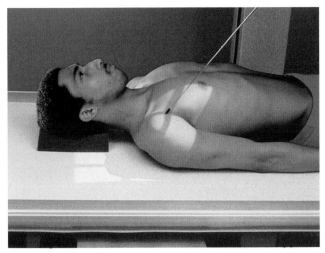

Fig. 5-43 AP axial shoulder joint.

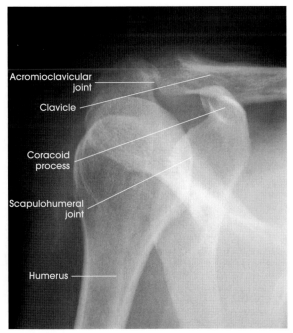
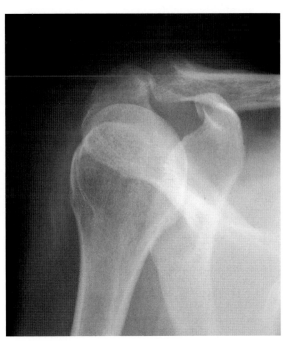

Fig. 5-44 AP axial shoulder joint.

Proximal Humerus
AP AXIAL PROJECTION
STRYKER NOTCH METHOD

Anterior dislocations of the shoulder frequently result in posterior defects involving the posterolateral head of the humerus. Such defects, called *Hill-Sachs defects,*[1] are often not shown using conventional radiographic positions. Hall et al.[2] described the notch projection, from ideas expressed by Stryker, as being useful to show this humeral defect.

Image receptor: 10 × 12 inch (24 × 30 cm)

Position of patient
- Place the patient on the radiographic table in the supine position.

---

[1]Hill H, Sachs M: The grooved defect of the humeral head: a frequently unrecognized complication of dislocations of the shoulder joint, *Radiology* 35:690, 1940.
[2]Hall RH et al: Dislocations of the shoulder with special reference to accompanying small fractures, *J Bone Joint Surg Am* 41:489, 1959.

Position of part
- With the coracoid process of the affected shoulder centered to the table, ask the patient to flex the arm slightly beyond 90 degrees and place the palm of the hand on top of the head with fingertips resting on the head. (This hand position places the humerus in a slight internal rotation position.) The body of the humerus is adjusted to be vertical so that it is parallel to the midsagittal plane of the body (Fig. 5-45).
- *Shield gonads.*
- *Respiration:* Suspend.

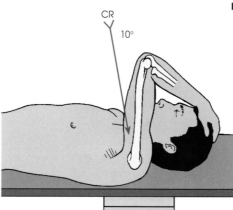

Fig. 5-45 AP axial humeral notch: Stryker notch method.

Central ray
- Angled 10 degrees cephalad, entering the coracoid process

Structures shown
The resulting image shows the posterosuperior and posterolateral areas of the humeral head (Figs. 5-46 and 5-47).

EVALUATION CRITERIA

The following should be clearly shown:
- Overlapping of coracoid process and clavicle
- Posterolateral lateral aspect of humeral head in profile
- Long axis of the humerus aligned with the long axis of the patient's body
- Bony trabeculation of the head of the humerus

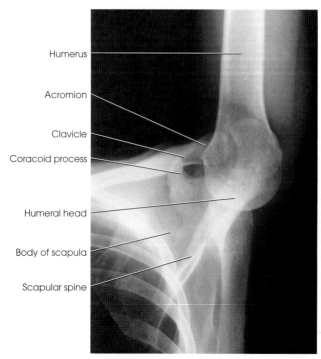

Fig. 5-46 AP axial humeral notch: Stryker notch method.

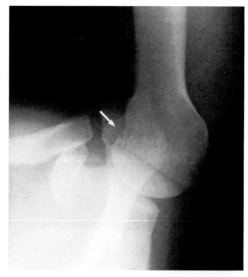

Fig. 5-47 Same projection as in Fig. 5-46 in a patient with small Hill-Sachs defect (*arrow*).

Glenoid Cavity

AP AXIAL OBLIQUE PROJECTION

GARTH METHOD

RPO or LPO position

This projection is recommended for acute shoulder trauma and for identifying posterior scapulohumeral dislocations, glenoid fractures, Hill-Sachs lesions, and soft tissue calcifications.[1]

Image receptor: 10 × 12 inch (24 × 30 cm) lengthwise

Position of patient

- Place the patient in the supine, seated, or upright position.

---

[1]Garth W et al: Roentgenographic demonstration of instability of the shoulder: the apical oblique projection, *J Bone Joint Surg Am* 66:1450, 1984.

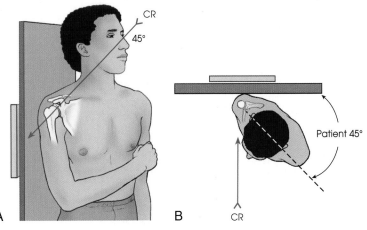

Fig. 5-48 A, AP axial oblique: Garth method, RPO position. Note 45-degree central ray (*CR*). **B,** Top view of same position as in **A.** Note 45-degree patient position.

Position of part

- Center the IR to the glenohumeral joint.
- Rotate the body approximately 45 degrees toward the affected side.
- The posterior surface of the affected side is closest to the IR.
- Flex the elbow of the affected arm and place arm across the chest (Fig. 5-48).
- *Shield gonads.*
- *Respiration:* Suspend.

Central ray

- Angled 45 degrees caudad through the scapulohumeral joint

Structures shown

The scapulohumeral joint, humeral head, coracoid process, and scapular head and neck are shown (Fig. 5-49).

EVALUATION CRITERIA

The following should be clearly shown:
- The scapulohumeral joint, humeral head, lateral angle, and scapular neck free of superimposition
- The coracoid process should be well visualized.
- Posterior dislocations project the humeral head *superiorly* from the glenoid cavity, and anterior dislocations project *inferiorly.*

RESEARCH: Catherine E. Hearty, MS, RT(R), performed the research and provided this new projection for this edition of the atlas.

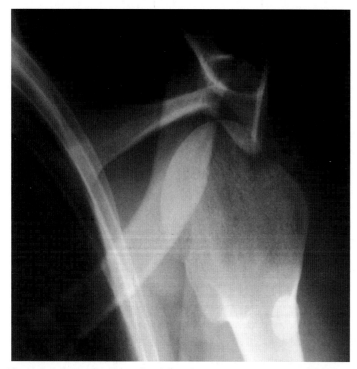

Fig. 5-49 AP axial oblique: Garth method showing anterior dislocation of proximal humerus. Humeral head is shown below coracoid process, a common appearance with anterior dislocation.

(Courtesy Bruce W. Long, MS, RT(R)(CV), and John A. Rafert, MS, RT(R).)

Intertubercular Groove
♠ TANGENTIAL PROJECTION
FISK MODIFICATION

In recent years, various modifications of the intertubercular groove image have been devised. In all cases, the central ray is aligned to be tangential to the intertubercular groove, which lies on the anterior surface of the humerus.[1]

The x-ray tube head assembly may limit the performance of this examination. Some radiographic units have large collimators or handles, or both, that limit flexibility in positioning. A mobile radiographic unit may be used to reduce this difficulty.

Image receptor: 8 × 10 inch (18 × 24 cm)

[1]Fisk C: Adaptation of the technique for radiography of the bicipital groove, *Radiol Technol* 34:47, 1965.

Position of patient
- Place the patient in the supine, seated, or standing position.
- To improve centering, extend the chin or rotate the head away from the affected side.

Position of part
- With the patient supine, palpate the anterior surface of the shoulder to locate the intertubercular groove.
- With the patient's hand in the supinated position, place the IR against the superior surface of the shoulder and immobilize the IR as shown in Fig. 5-50.
- *Shield gonads.*
- *Respiration:* Suspend.

Fisk modification Fisk first described this position with the patient standing at the end of the radiographic table. This employs a greater OID. The following steps are then taken with Fisk's technique:
- Instruct the patient to flex the elbow and lean forward far enough to place the posterior surface of the forearm on the table. The patient supports and grasps the IR as depicted in Fig. 5-51.
- For radiation protection and to reduce backscatter to the film from the forearm, place a lead shielding between the IR back and the forearm.
- Place a sandbag under the hand to place the IR horizontal.
- Have the patient lean forward or backward as required to place the vertical humerus at an angle of 10 to 15 degrees.

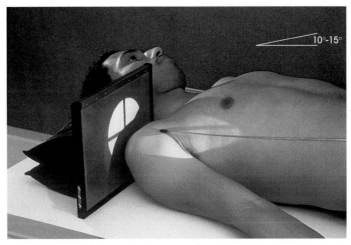

Fig. 5-50 Supine tangential intertubercular groove.

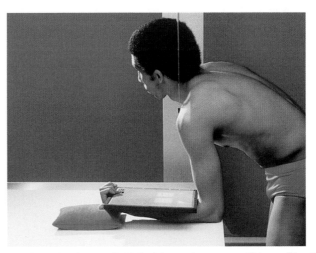

Fig. 5-51 Standing tangential intertubercular groove: Fisk modification.

Central ray
- Angled 10 to 15 degrees posterior (downward from horizontal) to the long axis of the humerus for the supine position (see Fig. 5-50)
  Fisk modification
- Perpendicular to the IR when the patient is leaning forward and the vertical humerus is positioned 10 to 15 degrees (see Fig. 5-51)

Collimation
- Adjust to 4 × 4 inches (10 × 10 cm) on the collimator.

Structures shown
The tangential image profiles the intertubercular groove free from superimposition of the surrounding shoulder structures (Figs. 5-52 and 5-53).

EVALUATION CRITERIA
The following should be clearly shown:
- Evidence of proper collimation
- Intertubercular groove in profile
- Soft tissue along with enhanced visibility of the intertubercular groove

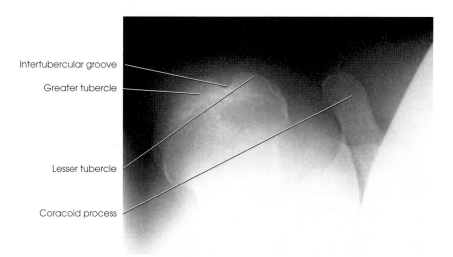

Intertubercular groove
Greater tubercle
Lesser tubercle
Coracoid process

Fig. 5-52 Supine tangential intertubercular groove.

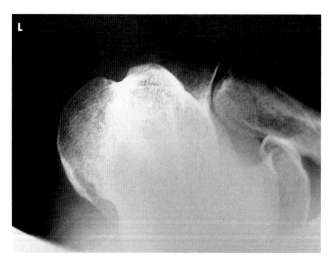

Fig. 5-53 Standing tangential intertubercular groove: Fisk modification.

AP PROJECTION
Bilateral
PEARSON METHOD

Image receptor: 7 × 17 inch (18 × 43 cm) or two 8 × 10 inch (18 × 24 cm), as needed to fit the patient

SID: 72 inches (183 cm). A longer SID reduces magnification, which enables both joints to be included on one image. It also reduces the distortion of the joint space resulting from central ray divergence.

Position of patient
• Place the patient in an upright body position, either seated or standing, because dislocation of the AC joint tends to reduce itself in the recumbent position. The positioning is easily modified to obtain a PA projection.

Position of part
• Place the patient in the upright position before a vertical grid device, and adjust the height of the IR so that the midpoint of the IR lies at the same level as the AC joints (Fig. 5-54).
• Center the midline of the body to the midline of the grid.
• Ensure that the weight of the body is equally distributed on the feet to avoid rotation.
• With the patient's arms hanging by the sides, adjust the shoulders to lie in the same horizontal plane. It is important that the arms hang unsupported.
• Make two exposures: one in which the patient is standing upright *without* weights attached, and a second in which the patient has *equal weights* (5 to 10 lb) affixed to each wrist.[1,2]
• After the first exposure, slowly affix the weights to the patient's wrist, using a band or strap.
• Instruct the patient not to favor (tense up) the injured shoulder.
• *Avoid having the patient hold weights in each hand*; this tends to make the shoulder muscles contract, reducing the possibility of showing a small AC separation (Fig. 5-55).
• *Shield gonads.* Also use a thyroid collar because the thyroid gland is exposed to the primary beam.
• *Respiration:* Suspend.

Central ray
• Perpendicular to the midline of the body at the level of the AC joints for a single projection; directed at each respective AC joint when two separate exposures are necessary for each shoulder in broad-shouldered patients

Collimation
• Single: to 6 × 8 inches (15 × 20 cm) (note 2 inches [5 cm] less than IR size).
• Double: to 6 × 17 inches (15 × 43 cm).

[1]Allman FL. Fractures and ligamentous injuries of the clavicle and its articulations, *J Bone Joint Surg Am* 49:774, 1967.
[2]Rockwood CA, Green DP: *Fractures in adults,* ed 7, Philadelphia, 2009, Lippincott.

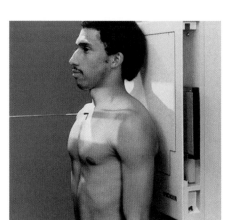

Fig. 5-54 Bilateral AP AC articulations.

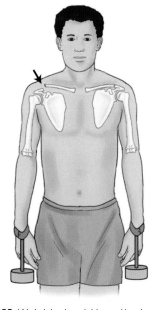

Fig. 5-55 Weights should be attached to wrists as shown and not held in hands. Note how separation of AC joint is shown by pulling of weights.

Acromioclavicular Articulations

Structures shown

Bilateral images of the AC joints are shown (Figs. 5-56 and 5-57). This projection is used to show dislocation, separation, and function of the joints.

EVALUATION CRITERIA

The following should be clearly shown:
- Evidence of proper collimation
- AC joints visualized with some soft tissue and without excessive density
- Both AC joints, with and without weights, entirely included on one or two single radiographs
- No rotation or leaning by the patient
- Right or left and weight or nonweight markers
- Separation, if done, clearly seen on the images with weights

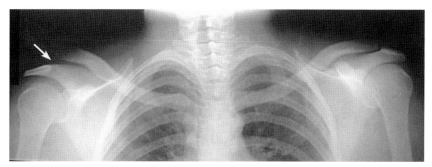

Fig. 5-56 Bilateral AP AC joints showing normal left joint and separation of right joint (*arrow*).

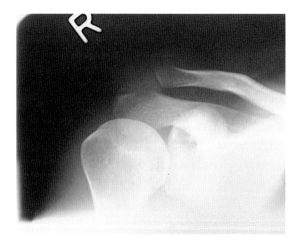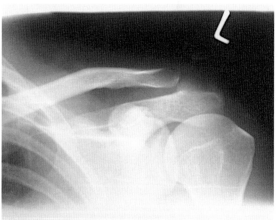

Fig. 5-57 Normal AC joints requiring two separate radiographs.

AP AXIAL PROJECTION
ALEXANDER METHOD

Alexander[1] suggested that AP and PA axial oblique projections be used in cases of suspected AC subluxation or dislocation. Each side is examined separately.

Image receptor: 8 × 10 inch (18 × 24 cm) lengthwise

---

[1]Alexander OM: Radiography of the acromioclavicular articulation, *Med Radiogr Photogr* 30:34, 1954.

Position of patient
- Place the patient in the upright position, either standing or seated.

Position of part
- Have the patient place the back against the vertical grid device and sit or stand upright.
- Center the affected shoulder under examination to the grid.
- Adjust the height of the IR so that the midpoint of the film is at the level of the AC joint.

- Adjust the patient's position to center the coracoid process to the IR (Fig. 5-58).
- *Shield gonads.*
- *Respiration:* Suspend.

Central ray
- Directed to the coracoid process at a cephalic angle of 15 degrees (Fig. 5-59). This angulation projects the AC joint above the acromion.

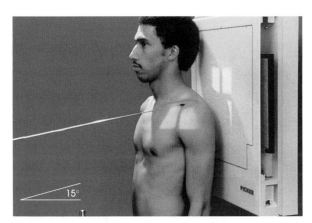

Fig. 5-58 Unilateral AP axial AC articulation: Alexander method.

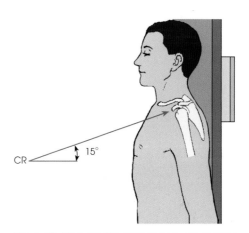

Fig. 5-59 AP axial AC articulation: Alexander method.

Structures shown

The resulting image shows the AC joint projected slightly superiorly compared with an AP projection (Fig. 5-60).

EVALUATION CRITERIA

The following should be clearly shown:

- AC joint and clavicle projected above the acromion
- AC joint visualized with some soft tissue and without excessive density

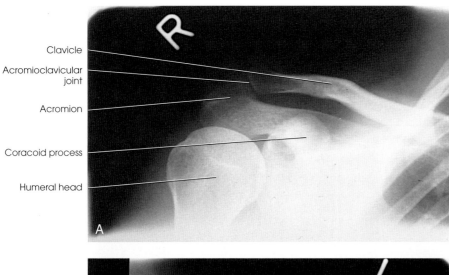

Clavicle
Acromioclavicular joint
Acromion
Coracoid process
Humeral head

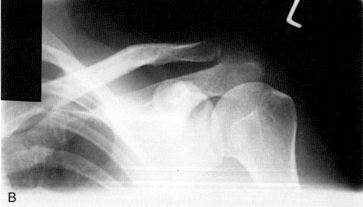

Fig. 5-60 AP axial AC articulation: Alexander method.

♠ AP PROJECTION

Image receptor: 10 × 12 inch (24 × 30 cm) crosswise

Position of patient
- Place the patient in the supine or upright position.
- If the clavicle is being examined for a fracture or a destructive disease, or if the patient cannot be placed in the upright position, use the supine position to reduce the possibility of fragment displacement or additional injury.

Position of part
- Adjust the body to center the clavicle to the midline of the table or vertical grid device.
- Place the arms along the sides of the body, and adjust the shoulders to lie in the same horizontal plane.
- Center the clavicle to the IR (Fig. 5-61).
- *Shield gonads.*
- *Respiration:* Suspend at the end of exhalation to obtain a more uniform-density image.

Central ray
- Perpendicular to the midshaft of the clavicle

Collimation
- Adjust to 8 × 12 inches (18 × 30 cm) on the collimator.

Structures shown
This projection shows a frontal image of the clavicle (Fig. 5-62).

EVALUATION CRITERIA
The following should be clearly shown:
- Evidence of proper collimation
- Entire clavicle centered on the image
- Uniform density
- Lateral half of the clavicle above the scapula, with the medial half superimposing the thorax

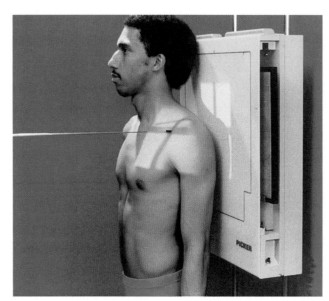

Fig. 5-61 AP clavicle.

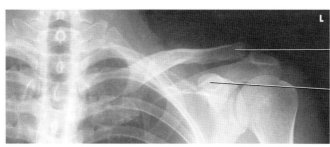

Clavicle

Coracoid process

Fig. 5-62 AP clavicle.

🌢 AP AXIAL PROJECTION
Lordotic position

NOTE: If the patient is injured or unable to assume the lordotic position, a slightly distorted image results when the tube is angled. An optional approach for improved recorded detail is the PA axial projection.

Image receptor: 10 × 12 inch (24 × 30 cm) crosswise

Position of patient

- Stand or seat the patient 1 ft in front of the vertical IR device, with the patient facing the x-ray tube.
- Alternatively, if the patient cannot stand and assume the lordotic position, place the patient supine on the table.

Position of part
Standing lordotic position

- Temporarily support the patient in the lordotic position to estimate the required central ray angulation, and have the patient reassume the upright position while the equipment is adjusted.

- Have the patient lean backward in a position of extreme lordosis, and rest the neck and shoulder against the vertical grid device. The neck is in extreme flexion (Figs. 5-63 and 5-64).
- Center the clavicle to the center of the IR (see Fig. 5-64).
  #### Supine position
- Center the IR to the clavicle.
- *Shield gonads.*
- *Respiration:* Suspend at the end of full inspiration to elevate and angle the clavicle further.

Central ray

- Directed to enter the midshaft of the clavicle
- Cephalic central ray angulation can vary from the long axis of the torso; thinner patients require more angulation to project the clavicle off the scapula and ribs
- For the *standing lordotic position*, 0 to 15 degrees is recommended (see Fig. 5-63).
- For the *supine position*, 15 to 30 degrees is recommended (see Fig. 5-64).

Collimation

- Adjust to 8 × 12 inches (18 × 30 cm) on the collimator.

Structures shown

An axial image of the clavicle is projected above the ribs (Fig. 5-65).

EVALUATION CRITERIA

The following should be clearly shown:
- Evidence of proper collimation
- Most of the clavicle projected above the ribs and scapula with the medial end overlapping the first or second rib
- Clavicle in a horizontal placement
- Entire clavicle along with the AC and SC joints

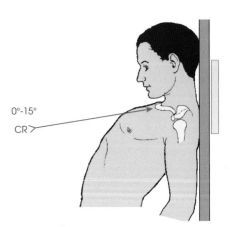

Fig. 5-63 AP axial clavicle, lordotic position.

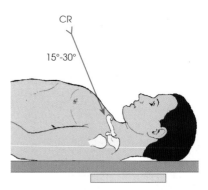

Fig. 5-64 AP axial clavicle.

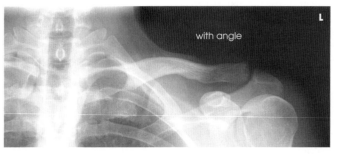

Fig. 5-65 AP axial clavicle. Same patient as Fig. 5-62. Note slightly different projection of the bone.

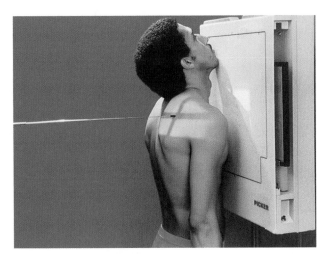

Fig. 5-66 PA clavicle.

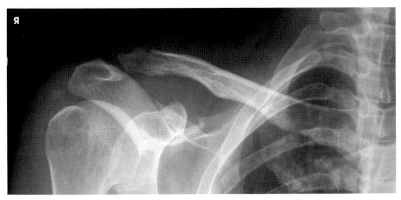

Fig. 5-67 PA clavicle.

♠ PA PROJECTION

The PA projection is generally well accepted by the patient who can stand, and it is most useful when improved recorded detail is desired. The advantage of the PA projection is that the clavicle is closer to the image receptor, reducing the OID. Positioning is similar to that of the AP projection. The differences are as follows:

- The patient is standing upright (back toward the x-ray tube) or prone (Fig. 5-66).
- The perpendicular central ray exits the midshaft of the clavicle (Fig. 5-67).

Structures shown and evaluation criteria are the same as for the AP projection.

♠ PA AXIAL PROJECTION

Positioning of the PA axial clavicle is similar to the AP axial projection described previously. The differences are as follows:

- The patient is prone or standing, facing the vertical grid device.
- The central ray is angled 15 to 30 degrees caudad (Fig. 5-68).

Structures shown and evaluation criteria are the same as for the AP axial projection described previously.

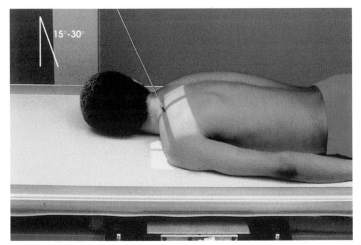

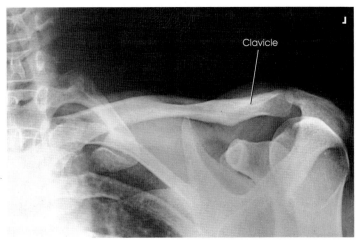

Clavicle

Fig. 5-68 PA axial clavicle.

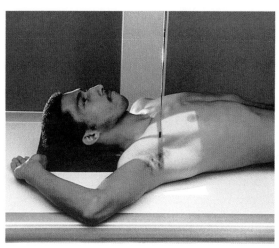

Fig. 5-69 AP scapula.

AP PROJECTION

Image receptor: 10 × 12 inch (24 × 30 cm) lengthwise

Position of patient
- Place the patient in the upright or supine position. The upright position is preferred if the shoulder is tender.

Position of part
- Adjust the patient's body, and center the affected scapula to the midline of the grid.
- Abduct the arm to a right angle with the body to draw the scapula laterally. Flex the elbow, and support the hand in a comfortable position.
- For this projection, do not rotate the body toward the affected side because the resultant obliquity would offset the effect of drawing the scapula laterally (Fig. 5-69).
- Position the top of the IR 2 inches (5 cm) above the top of the shoulder.
- *Shield gonads.*
- *Respiration:* Make this exposure during slow breathing to obliterate lung detail.

Central ray

- Perpendicular to the mid-scapular area at a point approximately 2 inches (5 cm) inferior to the coracoid process.

Collimation

- Adjust to 10 × 12 inches (24 × 30 cm) on the collimator.

Structures shown

An AP projection of the scapula is shown (Fig. 5-70).

EVALUATION CRITERIA

The following should be clearly shown:
- Evidence of proper collimation
- Lateral portion of the scapula free of superimposition from the ribs
- Scapula horizontal and not slanted
- Scapular detail through the superimposed lung and ribs (shallow breathing should help obliterate lung detail)
- Acromion process and inferior angle

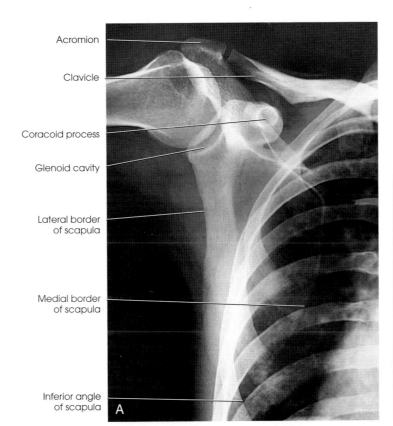

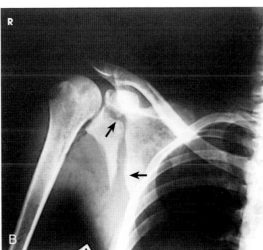

Acromion

Clavicle

Coracoid process

Glenoid cavity

Lateral border of scapula

Medial border of scapula

Inferior angle of scapula

Fig. 5-70 A, AP scapula. **B,** AP scapula showing fracture of scapula through glenoid cavity and extending inferiorly (*arrows*).

⬥ LATERAL PROJECTION
RAO or LAO body position

Image receptor: 10 × 12 inch (24 × 30 cm) lengthwise

Position of patient
- Place the patient in the upright position, standing or seated, facing a vertical grid device.
- The prone position can be used, but the projection is more difficult to perform. The supine position can also be used; however, the scapula is magnified.

Position of part
- Adjust the patient in RAO or LAO position, with the affected scapula centered to the grid. The average patient requires a 45- to 60-degree rotation from the plane of the IR. According to Johnston et al.,[1] the proper patient rotation is accomplished by orienting the plane through the superior angle of the scapula and acromial tip, perpendicular to the IR.
- Place the arm in one of two positions according to the area of the scapula to be shown.

[1] Johnston J et al: Landmarks for lateral scapula and scapular Y positioning, *Radiol Technol* 79:397, 2008.

- For delineation of the *acromion* and *coracoid processes* of the scapula, have the patient flex the elbow and place the back of the hand on the posterior thorax at a level sufficient to prevent the humerus from overlapping the scapula (Figs. 5-71 and 5-72). Mazujian[1] suggested that the patient place the arm across the upper chest by grasping the opposite shoulder, as shown in Fig. 5-73.
- To show the *body* of the scapula, ask the patient to extend the arm upward and rest the forearm on the head or across the upper chest by grasping the opposite shoulder (Fig. 5-74; see Fig. 5-73).
- After placing the arm in any of these positions, grasp the lateral and medial borders of the scapula between the thumb and index fingers of one hand. Make a final adjustment of the body rotation, placing the body of the scapula perpendicular to the plane of the IR.
- *Shield gonads.*
- *Respiration:* Suspend.

[1] Mazujian M: Lateral profile view of the scapula, *Xray Techn* 25:24, 1953.

Central ray
- Perpendicular to the mid-medial border of the protruding scapula (see Table 5-3)

Collimation
- Adjust to 12 inches (30 cm) in length and 1 inch (2.5 cm) from the lateral shadow.

⬛ COMPENSATING FILTER
Use of a specially designed compensating filter for the shoulder improves the quality of the image because of the large amount of primary beam radiation striking the IR. These filters are particularly useful when digital radiography (CR or DR) systems are used with this projection.

Structures shown
A lateral image of the scapula is shown by this projection. The placement of the arm determines the portion of the superior scapula that is superimposed over the humerus.

EVALUATION CRITERIA
The following should be clearly shown:
- Lateral and medial borders superimposed
- No superimposition of the scapular body on the ribs
- No superimposition of the humerus on the area of interest
- Inclusion of the acromion process and inferior angle
- Lateral thickness of scapula with proper density

NOTE: For trauma patients, this projection can be performed using the LPO or RPO position (see Fig. 13-42 in Volume 2).

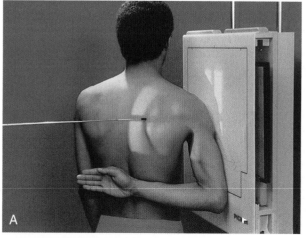
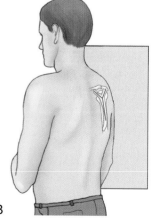

Fig. 5-71 A, Lateral scapula, RAO body position. **B,** Perspective from x-ray tube showing scapula centered in true lateral position.

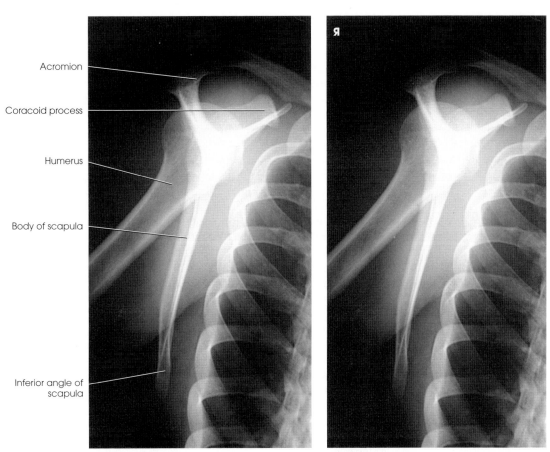

Acromion

Coracoid process

Humerus

Body of scapula

Inferior angle of scapula

Fig. 5-72 Lateral scapula with arm on posterior chest.

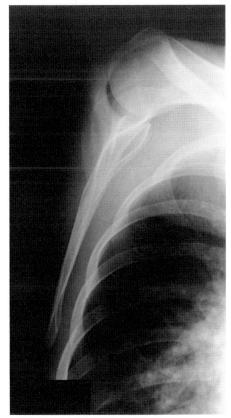

Fig. 5-73 Lateral scapula with arm across upper anterior thorax.

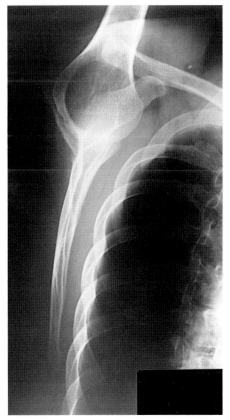

Fig. 5-74 Lateral scapula with arm extended above head.

AP OBLIQUE PROJECTION
RPO or LPO position

Image receptor: 10 × 12 inch (24 × 30 cm) lengthwise

Position of patient
- Place the patient in the supine or upright position.
- Use the upright position when the shoulder is painful unless contraindicated.

Position of part
- Align the body and center the affected scapula to the midline of the grid.
- For moderate AP oblique projection, ask the patient to extend the arm superiorly, flex the elbow, and place the supinated hand under the head, or have the patient extend the affected arm across the anterior chest.
- Have the patient turn away from the affected side enough to rotate the shoulder 15 to 25 degrees (Fig. 5-75).
- For a steeper oblique projection, ask the patient to extend the arm, rest the flexed elbow on the forehead, and rotate the body *away* from the affected side 25 to 35 degrees (Fig. 5-76).
- Grasp the lateral and medial borders of the scapula between the thumb and index fingers of one hand, and adjust the rotation of the body to project the scapula free of the rib cage.
- For a direct lateral projection of the scapula using this position, draw the arm across the chest, and adjust the body rotation to place the scapula perpendicular to the plane of the IR as previously described and shown in Figs. 5-71 to 5-74.
- *Shield gonads.*
- *Respiration:* Suspend.

Central ray
- Perpendicular to the lateral border of the rib cage at the mid-scapular area

Structures shown
This projection shows oblique images of the scapula, projected free or nearly free of rib superimposition (Figs. 5-77 and 5-78).

EVALUATION CRITERIA
The following should be clearly shown:
- Oblique scapula
- Lateral border adjacent to the ribs
- Acromion process and inferior angle

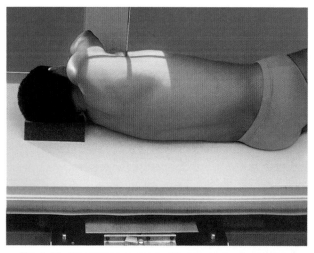

Fig. 5-75 AP oblique scapula, 20-degree body rotation.

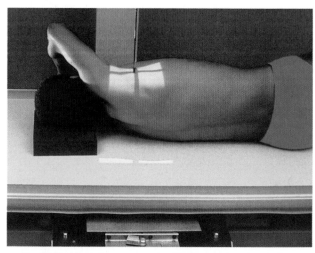

Fig. 5-76 AP oblique scapula, 35-degree body rotation.

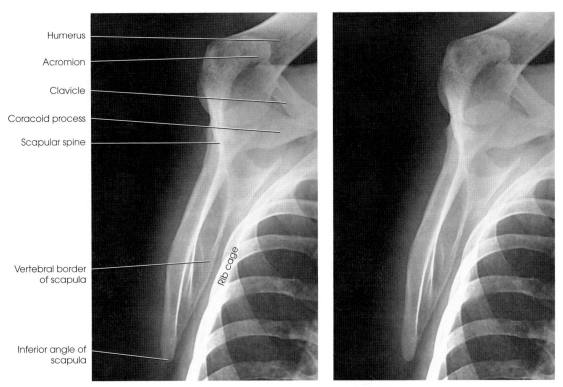

Humerus

Acromion

Clavicle

Coracoid process

Scapular spine

Vertebral border
of scapula

Rib cage

Inferior angle of
scapula

Fig. 5-77 AP oblique scapula, 15- to 25-degree body rotation.

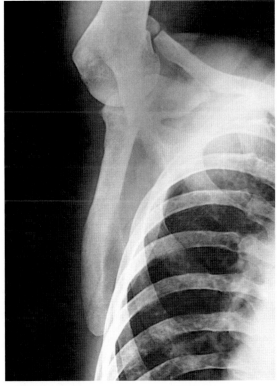

Fig. 5-78 AP oblique scapula, 25- to 30-degree body rotation.

Coracoid Process
AP AXIAL PROJECTION

Image receptor: 10 × 12 inch (24 × 30 cm) crosswise

Position of patient
• Place the patient in the supine position with the arms along the sides of the body.

Position of part
• Adjust the position of the body, and center the affected coracoid process to the midline of the grid.
• Position the IR so that the midpoint of the IR coincides with the central ray.
• Adjust the shoulders to lie in the same horizontal plane.

• Abduct the arm of the affected side slightly, and supinate the hand, immobilizing it with a sandbag across the palm (Fig. 5-79).
• *Shield gonads.*
• *Respiration:* Suspend at the end of exhalation for a more uniform density.

Central ray
• Directed to enter the coracoid process at an angle of 15 to 45 degrees cephalad. Kwak et al.[1] recommended an angle of 30 degrees. The degree of angulation depends on the shape of the patient's back. Round-shouldered patients require a greater angulation than patients with a straight back (Fig. 5-80).

[1]Kwak DL et al: Angled anteroposterior views of the shoulder, *Radiol Technol* 53:590, 1982.

Structures shown
A slightly elongated inferosuperior image of the coracoid process is illustrated (Fig. 5-81). Because the coracoid is curved on itself, it casts a small, oval shadow in the direct AP projection of the shoulder.

The following should be clearly shown:
■ Coracoid process with minimal self-superimposition
■ Clavicle slightly superimposing the coracoid process

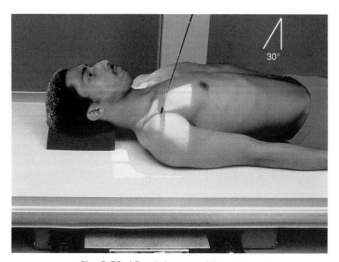

Fig. 5-79 AP axial coracoid process.

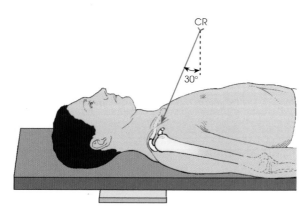

Fig. 5-80 AP axial coracoid process.

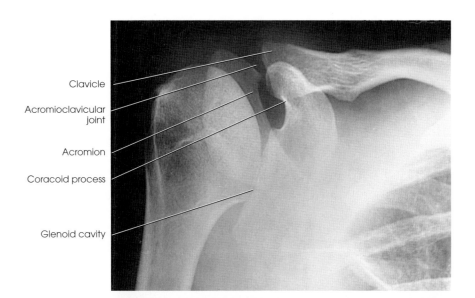

Clavicle
Acromioclavicular joint
Acromion
Coracoid process
Glenoid cavity

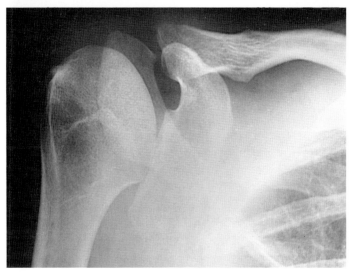

Fig. 5-81 AP axial coracoid process.

Scapular Spine

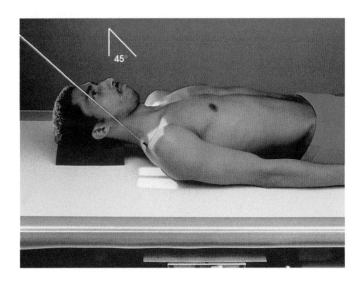

Fig. 5-82 Tangential scapular spine.

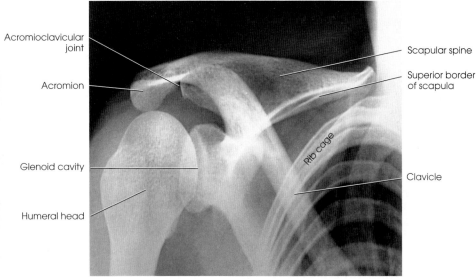

Acromioclavicular joint

Acromion

Glenoid cavity

Humeral head

Scapular spine

Superior border of scapula

Rib cage

Clavicle

Fig. 5-83 Tangential scapular spine image with 45-degree central ray angulation.

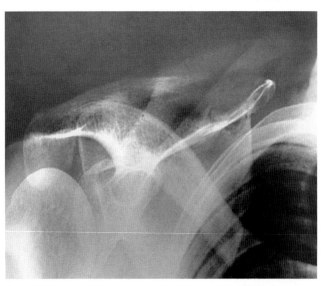

Fig. 5-84 Tangential scapular spine image with 30-degree central ray angulation.

TANGENTIAL PROJECTION
LAQUERRIÈRE-PIERQUIN METHOD

Image receptor: 8 × 10 inch (18 × 24 cm) crosswise

Position of patient
- As described by Laquerrière and Pierquin,[1] place the patient in the supine position.

Position of part
- Center the shoulder to the midline of the grid.
- Adjust the patient's rotation to place the body of the scapula in a horizontal position. When this requires elevation of the opposite shoulder, support it on sandbags or radiolucent sponges.
- Turn the head away from the shoulder being examined, enough to prevent superimposition (Fig. 5-82).
- *Shield gonads.*
- *Respiration:* Suspend.

Central ray
- Directed through the posterosuperior region of the shoulder at an angle of 45 degrees caudad. A 35-degree angulation suffices for obese and round-shouldered patients.
- After adjusting the x-ray tube, position the IR so that it is centered to the central ray.

Structures shown
The spine of the scapula is shown in profile and is free of bony superimposition except for the lateral end of the clavicle (Figs. 5-83 and 5-84).

EVALUATION CRITERIA
The following should be clearly shown:
- Scapular spine superior to the scapular body
- Scapular spine with some soft tissue around it and without excessive density

NOTE: When the shoulder is too painful to tolerate the supine position, this projection can be obtained with the patient in the prone or upright position.

[1]Laquerrière, Pierquin: De la nécessité d'employer une technique radiographique spéciale pour obtenir certains details squelettiques, *J Radiol Electr* 3:145, 1918.

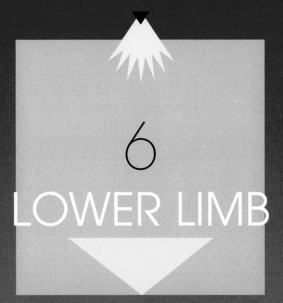

6
LOWER LIMB

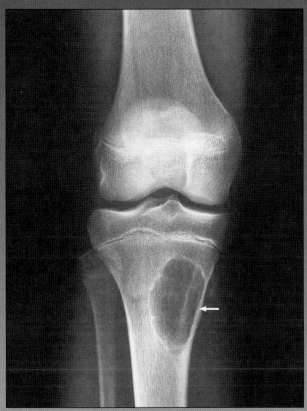

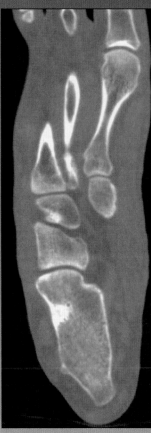

PROJECTIONS, POSITIONS, AND METHODS

Page	Essential	Anatomy	Projection	Position	Method
242	✦	Toes	AP or AP axial		
244		Toes	PA		
245	✦	Toes	AP oblique	Medial rotation	
246	✦	Toes	Lateral (mediolateral or lateromedial)		
250		Sesamoids	Tangential		LEWIS, HOLLY
252	✦	Foot	AP or AP axial		
256	✦	Foot	AP oblique	Medial rotation	
258		Foot	AP oblique	Lateral rotation	
260	✦	Foot	Lateral (mediolateral)		
262		Foot: *Longitudinal arch*	Lateral (lateromedial)	Standing	WEIGHT-BEARING
264		Feet	AP axial	Standing	WEIGHT-BEARING
265		Foot	AP axial	Standing	WEIGHT-BEARING COMPOSITE
267		Foot: *Congenital clubfoot*	AP		KITE
268		Foot: *Congenital clubfoot*	Lateral (mediolateral)		KITE
270		Foot: *Congenital clubfoot*	Axial (dorsoplantar)		KANDEL
271	✦	Calcaneus	Axial (plantodorsal)		
272		Calcaneus	Axial (dorsoplantar)		
273		Calcaneus	Axial (dorsoplantar)	Standing	WEIGHT-BEARING
274	✦	Calcaneus	Lateral (mediolateral)		
275		Calcaneus	Lateromedial oblique		WEIGHT-BEARING
276		Subtalar joint	Lateromedial oblique	Medial rotation foot	ISHERWOOD
277		Subtalar joint	AP axial oblique	Medial rotation ankle	ISHERWOOD
278		Subtalar joint	AP axial oblique	Lateral rotation ankle	ISHERWOOD
279	✦	Ankle	AP		
280	✦	Ankle	Lateral (mediolateral)		
282		Ankle	Lateral (lateromedial)		
283	✦	Ankle	AP oblique	Medial rotation	
284	✦	Ankle: *Mortise joint*	AP oblique	Medial rotation	
286		Ankle	AP oblique	Lateral rotation	
287	✦	Ankle	AP		STRESS
288		Ankles	AP	Standing	WEIGHT-BEARING
290	✦	Leg	AP		
292	✦	Leg	Lateral (mediolateral)		
294		Leg	AP oblique	Medial and lateral rotations	
296	✦	Knee	AP		
298		Knee	PA		

The icons in the Essential column indicate projections frequently performed in the United States and Canada. Students should become competent in these projections.

PROJECTIONS, POSITIONS, AND METHODS

Page	Essential	Anatomy	Projection	Position	Method
300	♠	Knee	Lateral (mediolateral)		
302	♠	Knees	AP	Standing	WEIGHT-BEARING
303		Knees	PA	Standing flexion	ROSENBERG, WEIGHT-BEARING
304	♠	Knee	AP oblique	Lateral rotation	
305	♠	Knee	AP oblique	Medial and lateral rotations	
306	♠	Intercondylar fossa	PA axial		HOLMBLAD
308	♠	Intercondylar fossa	PA axial		CAMP-COVENTRY
310		Intercondylar fossa	AP axial		BÉCLÈRE
311	♠	Patella	PA		
312	♠	Patella	Lateral (mediolateral)		
313		Patella and patello-femoral joint	Tangential		HUGHSTON
314		Patella and patello-femoral joint	Tangential		MERCHANT
316	♠	Patella and patello-femoral joint	Tangential		SETTEGAST
318	♠	Femur	AP		
320	♠	Femur	Lateral (mediolateral)		
322		Lower limbs: *Hips, knees, and ankles*	AP	Standing	WEIGHT-BEARING

Lower Limb

The lower limb, or extremity, and its girdle (considered in Chapter 7) are studied in four parts: (1) foot, (2) leg, (3) thigh, and (4) hip. The bones are composed, shaped, and placed so that they can carry the body in the upright position and transmit its weight to the ground with a minimal amount of stress to the individual parts.

Foot

The *foot* consists of 26 bones (Figs. 6-1 and 6-2):
- 14 phalanges (bones of the toes)
- 5 metatarsals (bones of the instep)
- 7 tarsals (bones of the ankle)

The bones of the foot are similar to the bones of the hand. Structural differences permit walking and support of the body's weight. For descriptive purposes, the foot is sometimes divided into the forefoot, midfoot, and hindfoot. The forefoot includes the metatarsals and toes. The midfoot includes five tarsals—the cuneiforms, navicular, and cuboid bones. The hindfoot includes the talus and calcaneus. The bones of the foot are shaped and joined together to form a series of longitudinal and transverse arches. The longitudinal arch functions as a shock absorber to distribute the weight of the body in all directions, which permits smooth walking (see Fig. 6-2). The transverse arch runs from side to side and assists in supporting the longitudinal arch. The superior surface of the foot is termed the *dorsum* or *dorsal surface,* and the inferior, or posterior, aspect of the foot is termed the *plantar surface.*

PHALANGES

Each foot has 14 *phalanges*—2 in the great toe and 3 in each of the other toes. The phalanges of the great toe are termed the *distal* and *proximal phalanges*. The phalanges of the other toes are termed the *proximal, middle,* and *distal phalanges*. Each phalanx is composed of a body and two expanded articular ends—the proximal *base* and the distal *head.*

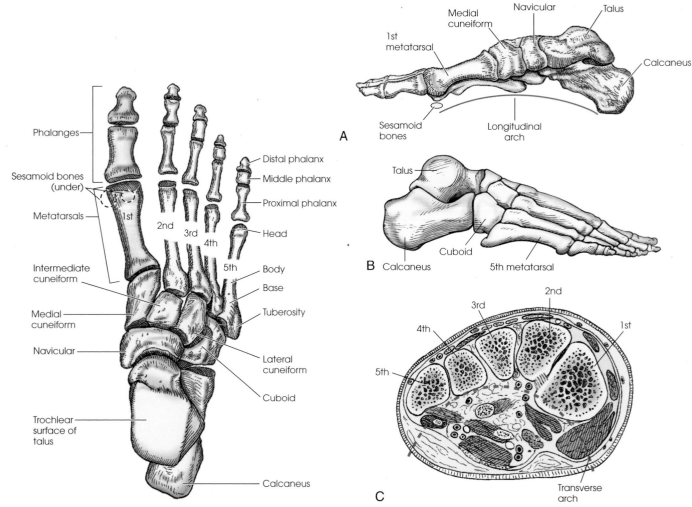

Fig. 6-1 Dorsal (superior) aspect of right foot.

Fig. 6-2 Right foot. **A,** Medial aspect. **B,** Lateral aspect. **C,** Coronal section near base of metatarsals. Transverse arch shown.

METATARSALS

The five *metatarsals* are numbered one to five beginning at the medial or great toe side of the foot. The metatarsals consist of a *body* and two articular ends. The expanded proximal end is called the *base*, and the small, rounded distal end is termed the *head*. The five heads form the "ball" of the foot. The first metatarsal is the shortest and thickest. The second metatarsal is the longest. The base of the fifth metatarsal contains a prominent *tuberosity*, which is a common site of fractures.

TARSALS

The proximal foot contains seven *tarsals* (see Fig. 6-1):
- Calcaneus
- Talus
- Navicular
- Cuboid
- Medial cuneiform
- Intermediate cuneiform
- Lateral cuneiform

Beginning at the medial side of the foot, the cuneiforms are described as *medial*, *intermediate*, and *lateral*.

The *calcaneus* is the largest and strongest tarsal bone (Fig. 6-3). Some texts refer to it as the *os calcis*. It projects posteriorly and medially at the distal part of the foot. The long axis of the calcaneus is directed inferiorly and forms an angle of approximately 30 degrees. The posterior and inferior portions of the calcaneus contain the posterior *tuberosity* for attachment of the Achilles tendon. Superiorly, three articular facets join with the talus. They are called the *anterior, middle,* and *posterior facets*. Between the middle and posterior talar articular facets is a groove, the calcaneal sulcus, which corresponds to a similar groove on the inferior surface of the talus. Collectively, these sulci constitute the *sinus tarsi*. The interosseous ligament passes through this sulcus. The medial aspect of the calcaneus extends outward as a shelflike overhang and is termed the *sustentaculum tali*. The lateral surface of the calcaneus contains the *trochlea*.

The *talus,* irregular in form and occupying the superiormost position of the foot, is the second largest tarsal bone (see Figs. 6-1 to 6-3). The talus articulates with four bones—tibia, fibula, calcaneus, and navicular bone. The superior surface, the *trochlear surface,* articulates with the tibia and connects the foot to the leg. The head of the talus is directed anteriorly and has articular surfaces that join the navicular bone and calcaneus. On the inferior surface is a groove, the *sulcus tali,* that forms the roof of the sinus tarsi. The inferior surface also contains three facets that align with the facets on the superior surface of the calcaneus.

The *cuboid* bone lies on the lateral side of the foot between the calcaneus and the fourth and fifth metatarsals (see Fig. 6-1). The *navicular* bone lies on the medial side of the foot between the talus and the three cuneiforms. The *cuneiforms* lie at the central and medial aspect of the foot between the navicular bone and the first, second, and third metatarsals. The *medial* cuneiform is the largest of the three cuneiform bones, and the *intermediate* cuneiform is the smallest.

The seven tarsals can be remembered using the following mnemonic:

Chubby	Calcaneus
Twisted,	Talus
Never	Navicular
Could	Cuboid
Cha	Cuneiform—medial
Cha	Cuneiform—intermediate
Cha	Cuneiform—lateral

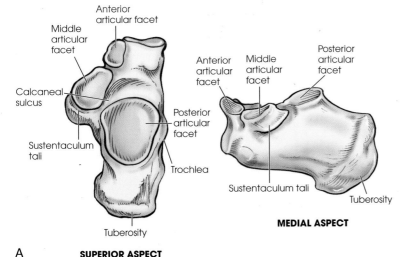
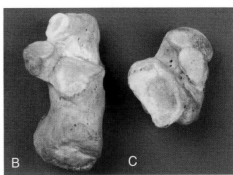

Fig. 6-3 A, Articular surfaces of right calcaneus. **B,** Photograph of superior aspect of right calcaneus. Note three articular facet surfaces. **C,** Photograph of inferior aspect of talus. Note three articular surfaces that articulate with superior calcaneus.

Labels for Figure A (SUPERIOR ASPECT):
- Middle articular facet
- Anterior articular facet
- Calcaneal sulcus
- Sustentaculum tali
- Posterior articular facet
- Trochlea
- Tuberosity
- A SUPERIOR ASPECT

Labels for MEDIAL ASPECT:
- Anterior articular facet
- Middle articular facet
- Posterior articular facet
- Sustentaculum tali
- Tuberosity
- MEDIAL ASPECT

B   C

SESAMOID BONES

Beneath the head of the first metatarsal are two small bones called *sesamoid* bones. They are detached from the foot and embedded within two tendons. These bones are seen on most adult foot radiographs. They are a common site of fractures and must be shown radiographically (see Fig. 6-2).

Leg

The leg has two bones: the *tibia* and *fibula*. The tibia, the second largest bone in the body, is situated on the medial side of the leg and is a weight-bearing bone. Slightly posterior to the tibia on the lateral side of the leg is the fibula. The fibula does not bear any body weight.

TIBIA

The *tibia* (Fig. 6-4) is the larger of the two bones of the leg and consists of one body and two expanded extremities. The proximal end of the tibia has two prominent processes—the *medial* and *lateral condyles*. The superior surfaces of the condyles form smooth facets for articulation with the condyles of the femur. These two flatlike superior surfaces are called the *tibial plateaus,* and they slope posteriorly about 10 to 20 degrees. Between the two articular surfaces is a sharp projection, the *intercondylar eminence,* which terminates in two peaklike processes called the *medial* and *lateral intercondylar tubercles.* The lateral condyle has a facet at its distal posterior surface for articulation with the *head* of the fibula. On the anterior surface of the tibia, just below the condyles, is a prominent process called the *tibial tuberosity,* to which the ligamentum patellae attach. Extending along the anterior surface of the tibial body, beginning at the tuberosity, is a sharp ridge called the *anterior crest.*

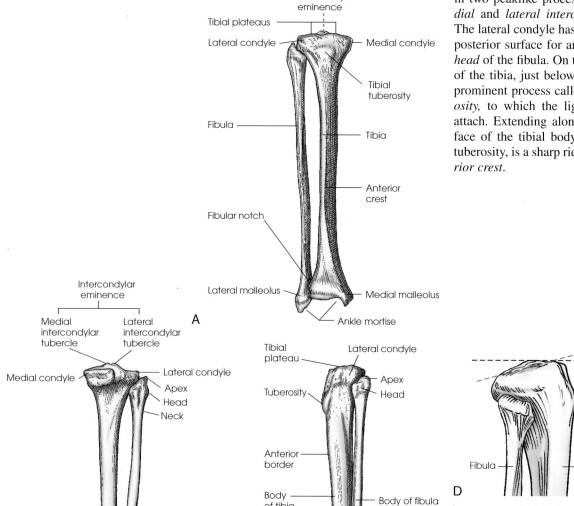

Fig. 6-4 Right tibia and fibula. **A,** Anterior aspect. **B,** Posterior aspect. **C,** Lateral aspect. **D,** Proximal end of tibia and fibula showing angle of tibial plateau. **E,** Photograph of superior and posterior aspect of the tibia.

Lower Limb

The distal end of the tibia (Fig. 6-5) is broad, and its medial surface is prolonged into a large process called the *medial malleolus.* Its anterolateral surface contains the *anterior tubercle,* which overlays the fibula. The lateral surface is flattened and contains the triangular *fibular notch* for articulation with the fibula. The surface under the distal tibia is smooth and shaped for articulation with the talus.

FIBULA

The *fibula* is slender compared with its length and consists of one *body* and two articular extremities. The proximal end of the fibula is expanded into a *head,* which articulates with the lateral condyle of the tibia. At the lateroposterior aspect of the head is a conic projection called the *apex.*

The enlarged distal end of the fibula is the *lateral malleolus.* The lateral malleolus is pyramidal and marked by several depressions at its inferior and posterior surfaces. Viewed axially, the lateral malleolus lies approximately 15 to 20 degrees more posterior than the medial malleolus (see Fig. 6-5, *C*).

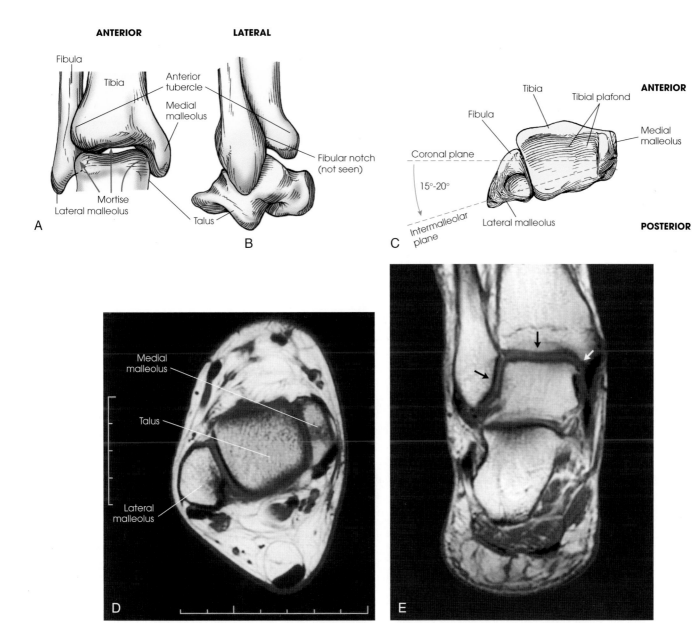

Fig. 6-5 Right distal tibia and fibula in true anatomic position. **A,** Mortise joint and surrounding anatomy. Note slight overlap of anterior tubercle of tibia and superolateral talus over fibula. **B,** Lateral aspect showing fibula positioned slightly posterior to tibia. **C,** Inferior aspect. Note lateral malleolus lies more posterior than medial malleolus. **D,** MRI axial plane of lateral and medial malleoli and talus. Lateral malleolus lies more posterior than medial malleolus. **E,** MRI coronal plane of ankle clearly showing ankle mortise joint (*arrows*).

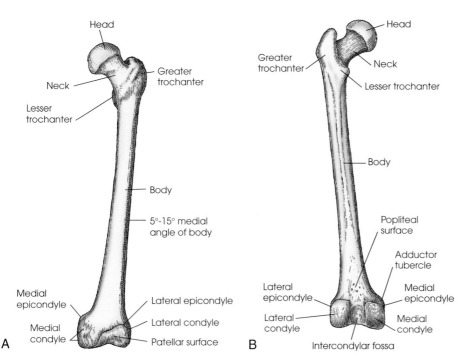

Femur

The *femur* is the longest, strongest, and heaviest bone in the body (Figs. 6-6 and 6-7). This bone consists of one body and two articular extremities. The *body* is cylindric, slightly convex anteriorly, and slants medially 5 to 15 degrees (see Fig. 6-6, *A*). The extent of medial inclination depends on the breadth of the pelvic girdle. When the femur is vertical, the medial condyle is lower than the lateral condyle (see Fig. 6-6, *C*). About a 5- to 7-degree difference exists between the two condyles. Because of this difference, on lateral radiographs of the knee the central ray is angled 5 to 7 degrees cephalad to "open" the joint space of the knee. The superior portion of the femur articulates with the acetabulum of the hip joint (considered with the pelvic girdle in Chapter 7).

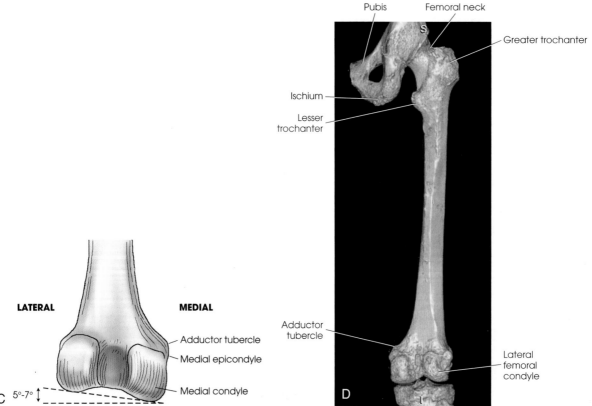

Fig. 6-6 A, Anterior aspect of left femur. **B,** Posterior aspect. **C,** Distal end of posterior femur showing 5- to 7-degree difference between medial and lateral condyle when femur is vertical. **D,** Three-dimensional CT scan showing posterior aspect and articulation with knee and hip.

The distal end of the femur is broadened and has two large eminences: the larger *medial condyle* and the smaller *lateral condyle*. Anteriorly, the condyles are separated by the *patellar surface*, a shallow, triangular depression. Posteriorly, the condyles are separated by a deep depression called the *intercondylar fossa*. A slight prominence above and within the curve of each condyle forms the *medial* and *lateral epicondyles*. The medial condyle contains the *adductor tubercle,* which is located on the posterolateral aspect. The tubercle is a raised bony area that receives the tendon of the adductor muscle. This tubercle is important to identify on lateral knee radiographs because it assists in identifying overrotation or underrotation. The triangular area superior to the intercondylar fossa on the posterior femur is the *trochlear groove,* over which the popliteal blood vessels and nerves pass.

The posterior area of the knee, between the condyles, contains a sesamoid bone in 3% to 5% of people. This sesamoid is called the *fabella* and is seen only on the lateral projection of the knee.

Patella

The *patella,* or knee cap (Fig. 6-8), is the largest and most constant sesamoid bone in the body (see Chapter 3). The patella is a flat, triangular bone situated at the distal anterior surface of the femur. The patella develops in the tendon of the quadriceps femoris muscle between 3 and 5 years of age. The *apex,* or tip, is directed inferiorly, lies ½ inch (1.3 cm) above the joint space of the knee, and is attached to the tuberosity of the tibia by the patellar ligament. The superior border of the patella is called the *base*.

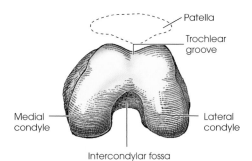

Fig. 6-7 Inferior aspect of left femur.

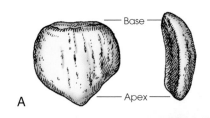

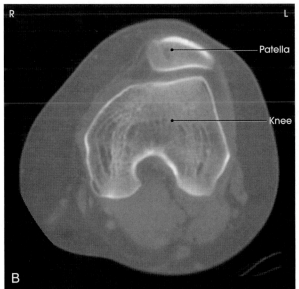

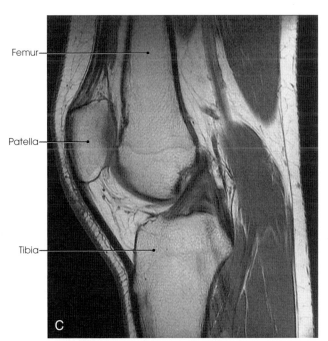

Fig. 6-8 **A,** Anterior and lateral aspects of patella. **B,** Axial CT scan of patella showing relationship to femur. **C,** Sagittal MRI showing patellar relationship to femur and knee joint. Apex of patella is ½ inch (1.2 cm) above knee joint.

(**B** and **C,** Modified from Kelley LL, Petersen CM: *Sectional anatomy for imaging professionals,* ed 2, St Louis, 2007, Mosby.)

Knee Joint

The knee joint is one of the most complex joints in the human body. The femur, tibia, fibula, and patella are held together by a complex group of ligaments. These ligaments work together to provide stability for the knee joint. Although radiographers do not produce images of these ligaments, they need to have a basic understanding of their positions and interrelationship. Many patients with knee injuries do not have fractures, but they may have torn one or more of these ligaments, which can cause great pain and may alter the position of the bones. Fig. 6-9 shows the following important ligaments of the knee:

- Posterior cruciate ligament
- Anterior cruciate ligament
- Tibial collateral ligament
- Fibular collateral ligament

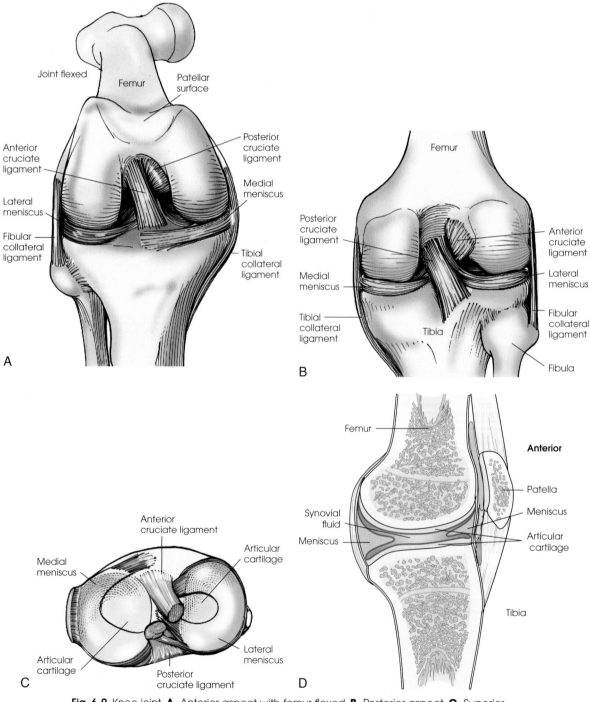

Fig. 6-9 Knee joint. **A,** Anterior aspect with femur flexed. **B,** Posterior aspect. **C,** Superior surface of tibia. **D,** Sagittal section.

The knee joint contains two fibrocartilage disks called the *lateral meniscus* and *medial meniscus* (Fig. 6-10; see Fig. 6-9). The circular menisci lie on the tibial plateaus. They are thick at the outer margin of the joint and taper off toward the center of the tibial plateau. The center of the tibial plateau contains cartilage that articulates directly with the condyles of the knee. The menisci provide stability for the knee and act as a shock absorber. The menisci are commonly torn during injury. Either a knee arthrogram or a magnetic resonance imaging (MRI) scan must be performed to visualize a meniscus tear.

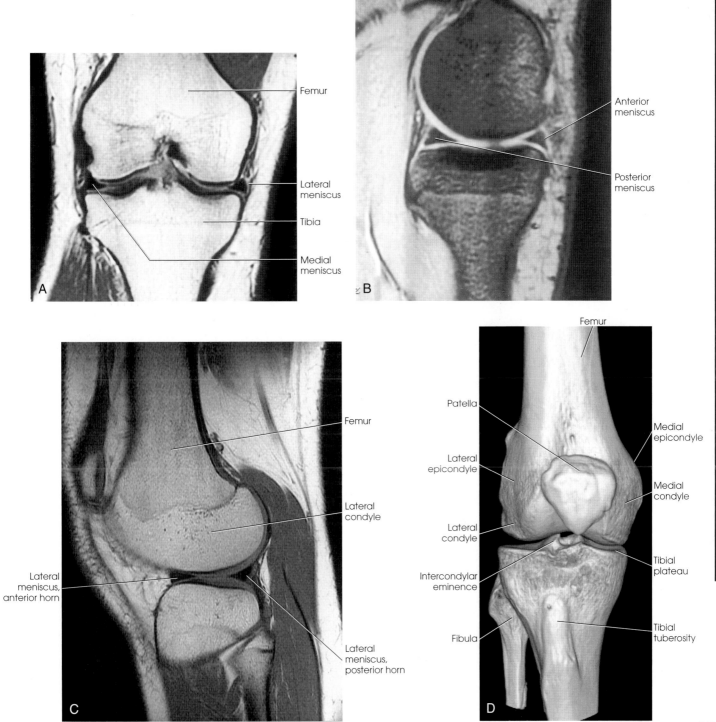

Fig. 6-10 **A,** MRI coronal plane. **B,** MRI sagittal plane. **C,** MRI oblique plane. **D,** Three-dimensional CT reformat of knee joint.

Lower Limb Articulations

The joints of the lower limb are summarized in Table 6-1 and shown in Figs. 6-11 and 6-12. Beginning with the distalmost portion of the lower limb, the articulations are as follows.

The *interphalangeal (IP) articulations,* between the phalanges, are *synovial hinges* that allow only flexion and extension. The joints between the distal and middle phalanges are the *distal interpha-* *langeal (DIP) joints.* Articulations between the middle and proximal phalanges are the *proximal interphalangeal (PIP) joints.* With only two phalanges in the great toe, the joint is known simply as the *IP joint.*

TABLE 6-1
Joints of the lower limb

Joint	Structural classification		Movement
	Tissue	Type	
Interphalangeal	Synovial	Hinge	Freely movable
Metatarsophalangeal	Synovial	Ellipsoidal	Freely movable
Intermetatarsal	Synovial	Gliding	Freely movable
Tarsometatarsal	Synovial	Gliding	Freely movable
Calcaneocuboid	Synovial	Gliding	Freely movable
Cuneocuboid	Synovial	Gliding	Freely movable
Intercuneiform	Synovial	Gliding	Freely movable
Cuboidonavicular	Fibrous	Syndesmosis	Slightly movable
Naviculocuneiform	Synovial	Gliding	Freely movable
Subtalar			
Talocalcaneal	Synovial	Gliding	Freely movable
Talocalcaneonavicular	Synovial	Ball and socket	Freely movable
Ankle mortise			
Talofibular	Synovial	Hinge	Freely movable
Tibiotalar	Synovial	Hinge	Freely movable
Tibiofibular			
Proximal	Synovial	Gliding	Freely movable
Distal	Fibrous	Syndesmosis	Slightly movable
Knee			
Patellofemoral	Synovial	Gliding	Freely movable
Femorotibial	Synovial	Hinge modified	Freely movable

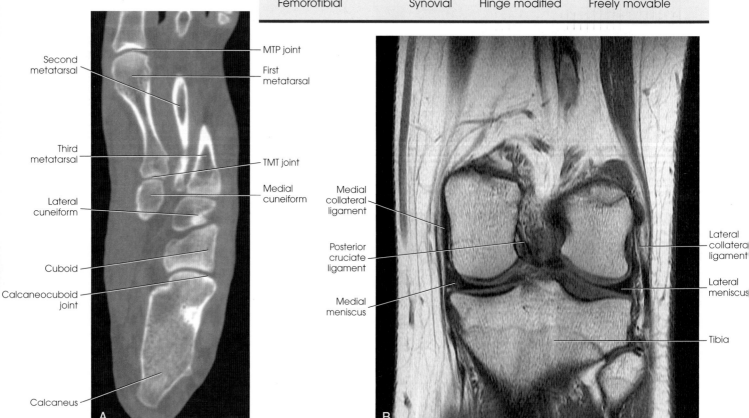

Fig. 6-11 A, Axial CT scan of foot and calcaneus. **B,** MRI coronal plane of knee joint. Joint spaces are clearly shown.

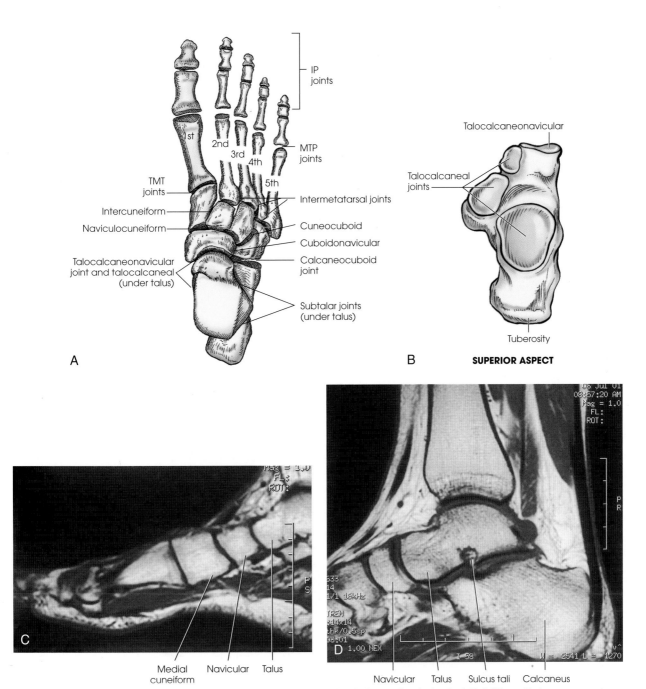

A

IP joints

MTP joints

1st   2nd   3rd   4th   5th

TMT joints

Intercuneiform

Naviculocuneiform

Talocalcaneonavicular joint and talocalcaneal (under talus)

Intermetatarsal joints

Cuneocuboid

Cuboidonavicular

Calcaneocuboid joint

Subtalar joints (under talus)

B   **SUPERIOR ASPECT**

Talocalcaneonavicular

Talocalcaneal joints

Tuberosity

C

Medial cuneiform   Navicular   Talus

D

Navicular   Talus   Sulcus tali   Calcaneus

Fig. 6-12 A and **B,** Joints of right foot. **C,** MRI sagittal plane of anterior foot. **D,** MRI sagittal plane of posterior foot and ankle. Joint spaces and articular surfaces are clearly shown.

The distal heads of the metatarsals articulate with the proximal ends of the phalanges at the *metatarsophalangeal* (MTP) articulations to form *synovial ellipsoidal* joints, which have movements of flexion, extension, and slight adduction and abduction. The proximal bases of the metatarsals articulate with one another (*intermetatarsal* articulations) and with the tarsals (*tarsometatarsal* [TMT] articulations) to form *synovial gliding* joints, which permit flexion, extension, adduction, and abduction movements.

The *intertarsal* articulations allow only slight gliding movements between the bones and are classified as *synovial gliding* or *synovial ball-and-socket* joints (see Table 6-1). The joint spaces are narrow and obliquely situated. When the joint surfaces of these bones are in question, it is necessary to angle the x-ray tube or adjust the foot to place the joint spaces parallel with the central ray.

The calcaneus supports the talus and articulates with it by an irregularly shaped, three-faceted joint surface, forming the *subtalar joint*. This joint is classified as a *synovial gliding* joint. Anteriorly, the calcaneus articulates with the cuboid at the calcaneocuboid joint. This joint is a synovial gliding joint. The talus rests on top of the calcaneus (see Fig. 6-12). It articulates with the navicular bone anteriorly, supports the tibia above, and articulates with

the malleoli of the tibia and fibula at its sides.

Each of the three parts of the subtalar joint is formed by reciprocally shaped facets on the inferior surface of the talus and the superior surface of the calcaneus. Study of the superior and medial aspects of the calcaneus (see Fig. 6-3) helps the radiographer to understand better the problems involved in radiography of this joint.

The intertarsal articulations are as follows:

- Calcaneocuboid
- Cuneocuboid
- Intercuneiform (two)
- Cuboidonavicular
- Naviculocuneiform
- Talocalcaneal
- Talocalcaneonavicular

The *ankle joint* is commonly called the *ankle mortise,* or *mortise joint.* It is formed by the articulations between the lateral malleolus of the fibula and the inferior surface and medial malleolus of the tibia (Fig. 6-13, *A*). The mortise joint is often divided specifically into the *talofibular* and *tibiofibular* joints. These form a socket type of structure that articulates with the superior portion of the talus. The talus fits inside the mortise. The articulation is a synovial hinge type of joint. The primary action of the ankle joint is dorsiflexion (flexion) and plantar flexion (extension); however, in full plantar flexion, a

small amount of rotation and abduction-adduction is permitted. The mortise joint also allows inversion and eversion of the foot. Other movements at the ankle largely depend on the gliding movements of the intertarsal joints, particularly the one between the talus and calcaneus.

The fibula articulates with the tibia at its distal and proximal ends. The *distal tibiofibular* joint is a *fibrous syndesmosis* joint allowing slight movement. The head of the fibula articulates with the posteroinferior surface of the lateral condyle of the tibia, which forms the *proximal tibiofibular* joint, which is a *synovial gliding* joint (see Fig. 6-13, *A*).

The patella articulates with the patellar surface of the femur and protects the front of the knee joint. This articulation is called the *patellofemoral joint;* when the knee is extended and relaxed, the patella is freely movable over the patellar surface of the femur. When the knee is flexed, which is also a *synovial gliding* joint, the patella is locked in position in front of the patellar surface. The knee joint, or *femorotibial* joint, is the largest joint in the body. It is called a *synovial modified-hinge joint.* In addition to flexion and extension, the knee joint allows slight medial and lateral rotation in the flexed position. The joint is enclosed in an articular capsule and held together by numerous ligaments (see Figs. 6-9 and 6-13, *B*).

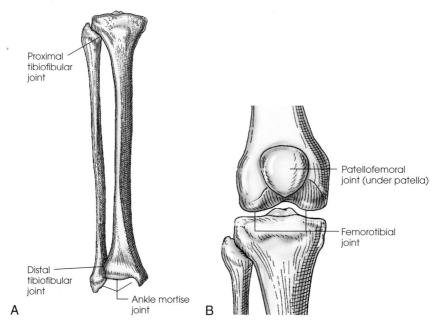

Fig. 6-13 A, Joints of right tibia and fibula. **B,** Joints of right knee.

SUMMARY OF ANATOMY

Foot
Phalanges
Metatarsals
Tarsals
Dorsum (dorsal surface)
Plantar surface

Phalanges (14)
Proximal phalanx
Middle phalanx
Distal phalanx
Body
Base
Head

Metatarsals (5)
First metatarsal
Second metatarsal
Third metatarsal
Fourth metatarsal
Fifth metatarsal
Body
Base
Head
Tuberosity (fifth)

Tarsals (7)
Calcaneus
Tuberosity
Anterior facet
Middle facet

Posterior facet
Calcaneal sulcus
Sinus tarsi
Sustentaculum tali
Trochlea
Talus
Trochlear surface
Sulcus tali
Posterior articular surface
Cuboid
Navicular
Medial cuneiform
Intermediate cuneiform
Lateral cuneiform

Others
Sesamoid bones

Leg
Tibia
Fibula

Tibia
Body
Medial condyle
Lateral condyle
Tibial plateau
Intercondylar eminence
Medial intercondylar
Tubercle
Lateral intercondylar

Tubercle
Tibial tuberosity
Anterior crest
Medial malleolus
Anterior tubercle
Fibular notch

Fibula
Body
Head
Apex
Lateral malleolus

Thigh
Femur
Body
Medial condyle
Lateral condyle
Trochlear groove
Intercondylar fossa
Medial epicondyle
Lateral epicondyle
Adductor tubercle
Popliteal surface
Fabella

Patella
Apex
Base

Knee joint
Posterior cruciate ligament
Anterior cruciate ligament
Tibial collateral ligament
Fibular collateral ligament
Lateral meniscus
Medial meniscus

Articulations
Interphalangeal
Metatarsophalangeal
Intermetatarsal
Tarsometatarsal
Intertarsal
Subtalar
    Talocalcaneonavicular
    Talocalcaneal
Calcaneocuboid
Cuneocuboid
Intercuneiform
Cuboidonavicular
Naviculocuneiform
Ankle mortise
    Talofibular
    Tibiotalar
Tibiofibular
    Proximal
    Distal
Knee
Patellofemoral
Femorotibial

Lower Limb Articulations

**ABBREVIATIONS USED
IN CHAPTER 6**

ASIS	Anterior superior iliac spine
DIP*	Distal interphalangeal
IP*	Interphalangeal
PIP*	Proximal interphalangeal
MTP	Metatarsophalangeal
TMT	Tarsometatarsal

See Addendum A for a summary of all abbreviations used in Volume 1.
*The same abbreviations are used for joints in the hand.

SUMMARY OF PATHOLOGY

Condition	Definition
Bone cyst	Fluid-filled cyst with a wall of fibrous tissue
Congenital clubfoot	Abnormal twisting of the foot, usually inward and downward
Dislocation	Displacement of a bone from the joint space
Fracture	Disruption in the continuity of bone
Pott	Avulsion fracture of the medial malleolus with loss of the ankle mortise
Jones	Avulsion fracture of the base of the fifth metatarsal
Gout	Hereditary form of arthritis in which uric acid is deposited in joints
Metastases	Transfer of a cancerous lesion from one area to another
Osgood-Schlatter disease	Incomplete separation or avulsion of the tibial tuberosity
Osteoarthritis or degenerative joint disease	Form of arthritis marked by progressive cartilage deterioration in synovial joints and vertebrae
Osteomalacia or rickets	Softening of the bones owing to vitamin D deficiency
Osteomyelitis	Inflammation of bone owing to a pyogenic infection
Osteopetrosis	Increased density of atypically soft bone
Osteoporosis	Loss of bone density
Paget disease	Chronic metabolic disease of bone marked by weakened, deformed, and thickened bone that fractures easily
Tumor	New tissue growth where cell proliferation is uncontrolled
Chondrosarcoma	Malignant tumor arising from cartilage cells
Enchondroma	Benign tumor consisting of cartilage
Ewing sarcoma	Malignant tumor of bone arising in medullary tissue
Osteochondroma or exostosis	Benign bone tumor projection with a cartilaginous cap
Osteoclastoma or giant cell tumor	Lucent lesion in the metaphysis, usually at the distal femur
Osteoid osteoma	Benign lesion of cortical bone
Osteosarcoma	Malignant, primary tumor of bone with bone or cartilage formation

EXPOSURE TECHNIQUE CHART ESSENTIAL PROJECTIONS

LOWER LIMB

Part	cm	kVp*	tm	mA	mAs	AEC	SID	IR	Dose† (mrad)
Toes—*All*‡	Ave	54	0.01	200s	2		40″	8 × 10 in-2	5
Foot—*AP, oblique, lateral*‡	Ave	60	0.01	200s	2		40″	24 × 30 cm-2	12
Calcaneus—*Axial*‡	Ave	65	0.03	200s	6		40″	8 × 10 in	42
Calcaneus—*Lateral*‡	Ave	60	0.01	200s	2		40″	8 × 10 in	12
Ankle—*AP*§	11	63	0.01	200s	2		40″	24 × 30 cm-2	4
Ankle—*Lateral*§	7	59	0.01	200s	2		40″	24 × 30 cm-2	4
Leg—*All*§	11	63	0.01	200s	2		40″	35 × 43 cm-2	4
Knee—*AP, oblique, lateral*‖	12	65		200s		◌◌●	40″	24 × 30 cm-2	28
Knees—*Standing*‖	12	65	0.06	200s	12		40″	35 × 43 cm-2	28
Intercondylar fossa§	14	70	0.02	200s	4		40″	8 × 10 in	9
Patella—*PA*‖	12	65		200s		◌◌●	40″	8 × 10 in	22
Patella—*Lateral*‖	12	65	0.01	200s	2		40″	8 × 10 in	22
Patella—*Tangential*§	12	65	0.01	200s	2		40″	24 × 30 cm-2	4
Femur—*AP, lateral*‖	15	70		200s		◌◌●	40″	35 × 43 cm-2	43
Femur—*Proximal*‖	19	65		200s		◌◌●	40″	35 × 43 cm-2	116

*kVp values are for a three-phase, 12-pulse generator or high frequency.
†Relative doses for comparison use. All doses are skin entrance for average adult at cm indicated.
‡Tabletop, extremity IR. Screen-film speed 100.
§Tabletop, standard IR. Screen-film speed 300 or equivalent CR.
‖Bucky, 16:1 grid. Screen-film speed 300.
s, small focal spot.

Radiation Protection

Protecting the patient from unnecessary radiation is a professional responsibility of the radiographer (see Chapter 1 for specific guidelines). In this chapter, the *Shield gonads* statement at the end of the *Position of part* sections indicates that the patient is to be protected from unnecessary radiation by restricting the radiation beam, using proper collimation, and placing lead shielding between the gonads and the radiation source.

PROJECTIONS REMOVED

Because of significant advances in MRI, CT, and CT three-dimensional reconstruction, the following projections have been removed from this edition of the atlas. The projections eliminated may be reviewed in their entirety in the 11th and all previous editions of this atlas.
Sesamoids
  • Tangential, Causton method
Foot
  • Lateral (lateromedial)
Patella
  • PA oblique, medial, and lateral rotation
  • PA axial oblique, lateral rotation, Kuchendorf method

Toes

✦ AP OR AP AXIAL PROJECTIONS

Because of the natural curve of the toes, the IP joint spaces are not best shown on the AP projection. When demonstration of these joint spaces is not critical, an AP projection may be performed (Figs. 6-14 and 6-15). An AP axial projection is recommended to open the joint spaces and reduce foreshortening (Figs. 6-16 and 6-17).

> **Image receptor:** 8 × 10 inch (18 × 24 cm) crosswise for two images on one IR

Position of patient

• Have the patient seated or placed supine on the radiographic table.

Position of part

• With the patient in the supine or seated position, flex the knees, separate the feet about 6 inches (15 cm), and touch the knees together for immobilization.
• Center the toes directly over one half of the IR (see Figs. 6-14 and 6-16), or place a 15-degree foam wedge well under the foot and rest the toes near the elevated base of the wedge (Fig. 6-18).
• Adjust the IR half with its midline parallel to the long axis of the foot, and center it to the third MTP joint.
• *Shield gonads.*

NOTE: Some institutions may show the entire foot, whereas others radiograph only the toe or toes of interest.

Central ray

• Perpendicular through the third MTP joint (see Fig. 6-14) when showing the joint spaces is not critical. To open the joint spaces, either direct the central ray 15 degrees posteriorly through the third MTP joint (see Fig. 6-16), or if the 15-degree foam wedge is used, direct the central ray perpendicularly (Fig. 6-19).

Collimation

• 1 inch (2.5 cm) on all sides of the toes, including 1 inch (2.5 cm) proximal to the MTP joint

Structures shown

Images show the 14 phalanges of the toes; the distal portions of the metatarsals; and, on the axial projections, the IP joints.

EVALUATION CRITERIA

The following should be clearly shown:
■ Evidence of proper collimation
■ No rotation of phalanges; soft tissue width and midshaft concavity equal on both sides
■ Open IP and MTP joint spaces on axial projections
■ Toes separated from each other
■ Distal ends of the metatarsals
■ Soft tissues and bony trabecular detail

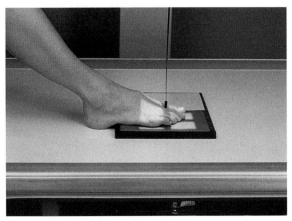

Fig. 6-14 AP toes, perpendicular central ray.

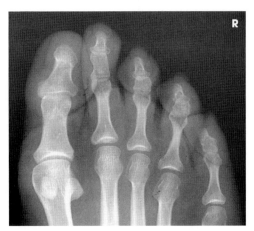

Fig. 6-15 AP toes, perpendicular central ray.

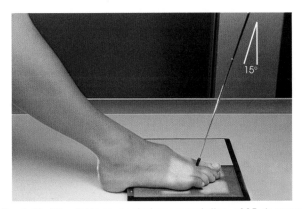

Fig. 6-16 AP axial toes, central ray angulation of 15 degrees.

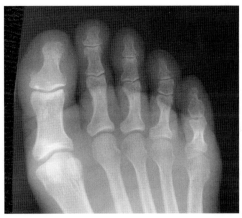

Fig. 6-17 AP axial toes, central ray angulation of 15 degrees.

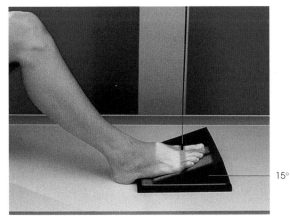

Fig. 6-18 AP axial, 15-degree foam wedge.

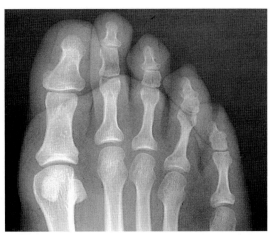

Fig. 6-19 AP axial, toes on 15-degree wedge.

Toes

PA PROJECTION

Image receptor: 8 × 10 inch (18 × 24 cm) crosswise for two images on one IR

Position of patient

- Have the patient lie prone on the radiographic table because this position naturally turns the foot over so that the dorsal aspect is in contact with the IR.

Position of part

- Place the toes in the appropriate position by elevating them on one or two small sandbags and adjusting the support to place the toes horizontal.
- Place the IR half under the toes with the midline of the side used parallel with the long axis of the foot, and center it to the third MTP joint (Fig. 6-20).

Central ray

- Perpendicular to the midpoint of the IR entering the third MTP joint (see Fig. 6-20). The IP joint spaces are shown well because the natural divergence of the x-ray beam coincides closely with the position of the toes (Fig. 6-21).

Structures shown

This projection shows the 14 phalanges of the toes, the IP joints, and the distal portions of the metatarsals.

EVALUATION CRITERIA

The following should be clearly shown:

- No rotation of phalanges; soft tissue width and midshaft concavity equal on both sides
- Open IP and MTP joint spaces
- Toes separated from each other
- Distal ends of the metatarsals
- Soft tissues and bony trabecular detail

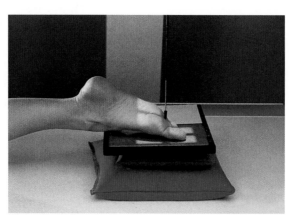

Fig. 6-20 PA toes.

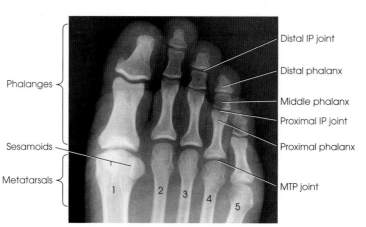

Fig. 6-21 PA toes.

♠ AP OBLIQUE PROJECTION
Medial rotation

Image receptor: 8 × 10 inch (18 × 24 cm) crosswise for two images on one IR

Position of patient
- Place the patient in the supine or seated position on the radiographic table.
- Flex the knee of the affected side enough to have the sole of the foot resting firmly on the table.

Position of part
- Position the IR half under the toes.
- Medially rotate the lower leg and foot, and adjust the plantar surface of the foot to form a 30- to 45-degree angle from the plane of the IR (Fig. 6-22).
- Center the toes to the IR.
- *Shield gonads.*

Central ray
- Perpendicular and entering the third MTP joint

Collimation
- 1 inch (2.5 cm) on all sides of the toes, including 1 inch (2.5 cm) proximal to the MTP joint

NOTE: Oblique projections of individual toes may be obtained by centering the affected toe to the portion of the IR being used and collimating closely. The foot may be placed in a medial oblique position for the first and second toes and in a lateral oblique position for the fourth and fifth toes. Either oblique position is adequate for the third (middle) toe.

Structures shown
An AP oblique projection of the phalanges shows the toes and the distal portion of the metatarsals rotated medially (Fig. 6-23).

EVALUATION CRITERIA
The following should be clearly shown:
- Evidence of proper collimation
- All phalanges
- Oblique toes; more soft tissue width and more midshaft concavity on side away from IR
- Open IP and second through fifth MTP joint spaces
- First MTP joint (not always opened)
- Toes separated from each other
- Distal ends of the metatarsals
- Soft tissue and bony trabecular detail

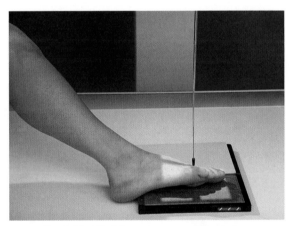

Fig. 6-22 AP oblique toes, medial rotation.

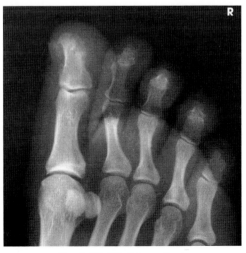

Fig. 6-23 AP oblique toes.

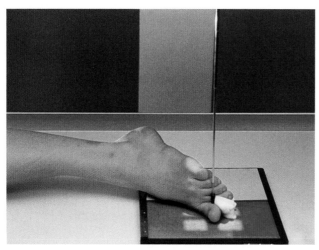

Fig. 6-24 Lateral great toe.

♠ LATERAL PROJECTIONS
Mediolateral or lateromedial

Image receptor: 8 × 10 inch (18 × 24 cm) crosswise for multiple exposures on one IR

Position of patient
- Have the patient lie in the lateral recumbent position.
- Support the affected limb on sandbags, and adjust it in a comfortable position.
- To prevent superimposition, tape the toes above the one being examined into a flexed position; a 4 × 4 inch gauze pad also may be used to separate the toes.

NOTE: Manipulate toes only if no deformity is apparent.

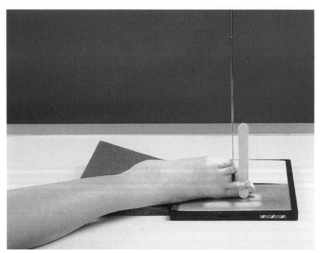

Fig. 6-25 Lateral second toe.

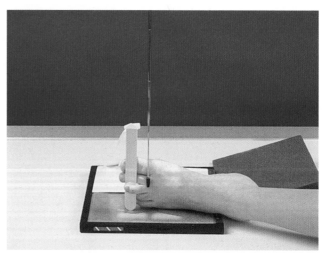

Fig. 6-26 Lateral third toe.

Position of part

Great toe, second toe

- Place the patient on the *unaffected* side for these two toes.
- Place an 8 × 10 inch (18 × 24 cm) IR under the toe, and center it to the proximal phalanx.
- Grasp the patient's limb by the heel and knee, and adjust its position to place the toe in a true lateral position (plane through MTP joints will be perpendicular to IR).
- Adjust the long axis of the IR so that it is parallel with the long axis of the toe (Figs. 6-24 and 6-25).

Third, fourth, fifth toes

- Place the patient on the *affected* side for these three toes.
- Select an 8 × 10 inch (18 × 24 cm) IR.
- Grasp patient's limb by heel and knee, and adjust its position to place the toes in a true lateral position (plane through MTP joints is perpendicular to IR).
- Adjust the position of the limb to place the toe of interest and the IR or film in a parallel position, placing the toe as close to the IR or film as possible.
- Support the elevated heel on a sandbag or sponge for immobilization (Figs. 6-26 to 6-28).
- *Shield gonads.*

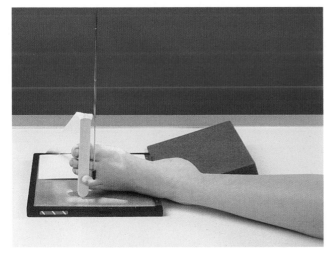

Fig. 6-27 Lateral fourth toe.

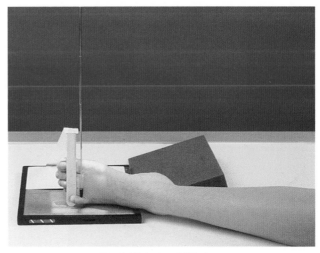

Fig. 6-28 Lateral fifth toe.

Central ray

- Perpendicular to the plane of the IR, entering the IP joint of the great toe or the proximal IP joint of the lesser toes

Collimation

- 1 inch (2.5 cm) on all sides of the toes, including 1 inch (2.5 cm) proximal to the MTP joint

Structures shown

Images show a lateral projection of the phalanges of the toe and the IP articulations projected free of the other toes (Figs. 6-29 to 6-33).

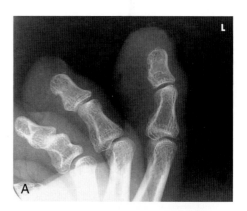

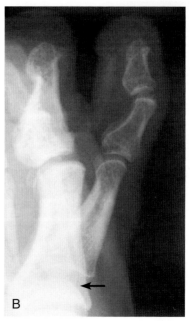

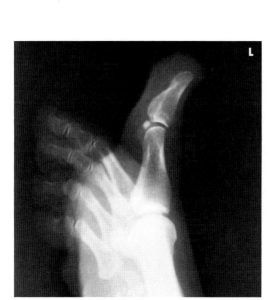

Fig. 6-29 Lateral great toe.

Fig. 6-30 A, Lateral second toe. **B,** Lateral second toe showing MTP joint (*arrow*).

EVALUATION CRITERIA

The following should be clearly shown:
- Evidence of proper collimation
- Phalanges in profile (toenail should appear lateral)
- Phalanx, without superimposition of adjacent toes; when superimposition cannot be avoided, the proximal phalanx must be shown
- Open IP joint spaces; the MTP joints are overlapped but may be seen in some patients
- Soft tissue and bony trabecular detail

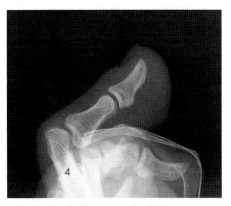

Fig. 6-32 Lateral fourth toe.

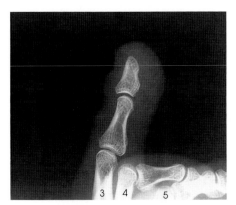

Fig. 6-31 Lateral third toe.

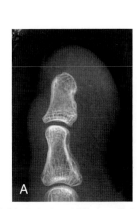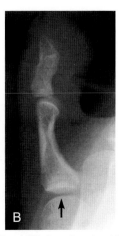

Fig. 6-33 A, Lateral fifth toe. **B,** Lateral fifth toe showing MTP joint (*arrow*). Note distal IP joint is fused.

Sesamoids

TANGENTIAL PROJECTION
LEWIS[1] AND HOLLY[2] METHODS

Image receptor: 8 × 10 inch (18 × 24 cm) crosswise for multiple exposures on one IR

---

[1]Lewis RW: Nonroutine views in roentgen examination of the extremities, *Surg Gynecol Obstet* 67:38, 1938.
[2]Holly EW: Radiography of the tarsal sesamoid bones, *Med Radiogr Photogr* 31:73, 1955.

Position of patient
- Place the patient in the prone position.
- Elevate the ankle of the affected side on sandbags for stability, if needed. A folded towel may be placed under the knee for comfort.

Position of part
- Rest the great toe on the table in a position of dorsiflexion, and adjust it to place the ball of the foot perpendicular to the horizontal plane.
- Center the IR to the second metatarsal (Fig. 6-34).
- *Shield gonads.*

Central ray
- Perpendicular and tangential to the first MTP joint

Structures shown
The resulting image shows a tangential projection of the metatarsal head in profile and the sesamoids (Fig. 6-35).

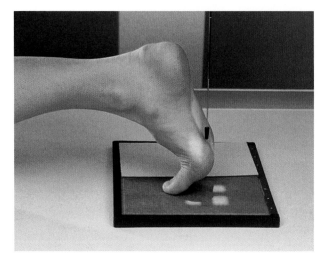

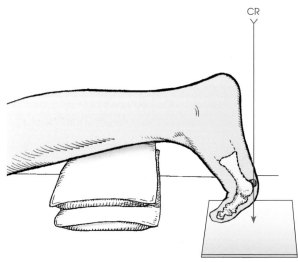

Fig. 6-34 Tangential sesamoids: Lewis method.

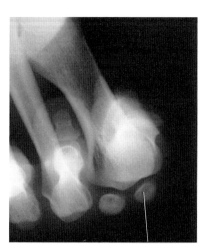

Sesamoid

Fig. 6-35 Tangential sesamoids: Lewis method with toes against IR.

Lower Limb

Sesamoids

The following should be clearly shown:
- Sesamoids free of any portion of the first metatarsal
- Metatarsal heads

NOTE: Holly[1] described a position that he believed was more comfortable for the patient. With the patient seated on the table, the foot is adjusted so that the medial border is vertical, and the plantar surface is at an angle of 75 degrees with the plane of the IR. The patient holds the toes in a flexed position with a strip of gauze bandage. The *central ray* is directed perpendicular to the head of the first metatarsal bone (Figs. 6-36 to 6-38).

---

[1]Holly EW: Radiography of the tarsal sesamoid bones, *Med Radiogr Photogr* 31:73, 1955.

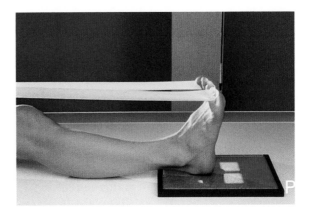

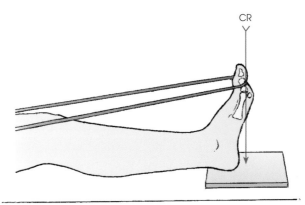

Fig. 6-36 Tangential sesamoids: Holly method.

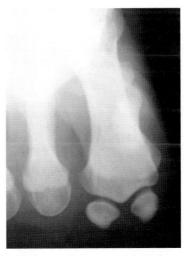

Fig. 6-37 Tangential sesamoids: Holly method with heel against IR.

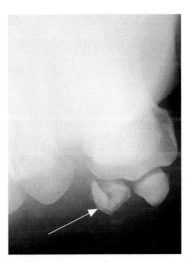

Fig. 6-38 Sesamoid with fracture (*arrow*).

🔷 AP OR AP AXIAL PROJECTION

Radiographs may be obtained by directing the central ray perpendicular to the plane of the IR or by angling the central ray 10 degrees posteriorly. When a 10-degree posterior angle is used, the central ray is perpendicular to the metatarsals, reducing foreshortening. The TMT joint spaces of the midfoot are also better shown (Figs. 6-39 and 6-40).

Image receptor: 10 × 12 inch (24 × 30 cm) lengthwise

Position of patient

- Place the patient in the supine or seated position.
- Flex the knee of the affected side enough to rest the sole of the foot firmly on the radiographic table.

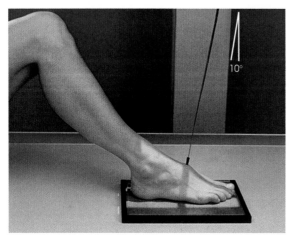

Fig. 6-39 AP axial foot with posterior angulation of 10 degrees.

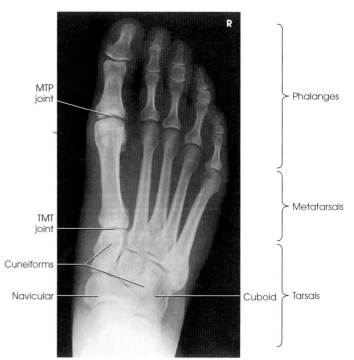

Fig. 6-40 AP axial foot with posterior angulation of 10 degrees.

Position of part

- Position the IR under the patient's foot, center it to the base of the third metatarsal, and adjust it so that its long axis is parallel with the long axis of the foot.
- Hold the leg in the vertical position by having the patient flex the opposite knee and lean it against the knee of the affected side.
- In this foot position, the entire plantar surface rests on the IR; it is necessary to take precautions against the IR slipping.
- Ensure that no rotation of the foot occurs.
- *Shield gonads.*

Central ray

- Directed one of two ways: (1) 10 degrees toward the heel entering the base of the third metatarsal (see Fig. 6-39) or (2) perpendicular to the IR and entering the base of the third metatarsal (Fig. 6-41). Palpating the prominent base of the fifth metatarsal assists in finding the third metatarsal. The third metatarsal base is in the midline, approximately 1 inch anterior (toward the toes) (Fig. 6-42).

Collimation

- 1 inch (2.5 cm) on the sides and 1 inch (2.5 cm) beyond the calcaneus and distal tip of the toes.

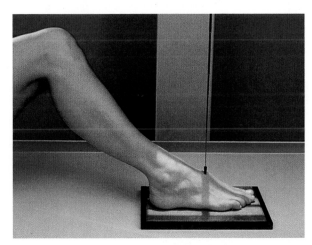

Fig. 6-41 AP foot with perpendicular central ray.

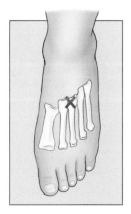

Fig. 6-42 Front view of foot in position showing central ray entrance point.

◤ COMPENSATING FILTER

This projection can be improved with the use of a wedge-type compensating filter because of the difference in thickness between the toe area and the much thicker tarsal area (see Fig. 6-44).

Structures shown

The resulting image shows an AP (dorsoplantar) projection of the tarsals anterior to the talus, metatarsals, and phalanges (Figs. 6-43 to 6-45). This projection is used for localizing foreign bodies, determining the location of fragments in fractures of the metatarsals and anterior tarsals, and performing general surveys of the bones of the foot.

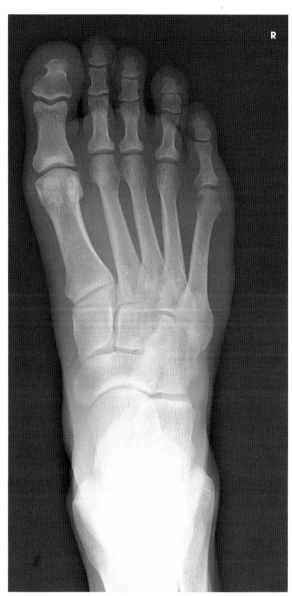

Fig. 6-44 AP foot with Ferlic compensating filter. Note how tarsal bones are better visualized.

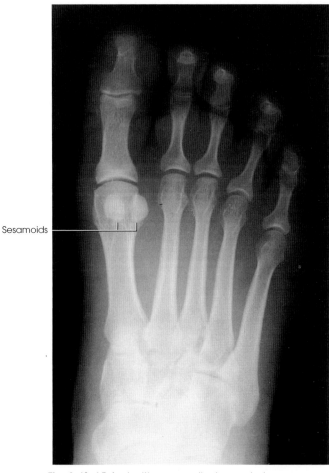

Sesamoids

Fig. 6-43 AP foot with perpendicular central ray.

Foot

EVALUATION CRITERIA

The following should be clearly shown:
- Evidence of proper collimation
- No rotation of the foot
- Equal amount of space between the adjacent midshafts of the second through fourth metatarsals
- Overlap of the second through fifth metatarsal bases
- Visualization of the phalanges and tarsals distal to the talus and the metatarsals
- Open joint space between medial and intermediate cuneiforms

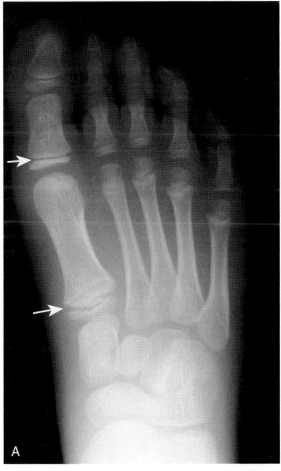
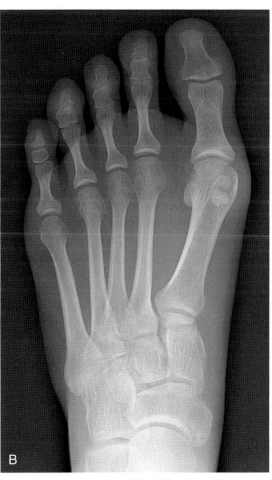

Fig. 6-45 A, AP foot of a 6-year-old patient. Note epiphyseal lines (*arrows*). **B,** AP foot showing well-penetrated tarsal bones.

255

♠ AP OBLIQUE PROJECTION
Medial rotation

Image receptor: 10 × 12 inch (24 × 30 cm) lengthwise

NOTE: The medial oblique is preferred over the lateral oblique because the plane through the metatarsals is more parallel to the IR, and it opens the lateral side joints of the midfoot and hindfoot better.

Position of patient
- Place the patient in the supine or seated position.
- Flex the knee of the affected side enough to have the plantar surface of the foot rest firmly on the radiographic table.

Position of part
- Place the IR under the patient's foot, parallel with its long axis, and center it to the midline of the foot at the level of the base of the third metatarsal.
- Rotate the patient's leg medially until the plantar surface of the foot forms an angle of 30 degrees to the plane of the IR (Fig. 6-46). If the angle of the foot is increased more than 30 degrees, the lateral cuneiform tends to be thrown over the other cuneiforms.[1]
- *Shield gonads.*

Central ray
- Perpendicular to the base of the third metatarsal

Collimation
- 1 inch (2.5 cm) on all sides and 1 inch (2.5 cm) beyond the calcaneus and distal tip of the toes

◥ COMPENSATING FILTER
This projection can be improved with the use of a wedge-type compensating filter because of the difference in thickness between the toe area and the much thicker tarsal area.

[1]Doub HP: A useful position for examining the foot, *Radiology* 16:764, 1931.

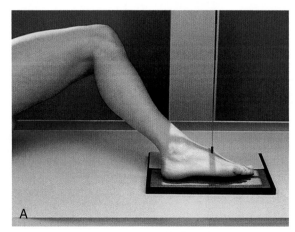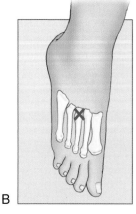

Fig. 6-46 A, AP oblique foot, medial rotation. **B,** Front view of oblique foot in position showing central ray entrance point.

Structures shown

The resulting image shows the interspaces between the following: the cuboid and the calcaneus, the cuboid and the fourth and fifth metatarsals, the cuboid and the lateral cuneiform, and the talus and the navicular bone. The cuboid is shown in profile. The sinus tarsi is also well shown (Fig. 6-47).

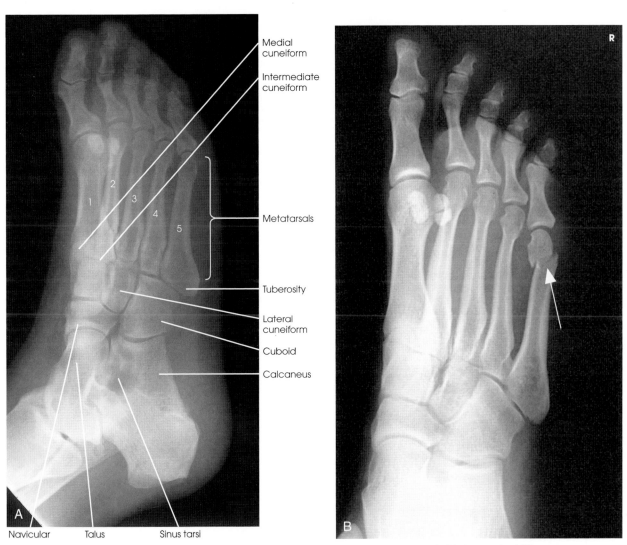

Fig. 6-47 A, AP oblique projection foot, medial rotation. **B,** Fracture of distal aspect of fifth metatarsal (*arrow*). Calcaneus was not included, and technique was adjusted to visualize distal foot better.

AP OBLIQUE PROJECTION
Lateral rotation

Image receptor: 10 × 12 inch (24 × 30 cm) lengthwise

Position of patient
- Place the patient in the supine position.
- Flex the knee of the affected side enough for the plantar surface of the foot to rest firmly on the radiographic table.

Position of part
- Place the IR under the patient's foot, parallel with its long axis, and center it to the midline of the foot at the level of the base of the third metatarsal.
- Rotate the leg laterally until the plantar surface of the foot forms an angle of 30 degrees to the IR.
- Support the elevated side of the foot on a 30-degree foam wedge to ensure consistent results (Fig. 6-48).
- *Shield gonads.*

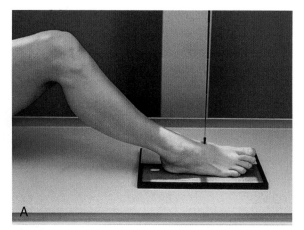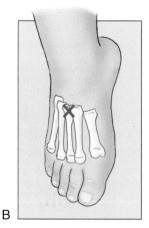

Fig. 6-48 A, AP oblique foot, lateral rotation. **B,** Front view of oblique foot in position showing central ray entrance point.

Lower Limb

Central ray

• Perpendicular to the base of the third metatarsal

Structures shown

The resulting image shows the interspaces between the first and second metatarsals and between the medial and intermediate cuneiforms (Fig. 6-49).

EVALUATION CRITERIA

The following should be clearly shown:

■ Separate first and second metatarsal bases
■ No superimposition of the medial and intermediate cuneiforms
■ Navicular bone more clearly shown than in the medial rotation
■ Sufficient density to show the phalanges, metatarsals, and tarsals

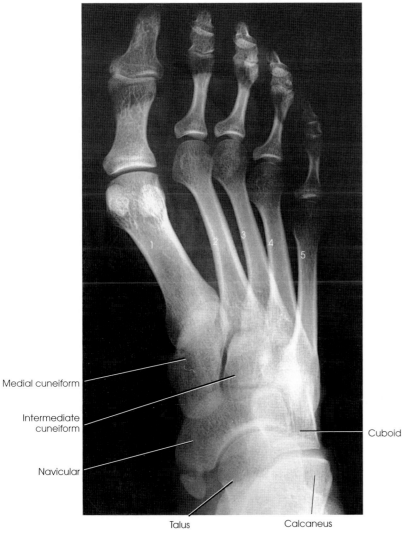
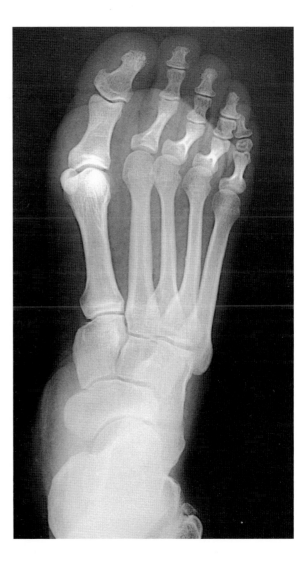

Medial cuneiform

Intermediate cuneiform

Navicular

Cuboid

Talus

Calcaneus

Fig. 6-49 AP oblique foot.

⚘ LATERAL PROJECTION
Mediolateral

The lateral (mediolateral) projection is routinely used in most radiology departments because it is the most comfortable position for the patient to assume.

Image receptor: 10 × 12 inch (24 × 30 cm) lengthwise

Position of patient
- Have the patient lie on the radiographic table and turn toward the affected side until the leg and foot are lateral.
- Place the opposite leg behind the affected leg.

Position of part
- Elevate the patient's knee enough to place the patella perpendicular to the horizontal plane, and adjust a sandbag support under the knee.
- Adjust the foot to place the plantar surface of the forefoot perpendicular to the IR (Fig. 6-50).
- Center the IR to the midfoot, and adjust it so that its long axis is parallel with the long axis of the foot.
- Dorsiflex the foot to form a 90-degree angle with the lower leg.
- *Shield gonads.*

Central ray
- Perpendicular to the base of the third metatarsal

Collimation
- 1 inch (2.5 cm) on all sides of the shadow of the foot including 1 inch (2.5 cm) above the medial malleolus

Structures shown
The resulting image shows the entire foot in profile, the ankle joint, and the distal ends of the tibia and fibula (Figs. 6-51 and 6-52).

EVALUATION CRITERIA

The following should be clearly shown:
- Evidence of proper collimation
- Metatarsals nearly superimposed
- Distal leg
- Fibula overlapping the posterior portion of the tibia
- Tibiotalar joint
- Sufficient density to show the superimposed tarsals and metatarsals

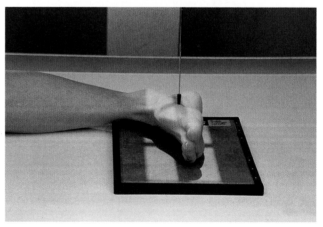

Fig. 6-50 Lateral foot.

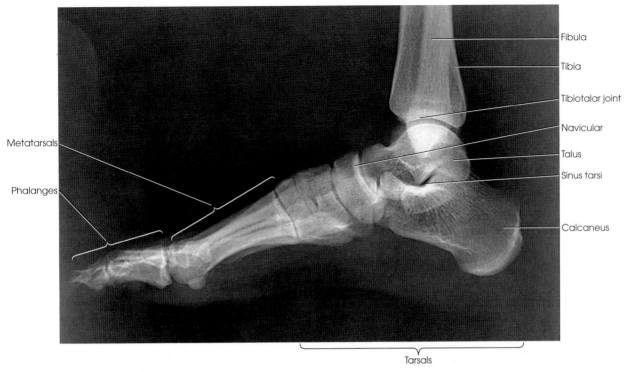

Fibula

Tibia

Tibiotalar joint

Navicular

Talus

Sinus tarsi

Calcaneus

Metatarsals

Phalanges

Tarsals

Fig. 6-51 Lateral (mediolateral) foot with anatomy identified.

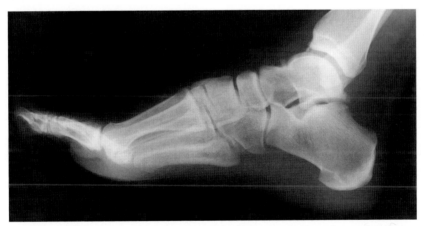

Fig. 6-52 Lateral (mediolateral foot) with foot not dorsiflexed completely.

Longitudinal Arch
LATERAL PROJECTION
Lateromedial
WEIGHT-BEARING METHOD
Standing

Image receptor: 10 × 12 inch (24 × 30 cm) lengthwise

Position of patient
- Place the patient in the upright position, preferably on a low riser that has an IR groove. If such a riser is unavailable, use blocks to elevate the feet to the level of the x-ray tube (Figs. 6-53 and 6-54).
- If needed, use a mobile unit to allow the x-ray tube to reach the floor level.

Position of part
- Place the IR in the IR groove of the stool or between blocks.
- Have the patient stand in a natural position, one foot on each side of the IR, with the weight of the body equally distributed on the feet.
- Adjust the IR so that it is centered to the base of the third metatarsal.
- After the exposure, replace the IR and position the new one to image the opposite foot.
- *Shield gonads.*

Central ray
- Perpendicular to a point just above the base of the third metatarsal

Structures shown
The resulting image shows a lateromedial projection of the bones of the foot with weight-bearing. The projection is used to show the structural status of the longitudinal arch. The right and left sides are examined for comparison (Figs. 6-55 and 6-56).

EVALUATION CRITERIA
The following should be clearly shown:
- Superimposed plantar surfaces of the metatarsal heads
- Entire foot and distal leg
- Fibula overlapping the posterior portion of the tibia
- Sufficient density to visualize the superimposed tarsals and metatarsals

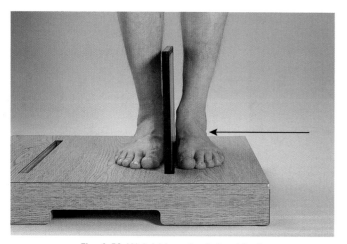

Fig. 6-53 Weight-bearing lateral foot.

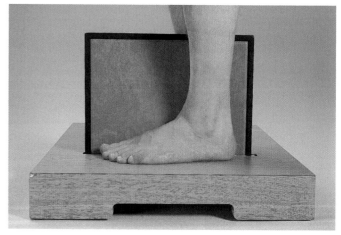

Fig. 6-54 Weight-bearing lateral foot.

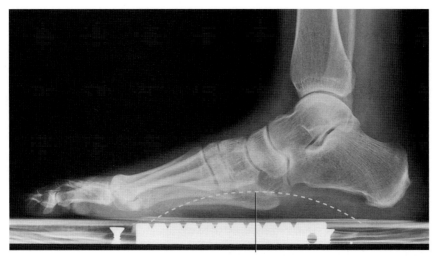

Longitudinal arch

Fig. 6-55 Weight-bearing lateral foot showing centimeter measuring scale built into standing platform.

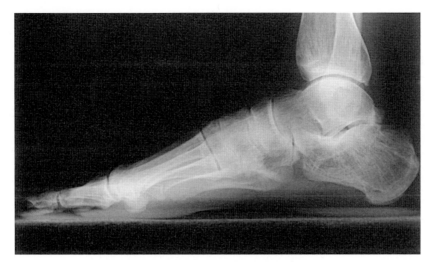

Fig. 6-56 Weight-bearing lateral foot.

AP AXIAL PROJECTION
WEIGHT-BEARING METHOD
Standing

Image receptor: 10 × 12 inch (24 × 30 cm) crosswise for both feet on one IR

SID: 48 inches (122 cm). This SID is used to reduce magnification and improve recorded detail in the image.

Position of patient
• Place the patient in the standing-upright position.

Position of part
• Place the IR on the floor, and have the patient stand on the IR with the feet centered on each side.

• Pull the patient's pant legs up to the knee level, if necessary.
• Ensure that right and left markers and an upright marker are placed on the IR.
• Ensure that the patient's weight is distributed equally on each foot (Fig. 6-57).
• The patient may hold the x-ray tube crane for stability.
• *Shield gonads.*

Central ray
• Angled 10 degrees toward the heel is optimal. A minimum of 15 degrees is usually necessary to have enough room to position the tube and allow the patient to stand. The central ray is positioned between the feet and at the level of the base of the third metatarsal.

Structures shown
The resulting image shows a weight-bearing AP axial projection of both feet, permitting an accurate evaluation and comparison of the tarsals and metatarsals (Fig. 6-58).

EVALUATION CRITERIA
The following should be clearly shown:
■ Both feet centered on one image
■ Phalanges, metatarsals, and distal tarsals
■ Correct right and left marker placement and a weight-bearing marker
■ Correct exposure technique to visualize all components

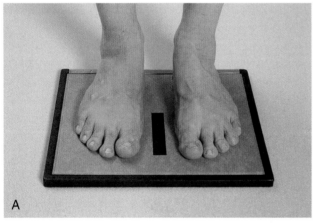 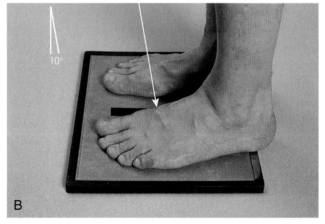

Fig. 6-57 Weight-bearing AP both feet, standing. **A,** Correct position of both feet on IR. **B,** Lateral perspective of same projection shows position of feet on IR and central ray.

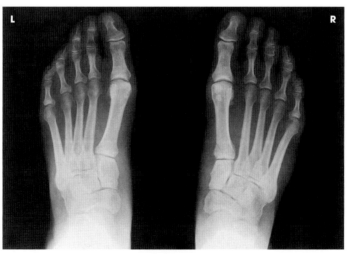

Fig. 6-58 Weight-bearing AP both feet, standing.

AP AXIAL PROJECTION
WEIGHT-BEARING COMPOSITE METHOD
Standing

Image receptor: 10 × 12 inch (24 × 30 cm) lengthwise

Position of patient
- Place the patient in the standing-upright position. The patient should stand at a comfortable height on a low stool or on the floor.

Position of part
- With the patient standing upright, adjust the IR under the foot and center its midline to the long axis of the foot.
- To prevent superimposition of the leg shadow on that of the ankle joint, have the patient place the opposite foot one step backward for the exposure of the forefoot and one step forward for the exposure of the hindfoot or calcaneus.
- *Shield gonads.*

Central ray
- To use the masking effect of the leg, direct the central ray along the plane of alignment of the foot in both exposures.
- With the tube in front of the patient and adjusted for a posterior angulation of 15 degrees, center the central ray to the base of the third metatarsal for the first exposure (Figs. 6-59 and 6-60).

- Caution the patient to maintain the position of the affected foot carefully and to place the opposite foot one step forward in preparation for the second exposure.
- Move the tube behind the patient, adjust it for an anterior angulation of 25 degrees, and direct the central ray to the posterior surface of the ankle. The central ray emerges on the plantar surface at the level of the lateral malleolus (Figs. 6-61 and 6-62). An increase in technical factors is recommended for this exposure.

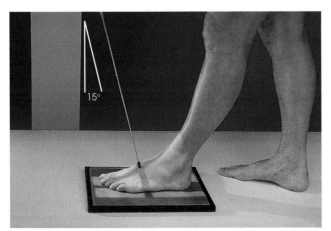

Fig. 6-59 Composite AP axial foot, posterior angulation of 15 degrees.

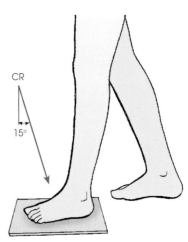

Fig. 6-60 Composite AP axial foot, posterior angulation of 15 degrees.

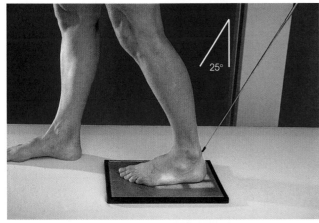

Fig. 6-61 Composite AP axial foot, anterior angulation of 25 degrees.

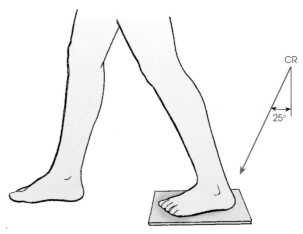

Fig. 6-62 Composite AP axial foot, anterior angulation of 25 degrees.

Structures shown

The resulting image shows a weight-bearing AP axial projection of all bones of the foot. The full outline of the foot is projected free of the leg (Fig. 6-63).

The following should be clearly shown:
- All tarsals
- Shadow of leg not overlapping the tarsals
- Foot not rotated
- Tarsals, metatarsals, and toes with similar densities

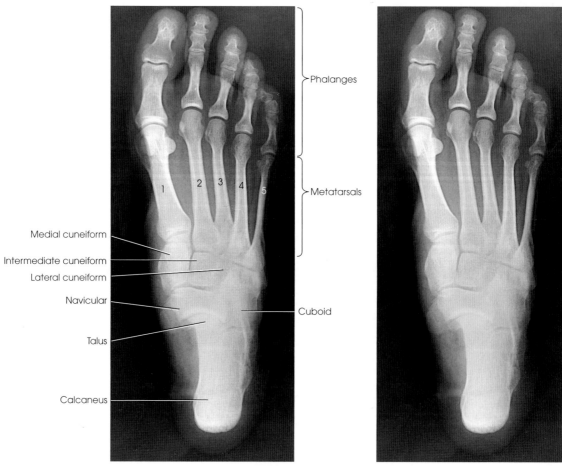

Fig. 6-63 Composite AP axial foot.

Phalanges

Metatarsals

Medial cuneiform

Intermediate cuneiform

Lateral cuneiform

Navicular

Talus

Cuboid

Calcaneus

Congenital Clubfoot
AP PROJECTION
KITE METHODS

The typical clubfoot, or *talipes equinovarus,* shows three deviations from the normal alignment of the foot in relation to the weight-bearing axis of the leg. These deviations are plantar flexion and inversion of the calcaneus (equinus), medial displacement of the forefoot (adduction), and elevation of the medial border of the foot (supination). The typical clubfoot has numerous variations. Each of the typical abnormalities just described has varying degrees of deformity.

The classic Kite methods[1,2]—exactly placed AP and lateral projections—for radiography of the clubfoot are used to show the anatomy of the foot and the bones or ossification centers of the tarsals and their relation to one another. *A primary objective makes it essential that no attempt be made to change the abnormal alignment of the foot when placing it on the IR.* Davis and Hatt[3] stated that even slight rotation of the foot can result in marked alteration in the radiographically projected relation of the ossification centers.

[1]Kite JH: Principles involved in the treatment of congenital clubfoot, *J Bone Joint Surg* 21:595, 1939.
[2]Kite JH: *The clubfoot,* New York, 1964, Grune & Stratton.
[3]Davis LA, Hatt WS: Congenital abnormalities of the feet, *Radiology* 64:818, 1955.

The AP projection shows the degree of adduction of the forefoot and the degree of inversion of the calcaneus.

Image receptor: 8 × 10 inch (18 × 24 cm)

Position of patient
- Place the infant in the supine position, with the hips and knees flexed to permit the foot to rest flat on the IR. Elevate the body on firm pillows to knee height to simplify gonad shielding and leg adjustment.

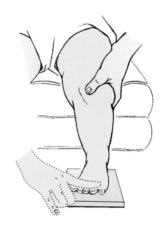

Fig. 6-64 AP foot to show clubfoot deformity.

Position of part
- Rest the feet flat on the IR with the ankles extended slightly to prevent superimposition of the leg shadow.
- Hold the infant's knees together or in such a way that the legs are exactly vertical (i.e., so that they do not lean medially or laterally).
- Using a lead glove, hold the infant's toes. When the adduction deformity is too great to permit correct placement of the legs and feet for bilateral images without overlap of the feet, they must be examined separately (Figs. 6-64 and 6-65).
- *Shield gonads.*

Central ray
- Perpendicular to the tarsals, midway between the tarsal areas for a bilateral projection
- An approximately 15-degree posterior angle is generally required for the central ray to be perpendicular to the tarsals.
- Kite[1,2] stressed the importance of directing the central ray vertically for the purpose of projecting the true relationship of the bones and ossification centers.

[1]Kite JH: Principles involved in the treatment of congenital clubfoot, *J Bone Joint Surg* 21:595, 1939.
[2]Kite JH: *The clubfoot,* New York, 1964, Grune & Stratton.

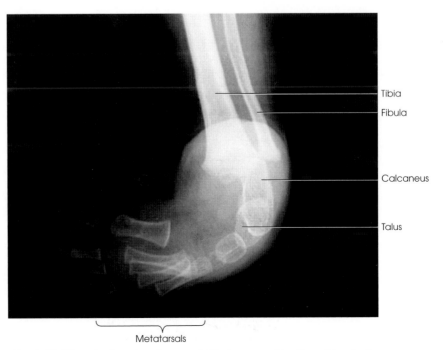

Fig. 6-65 AP projection showing nearly 90-degree adduction of forefoot.

Congenital Clubfoot
LATERAL PROJECTION
Mediolateral
KITE METHOD

The Kite method lateral radiograph shows the anterior talar subluxation and the degree of plantar flexion (equinus).

Position of patient
- Place the infant on his or her side in as near the lateral position as possible.
- Flex the uppermost limb, draw it forward, and hold it in place.

Position of part
- After adjusting the IR under the foot, place a support that has the same thickness as the IR under the infant's knee to prevent angulation of the foot and to ensure a lateral foot position.
- Hold the infant's toes in position with tape or a protected hand (Figs. 6-66 to 6-70).
- *Shield gonads.*

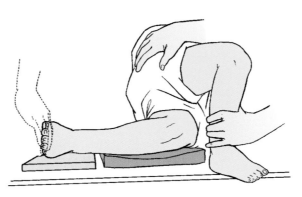

Fig. 6-66 Lateral foot.

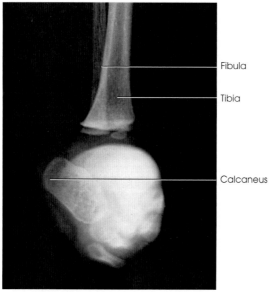

Fibula

Tibia

Calcaneus

Fig. 6-67 Lateral foot projection showing pitch of calcaneus. Other tarsals are obscured by adducted forefoot.

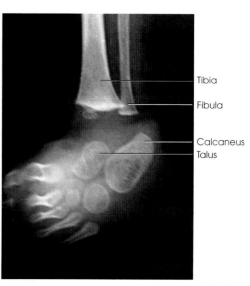

Tibia

Fibula

Calcaneus
Talus

Fig. 6-68 Nonroutine 45-degree medial rotation showing extent of talipes equinovarus.

Central ray

- Perpendicular to the midtarsal area

EVALUATION CRITERIA

The following should be clearly shown:

- No medial or lateral angulation of the leg
- Fibula in lateral projection overlapping the posterior half of the tibia
- The need for a repeat examination if slight variations in rotation are seen in either image compared with previous radiographs
- Sufficient density of the talus, calcaneus, and metatarsals to allow assessment of alignment variations

NOTE: Freiberger et al.[1] recommended that dorsiflexion of an infant's foot could be obtained by pressing a small plywood board against the sole of the foot. An older child or adult is placed in the upright position for a horizontal projection. With the upright position, the patient leans the leg forward to dorsiflex the foot.

NOTE: Conway and Cowell[2] recommended tomography to show coalition at the middle facet and particularly the hidden coalition involving the anterior facet.

[1]Freiberger RH et al: Roentgen examination of the deformed foot, *Semin Roentgenol* 5:341, 1970.
[2]Conway JJ, Cowell HR: Tarsal coalition: clinical significance and roentgenographic demonstration, *Radiology* 92:799, 1969.

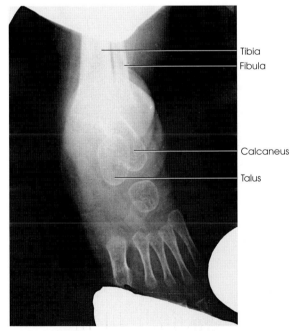

Fig. 6-69 AP projection after treatment (same patient as in Fig. 6-68).

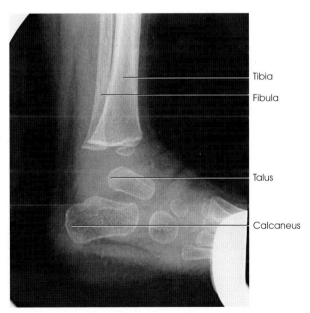

Fig. 6-70 Lateral projection after treatment (same patient as in Fig. 6-67).

Congenital Clubfoot

AXIAL PROJECTION

Dorsoplantar

KANDEL METHOD

Kandel[1] recommended the inclusion of a dorsoplantar axial projection in the examination of the patient with a clubfoot (Fig. 6-71).

[1]Kandel B: The suroplantar projection in the congenital clubfoot of the infant, *Acta Orthop Scand* 22:161, 1952.

For this method, the infant is held in a vertical or a bending-forward position. The plantar surface of the foot should rest on the IR, although a moderate elevation of the heel is acceptable when the equinus deformity is well marked. The central ray is directed 40 degrees anteriorly through the lower leg, as for the usual dorsoplantar projection of the calcaneus (Fig. 6-72).

Freiberger et al.[1] stated that sustentaculum talar joint fusion cannot be assumed on one projection because the central ray may not have been parallel with the articular surfaces. They recommended that three radiographs be obtained with varying central ray angulations (35, 45, and 55 degrees).

[1]Freiberger RH et al: Roentgen examination of the deformed foot, *Semin Roentgenol* 5:341, 1970.

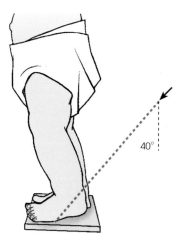

Fig. 6-71 Axial foot (dorsoplantar): Kandel method.

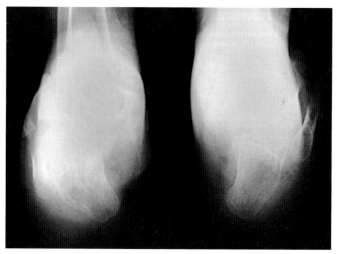

Fig. 6-72 Axial foot (dorsoplantar): Kandel method.

Calcaneus

 AXIAL PROJECTION
Plantodorsal

Image receptor: 8 × 10 inch (18 × 24 cm)

Position of patient
- Place the patient in the supine or seated position with the legs fully extended.

Position of part
- Place the IR under the patient's ankle, centered to the midline of the ankle (Figs. 6-73 and 6-74).
- Place a long strip of gauze around the ball of the foot. Have the patient grasp the gauze to hold the ankle in right-angle dorsiflexion.
- If the patient's ankles cannot be flexed enough to place the plantar surface of the foot perpendicular to the IR, elevate the leg on sandbags to obtain the correct position.
- *Shield gonads.*

Central ray
- Directed to the midpoint of the IR at a cephalic angle of 40 degrees to the long axis of the foot. The central ray enters the base of the third metatarsal.

Collimation
- 1 inch (2.5 cm) on three sides of the shadow of the calcaneus

 COMPENSATING FILTER

This projection can be improved significantly with the use of a compensating filter because of the increased density through the midportion of the foot.

Structures shown
The resulting image shows an axial projection of the calcaneus (Fig. 6-75).

EVALUATION CRITERIA
The following should be clearly shown:
- Evidence of proper collimation
- Calcaneus and subtalar joint
- No rotation of the calcaneus—the first or fifth metatarsals not projected to the sides of the foot
- Anterior portion of the calcaneus without excessive density over the posterior portion; otherwise, two images may be needed for the two regions of thickness

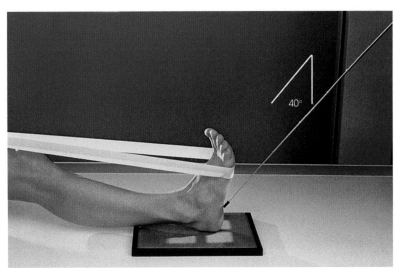

Fig. 6-73 Axial (plantodorsal) calcaneus.

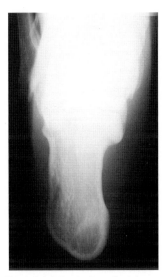

Fig. 6-74 Axial (plantodorsal) calcaneus. Note anterior calcaneus is not penetrated.

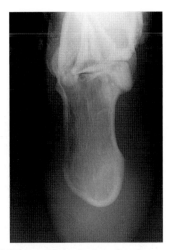

Fig. 6-75 Axial (plantodorsal) calcaneus. Image made using Ferlic swimmer's filter. Note penetration of anterior calcaneus and metatarsal joint spaces.

Calcaneus

AXIAL PROJECTION
Dorsoplantar

Image receptor: 8 × 10 inch (18 × 24 cm)

Position of patient
- Place the patient in the prone position.

Position of part
- Elevate the patient's ankle on sandbags.
- Adjust the height and position of the sandbags under the ankle in such a way that the patient can dorsiflex the ankle enough to place the long axis of the foot perpendicular to the tabletop.
- Place the IR against the plantar surface of the foot, and support it in position with sandbags or a portable IR holder (Figs. 6-76 and 6-77).
- *Shield gonads.*

Central ray
- Directed to the midpoint of the IR at a caudal angle of 40 degrees to the long axis of the foot. The central ray enters the dorsal surface of the ankle joint.

▼ COMPENSATING FILTER
This projection can be improved significantly with the use of a compensating filter because of the increased density through the midportion of the foot.

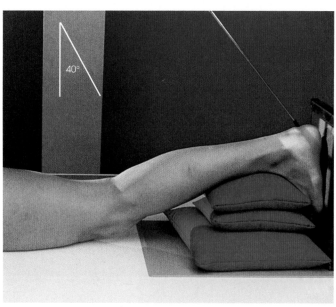

Fig. 6-76 Axial (dorsoplantar) calcaneus.

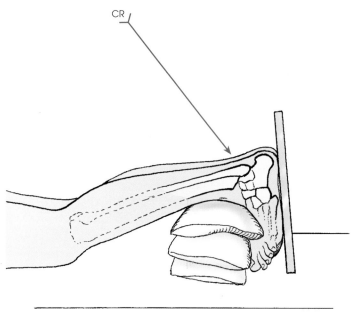

Fig. 6-77 Axial (dorsoplantar) calcaneus.

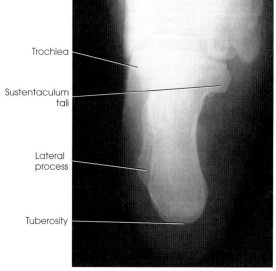
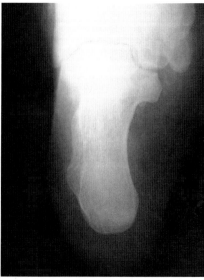

Trochlea

Sustentaculum tali

Lateral process

Tuberosity

Fig. 6-78 Axial (dorsoplantar) calcaneus.

Lower Limb

Calcaneus

Structures shown

The resulting image shows an axial projection of the calcaneus and the subtalar joint (Fig. 6-78). CT is often used to show this bone (Fig. 6-79).

EVALUATION CRITERIA

The following should be clearly shown:
- Calcaneus and the subtalar joint
- Sustentaculum tali
- Calcaneus not rotated—the first or fifth metatarsals not projected to the sides of the foot
- Anterior portion of the calcaneus without excessive density over posterior portion; otherwise, two images may be needed for the two regions of thickness

WEIGHT-BEARING COALITION METHOD

This weight-bearing method, described by Lilienfeld[1] (cit. Holzknecht), has come into use to show calcaneotalar coalition.[2-4] For this reason, it has been called the *coalition position*.

Position of patient

- Place the patient in the standing-upright position.

Position of part

- Center the IR to the long axis of the calcaneus, with the posterior surface of the heel at the edge of the IR.
- To prevent superimposition of the leg shadow, have the patient place the opposite foot one step forward (Fig. 6-80).

Central ray

- Angled exactly 45 degrees anteriorly and directed through the posterior surface of the flexed ankle to a point on the plantar surface at the level of the base of the fifth metatarsal

[1]Lilienfeld L: *Anordnung der normalisierten Röntgenaufnahmen des menschlichen Körpers*, ed 4, Berlin, 1927, Urban & Schwarzenberg.
[2]Harris RI, Beath T: Etiology of peroneal spastic flat foot, *J Bone Joint Surg Br* 30:624, 1948.
[3]Coventry MB: Flatfoot with special consideration of tarsal coalition, *Minn Med* 33:1091, 1950.
[4]Vaughan WH, Segal G: Tarsal coalition, with special reference to roentgenographic interpretation, *Radiology* 60:855, 1953.

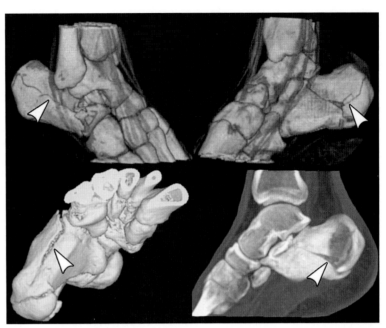

Fig. 6-79 CT images of calcaneal fracture with three-dimensional reconstruction. Conventional x-ray shows most fractures; however, complex regions, such as calcaneal-talar area, are best shown on CT. Note how bone (*arrows*) shows extent of fracture.

(From Jackson SA, Thomas RM: *Cross-sectional imaging made easy*, New York, 2004, Churchill Livingstone.)

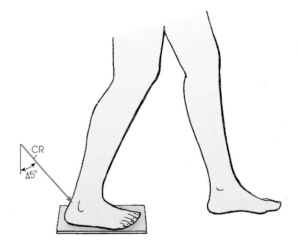

Fig. 6-80 Weight-bearing coalition method.

Calcaneus

♠ LATERAL PROJECTION
Mediolateral

Image receptor: 8 × 10 inch (18 × 24 cm)

Position of patient
• Have the supine patient turn toward the affected side until the leg is approximately lateral. A support may be placed under the knee.

Position of part
• Adjust the calcaneus to the center of the IR.
• Adjust the IR so that the long axis is parallel with the plantar surface of the heel (Fig. 6-81).
• *Shield gonads.*

Central ray
• Perpendicular to the calcaneus. Center about 1 inch (2.5 cm) distal to the medial malleolus. This places the central ray at the subtalar joint.

Collimation
• Adjust collimator to 1 inch (2.5 cm) past the posterior and inferior shadow of the heel. Include the medial malleolus and base of the fifth metatarsal.

Structures shown
The radiograph shows the ankle joint and the calcaneus in lateral profile (Fig. 6-82).

EVALUATION CRITERIA
The following should be clearly shown:
■ Evidence of proper collimation
■ No rotation of the calcaneus
■ Density of the sustentaculum tali, lateral tuberosity, and soft tissue
■ Sinus tarsi
■ Ankle joint and adjacent tarsals

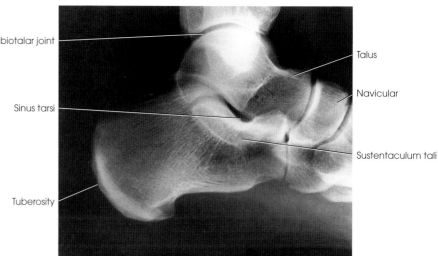

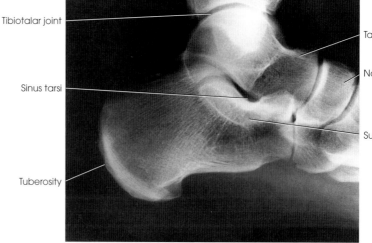

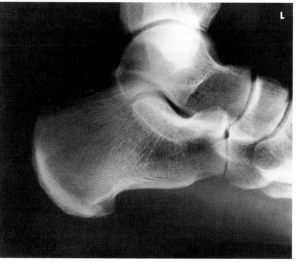

Fig. 6-82 Lateral calcaneus.

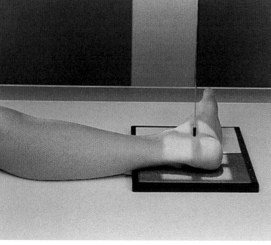

Fig. 6-81 Lateral calcaneus.

LATEROMEDIAL OBLIQUE PROJECTION
WEIGHT-BEARING METHOD

Image receptor: 8 × 10 inch (18 × 24 cm)

Position of patient
- Have the patient stand with the affected heel centered toward the lateral border of the IR (Fig. 6-83).
- A mobile radiographic unit may assist in this examination.

Position of part
- Adjust the patient's leg to ensure that it is exactly perpendicular.
- Center the calcaneus so that it is projected to the center of the IR.
- Center the lateral malleolus to the midline axis of the IR.
- *Shield gonads.*

Central ray
- Directed medially at a caudal angle of 45 degrees to enter the lateral malleolus.

Structures shown
The resulting image shows the calcaneal tuberosity and is useful in diagnosing stress fractures of the calcaneus or tuberosity (Fig. 6-84).

EVALUATION CRITERIA
The following should be clearly shown:
- Calcaneal tuberosity
- Sinus tarsi
- Cuboid

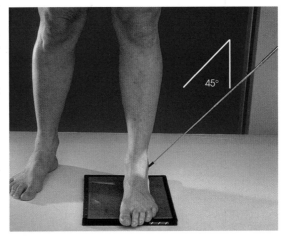

Fig. 6-83 Weight-bearing lateromedial oblique calcaneus.

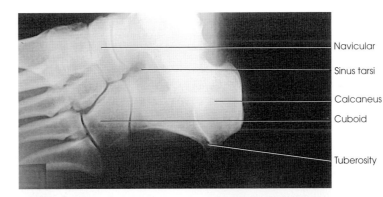

Navicular

Sinus tarsi

Calcaneus

Cuboid

Tuberosity

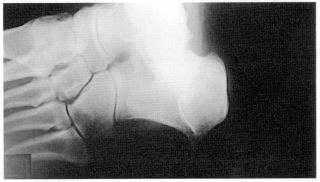

Fig. 6-84 Weight-bearing lateromedial oblique calcaneus.

LATEROMEDIAL OBLIQUE PROJECTION
ISHERWOOD METHOD
Medial rotation foot

Isherwood[1] devised a method for each of the three separate articulations of the subtalar joint: (1) a *medial rotation foot* position to show the anterior talar articulation, (2) a *medial rotation ankle* position to show the middle talar articulation, and (3) a *lateral rotation ankle* position to show the posterior talar articulation. Feist and Mankin[2] later described a similar position.

Image receptor: 8 × 10 inch (18 × 24 cm) for each position

Position of patient

- Place the patient in a semisupine or seated position, turned away from the side being examined.
- Ask the patient to flex the knee enough to place the ankle joint in nearly right-angle flexion and then to lean the leg and foot medially.

[1]Isherwood I: A radiological approach to the subtalar joint, *J Bone Joint Surg Br* 43:566, 1961.
[2]Feist JH, Mankin HJ: The tarsus: basic relationships and motions in the adult and definition of optimal recumbent oblique projection, *Radiology* 79:250, 1962.

Position of part

- With the medial border of the foot resting on the IR, place a 45-degree foam wedge under the elevated leg.
- Adjust the leg so that its long axis is in the same plane as the central ray.
- Adjust the foot to be at a right angle.
- Place a support under the knee (Fig. 6-85).
- *Shield gonads.*

Central ray

- Perpendicular to a point 1 inch (2.5 cm) distal and 1 inch (2.5 cm) anterior to the lateral malleolus

Structures shown

The resulting image shows the anterior subtalar articulation and an oblique projection of the tarsals (Fig. 6-86). The Feist-Mankin method produces a similar image representation.

EVALUATION CRITERIA

The following should be clearly shown:
- Anterior talar articular surface

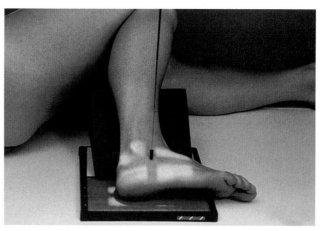

Fig. 6-85 Lateromedial oblique subtalar joint, medial rotation: Isherwood method.

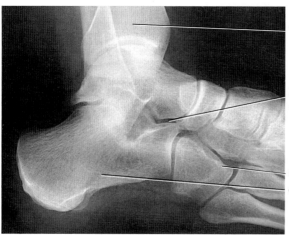
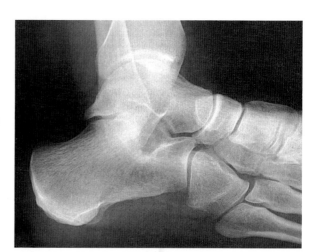

Tibia

Anterior talar articulation

Cuboid
Calcaneus

Fig. 6-86 Lateromedial oblique subtalar joint showing anterior articulation: Isherwood method.

AP AXIAL OBLIQUE PROJECTION
ISHERWOOD METHOD
Medial rotation ankle

Image receptor: 8 × 10 inch (18 × 24 cm)

Position of patient
- Have the patient assume a seated position on the radiographic table and turn with body weight resting on the flexed hip and thigh of the unaffected side.
- If a semilateral recumbent position is more comfortable, adjust the patient accordingly.

Position of part
- Ask the patient to rotate the leg and foot medially enough to rest the side of the foot and affected ankle on an optional 30-degree foam wedge (Fig. 6-87).
- Place a support under the knee. If the patient is recumbent, place another support under the greater trochanter.
- Dorsiflex the foot, then invert it if possible, and have the patient maintain the position by pulling on a strip of 2- or 3-inch (5- to 7.6-cm) bandage looped around the ball of the foot.
- *Shield gonads.*

Central ray
- Directed to a point 1 inch (2.5 cm) distal and 1 inch (2.5 cm) anterior to the lateral malleolus at an angle of 10 degrees cephalad

Structures shown
The resulting image shows the middle articulation of the subtalar joint and an "end-on" projection of the sinus tarsi (Fig. 6-88).

The following should be clearly shown:
- Middle (subtalar) articulation
- Open sinus tarsi

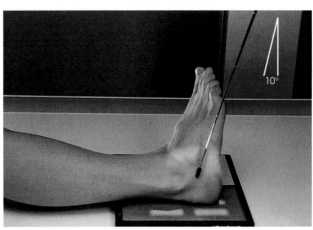

Fig. 6-87 AP axial oblique subtalar joint, medial rotation: Isherwood method.

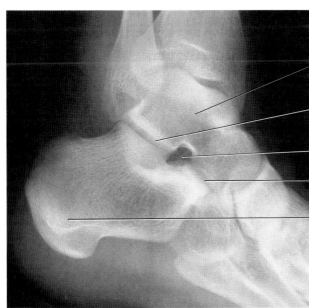
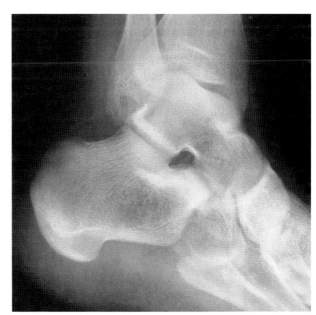

Talus

Posterior subtalar articulation

Sinus tarsi

Middle subtalar articulation

Calcaneus

Fig. 6-88 AP axial oblique subtalar joint: Isherwood method.

AP AXIAL OBLIQUE PROJECTION
ISHERWOOD METHOD
Lateral rotation ankle

Image receptor: 8 × 10 inch (18 × 24 cm)

Position of patient
- Place the patient in the supine or seated position.

Position of part
- Ask the patient to rotate the leg and foot laterally until the side of the foot and ankle rests against an optional 30-degree foam wedge.
- Dorsiflex the foot, evert it if possible, and have the patient maintain the position by pulling on a broad bandage looped around the ball of the foot (Fig. 6-89).
- *Shield gonads.*

Central ray
- Directed to a point 1 inch (2.5 cm) distal to the medial malleolus at an angle of 10 degrees cephalad

Structures shown
The resulting image shows the posterior articulation of the subtalar joint in profile (Fig. 6-90).

EVALUATION CRITERIA
The following should be clearly shown:
- Posterior subtalar articulation

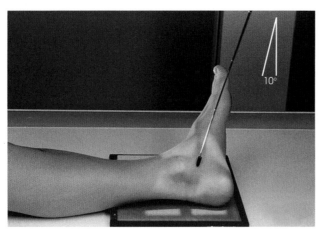

Fig. 6-89 AP axial oblique subtalar joint, lateral rotation: Isherwood method.

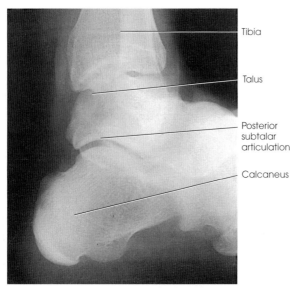
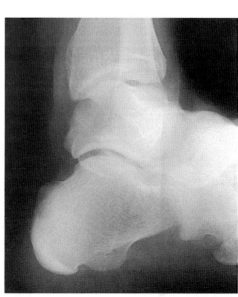

Tibia

Talus

Posterior subtalar articulation

Calcaneus

Fig. 6-90 AP oblique subtalar joint: Isherwood method.

Lower Limb

Ankle

🦅 AP PROJECTION

Image receptor: 8 × 10 inch (18 × 24 cm) lengthwise or 10 × 12 inch (24 × 30 cm) crosswise for two images on one IR

Position of patient

- Place the patient in the supine or seated position with the affected limb fully extended.

Position of part

- Adjust the ankle joint in the anatomic position (foot pointing straight up) to obtain a true AP projection. Flex the ankle and foot enough to place the long axis of the foot in the vertical position (Fig. 6-91).
- Ball and Egbert[1] stated that the appearance of the ankle mortise is not appreciably altered by moderate plantar flexion or dorsiflexion as long as the leg is rotated neither laterally nor medially.
- *Shield gonads.*

Central ray

- Perpendicular through the ankle joint at a point midway between the malleoli

Collimation

- 1 inch (2.5 cm) on the sides of the ankle and 8 inches (18 cm) lengthwise to include the heel

---

[1]Ball RP, Egbert EW: Ruptured ligaments of the ankle, *AJR Am J Roentgenol* 50:770, 1943.

Structures shown

The image shows a true AP projection of the ankle joint, the distal ends of the tibia and fibula, and the proximal portion of the talus.

NOTE: The inferior tibiofibular articulation and the talofibular articulation are not "open" or shown in profile in the true AP projection. This is a positive sign for the radiologist because it indicates that the patient has no ruptured ligaments or other type of separations. For this reason, it is important that the position of the ankle be anatomically "true" for the AP projection shown (Fig. 6-92).

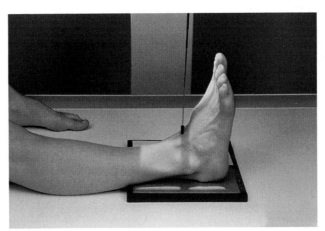

Fig. 6-91 AP ankle.

EVALUATION CRITERIA

The following should be clearly shown:

- Evidence of proper collimation
- Tibiotalar joint space
- Ankle joint centered to exposure area
- Normal overlapping of the tibiofibular articulation with the anterior tubercle slightly superimposed over the fibula
- Talus slightly overlapping the distal fibula
- No overlapping of the medial talomalleolar articulation
- Medial and lateral malleoli
- Talus with proper density
- Soft tissue

Ankle

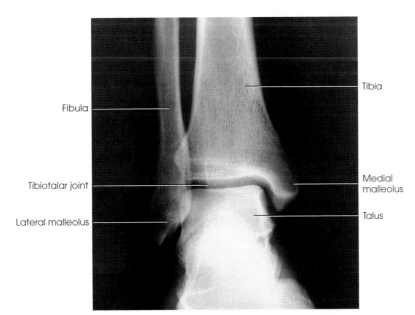

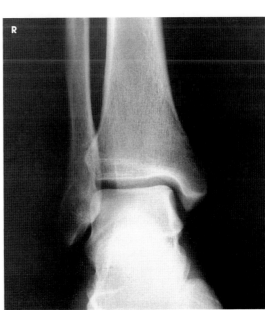

Fibula

Tibiotalar joint

Lateral malleolus

Tibia

Medial malleolus

Talus

Fig. 6-92 AP ankle.

♠ LATERAL PROJECTION
Mediolateral

Image receptor: 8 × 10 inch (18 × 24 cm)

Position of patient
- Have the supine patient turn toward the affected side until the ankle is lateral (Fig. 6-93).

Position of part
- Place the long axis of the IR parallel with the long axis of the patient's leg, and center it to the ankle joint.
- Ensure that the lateral surface of the foot is in contact with the IR.
- Dorsiflex the foot, and adjust it in the lateral position. Dorsiflexion is required to prevent lateral rotation of the ankle.
- *Shield gonads.*

Central ray
- Perpendicular to the ankle joint, entering the medial malleolus

Collimation
- 1 inch (2.5 cm) on the sides of the ankle and 8 inches (18 cm) lengthwise. Include the heel and fifth metatarsal base.

Structures shown
The resulting image shows a true lateral projection of the lower third of the tibia and fibula; the ankle joint; and the tarsals, including the base of the fifth metatarsal (Figs. 6-94 and 6-95).

EVALUATION CRITERIA
The following should be clearly shown:
- Evidence of proper collimation
- Ankle joint centered to exposure area
- Tibiotalar joint well visualized, with the medial and lateral talar domes superimposed
- Fibula over the posterior half of the tibia
- Distal tibia and fibula, talus, and adjacent tarsals
- Fifth metatarsal should be seen to check for Jones fracture
- Density of the ankle sufficient to see the outline of distal portion of the fibula

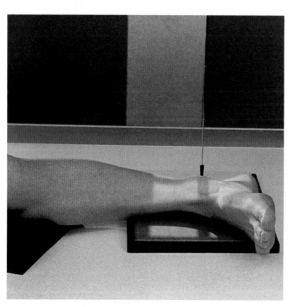

Fig. 6-93 Lateral ankle, mediolateral.

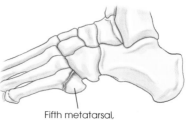

Fifth metatarsal,
Jones fracture

Fig. 6-94 Bones shown on lateral ankle. Including base of fifth metatarsal on lateral ankle projection can identify Jones fracture if present.

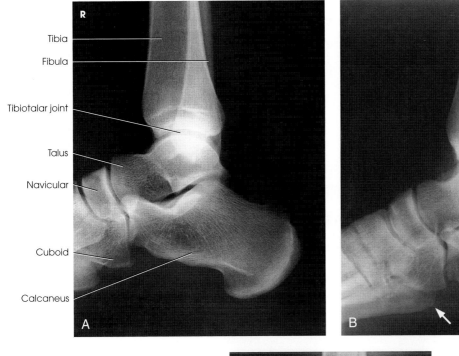

R

Tibia

Fibula

Tibiotalar joint

Talus

Navicular

Cuboid

Calcaneus

A

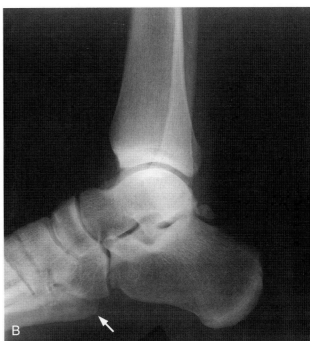

B

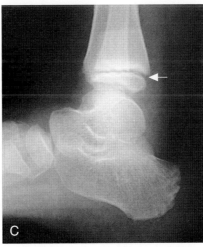

C

Fig. 6-95 A and **B,** Lateral ankle, mediolateral. Base of fifth metatarsal is seen. **C,** Lateral ankle of an 8-year-old child. Note tibial epiphysis (*arrow*).

LATERAL PROJECTION
Lateromedial

It is often recommended that the lateral projection of the ankle joint be made with the medial side of the ankle in contact with the IR. Exact positioning of the ankle is more easily and more consistently obtained when the limb is rested on its comparatively flat medial surface.

Image receptor: 8 × 10 inch (18 × 24 cm)

Position of patient

- Have the supine patient turn away from the affected side until the extended leg is placed laterally.

Position of part

- Center the IR to the ankle joint, and adjust the IR so that its long axis is parallel with the long axis of the leg.
- Adjust the foot in the lateral position.
- Have the patient turn anteriorly or posteriorly as required to place the patella perpendicular to the horizontal plane (Fig. 6-96).
- If necessary, place a support under the patient's knee.
- *Shield gonads.*

Central ray

- Perpendicular through the ankle joint, entering ½ inch (1.3 cm) superior to the lateral malleolus

Structures shown

The resulting image shows a lateral projection of the lower third of the tibia and fibula, the ankle joint, and the tarsals (Fig. 6-97).

The following should be clearly shown:

- Ankle joint centered to exposure area
- Tibiotalar joint well visualized, with the medial and lateral talar domes superimposed
- Fibula over the posterior half of the tibia
- Distal tibia and fibula, talus, and adjacent tarsals
- Density of the ankle sufficient to see the outline of distal portion of the fibula

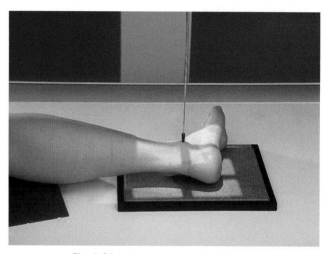

Fig. 6-96 Lateral ankle, lateromedial.

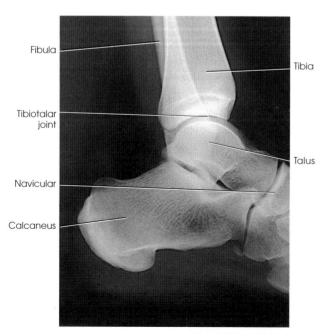
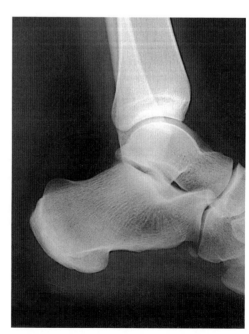

Fig. 6-97 Lateral ankle, lateromedial.

♠ AP OBLIQUE PROJECTION
Medial rotation

Image receptor: 8 × 10 inch (18 × 24 cm) lengthwise or 10 × 12 inch (24 × 30 cm) crosswise for two images on one IR

Position of patient
- Place the patient in the supine or seated position with the affected limb fully extended.

Position of part
- Center the IR to the ankle joint midway between the malleoli, and adjust the IR so that its long axis is parallel with the long axis of the leg.
- Dorsiflex the foot enough to place the ankle at nearly right-angle flexion (Fig. 6-98). The ankle may be immobilized with sandbags placed against the sole of the foot or by having the patient hold the ends of a strip of bandage looped around the ball of the foot.
- Rotate the patient's *leg* primarily and the *foot* for all oblique projections of the ankle. Because the knee is a hinge joint, rotation of the leg can come only from the hip joint. Positioning the ankle for the oblique projection requires that the *leg* and *foot* be medially rotated 45 degrees.
- Grasp the lower femur area with one hand and the foot with the other. Internally rotate the entire leg and foot together until the 45-degree position is achieved.
- The foot can be placed against a foam wedge for support.
- *Shield gonads.*

Central ray
- Perpendicular to the ankle joint, entering midway between the malleoli

Collimation
- 1 inch (2.5 cm) on the sides of the ankle and 8 inches (18 cm) lengthwise to include the heel.

Structures shown
The 45-degree medial oblique projection shows the distal ends of the tibia and fibula, parts of which are often superimposed over the talus. The tibiofibular articulation also should be shown (Fig. 6-99).

The following should be clearly shown:
- Evidence of proper collimation
- Distal tibia, fibula, and talus
- Distal tibia and fibula overlap some of the talus
- Talus and distal tibia and fibula adequately penetrated
- Tibiofibular articulation

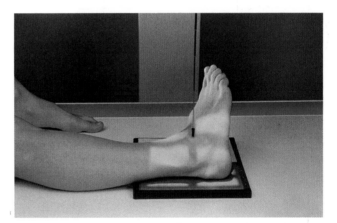

Fig. 6-98 AP oblique ankle, 45-degree medial rotation.

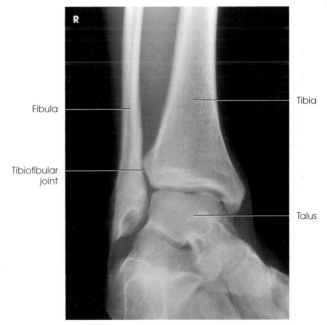

Fibula

Tibiofibular joint

Tibia

Talus

Fig. 6-99 AP oblique ankle, 45-degree medial rotation.

Mortise Joint[1]
▲ AP OBLIQUE
Medial rotation

Image receptor: 8 × 10 inch (18 × 24 cm) lengthwise or 10 × 12 inch (24 × 30 cm) crosswise for two images on one IR

Position of patient
- Place the patient in the supine or seated position.

[1]Frank ED et al: Radiography of the ankle mortise, *Radiol Technol* 62:354, 1991.

Position of part
- Center the patient's ankle joint to the IR.
- Grasp the distal femur area with one hand and the foot with the other. Assist the patient by internally rotating the *entire leg* and *foot* together 15 to 20 degrees until the intermalleolar plane is parallel with the IR (Fig. 6-100).

- The plantar surface of the foot should be placed at a right angle to the leg (Fig. 6-101).
- *Shield gonads.*

Central ray
- Perpendicular, entering the ankle joint midway between the malleoli

Collimation
- 1 inch (2.5 cm) on the sides of the ankle and 8 inches (18 cm) lengthwise to include the heel.

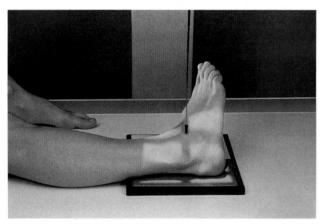

Fig. 6-100 AP oblique ankle, 15- to 20-degree medial rotation to show ankle mortise joint.

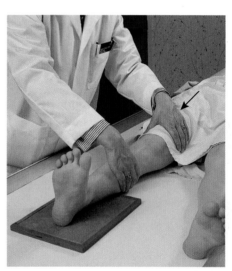

Fig. 6-101 Radiographer properly positioning the leg to show the ankle mortise joint. Note the action of the left hand (*arrow*) in turning the leg medially. Proper positioning requires turning the leg but not the foot.

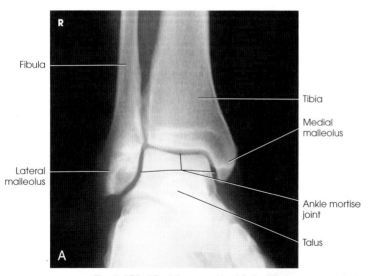

Fibula

Lateral malleolus

Tibia

Medial malleolus

Ankle mortise joint

Talus

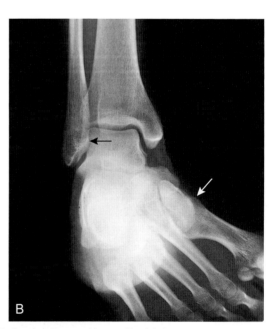

Fig. 6-102 AP oblique ankle, 15- to 20-degree medial rotation to show ankle mortise joint. **A,** Properly positioned leg to show mortise joint. **B,** Poorly positioned leg; radiograph had to be repeated. The foot was turned medially (*white arrow*), but the leg was not. Lateral mortise is closed (*black arrow*) because the "leg" was not medially rotated.

Structures shown

The entire ankle mortise joint should be shown in profile. The three sides of the mortise joint should be visualized (Figs. 6-102 and 6-103).

The following should be clearly shown:
- Evidence of proper collimation
- Entire ankle mortise joint
- No overlap of the anterior tubercle of the tibia and the superolateral portion of the talus with the fibula
- Talofibular joint space in profile
- Talus shown with proper density

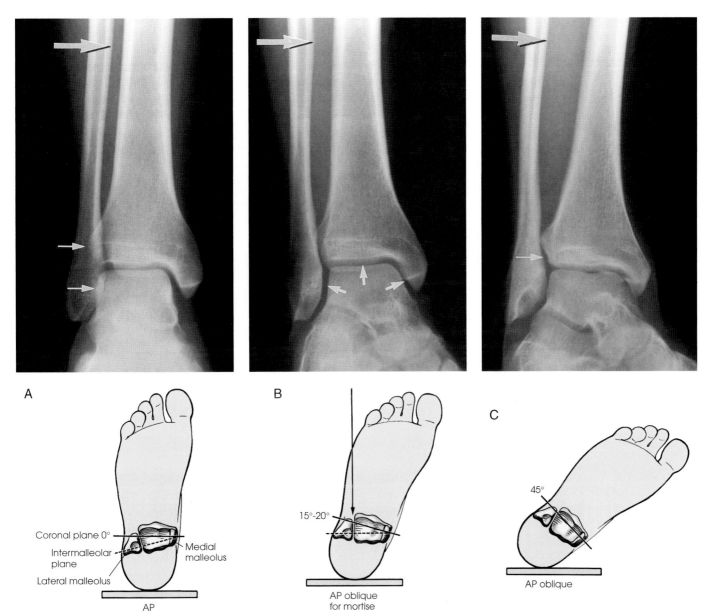

Fig. 6-103 Axial drawing of inferior surface of the tibia and fibula at the ankle joint along with matching radiographs. **A,** AP ankle position with no rotation of the leg and foot. Drawing shows lateral malleolus positioned posteriorly when leg is in true anatomic position. Radiograph shows normal overlap of anterior tubercle and superolateral talus over fibula (*arrows*). **B,** AP oblique ankle, 15- to 20-degree medial rotation to show ankle mortise. Drawing shows both malleoli parallel with IR. Radiograph clearly shows all three aspects of mortise joint (*arrows*). **C,** AP oblique ankle, 45-degree medial rotation. Radiograph shows tibiofibular joint (*arrow*) and entire distal fibula in profile. *Larger upper arrow* show wider space created between tibia and fibula as leg is turned medially for two AP oblique projections. This space should be observed when ankle radiographs are checked for proper positioning.

Ankle

AP OBLIQUE PROJECTION
Lateral rotation

Image receptor: 8 × 10 inch (18 × 24 cm)

Position of patient
- Seat the patient on the radiographic table with the affected leg extended.

Position of part
- Place the plantar surface of the patient's foot in the vertical position, and laterally rotate the *leg* and *foot* 45 degrees.
- Rest the foot against a foam wedge for support, and center the ankle joint to the IR (Fig. 6-104).
- *Shield gonads.*

Central ray
- Perpendicular, entering the ankle joint midway between the malleoli

Structures shown
The lateral rotation oblique projection is useful in determining fractures and showing the superior aspect of the calcaneus (Fig. 6-105).

EVALUATION CRITERIA

The following should be clearly shown:
- Subtalar joint
- Calcaneal sulcus (superior portion of calcaneus)

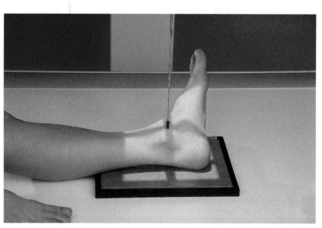

Fig. 6-104 AP oblique ankle, lateral rotation.

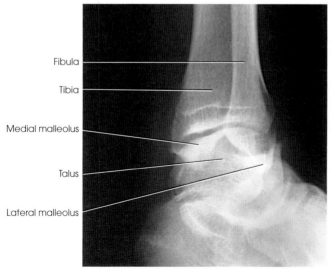
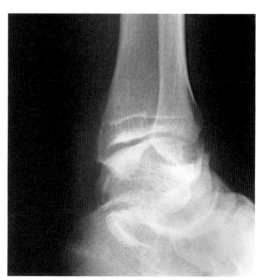

Fibula
Tibia
Medial malleolus
Talus
Lateral malleolus

Fig. 6-105 AP oblique ankle, lateral rotation.

✦ AP PROJECTION
STRESS METHOD

Stress studies of the ankle joint usually are obtained after an inversion or eversion injury to verify the presence of a ligamentous tear. Rupture of a ligament is shown by widening of the joint space on the side of the injury when, without moving or rotating the lower leg from the supine position, the foot is forcibly turned toward the opposite side.

When the injury is recent and the ankle is acutely sensitive to movement, the orthopedic surgeon may inject a local anesthetic into the sinus tarsi preceding the examination. The physician adjusts the foot when it must be turned into extreme stress and holds or straps it in position for the exposure. The patient usually can hold the foot in the stress position when the injury is not too painful or after he or she has received a local anesthetic by asymmetrically pulling on a strip of bandage looped around the ball of the foot (Figs. 6-106 to 6-108).

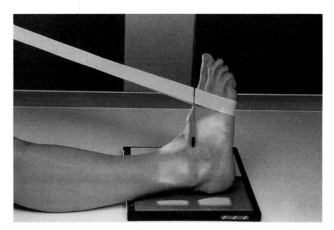

Fig. 6-106 AP ankle in neutral position. Use of lead glove and stress of the joint is required to obtain inversion and eversion radiographs (see Fig. 6-108).

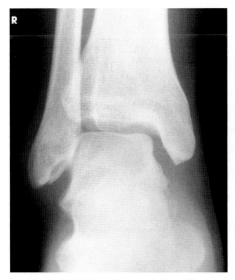

Fig. 6-107 AP ankle, neutral position.

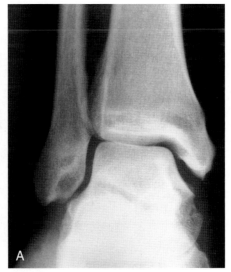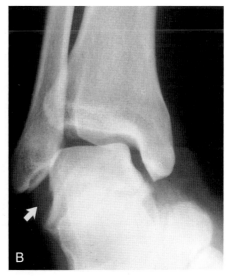

Fig. 6-108 A, Eversion stress. No damage to medial ligament is indicated. **B,** Inversion stress. Change in joint and rupture of lateral ligament (*arrow*) are seen.

AP PROJECTION
WEIGHT-BEARING METHOD
Standing
This projection is performed to identify ankle joint space narrowing with weight-bearing.

Image receptor: 10 × 12 inch (24 × 30 cm) crosswise

Position of patient
- Place the patient in the upright position, preferably on a low platform that has a cassette groove. If such a platform is unavailable, use blocks to elevate the feet to the level of the x-ray tube (Fig. 6-109).
- Ensure that the patient has proper support. Never stand the patient on the radiographic table.

Position of part
- Place the cassette in the cassette groove of the platform or between blocks.
- Have the patient stand with heels pushed back against the cassette and toes pointing straight ahead toward the x-ray tube.
- *Shield gonads.*

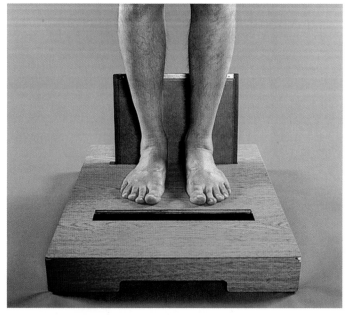

Fig. 6-109 AP weight-bearing ankles.

Central ray
- Perpendicular to the center of the cassette

TECHNICAL NOTE: If needed, use a mobile unit to allow the x-ray tube to reach the floor level.

Structures shown
The resulting image shows an AP projection of both ankle joints and the relationship of the distal tibia and fibula with weight-bearing. It also shows side-to-side comparison of the joint (Fig. 6-110).

EVALUATION CRITERIA

The following should be clearly shown:
- Both ankles centered on the image
- Medial mortise open
- Distal tibia and talus partially superimpose distal fibula
- Lateral mortise closed

RESEARCH: Catherine E. Hearty, MS, RT(R), performed the research and provided this new projection for the atlas.

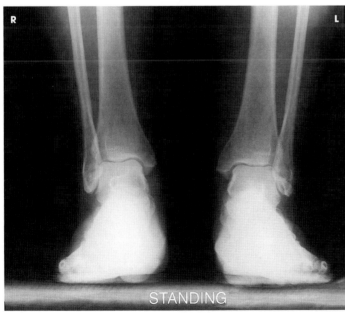

Fig. 6-110 AP weight-bearing ankles.

✿ AP PROJECTION

For this projection and the lateral and oblique projections described in the following sections, the long axis of the IR is placed parallel with the long axis of the leg and centered to the midshaft. Unless the leg is unusually long, the IR extends beyond the knee and ankle joints enough to prevent their being projected off the IR by the divergence of the x-ray beam. The IR must extend 1 to 1½ inches (2.5 to 3.8 cm) beyond the joints. When the leg is too long for these allowances, and the site of the lesion is unknown, two images should always be made. In these instances, the leg is imaged with the ankle joint, and a separate knee projection is performed. Diagonal use of a 14 × 17 inch (35 × 43 cm) IR is also an option if the leg is too long to fit lengthwise and if such use is permitted by the facility. The use of a 48-inch (122-cm) SID reduces the divergence of the x-ray beam, and more of the body part is included.

Image receptor: 7 × 17 inch (18 × 43 cm) or 14 × 17 inch (35 × 43 cm) for two images on one IR

Position of patient
- Place the patient in the supine position.

Position of part
- Adjust the patient's body so that the pelvis is not rotated.
- Adjust the leg so that the femoral condyles are parallel with the IR and the foot is vertical.
- Flex the ankle until the foot is in the vertical position.
- If necessary, place a sandbag against the plantar surface of the foot to immobilize it in the correct position (Fig. 6-111).
- *Shield gonads.*

Central ray
- Perpendicular to the center of the leg

Collimation
- 1 inch (2.5 cm) on the sides and 1½ inches (4 cm) beyond the ankle and knee joints

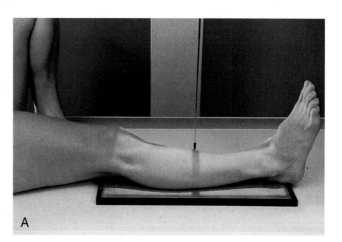

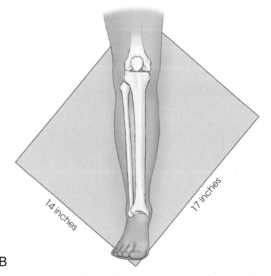

Fig. 6-111 A, AP tibia and fibula. **B,** Projection done on 14 × 17 inch (35 × 43 cm) IR diagonal to include knee and ankle joint.

Structures shown

The resulting image shows the tibia, fibula, and adjacent joints (Fig. 6-112).

The following should be clearly shown:

- Evidence of proper collimation
- Ankle and knee joints on one or more AP projections
- Ankle and knee joints without rotation
- Proximal and distal articulations of the tibia and fibula moderately overlapped
- Fibular midshaft free of tibial superimposition
- Trabecular detail and soft tissue for the entire leg

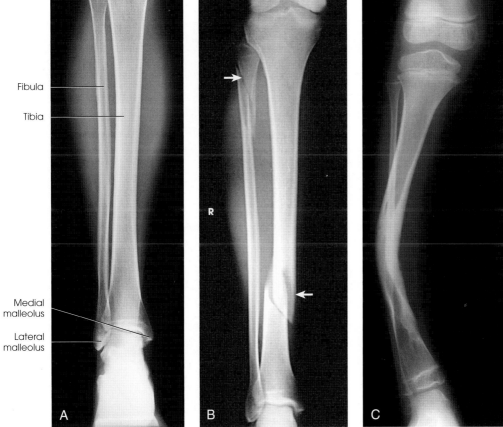

Fibula

Tibia

Medial malleolus

Lateral malleolus

Fig. 6-112 A, AP tibia and fibula. Long leg length prevented showing entire leg. A separate knee projection had to be performed on this patient. **B,** Short leg length allowed entire leg to be shown. Spiral fracture of distal tibia with accompanying spiral fracture of proximal fibula (*arrows*) is seen. This radiograph shows the importance of including the entire length of a long bone in trauma cases. **C,** AP tibia and fibula on a 4-year-old with neurofibromatosis.

♠ LATERAL PROJECTION
Mediolateral

Image receptor: 7 × 17 inch (18 × 43 cm) or 14 × 17 inch (35 × 43 cm) for two images on one IR

Position of patient
- Place the patient in the supine position.

Position of part
- Turn the patient toward the affected side with the leg on the IR.
- Adjust the rotation of the body to place the patella perpendicular to the IR, and ensure that a line drawn through the femoral condyles is also perpendicular.
- Place sandbag supports where needed for the patient's comfort and to stabilize the body position (Fig. 6-113, *A*).
- The knee may be flexed if necessary to ensure a true lateral position.
- The projection may be done with IR diagonal to include the ankle and knee joints (Fig. 6-113, *B*). Similar to the AP, if the leg is too long, it is imaged with the ankle joint, and a separate knee projection is performed.

Alternative method
- When the patient cannot be turned from the supine position, the lateromedial lateral projection may be taken cross-table using a horizontal central ray.
- Lift the leg enough for an assistant to slide a rigid support under the patient's leg.
- The IR may be placed between the legs, and the central ray may be directed from the lateral side.
- *Shield gonads.*

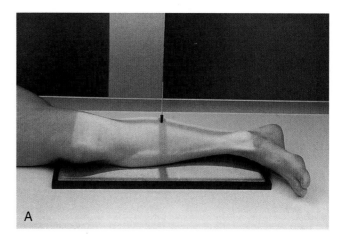

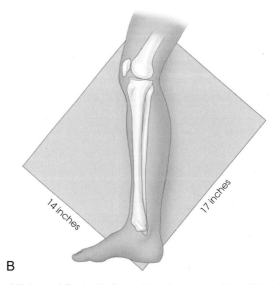

Fig. 6-113 A, Lateral tibia and fibula. **B,** Projection done on a 14 × 17 inch (35 × 43 cm) IR diagonal to include knee and ankle joint.

Central ray

• Perpendicular to the midpoint of the leg

Collimation

• 1 inch (2.5 cm) on the sides and 1½ inches (4 cm) beyond the ankle and knee joints

Structures shown

The resulting image shows the tibia, fibula, and adjacent joints (Fig. 6-114).

The following should be clearly shown:
■ Evidence of proper collimation
■ Ankle and knee joints on one or more images
■ Distal fibula lying over the posterior half of the tibia
■ Slight overlap of the tibia on the proximal fibular head
■ Ankle and knee joints not rotated
■ Possibly no superimposition of femoral condyles because of divergence of the beam
■ Moderate separation of the tibial and fibular bodies or shafts (except at their articular ends)
■ Trabecular detail and soft tissue

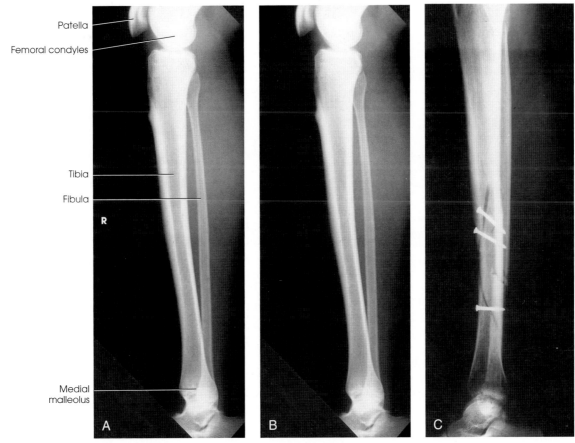

Patella
Femoral condyles
Tibia
Fibula
R
Medial malleolus
A
B
C

Fig. 6-114 A and **B,** Lateral tibia and fibula. **C,** Lateral postreduction tibia and fibula showing fixation device. The leg was too long to fit on one image.

AP OBLIQUE PROJECTIONS
Medial and lateral rotations

Image receptor: 7 × 17 inch (18 × 43 cm) or 14 × 17 inch (35 × 43 cm) for two exposures on one IR

Position of patient
- Place the patient in the supine position on the radiographic table.

Position of part
- Perform oblique projections of the leg by alternately rotating the limb 45 degrees medially (Fig. 6-115) or laterally (Fig. 6-116). For the medial rotation, ensure that the *leg* is turned inward and not just the foot.

- For the medial oblique projection, elevate the affected hip enough to rest the medial side of the foot and ankle against a 45-degree foam wedge, and place a support under the greater trochanter.
- *Shield gonads.*

Central ray
- Perpendicular to the midpoint of the IR

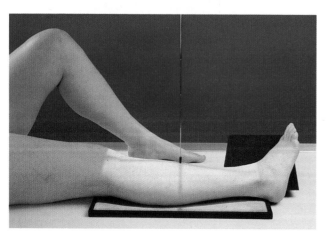

Fig. 6-115 AP oblique leg, medial rotation.

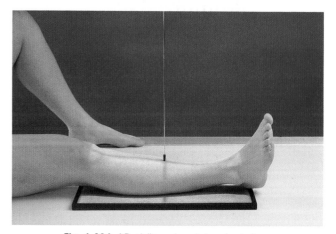

Fig. 6-116 AP oblique leg, lateral rotation.

Structures shown

The resulting image shows a 45-degree oblique projection of the bones and soft tissues of the leg and one or both of the adjacent joints (Figs. 6-117 and 6-118).

EVALUATION CRITERIA

The following should be clearly shown:

Medial rotation

- Proximal and distal tibiofibular articulations
- Maximum interosseous space between the tibia and fibula
- Ankle and knee joints

Lateral rotation

- Fibula superimposed by lateral portion of tibia
- Ankle and knee joints

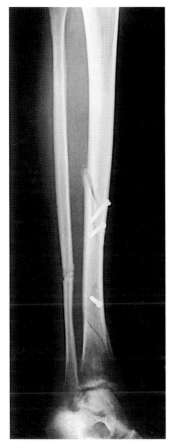

Fig. 6-117 AP oblique leg, medial rotation, showing fixation device.

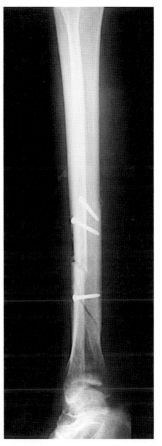

Fig. 6-118 AP oblique leg, lateral rotation, with fixation device in place.

♠ AP PROJECTION

Radiographs of the knee may be taken with or without use of a grid. The factors to consider in reaching a decision are the size of the patient's knee and the preference of the radiographer and physician.

Gonad shielding is needed during examinations of the lower limbs. (Lead shielding is not shown on illustrations of the patient model because it would obstruct demonstration of the body position.)

Image receptor: 10 × 12 inch (24 × 30 cm) lengthwise

Position of patient

- Place the patient in the supine position, and adjust the body so that the pelvis is not rotated.

Position of part

- With the IR under the patient's knee, flex the joint slightly, locate the apex of the patella, and as the patient extends the knee, center the IR about ½ inch (1.3 cm) below the patellar apex. This centers the IR to the joint space.
- Adjust the patient's leg by placing the femoral epicondyles parallel with the IR for a true AP projection (Fig. 6-119). The patella lies slightly off center to the medial side. If the knee cannot be fully extended, a curved IR may be used.
- *Shield gonads.*

Central ray

- Directed to a point ½ inch (1.3 cm) inferior to the patellar apex
- Variable, depending on the measurement between the anterior superior iliac spine (ASIS) and the tabletop (Fig. 6-120), as follows[1]:

<19 cm	3-5 degrees *caudad* (thin pelvis)
19-24 cm	0 degrees
>24 cm	3-5 degrees *cephalad* (large pelvis)

---

[1]Martensen KM: Alternate AP knee method assures open joint space, *Radiol Technol* 64:19, 1992.

Collimation

- Adjust to 10 × 12 inch (24 × 30 cm) size on the collimator.

Structures shown

The resulting image shows an AP projection of the knee structures (Fig. 6-121).

EVALUATION CRITERIA

The following should be clearly shown:

- Evidence of proper collimation
- Open femorotibial joint space, with interspaces of equal width on both sides if the knee is normal
- Knee fully extended if patient's condition permits
- Patella completely superimposed on the femur
- No rotation of the femur (femoral condyles symmetric) and tibia (intercondylar eminence centered)
- Slight superimposition of the fibular head if the tibia is normal
- Soft tissue around the knee joint
- Bony detail surrounding the patella on the distal femur

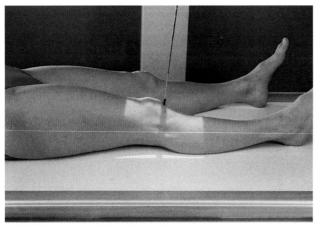

Fig. 6-119 AP knee.

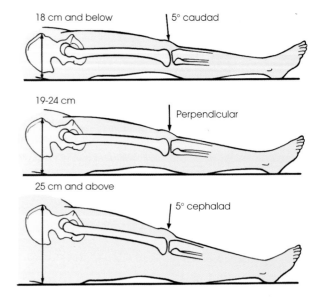

Fig. 6-120 Pelvic thickness and central ray angles for AP knee radiographs.

(Modified from Martensen KM: Alternate AP knee method assures open joint space, *Radiol Technol* 64:19, 1992.)

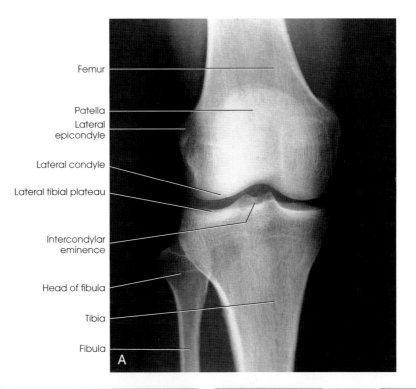

Femur
Patella
Lateral epicondyle
Lateral condyle
Lateral tibial plateau
Intercondylar eminence
Head of fibula
Tibia
Fibula

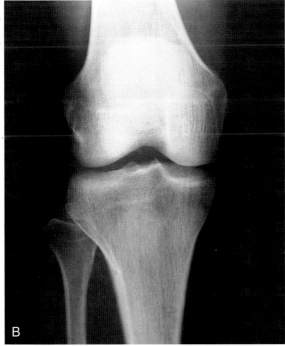

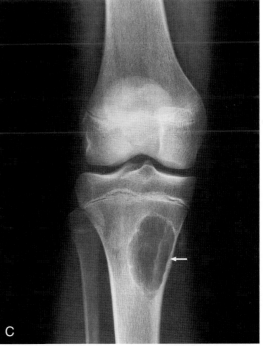

Fig. 6-121 A, AP knee with central ray (CR) angled 5 degrees cephalad. Patient's ASIS-to-tabletop distance was greater than 25 cm. **B,** Same patient as in **A** with CR perpendicular. Note joint space is not opened as well. **C,** AP knee on a 15-year-old. *Arrow* is pointing to a benign lesion in the tibia.

PA PROJECTION

Image receptor: 10 × 12 inch (24 × 30 cm) lengthwise

Position of patient

- Place the patient in the prone position with toes resting on the radiographic table, or place sandbags under the ankle for support.

Position of part

- Center a point ½ inch (1.3 cm) below the patellar apex to the center of the IR, and adjust the patient's leg so that the femoral epicondyles are parallel with the tabletop. Because the knee is balanced on the medial side of the obliquely located patella, care must be used in adjusting the knee (Fig. 6-122).
- *Shield gonads.*

Central ray

- Directed at an angle of 5 to 7 degrees caudad to exit a point ½ inch (1.3 cm) inferior to the patellar apex. Because the tibia and fibula are slightly inclined, the central ray is parallel with the tibial plateau. A perpendicular CR may be needed for patients with large thighs or when the foot is dorsiflexed.

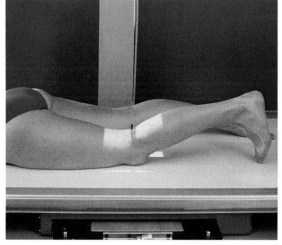

Fig. 6-122 PA knee.

Structures shown

The resulting image shows a PA projection of the knee (Fig. 6-123).

EVALUATION CRITERIA

The following should be clearly shown:
- Open femorotibial joint space with interspaces of equal width on both sides if the knee is normal
- Knee fully extended if the patient's condition permits
- No rotation of femur if tibia is normal
- Slight superimposition of the fibular head with the tibia
- Soft tissue around the knee joint
- Bony detail surrounding the patella

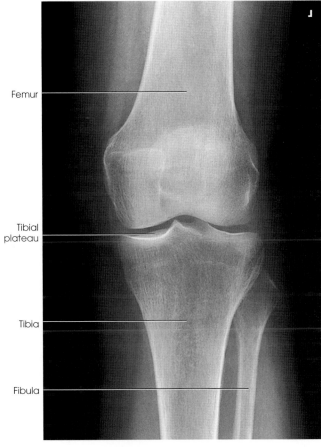

Femur

Tibial plateau

Tibia

Fibula

Fig. 6-123 PA knee.

Knee

✦ LATERAL PROJECTION
Mediolateral

Image receptor: 10 × 12 inch (24 × 30 cm) lengthwise

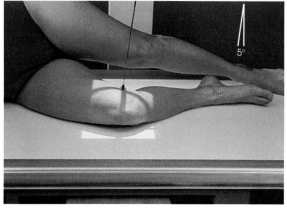

Fig. 6-124 Lateral knee showing 5 degree cephalad angulation of central ray.

Position of patient

- Ask the patient to turn onto the affected side. Ensure that the pelvis is not rotated.
- For a standard lateral projection, have the patient bring the affected knee forward and extend the other limb behind it (Fig. 6-124). The other limb may also be placed in front of the affected knee on a support block.

Position of part

- Flexion of 20 to 30 degrees is usually preferred because this position relaxes the muscles and shows the maximum volume of the joint cavity.[1]
- To prevent fragment separation in new or unhealed patellar fractures, the knee should not be flexed more than 10 degrees.
- Place a support under the ankle.
- Grasp the epicondyles and adjust them so that they are perpendicular to the IR (condyles superimposed). The patella is perpendicular to the plane of the IR (Fig. 6-125).
- *Shield gonads.*

[1]Sheller S: Roentgenographic studies on epiphyseal growth and ossification in the knee, *Acta Radiol* 195:12, 1960.

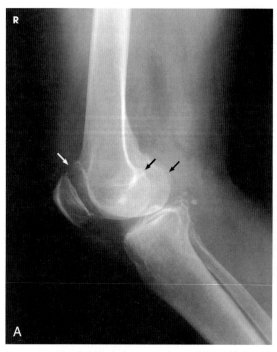
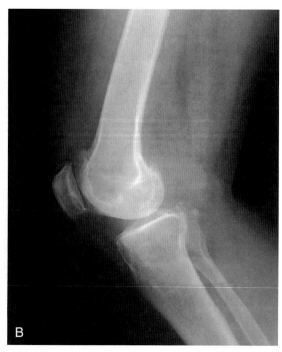

Fig. 6-125 A, Improperly positioned lateral knee. Note condyles are not superimposed (*black arrows*), and the patella is a closed joint (*white arrow*). **B,** Same patient as in **A** after correct positioning. Condyles are superimposed, and patellofemoral joint is open.

Central ray

- Directed to the knee joint 1 inch (2.5 cm) distal to the medial epicondyle at an angle of 5 to 7 degrees cephalad. This slight angulation of the central ray prevents the joint space from being obscured by the magnified image of the medial femoral condyle. In addition, in the lateral recumbent position, the medial condyle is slightly inferior to the lateral condyle.
- Center the IR to the central ray.

Collimation

- Adjust to 10 × 12 inches (24 × 30 cm) on the collimator.

Structures shown

The resulting radiograph shows a lateral image of the distal end of the femur, patella, knee joint, proximal ends of the tibia and fibula, and adjacent soft tissue (Fig. 6-126).

EVALUATION CRITERIA

The following should be clearly shown:
- Evidence of proper collimation
- Femoral condyles superimposed (locate the adductor tubercle on the posterior surface of the medial condyle to identify the medial condyle and to determine whether the knee is overrotated or underrotated)
- Open joint space between femoral condyles and tibia
- Patella in a lateral profile
- Open patellofemoral joint space
- Fibular head and tibia slightly superimposed (overrotation causes less superimposition, and underrotation causes more superimposition)
- Knee flexed 20 to 30 degrees
- All soft tissue around the knee
- Femoral condyles with proper density

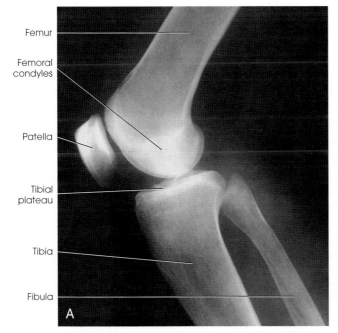
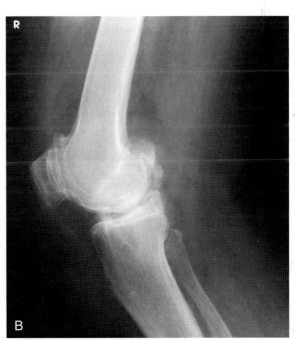

Femur

Femoral condyles

Patella

Tibial plateau

Tibia

Fibula

Fig. 6-126 A, Lateral knee. **B,** Lateral knee showing severe arthritis.

♠ AP PROJECTION
WEIGHT-BEARING METHOD
Standing

Leach et al.[1] recommended that a bilateral weight-bearing AP projection be routinely included in radiographic examination of arthritic knees. They found that a weight-bearing study often reveals narrowing of a joint space that appears normal on a non–weight-bearing study.

Image receptor: 14 × 17 inch (35 × 43 cm) crosswise for bilateral image

[1]Leach RE et al: Weight-bearing radiography in osteoarthritis of the knee, *Radiology* 97:265, 1970.

Position of patient
- Place the patient in the upright position with the back toward a vertical grid device.

Position of part
- Adjust the patient's position to center the knees to the IR.
- Place the toes straight ahead, with the feet separated enough for good balance.
- Ask the patient to stand straight with knees fully extended and weight equally distributed on the feet.
- Center the IR ½ inch (1.3 cm) below the apices of the patellae (Fig. 6-127).
- *Shield gonads.*

Central ray
- Horizontal and perpendicular to the center of the IR, entering at a point ½ inch (1.3 cm) below the apices of the patellae

Collimation
- Adjust to 14 × 17 inches (35 × 43 cm) on the collimator.

Structures shown
The resulting image shows the joint spaces of the knees. Varus and valgus deformities can also be evaluated with this procedure (Fig. 6-128).

EVALUATION CRITERIA
The following should be clearly shown:
- Evidence of proper collimation
- No rotation of the knees
- Both knees
- Knee joint space centered to the exposure area
- Adequate IR size to show the longitudinal axis of the femoral and tibial bodies or shafts

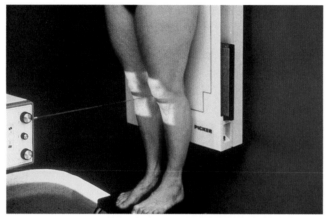

Fig. 6-127 AP bilateral weight-bearing knees.

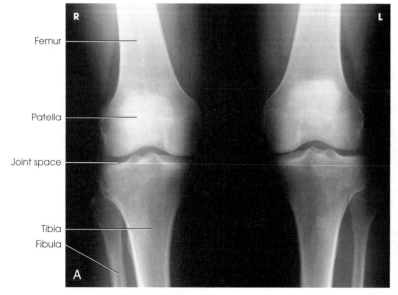

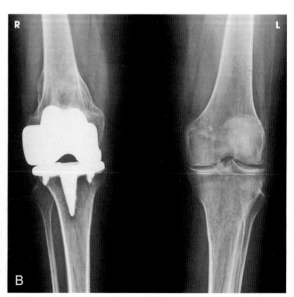

Femur
Patella
Joint space
Tibia
Fibula

Fig. 6-128 A, AP bilateral weight-bearing knees. **B,** Right knee has undergone total knee arthroplasty.

PA PROJECTION
ROSENBERG METHOD[1]
WEIGHT-BEARING
Standing flexion

Image receptor: 14 × 17 inch (35 × 43 cm) crosswise for bilateral knees

Position of patient
- Place the patient in the standing position with the anterior aspect of the knees centered to the vertical grid device.

Position of part
- For a direct PA projection, have the patient stand upright with the knees in contact with the vertical grid device.
- Center the IR at a level ½ inch (1.3 cm) below the apices of the patellae.
- Have the patient grasp the edges of the grid device and flex the knees to place the femora at an angle of 45 degrees (Fig. 6-129).
- *Shield gonads.*

Central ray
- Horizontal and perpendicular to the center of the IR. The central ray is perpendicular to the tibia and fibula. A 10-degree caudal angle is sometimes used.

Structures shown
The PA weight-bearing method is useful for evaluating joint space narrowing and showing articular cartilage disease (Fig. 6-130). The image is similar to images obtained when radiographing the intercondylar fossa.

EVALUATION CRITERIA
The following should be clearly shown:
- No rotation of the knees
- Both knees
- Knee joint centered to exposure area

NOTE: For a weight-bearing study of a single knee, the patient puts full weight on the affected side. The patient may balance with slight pressure on the toes of the unaffected side.

[1]Rosenberg TD et al: The forty-five degree posteroanterior flexion weight-bearing radiograph of the knee, *J Bone Joint Surg Am* 70:1479, 1988.

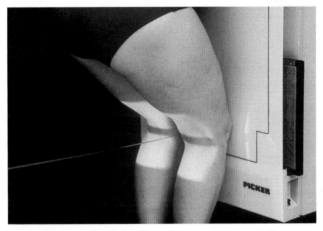

Fig. 6-129 PA projection with patient's knees flexed 45 degrees and using perpendicular central ray.

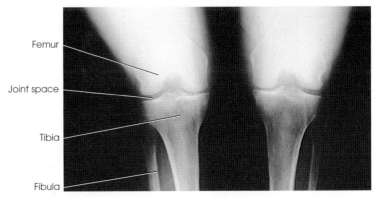

Femur

Joint space

Tibia

Fibula

Fig. 6-130 PA projection with knees flexed 45 degrees and central ray directed 10 degrees caudad.

AP OBLIQUE PROJECTION
Lateral rotation

Image receptor: 10 × 12 inch (24 × 30 cm) lengthwise

Position of patient
- Place the patient on the radiographic table in the supine position, and support the ankles.

Position of part
- If necessary, elevate the hip of the *unaffected* side enough to rotate the affected limb.
- Support the elevated hip and knee of the unaffected side (Fig. 6-131).
- Center the IR ½ inch (1.3 cm) below the apex of the patella.
- Externally rotate the limb 45 degrees.
- *Shield gonads.*

Central ray
- Directed ½ inch (1.3 cm) inferior to the patellar apex. The angle is variable, depending on measurement between the ASIS and the tabletop, as follows:

<19 cm	3-5 degrees *caudad*
19-24 cm	0 degrees
>24 cm	3-5 degrees *cephalad*

Collimation
- Adjust to 10 × 12 inches (24 × 30 cm) on the collimator.

Structures shown
The resulting image shows an AP oblique projection of the laterally rotated femoral condyles, patella, tibial condyles, and head of the fibula (Fig. 6-132).

EVALUATION CRITERIA
The following should be clearly shown:
- Evidence of proper collimation
- Medial femoral and tibial condyles
- Tibial plateaus
- Open knee joint
- Fibula superimposed over the lateral half of the tibia
- Margin of the patella projected slightly beyond the edge of the lateral femoral condyle
- Soft tissue around the knee joint
- Bony detail on the distal femur and proximal tibia

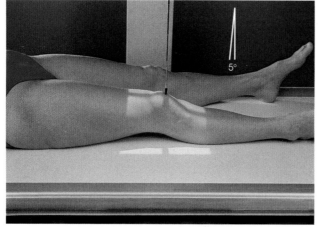

Fig. 6-131 AP oblique knee, lateral rotation.

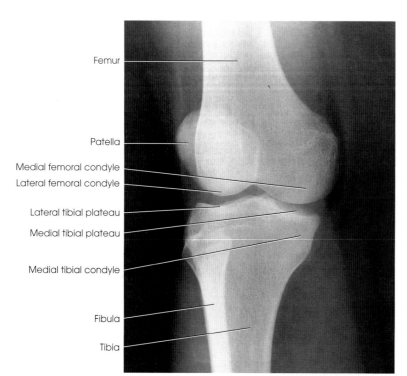
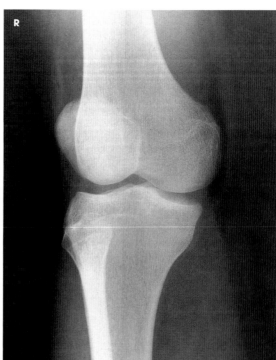

Femur
Patella
Medial femoral condyle
Lateral femoral condyle
Lateral tibial plateau
Medial tibial plateau
Medial tibial condyle
Fibula
Tibia

Fig. 6-132 AP oblique knee.

AP OBLIQUE PROJECTION
Medial rotation

Image receptor: 10 × 12 inch (24 × 30 cm) lengthwise

Position of patient
- Place the patient on the table in the supine position, and support the ankles.

Position of part
- Medially rotate the limb, and elevate the hip of the affected side enough to rotate the limb 45 degrees.

- Place a support under the hip, if needed (Fig. 6-133).
- *Shield gonads.*

Central ray
- Directed ½ inch (1.3 cm) inferior to the patellar apex; the angle is variable, depending on the measurement between the ASIS and the tabletop, as follows:

<19 cm	3-5 degrees *caudad*
19-24 cm	0 degrees
>24 cm	3-5 degrees *cephalad*

Collimation
- Adjust to 10 × 12 inches (24 × 30 cm) on the collimator.

Structures shown
The resulting image shows an AP oblique projection of the medially rotated femoral condyles, patella, tibial condyles, proximal tibiofibular joint, and head of the fibula (Fig. 6-134).

EVALUATION CRITERIA
The following should be clearly shown:
- Evidence of proper collimation
- Tibia and fibula separated at their proximal articulation
- Posterior tibia
- Lateral condyles of the femur and tibia
- Both tibial plateaus
- Open knee joint
- Margin of the patella projecting slightly beyond the medial side of the femoral condyle
- Soft tissue around the knee joint
- Bony detail on the distal femur and proximal tibia

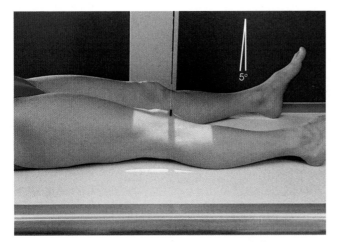

Fig. 6-133 AP oblique knee, medial rotation.

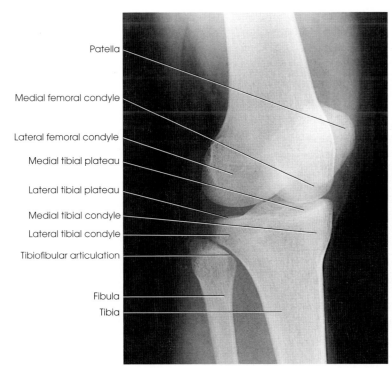
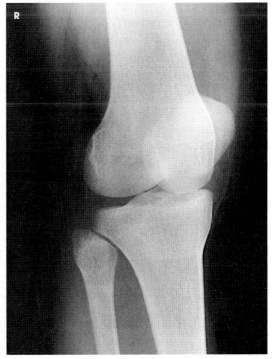

Patella

Medial femoral condyle

Lateral femoral condyle

Medial tibial plateau

Lateral tibial plateau

Medial tibial condyle

Lateral tibial condyle

Tibiofibular articulation

Fibula

Tibia

Fig. 6-134 AP oblique knee.

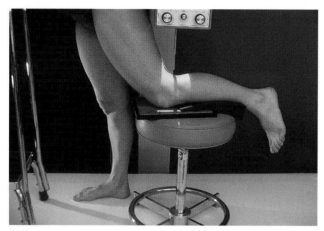

Fig. 6-135 PA axial intercondylar fossa, upright with knee on stool.

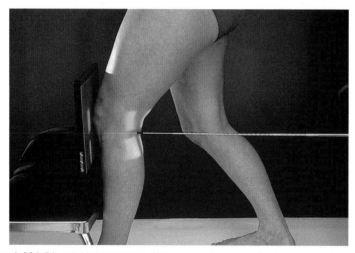

Fig. 6-136 PA axial intercondylar fossa, standing using horizontal central ray.

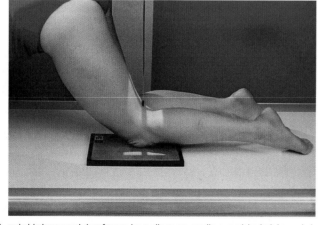

Fig. 6-137 PA axial intercondylar fossa, kneeling on radiographic table: original Holmblad method.

⚘ PA AXIAL PROJECTION
HOLMBLAD METHOD

The PA axial, or *tunnel,* projection, first described by Holmblad[1] in 1937, required that the patient assume a kneeling position on the radiographic table. In 1983, the Holmblad method[2] was modified so that if the patient's condition allowed, a standing position could be used.

Image receptor: 8 × 10 inch (18 × 24 cm)

Position of patient

- After consideration of the patient's safety, place the patient in one of three positions: (1) standing with the knee of interest flexed and resting on a stool at the side of the radiographic table (Fig. 6-135); (2) standing at the side of the radiographic table with the affected knee flexed and placed in contact with the front of the IR (Fig. 6-136); or (3) kneeling on the radiographic table as originally described by Holmblad, with the affected knee over the IR (Fig. 6-137). In all three approaches, the patient leans on the radiographic table for support.

---

[1]Holmblad EC: Postero-anterior x-ray view of the knee in flexion, *JAMA* 109:1196, 1937.
[2]Turner GW et al: Erect positions for "tunnel" views of the knee, *Radiol Technol* 55:640, 1983.

Position of part

- For all positions, place the IR against the anterior surface of the patient's knee, and center the IR to the apex of the patella. Flex the knee 70 degrees from full extension (20-degree difference from the central ray, as shown in Fig. 6-138).
- *Shield gonads.*

Central ray

- Perpendicular to the lower leg, entering the midpoint of the IR for all three positions

Collimation

- Adjust to 8 × 10 inches (18 × 24 cm) on the collimator.

Structures shown

The image shows the intercondylar fossa of the femur and the medial and lateral intercondylar tubercles of the intercondylar eminence in profile (Fig. 6-139). Holmblad[1] stated that the degree of flexion used in this position widens the joint space between the femur and tibia and gives an improved image of the joint and the surfaces of the tibia and femur.

---

[1]Holmblad EC: Posteroanterior x-ray view of the knee in flexion, *JAMA* 109:1196, 1937.

EVALUATION CRITERIA

The following should be clearly shown:
- Evidence of proper collimation
- Open fossa
- Posteroinferior surface of the femoral condyles
- Intercondylar eminence and knee joint space
- Apex of the patella not superimposing the fossa
- No rotation, evident by slight tibiofibular overlap
- Soft tissue in the fossa and interspaces
- Bony detail on the intercondylar eminence, distal femur, and proximal tibia

NOTE: The bilateral examination (Rosenberg method) is described on p. 303 (also see Fig. 6-130).

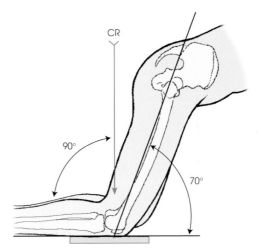

Fig. 6-138 Alignment relationship for any of three intercondylar fossa approaches: Holmblad method. Central ray (*CR*) is perpendicular to tibia-fibula.

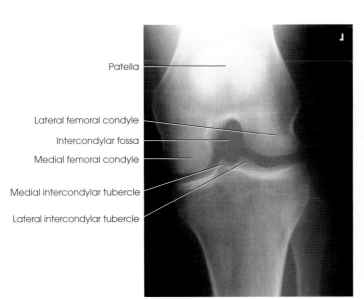
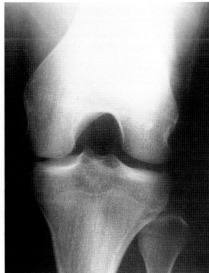

Patella
Lateral femoral condyle
Intercondylar fossa
Medial femoral condyle
Medial intercondylar tubercle
Lateral intercondylar tubercle

Fig. 6-139 PA axial (tunnel) intercondylar fossa: Holmblad method.

♠ PA AXIAL PROJECTION
CAMP-COVENTRY METHOD[1]

Image receptor: 8 × 10 inch (18 × 24 cm) lengthwise

Position of patient
- Place the patient in the prone position, and adjust the body so that it is not rotated.

[1]Camp JD, Coventry MB: Use of special views in roentgenography of the knee joint, *US Naval Med Bull* 42:56, 1944.

Position of part
- Flex the patient's knee to a 40- or 50-degree angle, and rest the foot on a suitable support.
- Center the upper half of the IR to the knee joint; the central ray angulation projects the joint to the center of the IR (Figs. 6-140 and 6-141).
- A protractor may be used beside the leg to determine the correct leg angle.
- Adjust the leg so that the knee has no medial or lateral rotation.
- *Shield gonads.*

Central ray
- Perpendicular to the long axis of the lower leg and centered to the knee joint (i.e., over the popliteal depression)
- Angled 40 degrees when the knee is flexed 40 degrees and 50 degrees when the knee is flexed 50 degrees

Collimation
- Adjust to 8 × 10 inches (18 × 24 cm) on the collimator.

Structures shown
This axial image shows an unobstructed projection of the intercondyloid fossa and the medial and lateral intercondylar tubercles of the intercondylar eminence (Figs. 6-142 and 6-143).

The following should be clearly shown:
- Evidence of proper collimation
- Open fossa
- Posteroinferior surface of the femoral condyles
- Intercondylar eminence centered in open femorotibial joint space
- Apex of the patella not superimposing the fossa
- No rotation, evident by slight tibiofibular overlap
- Soft tissue in the fossa and interspaces
- Bony detail on the intercondylar eminence, distal femur, and proximal tibia

NOTE: In routine examinations of the knee joint, an intercondylar fossa projection is usually included to detect loose bodies ("joint mice"). This projection is also used in evaluating split and displaced cartilage in osteochondritis dissecans and flattening, or underdevelopment, of the lateral femoral condyle in congenital slipped patella.

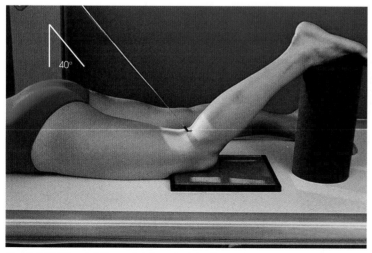

Fig. 6-140 PA axial (tunnel) intercondylar fossa: Camp-Coventry method.

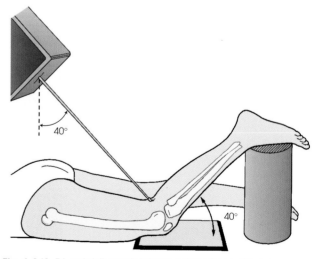

Fig. 6-141 PA axial (tunnel) intercondylar fossa: Camp-Coventry method.

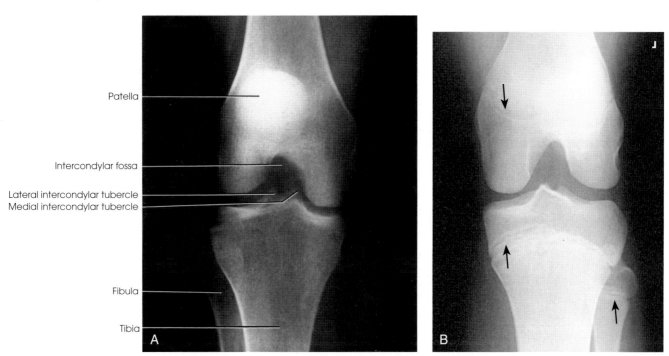

Patella

Intercondylar fossa

Lateral intercondylar tubercle
Medial intercondylar tubercle

Fibula

Tibia

A

B

Fig. 6-142 Camp-Coventry method. **A,** Flexion of knee at 40 degrees. **B,** Flexion of knee at 40 degrees in a 13-year-old patient. Note epiphyses (*arrows*).

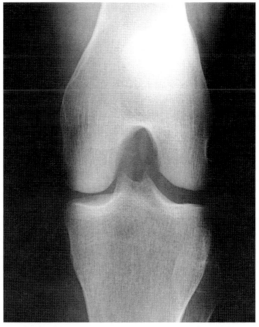

Fig. 6-143 Flexion of knee at 50 degrees (same patient as in Fig. 6-142): Camp-Coventry method.

Intercondylar Fossa

AP AXIAL PROJECTION
BÉCLÈRE METHOD

Image receptor: 8 × 10 inch (18 × 24 cm) crosswise

Position of patient
- Place the patient in the supine position, and adjust the body so that it is not rotated.

Position of part
- Flex the affected knee enough to place the long axis of the femur at an angle of 60 degrees to the long axis of the tibia.
- Support the knee on sandbags (Fig. 6-144).

- Place the IR under the knee, and position the IR so that the center point coincides with the central ray.
- Adjust the leg so that the femoral condyles are equidistant from the IR. Immobilize the foot with sandbags.
- *Shield gonads.*

Central ray
- Perpendicular to the long axis of the lower leg, entering the knee joint ½ inch (1.3 cm) below the patellar apex

Structures shown
The resulting image shows the intercondylar fossa, intercondylar eminence, and knee joint (Fig. 6-145).

The following should be clearly shown:
- Open intercondylar fossa
- Posteroinferior surface of the femoral condyles
- Intercondylar eminence and knee joint space
- No superimposition of the fossa by the apex of the patella
- No rotation, evident by slight tibiofibular overlap
- Soft tissue in the fossa and interspaces
- Bony detail on the intercondylar eminence, distal femur, and proximal tibia

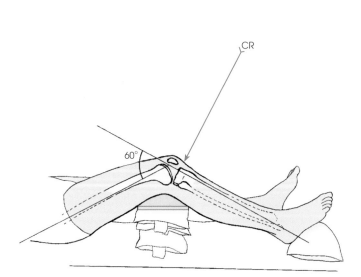

Fig. 6-144 AP axial intercondylar fossa with transverse IR: Béclère method.

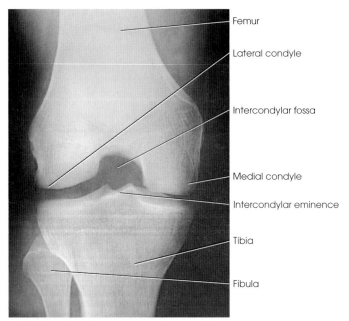

Femur

Lateral condyle

Intercondylar fossa

Medial condyle

Intercondylar eminence

Tibia

Fibula

Fig. 6-145 AP axial intercondylar fossa: Béclère method with identified anatomy.

Patella

☀ PA PROJECTION

Image receptor: 8 × 10 inch (18 × 24 cm) lengthwise

Position of patient
- Place the patient in the prone position.
- If the knee is painful, place one sand-bag under the thigh and another under the leg to relieve pressure on the patella.

Position of part
- Center the IR to the patella.
- Adjust the position of the leg to place the patella parallel with the plane of the IR. This usually requires that the heel be rotated 5 to 10 degrees laterally (Fig. 6-146).
- *Shield gonads.*

Central ray
- Perpendicular to the mid-popliteal area exiting the patella
- Collimate closely to the patellar area.

Collimation
- Adjust to 6 × 6 inches (15 × 15 cm) on the collimator.

Structures shown
The PA projection of the patella provides sharper recorded detail than in the AP projection because of a closer object-to-IR distance (OID) (Figs. 6-147 and 6-148).

EVALUATION CRITERIA
The following should be clearly shown:
- Evidence of proper collimation
- Patella completely superimposed by the femur
- Adequate penetration for visualization of the patella clearly through the super-imposing femur
- No rotation

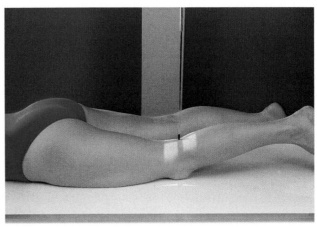

Fig. 6-146 PA patella.

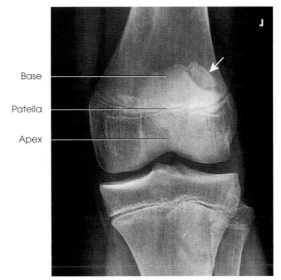

Base
Patella
Apex

Fig. 6-147 AP patella showing fracture (*arrow*).

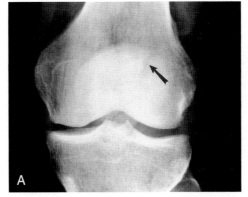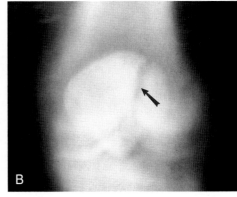

Fig. 6-148 A, Conventional PA projection of patella shows vertical radiolucent line (*arrow*) passing through junction of lateral and middle third of patella. **B,** On tomography this defect extends from superior to inferior margin of patella. It is a bipartite patella and not a fracture.

♠ LATERAL PROJECTION
Mediolateral

Image receptor: 8 × 10 inch (18 × 24 cm) lengthwise

Position of patient
• Place the patient in the lateral recumbent position.

Position of part
• Ask the patient to turn onto the affected hip. A sandbag may be placed under the ankle for support.
• Have the patient flex the unaffected knee and hip, and place the unaffected foot in front of the affected limb for stability.
• Flex the affected knee approximately 5 to 10 degrees. Increasing the flexion reduces the patellofemoral joint space.
• Adjust the knee in the lateral position so that the femoral epicondyles are superimposed, and the patella is perpendicular to the IR (Fig. 6-149).
• *Shield gonads.*
• Center the IR to the patella.

Central ray
• Perpendicular to the IR, entering the knee at the mid-patellofemoral joint
• Collimate closely to the patellar area.

Collimation
• Adjust to 4 × 4 inches (10 × 10 cm) on the collimator.

Structures shown
The resulting image shows a lateral projection of the patella and patellofemoral joint space (Figs. 6-150 and 6-151).

EVALUATION CRITERIA
The following should be clearly shown:
■ Evidence of proper collimation
■ Knee flexed 5 to 10 degrees
■ Open patellofemoral joint space
■ Patella in lateral profile
■ Close collimation

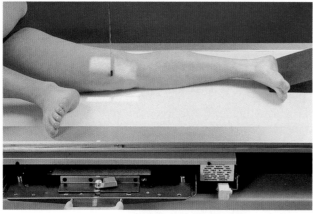

Fig. 6-149 Lateral patella, mediolateral.

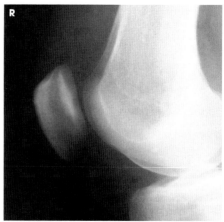

Fig. 6-150 Lateral patella, mediolateral.

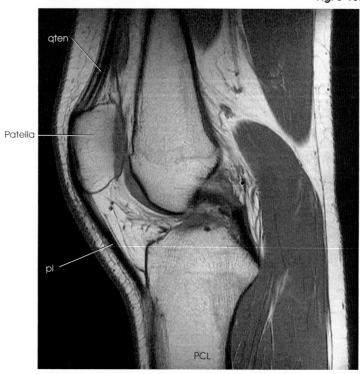

Fig. 6-151 Sagittal MRI shows patella, patellofemoral joint and surrounding soft tissues. Quadriceps tendon (*qten*) and patellar ligament (*pl*) are shown on this image.

Lower Limb

TANGENTIAL PROJECTION
HUGHSTON METHOD[1,2]

Radiography of the patella has been the topic of hundreds of articles. For a tangential radiograph, the patient may be placed in any of the following body positions: prone, supine, lying on the side, seated on the table, seated on the radiographic table with the leg hanging over the edge, or standing.

Various authors have described the degree of flexion of the knee joint as ranging from 20 to 120 degrees. Laurin[3] reported that patellar subluxation is easier to show when the knee is flexed 20 degrees and noted a limitation of using this small angle. Modern radiographic equipment often does not permit such small angles because of the large size of the collimator.

Fodor et al.[4] and Merchant et al.[5] recommended a 45-degree flexion of the knee, and Hughston[6] recommended an approximately 55-degree angle with the central ray angled 45 degrees. In addition, Merchant et al.[5] stated that relaxation of the quadriceps muscles is required to show patellar subluxation.

Image receptor: 8 × 10 inch (18 × 24 cm) for unilateral examination; 10 × 12 inch (24 × 30 cm) crosswise for bilateral examination

Position of patient
- Place the patient in a prone position with the foot resting on the radiographic table.
- Adjust the body so that it is not rotated.

[1]Hughston JC: Subluxation of the patella, *J Bone Joint Surg Am* 50:1003, 1968.
[2]Kimberlin GE: Radiological assessment of the patellofemoral articulation and subluxation of the patella, *Radiol Technol* 45:129, 1973.
[3]Laurin CA: The abnormal lateral patellofemoral angle, *J Bone Joint Surg Am* 60:55, 1968.
[4]Fodor J et al: Accurate radiography of the patellofemoral joint, *Radiol Technol* 53:570, 1982.
[5]Merchant AC et al: Roentgenographic analysis of patellofemoral congruence, *J Bone Joint Surg Am* 56:1391, 1974.
[6]Hughston JC: Subluxation of the patella, *J Bone Joint Surg Am* 50:1003, 1968.

Position of part
- Place the IR under the patient's knee, and slowly flex the affected knee so that the tibia and fibula form a 50- to 60-degree angle from the table.
- Rest the foot against the collimator, or support it in position (Fig. 6-152).
- Ensure that the collimator surface is not hot because this could burn the patient.
- Adjust the patient's leg so that it is not rotated medially or laterally from the vertical plane.
- *Shield gonads.*

Central ray
- Angled 45 degrees cephalad and directed through the patellofemoral joint

Structures shown

The tangential image shows subluxation of the patella and patellar fractures and allows radiologic assessment of the femoral condyles. Hughston recommended that both knees be examined for comparison (Fig. 6-153).

EVALUATION CRITERIA

The following should be clearly shown:
- Patella in profile
- Open patellofemoral articulation
- Surfaces of femoral condyles
- Soft tissue of the femoropatellar articulation
- Bony recorded detail on the patella and femoral condyles

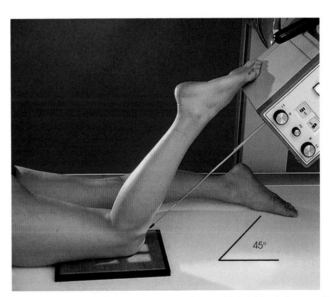

Fig. 6-152 Tangential patella and patellofemoral joint: Hughston method.

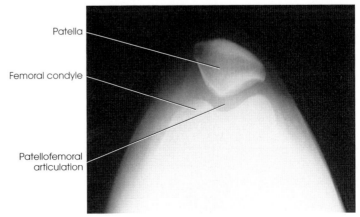

Patella

Femoral condyle

Patellofemoral articulation

Fig. 6-153 Tangential patellofemoral joint: Hughston method.

TANGENTIAL PROJECTION
MERCHANT METHOD[1]

Image receptor: 10 × 12 inch (24 × 30 cm) crosswise for bilateral examination

SID: A 6-ft (2-m) SID is recommended to reduce magnification.

Position of patient
- Place the patient supine with both knees at the end of the radiographic table.
- Support the knees and lower legs with an adjustable IR-holding device (Axial Viewer).[2]
- To increase comfort and relaxation of the quadriceps femoris, place pillows or a foam wedge under the patient's head and back.

[1]Merchant AC et al: Roentgenographic analysis of patellofemoral congruence, *J Bone Joint Surg Am* 56:1391, 1974.
[2]Merchant AC: The Axial Viewer, Orthopedic Products, 2500 Hospital Dr., Bldg. 7, Mountain View, CA 94040.

Position of part
- Using the Axial Viewer device, elevate the patient's knees approximately 2 inches to place the femora parallel with the tabletop (Figs. 6-154 and 6-155).
- Adjust the angle of knee flexion to 40 degrees. (Merchant reported that the degree of angulation may be varied between 30 degrees and 90 degrees to show various patellofemoral disorders.)
- Strap both legs together at the calf level to control leg rotation and allow patient relaxation.

- Place the IR perpendicular to the central ray and resting on the patient's shins (a thin foam pad aids comfort) approximately 1 ft distal to the patellae.
- Ensure that the patient is able to relax. Relaxation of the quadriceps femoris is crucial for an accurate diagnosis. If these muscles are not relaxed, a subluxated patella may be pulled back into the intercondylar sulcus, showing a false normal appearance.
- Record the angle of knee flexion for reproducibility during follow-up examinations because the severity of patella subluxation commonly changes inversely with the angle of knee flexion.
- *Shield gonads.*

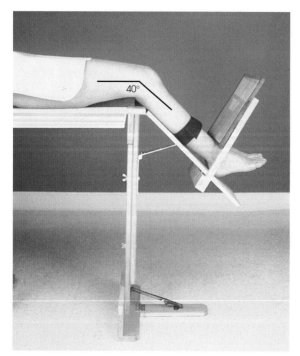

Fig. 6-154 Tangential patella and patellofemoral joint: Merchant method. Note use of Axial Viewer device.

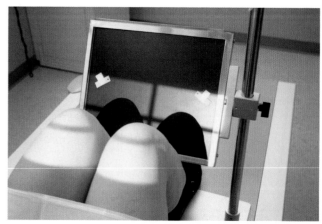

Fig. 6-155 Tabletop IR holder. Note how shadow of knees is used to position patella on IR.

Lower Limb

Central ray

- Perpendicular to the IR
- With 40-degree knee flexion, angle the central ray 30 degrees caudad from the horizontal plane (60 degrees from vertical) to achieve a 30-degree central ray–to–femur angle. The central ray enters midway between the patellae at the level of the patellofemoral joint.

Structures shown

The bilateral tangential image shows an axial projection of the patellae and patellofemoral joints (Fig. 6-156). Because of the right-angle alignment of the IR and central ray, the patellae are seen as nondistorted, albeit slightly magnified, images.

The following should be clearly shown:
- Patellae in profile
- Femoral condyles and intercondylar sulcus
- Open patellofemoral articulations

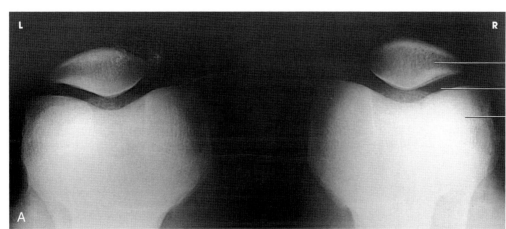

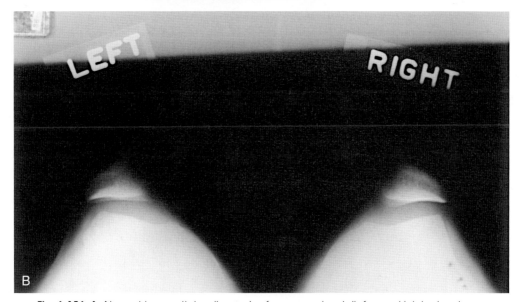

Fig. 6-156 A, Normal tangential radiograph of congruent patellofemoral joints, showing patellae to be well centered with normal trabecular pattern. **B,** Abnormal tangential radiograph showing abnormally shallow intercondylar sulci, misshapen and laterally subluxated patellae, and incongruent patellofemoral joints (left worse than right).

(Courtesy Alan J. Merchant.)

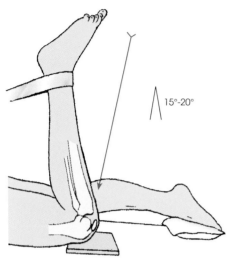

Fig. 6-157 Tangential patella and patello-femoral joint: Settegast method.

⚘ TANGENTIAL PROJECTION
SETTEGAST METHOD

Because of the danger of fragment displacement by the acute knee flexion required for this procedure, this projection should not be attempted until a transverse fracture of the patella has been ruled out with a lateral image, or if the patient is in pain.

Image receptor: 8 × 10 inch (18 × 24 cm)

Position of patient

- Place the patient in the supine or prone position. The latter is preferable because the knee can usually be flexed to a greater degree, and immobilization is easier (Figs. 6-157 and 6-158).

- If the patient is seated on the radiographic table, hold the IR securely in place (Fig. 6-159). Alternative positions are shown in Figs. 6-160 and 6-161.

Position of part

- Flex the patient's knee slowly as much as possible or until the patella is perpendicular to the IR if the patient's condition permits. With *slow, even flexion,* the patient should be able to tolerate the position, whereas quick, uneven flexion may cause too much pain.

- If desired, loop a long strip of bandage around the patient's ankle or foot. Have the patient grasp the ends over the shoulder to hold the leg in position. Gently adjust the leg so that its long axis is vertical.

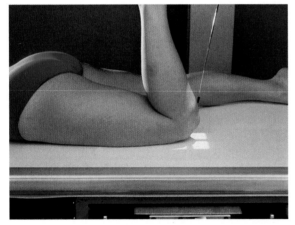

Fig. 6-158 Tangential patella and patellofemoral joint: Settegast method.

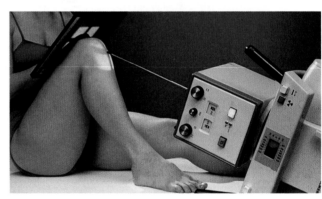

Fig. 6-159 Tangential patella and patellofemoral joint: Settegast method.

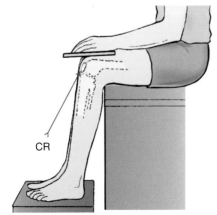

Fig. 6-160 Tangential patella and patellofemoral joint: patient seated.

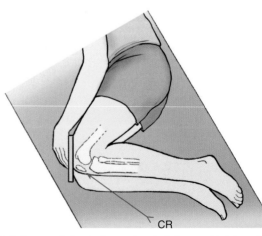

Fig. 6-161 Tangential patella and patellofemoral joint: patient lateral.

Lower Limb

- Place the IR transversely under the knee, and center it to the joint space between the patella and the femoral condyles.
- *Shield gonads.*
- By maintaining the same OID and SID relationships, this position can be obtained with the patient in a lateral or seated position (see Figs. 6-160 and 6-161).

NOTE: When the central ray is directed toward the patient's upper body (see Figs. 6-159 and 6-160), the thorax and thyroid should be shielded. *Gonad shielding* (not shown) should be used in all patients.

Central ray

- Perpendicular to the joint space between the patella and the femoral condyles when the joint is perpendicular. When the joint is not perpendicular, the degree of central ray angulation depends on the degree of flexion of the knee. The angulation typically is 15 to 20 degrees.
- Close collimation is recommended.

Collimation

- Adjust to 4×4 inches (10×10 cm) on the collimator for a single-side image and 4×10 inches (10×24 cm) size for a bilateral examination.

Structures shown

The image shows vertical fractures of bone and the articulating surfaces of the patellofemoral articulation (Figs. 6-162 and 6-163).

The following should be clearly shown:
- Evidence of proper collimation
- Patella in profile
- Open patellofemoral articulation
- Surfaces of the femoral condyles
- Soft tissue of the patellofemoral articulation
- Bony detail on the patella and femoral condyles

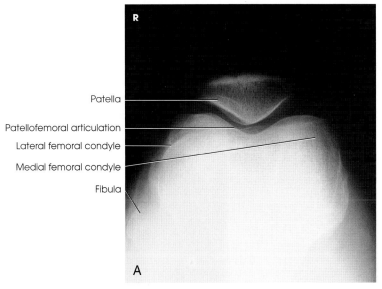
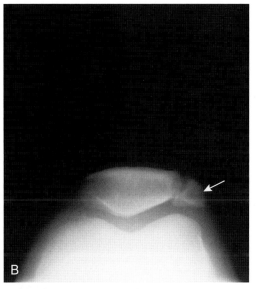

Patella
Patellofemoral articulation
Lateral femoral condyle
Medial femoral condyle
Fibula

Fig. 6-162 A, Tangential patella and patellofemoral joint: Settegast method. **B,** Fracture (*arrow*).

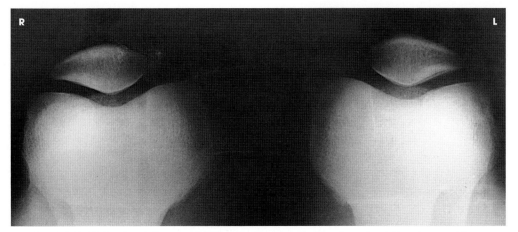

Fig. 6-163 Bilateral patella examination. For this examination, legs should be strapped together at the level of the calf, using appropriate binding to control femoral rotation.

Femur

♠ AP PROJECTION

If the femoral heads are separated by an unusually broad pelvis, the bodies (shafts) are more strongly angled toward the midline.

Image receptor: 7 × 17 inch (18 × 43 cm) or 14 × 17 inch (35 × 43 cm)

Position of patient

- Place the patient in the supine position.
- Check the pelvis to ensure it is not rotated.

Position of part

- Center the affected thigh to the midline of the IR. When the patient is too tall to include the entire femur, include the joint closest to the area of interest on one image (Fig. 6-164).

With the knee included

- For projection of the *distal* femur, rotate the patient's limb internally to place it in true anatomic position. The limb is naturally turned externally when laying on the table. Ensure that the epicondyles are parallel with the IR.
- Place the bottom of the IR 2 inches (5 cm) below the knee joint.

With the hip included

- For projection of the *proximal* femur, which must include the hip joint, place the top of the IR at the level of the ASIS.
- Rotate the limb internally 10 to 15 degrees to place the femoral neck in profile.
- *Shield gonads.*

Central ray

- Perpendicular to the mid-femur and the center of the IR

Collimation

- 1 inch (2.5 cm) on the sides of the shadow of the femur and 17 inches (43 cm) in length.

Structures shown

The resulting image shows an AP projection of the femur, including the knee joint or hip or both (Figs. 6-165 and 6-166).

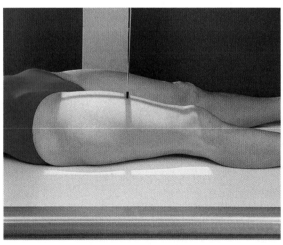

Fig. 6-164 AP distal femur.

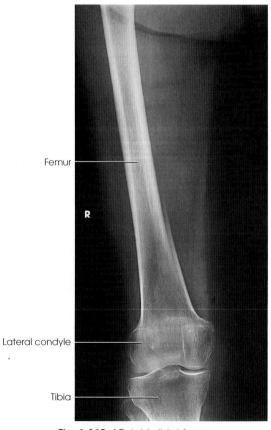

Fig. 6-165 AP right distal femur.

EVALUATION CRITERIA

The following should be clearly shown:
- Evidence of proper collimation
- Most of the femur and the joint nearest to the pathologic condition or site of injury (a second projection of the other joint is recommended)
- Femoral neck not foreshortened on the proximal femur
- Lesser trochanter not seen beyond the medial border of the femur or only a very small portion seen on the proximal femur
- No knee rotation on the distal femur
- Gonad shielding when indicated, but without the shield covering proximal femur
- Any orthopedic appliance in its entirety
- Trabecular recorded detail on the femoral shaft

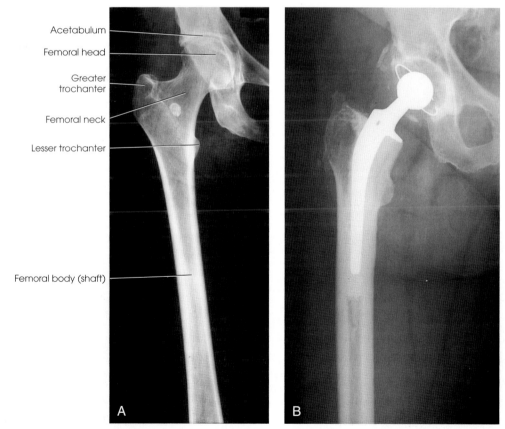

Acetabulum
Femoral head
Greater trochanter
Femoral neck
Lesser trochanter
Femoral body (shaft)

A

B

Fig. 6-166 A, AP proximal femur. **B,** AP proximal femur showing "total hip" arthroplasty procedure.

♠ LATERAL PROJECTION
Mediolateral

Image receptor: 7 × 17 inch (18 × 43 cm) or 14 × 17 inch (35 × 43 cm) lengthwise

Position of patient
- Ask the patient to turn onto the affected side.
- Adjust the body position, and center the affected thigh to the midline of the grid.

Position of part
With the knee included
- For projection of the *distal* femur, draw the patient's uppermost limb forward and support it at hip level on sandbags.
- Adjust the pelvis in a true lateral position (Fig. 6-167).
- Flex the affected knee about 45 degrees, place a sandbag under the ankle, and adjust the body rotation to place the epicondyles perpendicular to the table-top.
- Adjust the position of the Bucky tray so that the IR projects approximately 2 inches (5 cm) beyond the knee to be included.

NOTE: This radiograph can also be accomplished using the part positions for "with the hip included."

With the hip included
- For projection of the *proximal* femur, place the top of the IR at the level of the ASIS.
- Draw the upper limb posteriorly, and support it.
- Adjust the pelvis so that it is rolled posteriorly just enough to prevent superimposition; 10 to 15 degrees from the lateral position is sufficient (Fig. 6-168).
- *Shield gonads.*

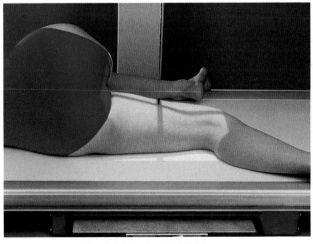

Fig. 6-167 Lateral distal femur.

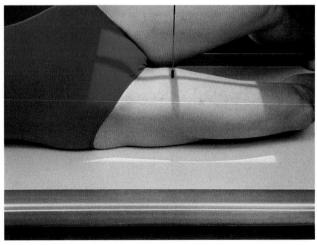

Fig. 6-168 Lateral proximal femur.

Lower Limb

Central ray

• Perpendicular to the mid-femur and the center of the IR

Collimation

• 1 inch (2.5 cm) on the sides of the shadow of the femur and 17 inches (43 cm) in length

Structures shown

The image shows a lateral projection of about three fourths of the femur and the adjacent joint. If needed, use two IRs to show the entire length of the adult femur (Figs. 6-169 and 6-170).

EVALUATION CRITERIA

The following should be clearly shown:
■ Evidence of proper collimation
■ Most of the femur and the joint nearest to the pathologic condition or site of injury (a second radiograph of the other end of the femur is recommended)
■ Any orthopedic appliance in its entirety
■ Trabecular detail on the femoral body

With the knee included
■ Superimposed anterior surface of the femoral condyles
■ Patella in profile
■ Open patellofemoral space

■ Inferior surface of the femoral condyles not superimposed because of divergent rays

With the hip included
■ Opposite thigh not over area of interest
■ Greater and lesser trochanters not prominent

NOTE: Because of the danger of fragment displacement, the aforementioned position is not recommended for patients with fracture or patients who may have destructive disease. Patients with these conditions should be examined in the supine position by placing the IR vertically along the medial or lateral aspect of the thigh and knee and then directing the central ray horizontally. A wafer grid or a grid-front IR should be used to minimize scattered radiation.

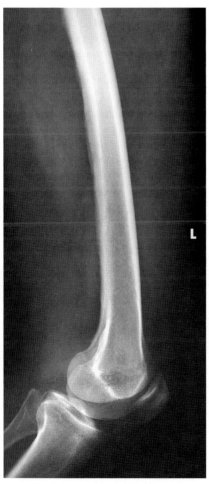

Fig. 6-169 Lateral distal femur.

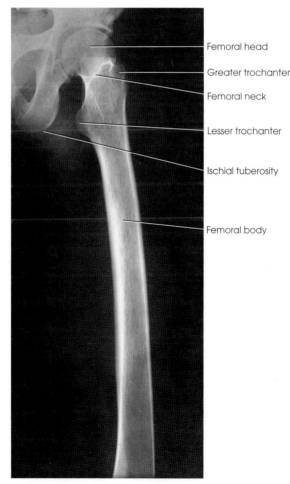

Femoral head

Greater trochanter

Femoral neck

Lesser trochanter

Ischial tuberosity

Femoral body

Fig. 6-170 Lateral proximal femur.

Lower Limb

Hips, Knees, and Ankles
AP PROJECTION
WEIGHT-BEARING METHOD[1,2]
Standing

NOTE: A specially built, long grid holder consisting of three grids, each 17 inches (43 cm) long, is required to hold the 51-inch (130-cm) IR and its trifold film. With computed radiography (CR), three separate 14- × 17-inch (35- × 43-cm) plates are held in a special long holder. The three individual images are "stitched" together using computer software.

Image receptor: 14 × 51 inch (31 × 130 cm) lengthwise

SID: 8 ft (244 cm). This minimum-length SID is required to open the collimators wide enough to expose the entire 51-inch (130-cm) length of the IR.

---

[1]Krushell R et al: A comparison of the mechanical and anatomical axes in arthritic knees. In *Proceedings of the Knee Society, 1985-1986,* Aspen, CO, 1987.
[2]Peterson TD, Rohr W: Improved assessment of lower extremity alignment using new roentgenographic techniques, *Clin Orthop Rel Res* (219):112, 1987.

Position of patient
- Stand the patient with the back against the upright grid unit.

Position of part
- Have the patient stand on a 2-inch (5-cm) riser so that the ankle joint is visible on the image. The bottom of the grid unit is positioned behind and below the riser.
- Measure both lateral malleoli, and position the legs so that they are exactly *20 cm* apart. If this distance cannot be achieved, measure the width of the malleoli and indicate this number on the request form. This image must be performed the same way for each return visit by the patient.
- Ensure that the patient's toes are positioned straight forward in the anatomic position (Fig. 6-171).
- Ensure that the patient is distributing weight equally on both feet.
- Mark with a right-side or left-side marker, and place a magnification marker in the area of the knee.
- *Shield gonads.*
- *Respiration:* Suspend.

NOTE: A graduated speed screen (three sections and three speeds) may be used in place of a wedge filter.

Central ray
- Perpendicular to the IR, entering midway between the knees at the level of the *knee joint*
- Collimate appropriately, and ensure that the hip joints and ankle joints are seen on the image.

◥ COMPENSATING FILTER
A compensating filter must be used for this projection (Fig. 6-172) because of the extreme difference between the hip joints and the ankle joints.

Structures shown
This projection shows the entire right and left limbs from the hip joint to the ankle joint (Fig. 6-173).

EVALUATION CRITERIA
The following should be clearly shown:
- Appropriate density to visualize the hips to the ankles
- Both feet in anatomic position
- Hips, knees, and ankles
- Right or left marker and a magnification marker near the knee

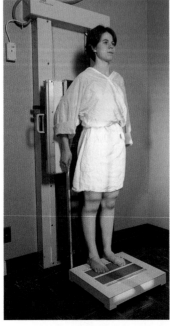

Fig. 6-171 Patient in position for radiograph of lower limbs: hips, knees, and ankles. The patient is placed in the anatomic position. The patient is standing on a raised platform so that the ankles are shown.

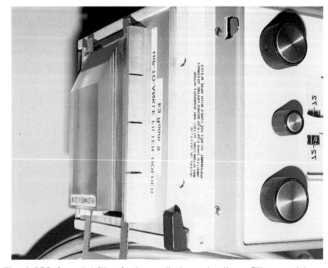

Fig. 6-172 Special filter for lower limb projections. Filter enables hips, knees, and ankles to be shown on one radiograph.

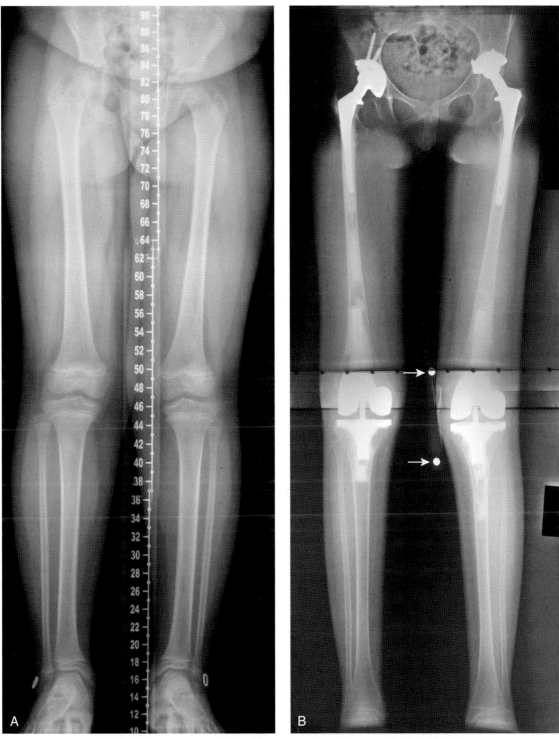

Fig. 6-173 Lower limbs: hips, knees, and ankles. **A,** Computed radiography (CR) "stitched" image. Computer created one image from three separate CR plates within a 51-inch (130-cm) IR. Note centimeter scale created within the image. **B,** A 51-inch (130-cm) radiographic film image. *Arrows* point to magnification marker taped to knee for measurements.

7

PELVIS AND UPPER FEMORA

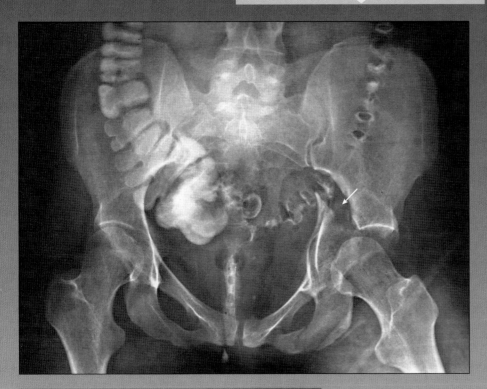

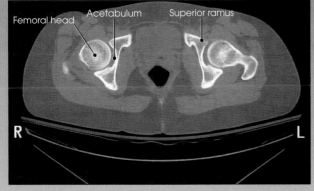

Femoral head   Acetabulum   Superior ramus

R   L

SUMMARY OF PROJECTIONS

PROJECTIONS, POSITIONS, AND METHODS

Page	Essential	Anatomy	Projection	Position	Method
337	✦	Pelvis and upper femora	AP		
340		Pelvis and upper femora	Lateral	R or L	
342	✦	Femoral necks	AP oblique		MODIFIED CLEAVES
344		Femoral necks	Axiolateral		ORIGINAL CLEAVES
346	✦	Hip	AP		
348	✦	Hip	Lateral (mediolateral)		LAUENSTEIN, HICKEY
350	✦	Hip	Axiolateral		DANELIUS-MILLER
352		Hip	Modified axiolateral		CLEMENTS-NAKAYAMA
354		Acetabulum	PA axial oblique	RAO or LAO	TEUFEL
356	✦	Acetabulum	AP oblique	RPO or LPO	JUDET, MODIFIED JUDET
358		Anterior pelvic bones	PA		
359		Anterior pelvic bones	AP axial (outlet)		TAYLOR
360		Anterior pelvic bones	Superoinferior axial (inlet)		BRIDGEMAN
361		Ilium	AP and PA oblique	RPO and LPO, RAO and LAO	

The icons in the Essential column indicate projections frequently performed in the United States and Canada. Students should become competent in these projections.

The *pelvis* serves as a base for the trunk and a girdle for the attachment of the lower limbs. The pelvis consists of four bones: two *hip bones,* the *sacrum,* and the *coccyx.* The *pelvic girdle* is composed of only the two hip bones.

Hip Bone

The *hip bone* is often referred to as the *os coxae,* and some textbooks continue to refer to it as the *innominate bone.* The most widely used term is hip bone.

The hip bone consists of the *ilium, pubis,* and *ischium* (Figs. 7-1 and 7-2). These three bones join together to form the *acetabulum,* the cup-shaped socket that re-ceives the head of the femur. The ilium, pubis, and ischium are separated by carti-lage in children but become fused into one bone in adults.

The hip bone is divided further into two distinct areas: the *iliopubic column* and the *ilioischial column* (see Fig. 7-2, *C*). These columns are used to identify frac-tures around the acetabulum.

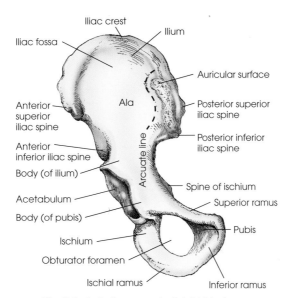

Fig. 7-1 Anterior aspect of right hip bone.

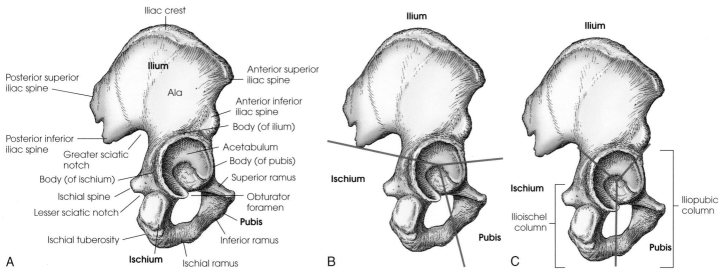

Fig. 7-2 A, Lateral aspect of right hip bone. **B,** Lateral aspect of right hip bone showing its three parts. **C,** Lateral aspect of hip bone showing ilioischial and iliopubic columns.

ILIUM

The *ilium* consists of a *body* and a broad, curved portion called the *ala*. The body of the ilium forms approximately two fifths of the acetabulum superiorly (Fig. 7-3). The ala projects superiorly from the body to form the prominence of the hip. The ala has three borders: anterior, posterior, and superior. The anterior and posterior borders present four prominent projections:
• Anterior superior iliac spine
• Anterior inferior iliac spine
• Posterior superior iliac spine
• Posterior inferior iliac spine

The *anterior superior iliac spine* (ASIS) is an important and frequently used radiographic positioning reference point. The superior margin extending from the ASIS to the posterior superior iliac spine is called the *iliac crest*. The medial surface of the wing contains the *iliac fossa* and is separated from the body of the bone by a smooth, arc-shaped ridge, the *arcuate line*, which forms a part of the circumference of the pelvic brim. The arcuate line passes obliquely, inferiorly, and medially to its junction with the pubis. The inferior and posterior portions of the wing present a large, rough surface—the *auricular surface*—for articulation with the sacrum. This articular surface and the articular surface of the adjacent sacrum have irregular elevations and depressions that cause a partial interlock of the two bones. The ilium curves inward below this surface, forming the *greater sciatic notch*.

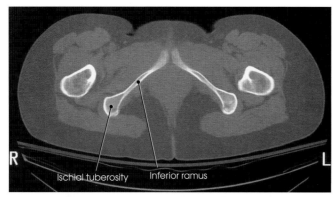

Fig. 7-3 Axial CT image of inferior ramus and ischial tuberosity.

(Modified from Kelley L, Petersen CM: *Sectional anatomy for imaging professionals*, ed 2, St Louis, 2007, Mosby.)

PUBIS

The *pubis* consists of a *body*, the *superior ramus*, and the *inferior ramus*. The body of the pubis forms approximately one fifth of the acetabulum anteriorly (see Fig. 7-2). The superior ramus projects inferiorly and medially from the acetabulum to the midline of the body. There the bone curves inferiorly and then posteriorly and laterally to join the ischium. The lower prong is termed the *inferior ramus*.

ISCHIUM

The *ischium* consists of a *body* and the *ischial ramus*. The body of the ischium forms approximately two fifths of the acetabulum posteriorly (see Figs. 7-2 and 7-3). It projects posteriorly and inferiorly from the acetabulum to form an expanded portion called the *ischial tuberosity*. When the body is in a seated-upright position, its weight rests on the two ischial tuberosities. The ischial ramus projects anteriorly and medially from the tuberosity to its junction with the inferior ramus of the pubis. By this posterior union the rami of the pubis and ischium enclose the *obturator foramen*. At the superoposterior border of the body is a prominent projection called the *ischial spine*. An indentation, the *lesser sciatic notch*, is just below the ischial spine.

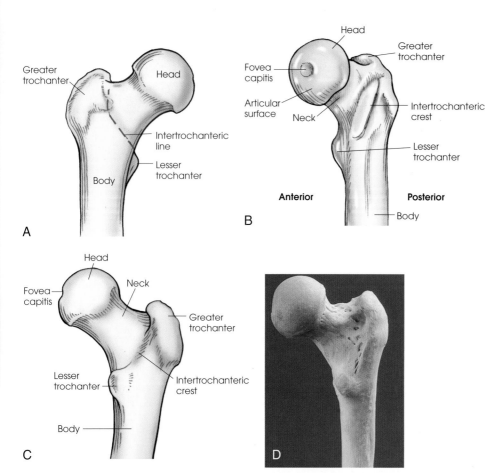

Fig. 7-4 Proximal right femur. **A,** Anterior aspect. **B,** Medial aspect. The body is positioned 15 to 20 degrees posterior from head. **C,** Posterior aspect. **D,** Posterior aspect of right proximal human femur. Note anatomic details and compare with **C.**

Proximal Femur

The *femur* is the longest, strongest, and heaviest bone in the body. The proximal end of the femur consists of a *head,* a *neck,* and two large processes: the *greater* and *lesser trochanters* (Fig. 7-4). The smooth, rounded head is connected to the femoral body by a pyramid-shaped neck and is received into the acetabular cavity of the hip bone. A small depression at the center of the head, the *fovea capitis,* at-taches to the ligamentum capitis femoris (Fig. 7-5; see Fig. 7-4). The neck is con-stricted near the head but expands to a broad base at the *body* of the bone. The neck projects medially, superiorly, and anteriorly from the body. The trochanters are situated at the junction of the body and the base of the neck. The greater trochan-ter is at the superolateral part of the femo-ral body, and the lesser trochanter is at the posteromedial part. The prominent ridge extending between the trochanters at the base of the neck on the posterior surface of the body is called the *intertrochanteric crest.* The less prominent ridge connect-ing the trochanters anteriorly is called the *intertrochanteric line.* The femoral neck and the intertrochanteric crest are two common sites of fractures in elderly adults. The superior portion of the greater trochanter projects above the neck and curves slightly posteriorly and medially.

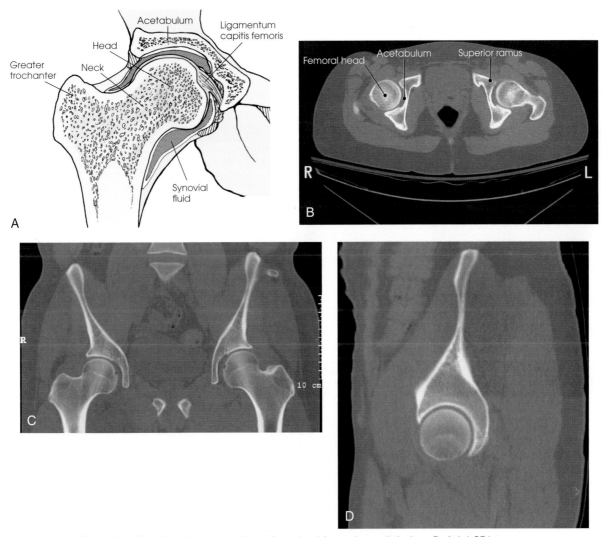

Fig. 7-5 A, Hip joint. Coronal section of proximal femur in acetabulum. **B,** Axial CT image of hip joint showing acetabulum, head of femur, and superior ramus. **C,** Coronal CT im-age of both hip joints. **D,** Sagittal CT image of the right hip joint.

(Modified from Kelley L, Petersen CM: *Sectional anatomy for imaging professionals,* ed 2, St Louis, 2007, Mosby.)

The angulation of the neck of the femur varies considerably with age, sex, and stature. In the average adult, the neck projects anteriorly from the body at an angle of approximately 15 to 20 degrees and superiorly at an angle of approximately 120 to 130 degrees to the long axis of the femoral body (Fig. 7-6). The longitudinal plane of the femur is angled about 10 degrees from vertical. In children, the latter angle is wider—that is, the neck is more vertical in position. In wide pelves, the angle is narrower, placing the neck in a more horizontal position.

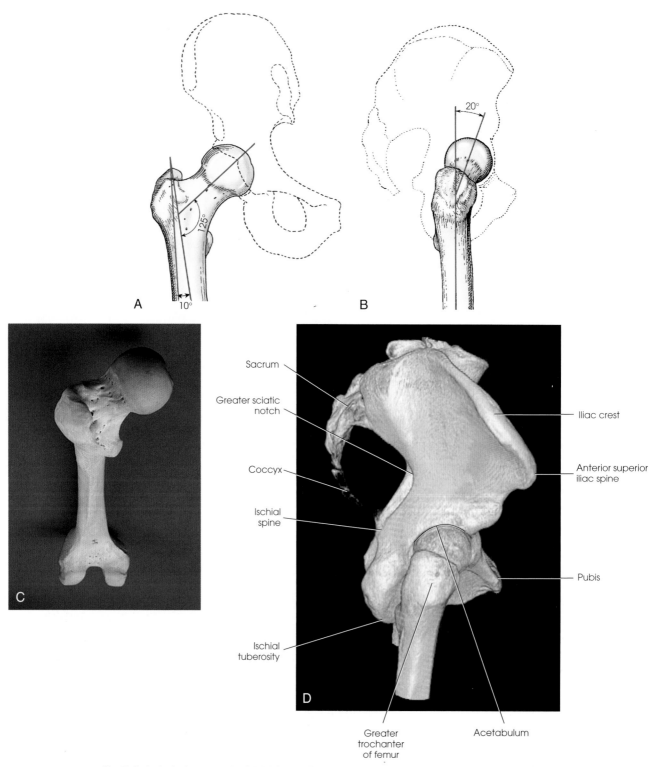

Fig. 7-6 A, Anterior aspect of right femur. **B,** Lateral aspect of right femur. **C,** Superoinferior view of posterior aspect of a human femur showing 15- to 20-degree anterior angle of femoral neck. **D,** Three-dimensional CT scan of lateral hip bone and proximal femur.

Articulations of the Pelvis

Table 7-1 and Fig. 7-7 provide a summary of the three joints of the pelvis and upper femora. The articulation between the acetabulum and the head of the femur (the hip joint) is a *synovial ball-and-socket* joint that permits free movement in all directions. The knee and ankle joints are hinge joints; the wide range of motion of the lower limb depends on the ball-and-socket joint of the hip. Because the knee and ankle joints are hinge joints, medial and lateral rotations of the foot cause rotation of the entire limb, which is centered at the hip joint.

The pubes of the hip bones articulate with each other at the anterior midline of the body, forming a joint called the *pubic symphysis*. The pubic symphysis is a *cartilaginous symphysis* joint.

The right and left ilia articulate with the sacrum posteriorly at the *sacroiliac* (SI) joints. These two joints angle 25 to 30 degrees relative to the midsagittal plane (see Fig. 7-7, *B*). The SI articulations are *synovial irregular gliding* joints. Because the bones of the SI joints interlock, movement is limited or nonexistent.

TABLE 7-1

Joints of the pelvis and upper femora

| Joint | Structural classification | | Movement |
	Tissue	Type	
Hip joint	Synovial	Ball and socket	Freely movable
Pubic symphysis	Cartilaginous	Symphysis	Slightly movable
Sacroiliac	Synovial	Irregular gliding*	Slightly movable

*Some anatomists term this a synovial fibrous joint.

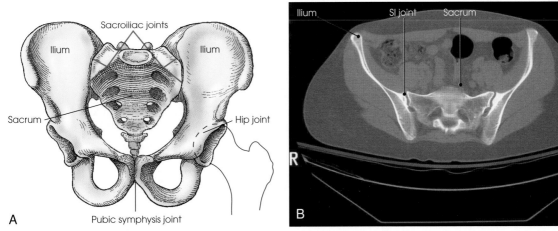

Fig. 7-7 A, Joints of pelvis and upper femora. **B,** Axial CT image of pelvis showing SI joints. Note 25- to 30-degree angulation of joint.

(**B,** Modified from Kelley L, Petersen CM: *Sectional anatomy for imaging professionals,* ed 2, St Louis, 2007, Mosby.)

TABLE 7-2

Female and male pelvis characteristics

Feature	Female	Male
Shape	Wide, shallow	Narrow, deep
Bony structure	Light	Heavy
Superior aperture (inlet)	Oval	Round
Inferior aperture (outlet)	Wide	Narrow

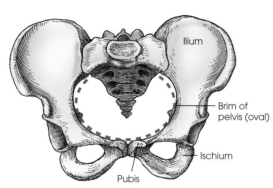

Fig. 7-8 Female pelvis.

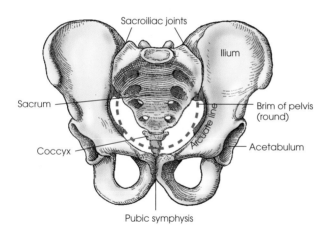

Fig. 7-9 Male pelvis.

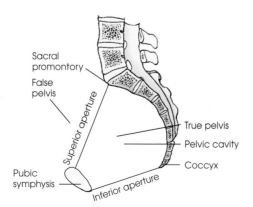

Fig. 7-10 Midsagittal section showing inlet and outlet of true pelvis.

Pelvis

The female pelvis (Fig. 7-8) is lighter in structure than the male pelvis (Fig. 7-9). It is wider and shallower, and the inlet is larger and more oval-shaped. The sacrum is wider, it curves more sharply posteriorly, and the sacral promontory is flatter. The width and depth of the pelvis vary with stature and gender (Table 7-2). The female pelvis is shaped for childbearing and delivery.

The pelvis is divided into two portions by an oblique plane that extends from the upper anterior margin of the sacrum to the upper margin of the pubic symphysis. The boundary line of this plane is called the *brim of the pelvis* (see Figs. 7-8 and 7-9). The region above the brim is called the *false* or *greater pelvis,* and the region below the brim is called the *true* or *lesser pelvis.*

The brim forms the *superior aperture,* or *inlet,* of the true pelvis. The *inferior aperture,* or *outlet,* of the true pelvis is measured from the tip of the coccyx to the inferior margin of the pubic symphysis in the anteroposterior direction and between the ischial tuberosities in the horizontal direction. The region between the inlet and the outlet is called the *pelvic cavity* (Fig. 7-10).

When the body is in the upright or seated position, the brim of the pelvis forms an angle of approximately 60 degrees to the horizontal plane. This angle varies with other body positions; the degree and direction of the variation depend on the lumbar and sacral curves.

Localizing Anatomic Structures

The bony landmarks used in radiography of the pelvis and hips are as follows:

- Iliac crest
- ASIS
- Pubic symphysis
- Greater trochanter of the femur
- Ischial tuberosity
- Tip of the coccyx

Most of these points are easily palpable, even in hypersthenic patients (Fig. 7-11). Because of the heavy muscles immediately above the iliac crest, care must be exercised in locating this structure to avoid *centering errors*. Having the patient inhale deeply is advisable; while the muscles are relaxed during expiration, the radiographer should palpate for the highest point of the iliac crest.

The highest point of the greater trochanter, which can be palpated immediately below the depression in the soft tissues of the lateral surface of the hip, is in the same horizontal plane as the midpoint of the hip joint and the coccyx. The most prominent point of the greater trochanter is in the same horizontal plane as the pubic symphysis (see Fig. 7-11).

The greater trochanter is most prominent laterally and more easily palpated when the lower leg is medially rotated. When properly used, medial rotation assists in localization of hip and pelvis centering points and avoids distortion of the proximal end of the femur during radiography. Improper rotation of the lower leg

can rotate the pelvis. Consequently, positioning of the lower leg is important in radiographing the hip and pelvis; the feet must be immobilized in the correct position to avoid distortion of the image. Traumatic injuries or pathologic conditions of the pelvis or lower limb may rule out the possibility of medial rotation.

The pubic symphysis can be palpated on the midsagittal plane and on the same horizontal plane as the greater trochanters. By placing the fingertips at this location and performing a brief downward palpation with the hand flat, palm down, and fingers together, the radiographer can locate the superior margin of the pubic symphysis. *To avoid possible embarrassment or misunderstanding, the radiographer should advise the patient in advance that this and other palpations of pelvic landmarks are part of normal procedure and necessary for an accurate examination.* When performed in an efficient and professional manner with respect for the patient's condition, such palpations are generally well tolerated.

The hip joint can be located by palpating the ASIS and the superior margin of the pubic symphysis (Fig. 7-12). The mid-

point of a line drawn between these two points is directly above the center of the dome of the acetabular cavity. A line drawn at right angles to the midpoint of the first line lies parallel to the long axis of the femoral neck of an average adult in the anatomic position. The femoral head lies 1½ inches (3.8 cm) distal, and the femoral neck is 2½ (6.4 cm) distal to this point.

For accurate localization of the femoral neck in atypical patients or in patients in whom the limb is not in the anatomic position, a line is drawn between the ASIS and the superior margin of the pubic symphysis, and a second line is drawn from a point 1 inch (2.5 cm) inferior to the greater trochanter to the midpoint of the previously marked line. The femoral head and neck lies along this line (see Fig. 7-12).

ALTERNATIVE POSITIONING LANDMARK

Bello[1] described an alternative positioning landmark for the pelvis and hip.

[1]Bello A: An alternative positioning landmark, *Radiol Technol* 5:477, 1999.

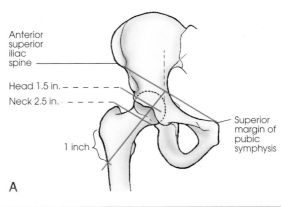

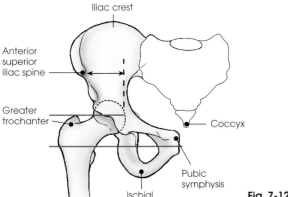

Fig. 7-11 Bony landmarks and localization planes of pelvis.

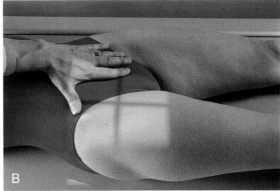

Fig. 7-12 A, Method of localizing right hip joint and long axis of femoral neck. **B,** Suggested method of localizing right hip. Left thumb is on ASIS, and second finger is on superior margin of pubic symphysis. Central ray is positioned 1.5 inches distal to center of line drawn between ASIS and pubic symphysis.

SUMMARY OF ANATOMY

Pelvis
Hip bones (two)
Sacrum
Coccyx
Pelvic girdle

Hip bone
Ilium
Pubis
Ischium
Acetabulum

Ilium
Body
Wing
Superior spine
Inferior spine

Anterior superior iliac spine
  (ASIS)
Anterior inferior iliac spine
Posterior superior iliac spine
Posterior inferior iliac spine
Iliac crest
Iliac fossa
Arcuate line
Auricular surface
Greater sciatic notch

Pubis
Body
Superior ramus
Inferior ramus
Iliopubic column

Ischium
Body
Ischial ramus
Ischial tuberosity
Obturator foramen
Ischial spine
Lesser sciatic notch
Ilioischial column

Femur (proximal aspect)
Head
Neck
Body
Fovea capitis
Greater trochanter
Lesser trochanter

Intertrochanteric crest
Intertrochanteric line

Articulations
Hip
Pubic symphysis
Sacroiliac joints

Pelvis
Brim of the pelvis
Greater or false pelvis
Lesser or true pelvis
Superior aperture or inlet
Inferior aperture or outlet
Pelvic cavity

ABBREVIATIONS USED IN CHAPTER 7

ASIS	Anterior superior iliac spine
SI	Sacroiliac

See Addendum A for a summary of all abbreviations used in Volume 1.

SUMMARY OF PATHOLOGY

Condition	Definition
Ankylosing spondylitis	Rheumatoid arthritis variant involving the SI joints and spine
Congenital hip dysplasia	Malformation of the acetabulum causing displacement of the femoral head
Dislocation	Displacement of a bone from the joint space
Fracture	Disruption in the continuity of bone
Legg-Calvé-Perthes disease	Flattening of the femoral head owing to vascular interruption
Metastases	Transfer of a cancerous lesion from one area to another
Osteoarthritis or degenerative joint disease	Form of arthritis marked by progressive cartilage deterioration in synovial joints and vertebrae
Osteopetrosis	Increased density of atypically soft bone
Osteoporosis	Loss of bone density
Paget disease	Thick, soft bone marked by bowing and fractures
Slipped epiphysis	Proximal portion of femur dislocated from distal portion at the proximal epiphysis
Tumor	New tissue growth where cell proliferation is uncontrolled
Chondrosarcoma	Malignant tumor arising from cartilage cells
Multiple myeloma	Malignant neoplasm of plasma cells involving the bone marrow and causing destruction of the bone

EXPOSURE TECHNIQUE CHART ESSENTIAL PROJECTIONS

PELVIS AND UPPER FEMORA

Part	cm	kVp*	tm	mA	mAs	AEC	SID	IR	Dose[†] (mrad)
Pelvis and upper femora—AP[‡]	19	70		200s		●● ○	40"	35 × 43 cm	135
Femoral necks—AP oblique[‡]	19	70		200s		●● ○	40"	35 × 43 cm	135
Hip—AP[‡]	18	65		200s		○○ ●	40"	24 × 30 cm	118
Hip—Lateral (Lauenstein-Hickey)[‡]	18	65		200s		○○ ●	40"	24 × 30 cm	118
Hip—Axiolateral (Danelius-Miller)[§]	24	80	0.80	200s	160		40"	24 × 30 cm	347

*kVp values are for a three-phase, 12-pulse generator or high frequency.
[†]Relative doses for comparison use. All doses are skin entrance for average adult at cm indicated.
[‡]Bucky, 16:1 grid. Screen-film speed 300 or equivalent CR.
[§]Tabletop, 8:1 grid. Screen-film speed 300.
s, small focal spot.

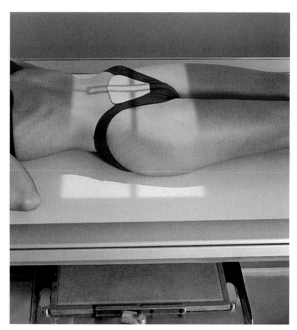

Fig. 7-13 Female AP pelvis with gonad shield.

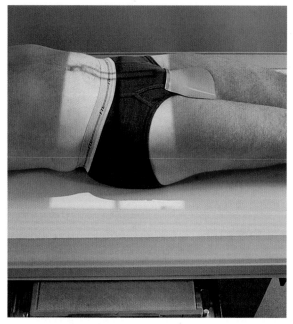

Fig. 7-14 Male AP pelvis with gonad shield.

Radiation Protection

Protection of the patient from unnecessary radiation is a professional responsibility of the radiographer (see Chapter 1 for specific guidelines). In this chapter, the *Shield gonads* statement at the end of the *Position of part* section indicates that the patient is to be protected from unnecessary radiation by restricting the radiation beam using proper collimation. In addition, placing lead shielding between the gonads and the radiation source is appropriate when the clinical objectives of the examination are not compromised (Figs. 7-13 and 7-14).

▲ AP PROJECTION

Image receptor: 14 × 17 inch (35 × 43 cm) crosswise

Position of patient
- Place the patient on the table in the supine position.

Position of part
- Center the midsagittal plane of the body to the midline of the grid, and adjust it in a true supine position.
- Unless contraindicated because of trauma or pathologic factors, medially rotate the feet and lower limbs about 15 to 20 degrees to place the femoral necks parallel with the plane of the image receptor (IR) (Figs. 7-15 and 7-16). Medial rotation is easier for the patient to maintain if the knees are supported. The heels should be placed about 8 to 10 inches (20 to 24 cm) apart.
- Immobilize the legs with a sandbag across the ankles, if necessary.
- Check the distance from ASIS to the tabletop on each side to be sure that the pelvis is not rotated.

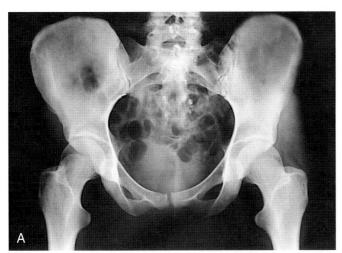
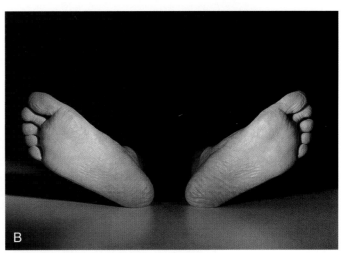

Fig. 7-15 A, AP pelvis with femoral necks and trochanters poorly positioned because of lateral rotation of limbs. **B,** Feet and lower limbs in natural, laterally rotated tabletop position, causing poor profile of proximal femora in **A.**

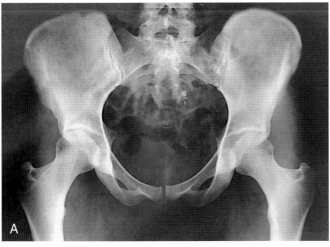
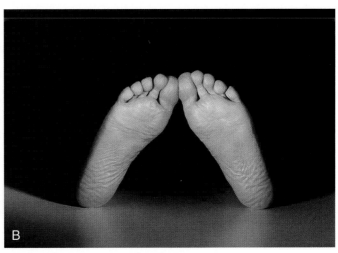

Fig. 7-16 A, AP pelvis with femoral necks and trochanters in correct position. **B,** Feet and lower limbs medially rotated 15 to 20 degrees, correctly placed with upper femora in correct profile in **A.**

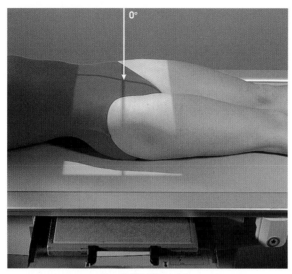

Fig. 7-17 AP pelvis.

- Center the IR midway between ASIS and pubic symphysis. In average-sized patients, the center of the IR is about 2 inches (5 cm) inferior to ASIS and 2 inches (5 cm) superior to pubic symphysis (Fig. 7-17).
- If the pelvis is deep, palpate for the iliac crest and adjust the position of the IR so that its upper border projects 1 to 1½ inches (2.5 to 3.8 cm) above the crest.
- *Shield gonads.*
- *Respiration:* Suspend.

Central ray
- Perpendicular to the midpoint of the IR

Collimation
- Adjust to 14 × 17 inches (35 × 43 cm) on the collimator.

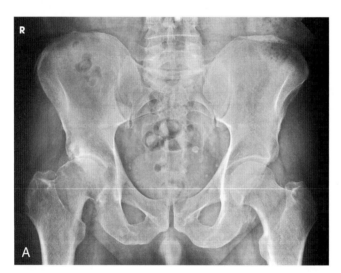

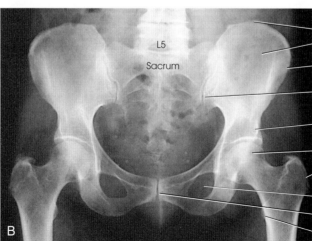

Iliac crest
Ala
Anterior superior iliac spine
Sacroiliac joint
Anterior inferior iliac spine
Femoral head
Greater trochanter
Obturator foramen
Pubic symphysis
Lesser trochanter

L5
Sacrum

Fig. 7-18 A, Male AP pelvis. **B,** Female AP pelvis.

Structures shown

The image shows an AP projection of the pelvis and of the head, neck, trochanters, and proximal one third or one fourth of the shaft of the femora (Fig. 7-18).

EVALUATION CRITERIA

The following should be clearly shown:
- Evidence of proper collimation
- Entire pelvis along with the proximal femora
- Lesser trochanters, if seen, shown on the medial border of the femora
- Femoral necks in their full extent without superimposition
- Greater trochanters in profile
- Both ilia equidistant to the edge of the radiograph
- Both greater trochanters equidistant to the edge of the radiograph
- Lower vertebral column centered to the middle of the radiograph
- Symmetric obturator foramina
- Ischial spines equally shown
- Symmetric ilia alae
- Sacrum and coccyx aligned with the pubic symphysis

Congenital dislocation of the hip

Martz and Taylor[1] recommended two AP projections of the pelvis to show the relationship of the femoral head to the acetabulum in patients with congenital dislocation of the hip. The first projection is obtained with the central ray directed perpendicular to the pubic symphysis to detect any lateral or superior displacement of the femoral head. The second projection is obtained with the central ray directed to the pubic symphysis at a cephalic angulation of 45 degrees (Fig. 7-19). This angulation casts the shadow of an anteriorly displaced femoral head above that of the acetabulum and the shadow of a posteriorly displaced head below that of the acetabulum.

[1]Martz CD, Taylor CC: The 45-degree angle roentgenographic study of the pelvis in congenital dislocation of the hip, *J Bone Joint Surg Am* 36:528, 1954.

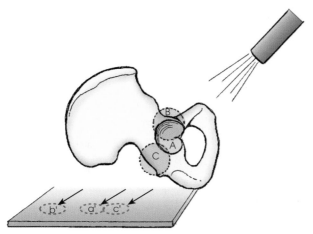

Fig. 7-19 Special projection taken for congenital dislocation of hip.

LATERAL PROJECTION
Right or left position

Image receptor: 14 × 17 inch (35 × 43 cm) lengthwise

Position of patient
• Place the patient in the lateral recumbent, dorsal decubitus, or upright position.

Position of part
Recumbent position
• When the patient can be placed in the lateral position, center the midcoronal plane of the body to the midline of the grid.
• Extend the thighs enough to prevent the femora from obscuring the pubic arch.
• Place a support under the lumbar spine, and adjust it to place the vertebral column parallel with the tabletop (Fig. 7-20). If the vertebral column is allowed to sag, it tilts the pelvis in the longitudinal plane.

• Adjust the pelvis in a true lateral position, with ASIS lying in the same vertical plane.
• Place one knee directly over the other knee. A pillow or other support between the knees promotes stabilization and patient comfort.
• Berkebile et al.[1] recommended a dorsal decubitus lateral projection of the pelvis to show the "gull-wing" sign in cases of fracture-dislocation of the acetabular rim and posterior dislocation of the femoral head.

---

[1]Berkebile RD et al: The gull-wing sign: value of the lateral view of the pelvis in fracture dislocation of the acetabular rim and posterior dislocation of the femoral head, *Radiology* 84:937, 1965.

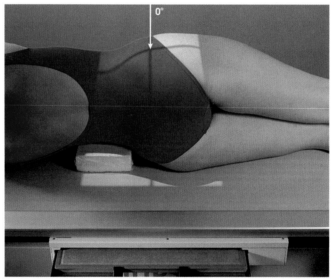

Fig. 7-20 Lateral pelvis.

Upright position
- Place the patient in the lateral position in front of a vertical grid device, and center the midcoronal plane of the body to the midline of the grid.
- Have the patient stand straight, with the weight of the body equally distributed on the feet so that the midsagittal plane is parallel with the plane of the IR.
- If the limbs are of unequal length, place a support of suitable height under the foot of the short side.
- Have the patient grasp the side of the stand for support.
- *Shield gonads.*
- *Respiration:* Suspend.

Central ray
- Perpendicular to a point centered at the level of the soft tissue depression just above the greater trochanter (approximately 2 inches [5 cm]) and to the midpoint of the image receptor
- Center the IR to the central ray.

Structures shown
The resulting image shows a lateral radiograph of the lumbosacral junction, sacrum, coccyx, and superimposed hip bones and upper femora (Fig. 7-21).

The following should be clearly shown:
- Entire pelvis and the proximal femora
- Sacrum and coccyx
- Superimposed posterior margins of the ischium and ilium
- Superimposed femora
- Superimposed acetabular shadows. The larger circle of the fossa (farther from the IR) is equidistant from the smaller circle of the fossa nearer the *IR* throughout their circumference.
- Pubic arch unobscured by the femora

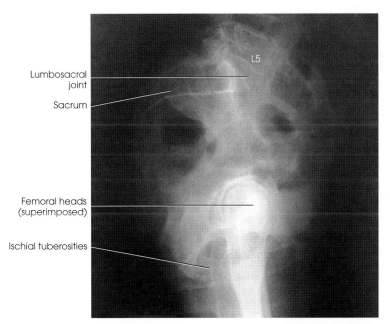
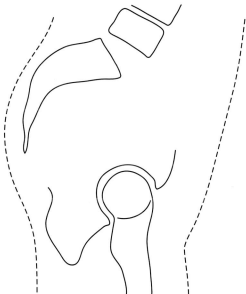

Lumbosacral joint
Sacrum
Femoral heads (superimposed)
Ischial tuberosities
L5

Fig. 7-21 Lateral pelvis.

AP OBLIQUE PROJECTION
MODIFIED CLEAVES METHOD

Image receptor: 14 × 17 inch (35 × 43 cm) crosswise

This projection is often called the bilateral *frog leg* position.

NOTE: This examination is contraindicated for a patient suspected to have a fracture or other pathologic disease.

Position of patient
• Place the patient in the supine position.

Position of part
• Center the midsagittal plane of the body to the midline of the grid.
• Flex the patient's elbows, and rest the hands on the upper chest.
• Adjust the patient so that the pelvis is not rotated. This position can be achieved by placing the two ASIS equidistant from the radiographic table.
• Place a compression band across the patient well above the hip joints for stability, if necessary.

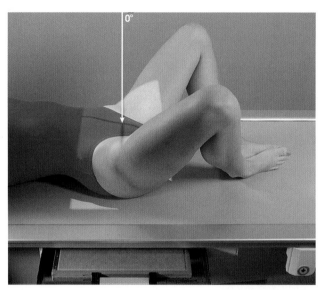

Fig. 7-22 AP oblique femoral necks with perpendicular central ray: modified Cleaves method.

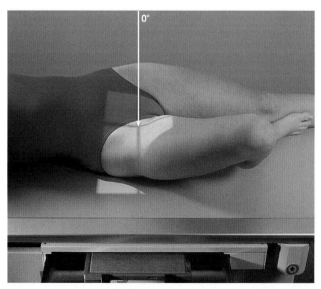

Fig. 7-23 Unilateral AP oblique femoral neck: modified Cleaves method.

Bilateral projection
Step 1
• Have the patient flex the hips and knees and draw the feet up as much as possible (i.e., enough to place the femora in a nearly vertical position if the affected side permits).
• Instruct the patient to hold this position, which is relatively comfortable, while the x-ray tube and IR are adjusted.
Step 2
• Center the IR 1 inch (2.5 cm) superior to the pubic symphysis.
Step 3
• Abduct the thighs as much as possible, and have the patient turn the feet inward to brace the soles against each other for support. According to Cleaves, the angle may vary between 25 degrees and 45 degrees, depending on how vertical the femora can be placed.
• Center the feet to the midline of the grid (Fig. 7-22).
• If possible, abduct the thighs approximately 45 degrees from the vertical plane to place the long axes of the femoral necks parallel with the plane of the IR.
• Check the position of the thighs, being careful to abduct them to the same degree.

Unilateral projection
• Adjust the body position to center ASIS of the affected side to the midline of the grid.
• Have the patient flex the hip and knee of the affected side and draw the foot up to the opposite knee as much as possible.
• After adjusting the perpendicular central ray and positioning the IR tray, have the patient brace the sole of the foot against the opposite knee and abduct the thigh laterally approximately 45 degrees (Fig. 7-23). The pelvis may rotate slightly.
• *Shield gonads.*
• *Respiration:* Suspend.

Femoral Necks

Central ray
- Perpendicular to enter the patient's midsagittal plane at the level 1 inch (2.5 cm) superior to the pubic symphysis. For the unilateral position, direct the central ray to the femoral neck (see Fig. 7-12).

Collimation
- Adjust to 14 × 17 inches (35 × 43 cm) on the collimator. If the patient is smaller than average, collimate smaller.

Structures shown
The bilateral image shows an AP oblique projection of the femoral heads, necks, and trochanteric areas projected onto one radiograph for comparison (Figs. 7-24 to 7-26).

EVALUATION CRITERIA
The following should be clearly shown:
- Evidence of proper collimation
- No rotation of the pelvis, as evidenced by a symmetric appearance
- Acetabulum, femoral head, and femoral neck
- Lesser trochanter on the medial side of the femur
- Femoral neck without superimposition by the greater trochanter; excess abduction causes the greater trochanter to obstruct the neck.
- Femoral axes extended from the hip bones at equal angles

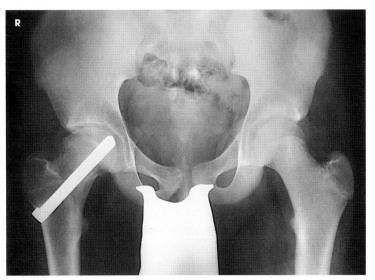

Fig. 7-24 AP femoral necks. Note fixation device in right hip and male gonad shield.

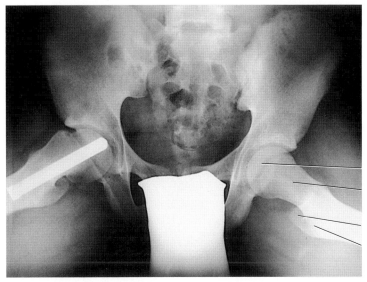

Femoral head

Femoral neck

Greater trochanter

Lesser trochanter

Fig. 7-25 AP oblique femoral necks: modified Cleaves method (same patient as in Fig. 7-24).

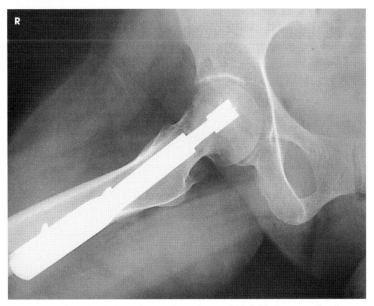

Fig. 7-26 AP oblique femoral neck: modified Cleaves method.

AXIOLATERAL PROJECTION
ORIGINAL CLEAVES METHOD[1]

NOTE: This examination is contraindicated for patients with suspected fracture or pathologic condition.

Image receptor: 14 × 17 inch (35 × 43 cm) crosswise

[1]Cleaves EN: Observations on lateral views of the hip, *AJR Am J Roentgenol* 34:964, 1938.

Position of patient
- Place the patient in the supine position.

Position of part

NOTE: This is the same part position as the modified Cleaves method previously described. The projection can be performed unilaterally or bilaterally.

- Before having the patient abduct the thighs (described in step 3 on p. 342), direct the x-ray tube parallel to the long axes of the femoral shafts (Fig. 7-27).
- Adjust the IR so that the midpoint coincides with the central ray.
- *Shield gonads.*
- *Respiration:* Suspend.

Central ray
- Parallel with the femoral shafts. According to Cleaves,[1] the angle may vary between 25 degrees and 45 degrees, depending on how vertical the femora can be placed.

[1]Cleaves EN: Observations on lateral views of the hip, *AJR Am J Roentgenol* 34:964, 1938.

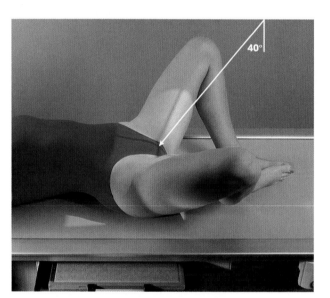

Fig. 7-27 Axiolateral femoral necks: Cleaves method.

Structures shown

The resulting image shows an axiolateral projection of the femoral heads, necks, and trochanteric areas (Fig. 7-28).

EVALUATION CRITERIA

The following should be clearly shown:
- Axiolateral projections of the femoral necks
- Femoral necks without overlap from the greater trochanters
- Small parts of the lesser trochanters on the posterior surfaces of the femora
- Small amount of the greater trochanters on the posterior and anterior surfaces of the femora
- Both sides equidistant from the edge of the radiograph
- Greater amount of the proximal femur on a unilateral examination
- Femoral neck angles approximately 15 to 20 degrees superior to the femoral bodies

Congenital dislocation of the hip

The diagnosis of congenital dislocation of the hip in newborns has been discussed in numerous articles. Andren and von Rosén[1] described a method that is based on certain theoretic considerations. Their method requires accurate and judicious application of the positioning technique to make an accurate diagnosis. The Andren-von Rosén approach involves taking a bilateral hip projection with both legs forcibly abducted to at least 45 degrees with appreciable inward rotation of the femora. Knake and Kuhns[2] described the construction of a device that controlled the degree of abduction and rotation of both limbs. They reported that the device essentially eliminated and greatly simplified the positioning difficulties, reducing the number of repeat examinations.

[1]Andren L, von Rosén S: The diagnosis of dislocation of the hip in newborns and the primary results of immediate treatment, *Acta Radiol* 49:89, 1958.
[2]Knake JE, Kuhns LR: A device to aid in positioning for the Andren-von Rosén hip view, *Radiology* 117:735, 1975.

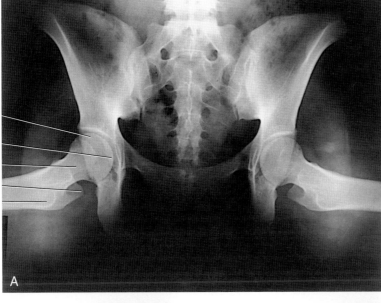

Femoral head
Femoral head within acetabulum
Femoral neck
Greater trochanter
Lesser trochanter

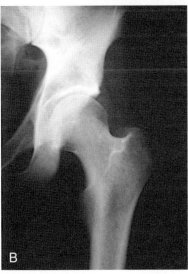

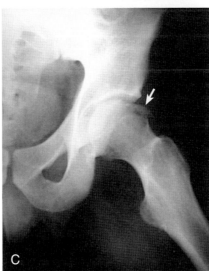

Fig. 7-28 Axiolateral femoral necks: Cleaves method. **A,** Bilateral examination. **B** and **C,** Unilateral hip examination of a patient who fell. No fractures were seen on initial AP hip radiograph (**B**), and a second projection using the Cleaves method was performed. Chip fracture of femoral head (*arrow*) was seen (**C**). At least two projections are required in trauma diagnoses.

♠ AP PROJECTION

Image receptor: 10 × 12 inch (24 × 30 cm) lengthwise

Position of patient
- Place the patient in the supine position.

Position of part
- Adjust the patient's pelvis so that it is not rotated. This is accomplished by placing ASIS equidistant from the table (Figs. 7-29 and 7-30).
- Place the patient's arms in a comfortable position.
- Medially rotate the lower limb and foot approximately 15 to 20 degrees to place the femoral neck parallel with the plane of the IR, unless this maneuver is contraindicated or other instructions are given.
- Place a support under the knee and a sandbag across the ankle. This makes it easier for the patient to maintain this position.
- *Shield gonads.*
- *Respiration:* Suspend.

Central ray
- Perpendicular to the femoral neck. Using the localizing technique previously described (see Fig. 7-12), place the central ray approximately 2½ inches (6.4 cm) distal on a line drawn perpendicular to the midpoint of a line between ASIS and pubic symphysis (see Fig. 7-30, *B*).
- Center the IR to the central ray.
- Make any necessary adjustments in the IR size and central ray point when an entire orthopedic device is to be shown on one image.

Collimation
- Adjust to 10 × 12 inches (24 × 30 cm) on the collimator.

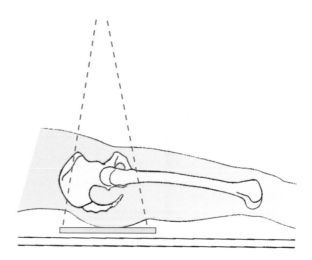

A

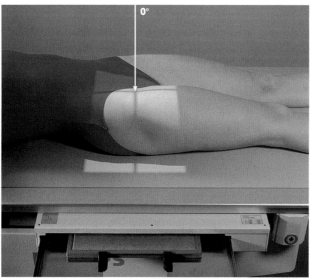

Fig. 7-29 AP hip.

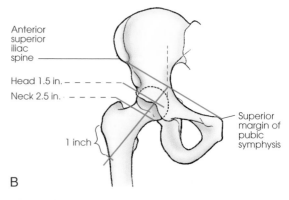

B

Fig. 7-30 A, AP hip. **B,** Localization planes of pelvis.

Structures shown

The resulting image shows the head, neck, trochanters, and proximal one third of the body of the femur (Fig. 7-31). In the initial examination of a hip lesion, whether traumatic or pathologic in origin, the AP projection is often obtained using an IR large enough to include the entire pelvic girdle and upper femora. Progress studies may be restricted to the affected side.

The following should be clearly shown:
- Evidence of proper collimation
- Femoral head, penetrated and seen through the acetabulum
- Regions of the ilium and pubic bones adjoining the pubic symphysis
- Any orthopedic appliance in its entirety
- Hip joint
- Greater trochanter in profile
- Entire long axis of the femoral neck not foreshortened
- Proximal one third of the femur

- Lesser trochanter is usually not projected beyond the medial border of the femur, or only a very small amount of the trochanter is seen.

NOTE: Trauma patients who have sustained severe injury are not usually transferred to the radiographic table but are radiographed on the stretcher or bed. After the localization point has been established and marked, one assistant should be on each side of the stretcher to grasp the sheet and lift the pelvis just enough for placement of the IR, while a third person supports the injured limb. Any necessary manipulation of the limb must be made by a physician.

Ilium
Acetabulum
Femoral head
Greater trochanter
Femoral neck
Pubic symphysis
Lesser trochanter
Femoral body

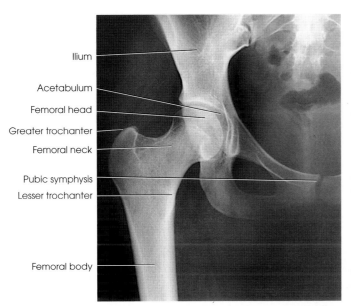 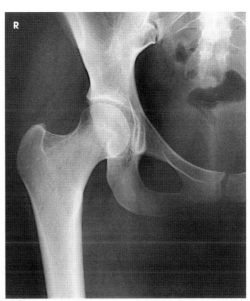

Fig. 7-31 AP hip.

✷ LATERAL PROJECTION
Mediolateral
LAUENSTEIN AND HICKEY METHODS

NOTE: This examination is contraindicated for patients with a suspected fracture or pathologic condition.

The Lauenstein and Hickey methods are used to show the hip joint and the relationship of the femoral head to the acetabulum. This position is similar to the previously described modified Cleaves method.

Image receptor: 10 × 12 inch (24 × 30 cm) crosswise

Position of patient
- From the supine position, rotate the patient slightly toward the affected side to an oblique position. The degree of obliquity depends on how much the patient can abduct the leg.

Position of part
- Adjust the patient's body, and center the affected hip to the midline of the grid.
- Ask the patient to flex the affected knee and draw the thigh up to a position at nearly a right angle to the hip bone.
- Keep the body of the affected femur parallel to the table.
- Extend the opposite limb and support it at hip level and under the knee.
- Rotate the pelvis no more than necessary to accommodate flexion of the thigh and to avoid superimposition of the affected side (Fig. 7-32).
- *Shield gonads.*
- *Respiration:* Suspend.

Central ray
- Perpendicular through the hip joint, which is located midway between ASIS and pubic symphysis for the Lauenstein method (Fig. 7-33) and at a cephalic angle of 20 to 25 degrees for the Hickey method (Fig. 7-34)
- Center the IR to the central ray.

Collimation
- Adjust to 10 × 12 inches (24 × 30 cm) on the collimator.

Structures shown
The resulting image shows a lateral projection of the hip including the acetabulum, proximal end of the femur, and relationship of the femoral head to the acetabulum (see Figs. 7-33 and 7-34).

EVALUATION CRITERIA
The following should be clearly shown:
- Evidence of proper collimation
- Hip joint centered to the radiograph
- Hip joint, acetabulum, and femoral head
- Femoral neck overlapped by the greater trochanter in the Lauenstein method
- With cephalic angulation in the Hickey method, the femoral neck free of superimposition

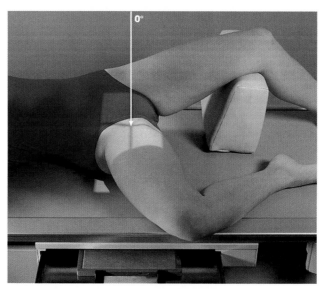

Fig. 7-32 Mediolateral hip: Lauenstein method.

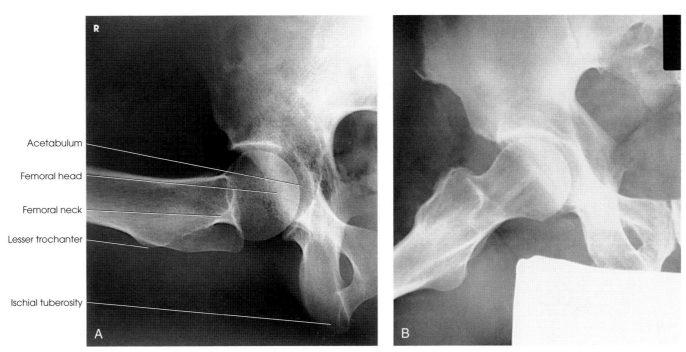

Acetabulum

Femoral head

Femoral neck

Lesser trochanter

Ischial tuberosity

Fig. 7-33 A, Mediolateral hip with perpendicular central ray: Lauenstein method. **B,** Mediolateral hip with perpendicular central ray using male gonad (contact) shield.

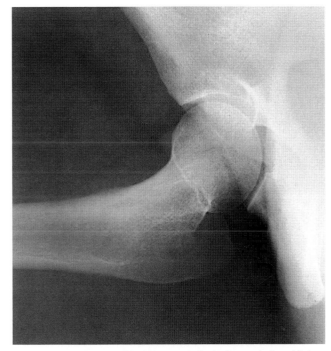

Fig. 7-34 Mediolateral hip with 20-degree cephalad angulation: Hickey method.

⚜ AXIOLATERAL PROJECTION
DANELIUS-MILLER METHOD

This projection is often called the *cross-table* or *surgical-lateral* projection.

Image receptor: 10 × 12 inch (24 × 30 cm) lengthwise or 10 × 12 inch (25 × 30 cm) grid cassette

Position of patient
- Place the patient in the supine position.

Position of part
- When examining a patient who is thin or who is lying on a soft bed, elevate the pelvis on a firm pillow or folded sheets sufficiently to center the most prominent point of the greater trochanter to the midline of the IR. The support must not extend beyond the lateral surface of the body; otherwise, it would interfere with the placement of the IR.
- When the pelvis is elevated, support the affected limb at hip level on sandbags or firm pillows.

- Flex the knee and hip of the unaffected side to elevate the thigh in a vertical position.
- Rest the unaffected leg on a suitable support that does not interfere with the central ray. Special support devices are available. *Do not rest the foot on the x-ray tube or collimator.*
- Adjust the pelvis so that it is not rotated (Figs. 7-35 and 7-36).
- Unless contraindicated, grasp the heel and medially rotate the foot and lower limb of the affected side about 15 or 20 degrees. A sandbag may be used to hold the leg and foot in this position, and a small support can be placed under the knee. The manipulation of patients with unhealed fractures should be performed by a physician.

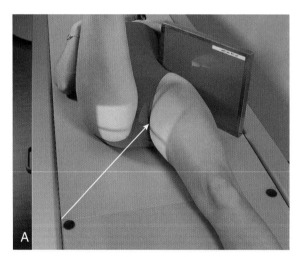

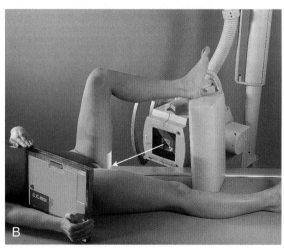

Fig. 7-35 A, Axiolateral hip: Danelius-Miller method, IR supported with sandbags. **B,** Same projection, patient holding IR. Foot is on a footrest.

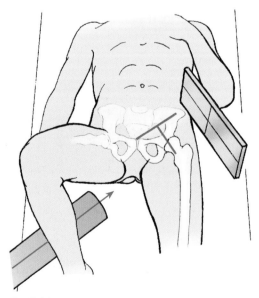

Fig. 7-36 Axiolateral hip: Danelius-Miller method.

Position of IR

- Place the IR in the vertical position with its upper border in the crease above the iliac crest.
- Angle the lower border away from the body until the IR is exactly parallel with the long axis of the femoral neck.
- Support the IR in this position with sandbags or a vertical IR holder. These are the preferred methods. Alternatively, the patient may support the IR with the hand.
- Be careful to position the grid so that the lead strips are in the horizontal position.
- *Shield gonads.*
- *Respiration:* Suspend.

Central ray

- Perpendicular to the long axis of the femoral neck. The central ray enters at the mid-thigh and passes through the femoral neck about 2½ inches (6.4 cm) below the point of intersection of the localization lines described previously (see Fig. 7-12).

Collimation

- Adjust to 10 × 12 inches (24 × 30 cm) on the collimator.

◤ COMPENSATING FILTER

This projection is improved dramatically and can be performed with one exposure with the use of a specially designed compensating filter (see Fig. 2-9 in Chapter 2).

Structures shown

The resulting image shows the acetabulum, head, neck, and trochanters of the femur (Fig. 7-37).

EVALUATION CRITERIA

The following should be clearly shown:
- Femoral neck without overlap from the greater trochanter
- Small amount of the lesser trochanter on the posterior surface of the femur
- Small amount of the greater trochanter on the anterior and posterior surfaces of the proximal femur when the femur is properly inverted
- Soft tissue shadow of the unaffected thigh not overlapping the hip joint or proximal femur
- Hip joint with the acetabulum
- Any orthopedic appliance in its entirety
- Ischial tuberosity below the femoral head

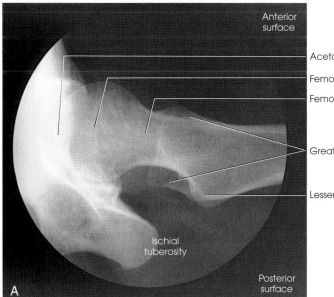

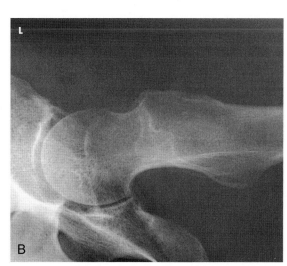

Fig. 7-37 A, Axiolateral hip: Danelius-Miller method. **B,** Same projection with use of compensating filter. Note excellent detail of acetabular area and femur.

MODIFIED AXIOLATERAL PROJECTION
CLEMENTS-NAKAYAMA MODIFICATION

When the patient has bilateral hip fractures, bilateral hip arthroplasty (plastic surgery of the hip joints), or limitation of movement of the unaffected leg, the Danelius-Miller method cannot be used. Clements and Nakayama[1] described a modification using a 15-degree posterior angulation of the central ray (Fig. 7-38).

---

[1]Clements RS, Nakayama HK: Radiographic methods in total hip arthroplasty, *Radiol Technol* 51:589, 1980.

Image receptor: 10 × 12 inch (24 × 30 cm) lengthwise or 10 × 12 inch (25 × 30 cm) grid cassette

Position of patient
- Position the patient supine on the radiographic table with the affected side near the edge of the table.

Position of part
- For this position, do not rotate the lower limb internally. Instead, the limb remains in a neutral or slightly externally rotated position.
- Support a grid IR on the Bucky tray so that its lower margin is below the patient. Position the grid so that the lines run parallel with the floor.
- Adjust the grid parallel to the axis of the femoral neck, and tilt its top back 15 degrees.
- *Shield gonads.*
- *Respiration:* Suspend.

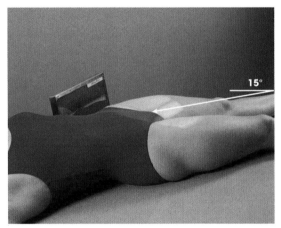

Fig. 7-38 Axiolateral hip: Clements-Nakayama method.

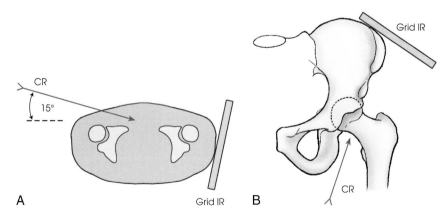

Fig. 7-39 Central ray (*CR*) angles for Clements-Nakayama method. **A,** 15 degrees posteriorly. Note grid IR tilted 15 degrees. **B,** Perpendicular to femoral neck and grid IR.

Central ray

• Directed 15 degrees posteriorly and aligned perpendicular to the femoral neck and grid IR (Fig. 7-39)

Structures shown

This leg position shows a lateral hip image because the central ray is angled 15 degrees posterior instead of the toes being medially rotated. The resulting image shows the acetabulum and the proximal femur including the head, neck, and trochanters in lateral profile. The Clements-Nakayama modification (Fig. 7-40) can be compared with the Danelius-Miller approach described previously (Fig. 7-41).

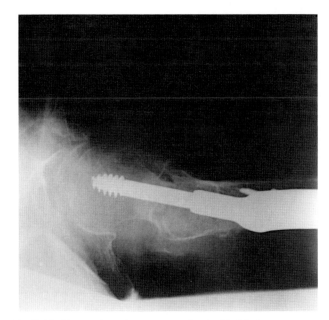

Fig. 7-40 Clements-Nakayama method with 15-degree central ray angulation in same patient as in Fig. 7-41.

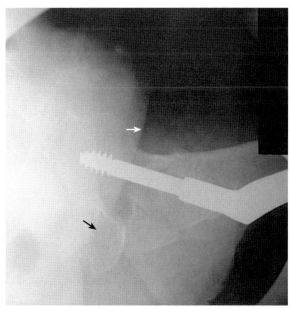

Fig. 7-41 Postoperative Danelius-Miller method used for a patient who was unable to flex unaffected hip. Contralateral thigh (arrows) is obscuring femoral head and acetabular area.

PA AXIAL OBLIQUE PROJECTION
TEUFEL METHOD
RAO or LAO position

Image receptor: 8 × 10 inch (18 × 24 cm) lengthwise

Position of patient
- Have the patient lie in a semiprone position on the affected side.

Position of part
- Align the body, and center the hip being examined to the midline of the grid.
- Elevate the unaffected side so that the anterior surface of the body forms a 38-degree angle from the table (Fig. 7-42).

- Have the patient support the body on the forearm and flexed knee of the elevated side.
- With the IR in the Bucky tray, adjust the position of the IR so that its midpoint coincides with the central ray.
- *Shield gonads.*
- *Respiration:* Suspend.

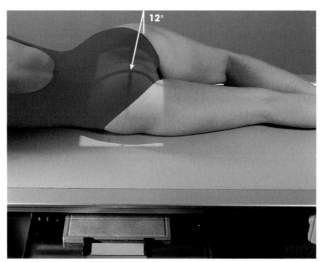

Fig. 7-42 PA axial oblique acetabulum: Teufel method.

Central ray

- Directed through the acetabulum at an angle of 12 degrees cephalad. The central ray enters the body at the inferior level of the coccyx and approximately 2 inches (5 cm) lateral to the midsagittal plane toward the side being examined.

Structures shown

The resulting image shows the fovea capitis and particularly the superoposterior wall of the acetabulum (Fig. 7-43).

The following should be clearly shown:

- Hip joint and acetabulum near the center of the radiograph
- Femoral head in profile to show the concave area of the fovea capitis
- Superoposterior wall of the acetabulum

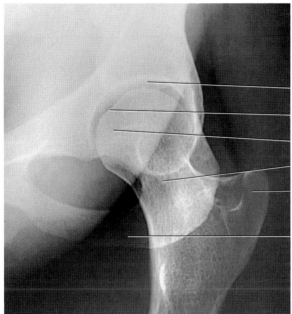 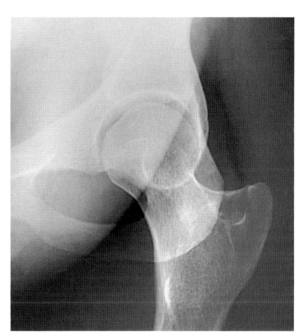

Acetabulum

Fovea capitis

Femoral head

Femoral neck

Greater trochanter

Ischium

Fig. 7-43 PA axial oblique acetabulum: Teufel method.

AP OBLIQUE PROJECTION
JUDET METHOD[1]
MODIFIED JUDET METHOD[2]
RPO or LPO position

Judet et al.[1] described two 45-degree posterior oblique positions that are useful in diagnosing fractures of the acetabulum: the internal oblique position (affected side up) and the external oblique position (affected side down).

Image receptor: 10 × 12 inch (24 × 30 cm) lengthwise

Internal oblique

The internal oblique position is for a patient with a suspected fracture of the *iliopubic column* (anterior) and the posterior rim of the acetabulum.

---

[1]Judet R et al: Fractures of the acetabulum: classification and surgical approaches for open reduction, *J Bone Joint Surg Am* 46:1615, 1964.

[2]Rafert JA, Long BW: Showing acetabular trauma with more clarity, less pain, *Radiol Technol* 63:93, 1991.

NOTE: *Iliopubic column* (anterior)—composed of a short segment of the ilium and the pubis; extends up as far as the anterior spine of the ilium and extends from the symphysis pubis and obturator foramen through acetabulum to ASIS.

Position of patient
- Place the patient in a semisupine position with the affected hip *up*.

Position of part
- Align the body, and center the hip being examined to the middle of the IR.
- Elevate the affected side so that the anterior surface of the body forms a 45-degree angle from the table (Fig. 7-44, *A*).
- *Shield gonads.*
- *Respiration:* Suspend.

Central ray
- Perpendicular to the IR and entering 2 inches (5 cm) inferior to ASIS of the affected side

External oblique

The external oblique is for a patient with a suspected fracture of the *ilioischial column* (posterior) and the anterior rim of the acetabulum.

Position of patient
- Place the patient in a semisupine position with the affected hip *down*.

Position of part
- Align the body, and center the hip being examined to the middle of the IR.
- Elevate the affected side so that the anterior surface of the body forms a 45-degree angle from the table (Fig. 7-44, *B*).
- *Shield gonads.*
- *Respiration:* Suspend.

Central ray
- Perpendicular to the IR and entering at the pubic symphysis

Collimation
- Adjust to 10 × 12 inches (24 × 30 cm) on the collimator.

Structures shown

The resulting image shows the acetabular rim (Fig. 7-45).

NOTE: *Ilioischial column* (posterior)—composed of the vertical portion of the ischium and the portion of the ilium immediately above the ischium and extends from the obturator foramen through the posterior aspect of the acetabulum.

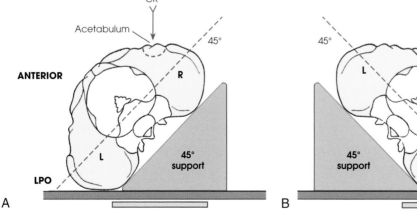

Fig. 7-44 AP oblique projection, Judet method for right hip. **A,** LPO places right hip in *internal* oblique position. **B,** RPO places right hip in *external* oblique position.

Acetabulum

EVALUATION CRITERIA

The following should be clearly shown:

- Evidence of proper collimation
- Acetabulum centered to the IR
- The iliopubic column and the posterior rim of the affected acetabulum on the internal oblique
- The ilioischial column and the anterior rim of the acetabulum on the external oblique

NOTE: Rafert and Long[1] described a modification of the Judet method on trauma patients. The patient is not required to lie on the affected side for the external oblique (Fig. 7-46).

RESEARCH: Catherine E. Hearty, MS, RT(R), performed the research and provided this new projection for this edition of the atlas.

---

[1]Rafert JA, Long BW: Showing acetabular trauma with more clarity, less pain, *Radiol Technol* 63:93, 1991.

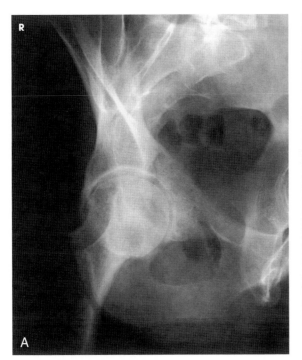
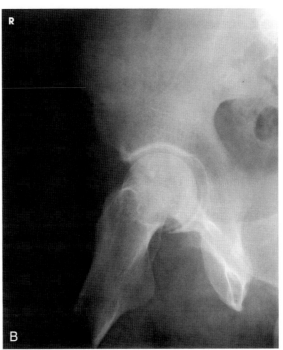

Fig. 7-45 AP oblique projection, Judet method, right hip. **A,** LPO. **B,** RPO.

(From Long BW, Rafert JA: *Orthopedic radiography,* Philadelphia, 1995, Saunders.)

Fig. 7-46 AP oblique projection, *modified Judet method* for right hip on a trauma patient. *External* oblique projection is obtained using cross-table central ray (*CR*) and grid IR. *Internal oblique* is obtained on a trauma patient in same position using vertical CR (same as Fig. 7-44, A).

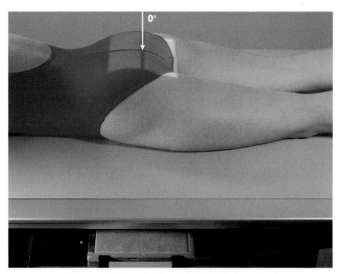

Fig. 7-47 PA pelvic bones.

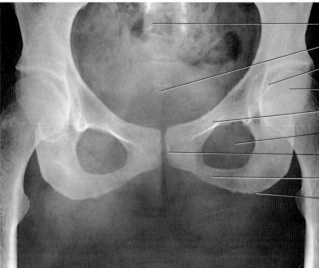

Sacrum
Coccyx
Acetabulum
Femoral head
Superior pubic ramus
Obturator foramen
Pubic symphysis
Inferior pubic ramus
Ischial tuberosity

PA PROJECTION

Image receptor: 8 × 10 inch (18 × 24 cm) crosswise

Position of patient
- Place the patient in the prone position, and center the midsagittal plane of the body to the midline of the grid.

Position of part
- With the IR in the Bucky tray, center the IR at the level of the greater trochanters. This positioning also centers the IR to the pubic symphysis (Fig. 7-47).
- *Shield gonads.*
- *Respiration:* Suspend.

Central ray
- Perpendicular to the midpoint of the IR. The central ray enters the distal coccyx and exits the pubic symphysis.

Structures shown
This image shows a PA projection of the pubic symphysis and ischia including the obturator foramina (Fig. 7-48).

EVALUATION CRITERIA
The following should be clearly shown:
- Pubic and ischial bones not magnified or superimposing the sacrum or coccyx
- Pubic and ischial bones near the center of the radiograph
- Hip joints
- Symmetric obturator foramina

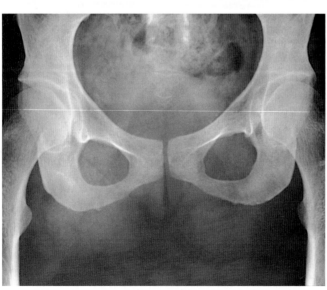

Fig. 7-48 PA pelvic bones.

Pelvis and Upper Femora

AP AXIAL OUTLET PROJECTION
TAYLOR METHOD[1]

Image receptor: 24 × 30 inch (24 × 30 cm) crosswise

Position of patient
- Place the patient in the supine position.

Position of part
- Center the midsagittal plane of the patient's body to the midline of the grid, and adjust the pelvis so that it is not rotated. ASIS should be equidistant from the table (Fig. 7-49).
- Flex the knees slightly with a support underneath if the patient is uncomfortable.
- With the IR in the Bucky tray, adjust the tray's position so that the midpoint of the IR coincides with the central ray.
- *Shield gonads.*
- *Respiration:* Suspend.

Central ray
Men
- Directed 20 to 35 degrees cephalad and centered to a point 2 inches (5 cm) distal to the superior border of the pubic symphysis

Women
- Directed 30 to 45 degrees cephalad and centered to a point 2 inches (5 cm) distal to the superior border of the pubic symphysis

Structures shown
The resulting image shows the superior and inferior rami without the foreshortening seen in a PA or AP projection owing to the central ray being more perpendicular to the rami (Figs. 7-50 and 7-51).

EVALUATION CRITERIA
The following should be clearly shown:
- Pubic and ischial bones magnified with pubic bones superimposed over the sacrum and coccyx
- Symmetric obturator foramina
- Pubic and ischial rami near the center of the radiograph
- Hip joints

[1]Taylor R: Modified anteroposterior projection of the anterior bones of the pelvis, *Radiog Clin Photog* 17:67, 1941.

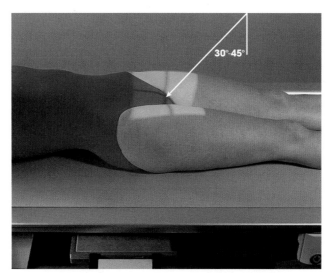

Fig. 7-49 AP axial pelvic bones: Taylor method.

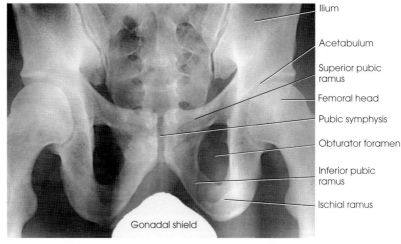

Ilium
Acetabulum
Superior pubic ramus
Femoral head
Pubic symphysis
Obturator foramen
Inferior pubic ramus
Ischial ramus
Gonadal shield

Fig. 7-50 Male AP axial pelvic bones: Taylor method.

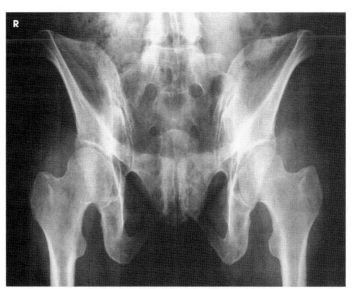

Fig. 7-51 Female AP axial pelvic bones: Taylor method.

SUPEROINFERIOR AXIAL INLET PROJECTION
BRIDGEMAN METHOD[1]

Image receptor: 8 × 10 inch (18 × 24 cm) crosswise

[1]Bridgeman CF: Radiography of the hip bone, *Med Radiog Photog* 28:41, 1952.

Position of patient
• Place the patient on the radiographic table in the supine position.

Position of part
• Center the midsagittal plane of the patient's body to the midline of the grid.
• Flex the knees slightly and support them to relieve strain.
• Adjust the pelvis so that ASIS are equidistant from the table.
• With the IR in the Bucky tray, center it at the level of the greater trochanters (Fig. 7-52).
• *Shield gonads.*
• *Respiration:* Suspend.

Central ray
• Directed 40 degrees caudad, entering at the level of ASIS

Structures shown
The resulting image shows an axial projection of the pelvic ring, or inlet, in its entirety (Fig. 7-53).

EVALUATION CRITERIA
The following should be clearly shown:
■ Medially superimposed superior and inferior rami of the pubic bones
■ Nearly superimposed lateral two thirds of the pubic and ischial bones
■ Symmetric pubes and ischial spines
■ Hip joints
■ Anterior pelvic bones

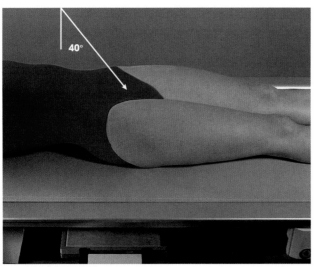

Fig. 7-52 AP axial pelvic bones: Bridgeman method.

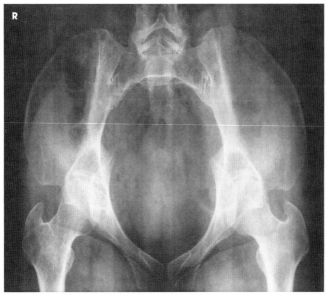

Fig. 7-53 AP axial inlet projection.

AP AND PA OBLIQUE PROJECTIONS

Image receptor: 10 × 12 inch (24 × 30 cm) lengthwise

RPO and LPO positions
Position of patient
- Place the patient in the supine position.

Position of part
- Center the sagittal plane passing through the hip joint of the affected side to the midline of the grid.
- Elevate the unaffected side approximately 40 degrees to place the broad surface of the wing of the affected ilium parallel with the plane of the IR.
- Support the elevated shoulder, hip, and knee on sandbags.
- Adjust the position of the uppermost limb to place ASIS in the same transverse plane (Fig. 7-54).
- Center the IR at the level of ASIS.

- *Shield gonads.*
- *Respiration:* Suspend.

RAO and LAO positions

Position of patient
- Place the patient in the prone position.

Position of part
- Center the sagittal plane passing through the hip joint of the affected side to the midline of the grid.
- Elevate the unaffected side about 40 degrees to place the affected ilium perpendicular to the plane of the IR.
- Have the patient rest on the forearm and flexed knee of the elevated side.
- Adjust the position of the uppermost thigh to place the iliac crests in the same horizontal plane.
- Center the IR at the level of ASIS (Fig. 7-55).
- *Shield gonads.*
- *Respiration:* Suspend.

Central ray
- Perpendicular to the midpoint of the IR

Structures shown
AP oblique image shows an unobstructed projection of the ala and sciatic notches and a profile image of the acetabulum (Fig. 7-56). PA oblique image shows the ilium in profile and the femoral head within the acetabulum (Fig. 7-57).

EVALUATION CRITERIA
The following should be clearly shown:
- Entire ilium
- Hip joint, proximal femur, and SI joint
  AP oblique projection
- Broad surface of the iliac wing without rotation
  PA oblique projection
- Ilium in profile

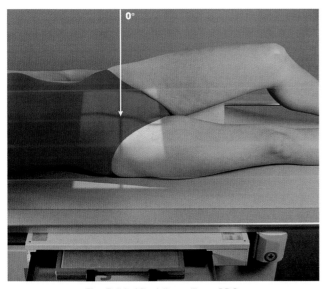

Fig. 7-54 AP oblique ilium, RPO.

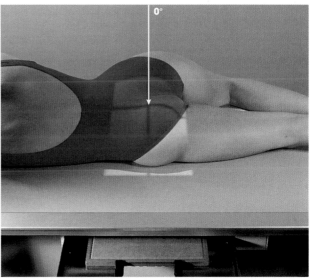

Fig. 7-55 PA oblique ilium, LAO.

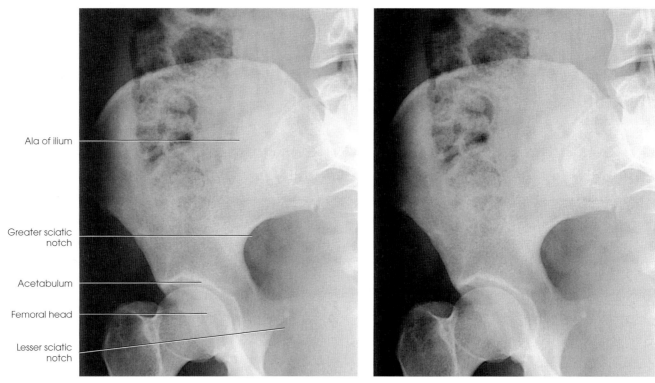

Ala of ilium

Greater sciatic notch

Acetabulum

Femoral head

Lesser sciatic notch

Fig. 7-56 AP oblique ilium, RPO.

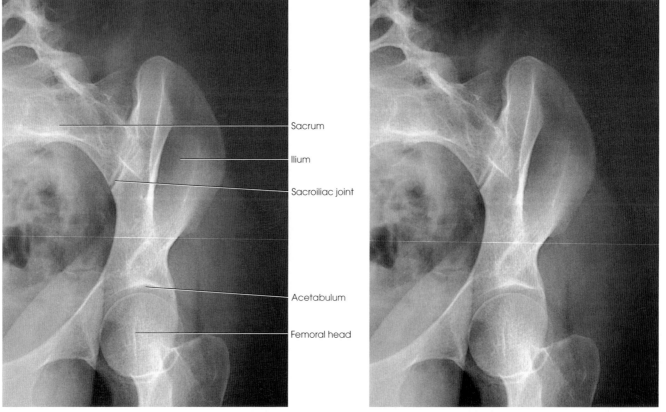

Sacrum

Ilium

Sacroiliac joint

Acetabulum

Femoral head

Fig. 7-57 PA oblique ilium, LAO.

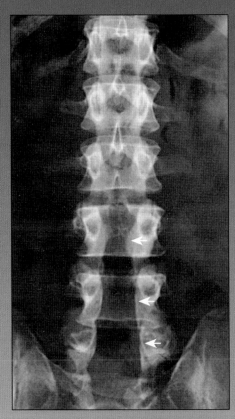

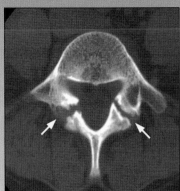

8
VERTEBRAL COLUMN

PROJECTIONS, POSITIONS, AND METHODS

Page	Essential	Anatomy	Projection	Position	Method
382	✦	Dens	AP		FUCHS
383	✦	Atlas and axis	AP	Open mouth	
385		Atlas and axis	Lateral	R or L	
386	✦	Cervical vertebrae	AP axial		
388	✦	Cervical vertebrae	Lateral	R or L	GRANDY
390	✦	Cervical vertebrae	Lateral	R or L hyperflexion and hyperextension	
392	✦	Cervical intervertebral foramina	AP axial oblique	RPO and LPO	
393		Cervical intervertebral foramina	AP oblique	Hyperflexion and hyperextension	
394	✦	Cervical intervertebral foramina	PA axial oblique	RAO and LAO	
396		Cervical vertebrae	AP		OTTONELLO
398		Cervical and upper thoracic vertebrae: *vertebral arch (pillars)*	AP axial		
400		Cervical and upper thoracic vertebrae: *vertebral arch (pillars)*	AP axial oblique	R and L head rotations	
401	✦	Cervicothoracic region	Lateral	R or L	SWIMMER'S TECHNIQUE
403	✦	Thoracic vertebrae	AP		
406	✦	Thoracic vertebrae	Lateral	R or L	
409		Zygapophyseal joints	AP, PA oblique	RAO and LAO, RPO and LPO	

Icons in the Essential column indicate projections that are frequently performed in the United States and Canada. Students should be competent in these projections.

Page	Essential	Anatomy	Projection	Position	Method
412	⚜	Lumbar-lumbosacral vertebrae	AP		
412		Lumbar-lumbosacral vertebrae	PA		
416	⚜	Lumbar-lumbosacral vertebrae	Lateral	R or L	
418	⚜	L5-S1 lumbosacral junction	Lateral	R or L	
420	⚜	Zygapophyseal joints	AP oblique	RPO and LPO	
422		Zygapophyseal joints	PA oblique	RAO and LAO	
424	⚜	Lumbosacral junction and sacroiliac joints	AP, PA axial		FERGUSON
426	⚜	Sacroiliac joints	AP oblique	RPO and LPO	
428		Sacroiliac joints	PA oblique	RAO and LAO	
430	⚜	Sacrum and coccyx	AP, PA axial		
432	⚜	Sacrum and coccyx	Lateral	R or L	
434		Lumbar intervertebral disks	PA	R and L bending	WEIGHT-BEARING
436	⚜	Thoracolumbar spine: scoliosis	PA, lateral		FRANK ET AL.
438	⚜	Thoracolumbar spine: scoliosis	PA		FERGUSON
440		Lumbar spine: spinal fusion	AP	R and L bending	
442		Lumbar spine: spinal fusion	Lateral	R or L hyperflexion and hyperextension	

Vertebral Column

The *vertebral column,* or *spine,* forms the central axis of the skeleton and is centered in the midsagittal plane of the posterior part of the trunk. The vertebral column has many functions: It encloses and protects the spinal cord, acts as a support for the trunk, supports the skull superiorly, and provides for attachment for the deep muscles of the back and the ribs laterally. The upper limbs are supported indirectly via the ribs, which articulate with the sternum. The sternum articulates with the shoulder girdle. The vertebral column articulates with each hip bone at the sacroiliac joints. This articulation supports the vertebral column and transmits the weight of the trunk through the hip joints and to the lower limbs.

The vertebral column is composed of small segments of bone called *vertebrae.* Disks of fibrocartilage are interposed between the vertebrae and act as cushions. The vertebral column is held together by ligaments, and it is jointed and curved so that it has considerable flexibility and resilience.

In early life, the vertebral column usually consists of 33 small, irregularly shaped bones. These bones are divided into five groups and named according to the region they occupy (Fig. 8-1). The superiormost seven vertebrae occupy the region of the neck and are termed *cervical vertebrae.* The succeeding 12 bones lie in the dorsal, or posterior, portion of the thorax and are called the *thoracic vertebrae.*

The five vertebrae occupying the region of the loin are termed *lumbar vertebrae.* The next five vertebrae, located in the pelvic region, are termed *sacral vertebrae.* The terminal vertebrae, also in the pelvic region, vary from three to five in number in adults and are termed the *coccygeal vertebrae.*

The 24 vertebral segments in the upper three regions remain distinct throughout life and are termed the *true* or movable vertebrae. The pelvic segments in the two lower regions are called *false* or fixed vertebrae because of the change they undergo in adults. The sacral segments usually fuse into one bone called the *sacrum,* and the coccygeal segments, referred to as the *coccyx,* also fuse into one bone.

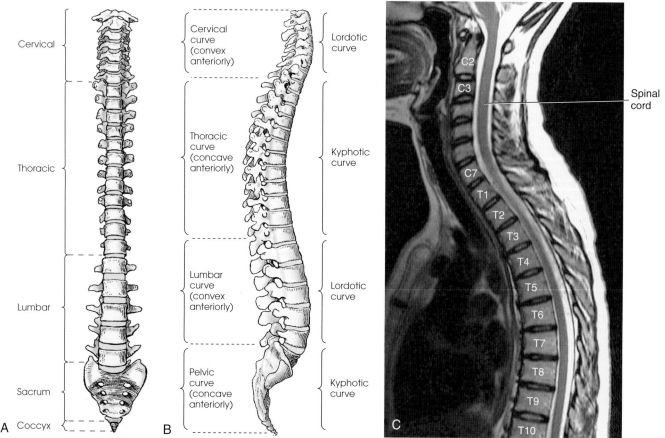

Fig. 8-1 A, Anterior aspect of vertebral column. **B,** Lateral aspect of vertebral column, showing regions and curvatures. **C,** Midsagittal MRI scan of cervical and thoracic spine. Note curves and spinal cord protected by vertebrae.

Vertebral Curvature

Viewed from the side, the vertebral column has four curves that arch anteriorly and posteriorly from the midcoronal plane of the body. The *cervical, thoracic, lumbar,* and *pelvic* curves are named for the regions they occupy.

In this text, the vertebral curves are discussed in reference to the *anatomic position* and are referred to as "convex anteriorly" or "concave anteriorly." Because physicians and surgeons evaluate the spine from the posterior aspect of the body, *convex* and *concave* terminology can be the exact opposites. When viewed posteriorly, the normal lumbar curve can correctly be referred to as "concave posteriorly." Whether the curve is described as "convex anteriorly" or "concave posteriorly," the curvature of the patient's spine is the same. The cervical and lumbar curves, which are convex anteriorly, are called *lordotic* curves. The thoracic and pelvic curves are concave anteriorly and are called *kyphotic* curves (see Fig. 8-1, *B*).

The cervical and thoracic curves merge smoothly.

The lumbar and pelvic curves join at an obtuse angle termed the *lumbosacral angle*. The acuity of the angle in the junction of these curves varies among patients. The thoracic and pelvic curves are called *primary curves* because they are present at birth. The cervical and lumbar curves are called *secondary* or *compensatory curves* because they develop after birth. The cervical curve, which is the least pronounced of the curves, develops when an infant begins to hold the head up at about 3 or 4 months of age and begins to sit alone at about 8 or 9 months of age. The lumbar curve develops when the child begins to walk at about 1 to 1½ years of age. The lumbar and pelvic curves are more pronounced in females, who have a more acute angle at the lumbosacral junction.

Any abnormal increase in the anterior concavity (or posterior convexity) of the thoracic curve is termed *kyphosis* (Fig.

8-2, *B*). Any abnormal increase in the anterior convexity (or posterior concavity) of the lumbar or cervical curve is termed *lordosis*.

In frontal view, the vertebral column varies in width in several regions (see Fig. 8-1). Generally, the width of the spine gradually increases from the second cervical vertebra to the superior part of the sacrum and then decreases sharply. A *slight* lateral curvature is sometimes present in the upper thoracic region. The curve is to the right in right-handed persons and to the left in left-handed persons. For this reason, lateral curvature of the vertebral column is believed to be the result of muscle action and to be influenced by occupation. An abnormal lateral curvature of the spine is called *scoliosis*. This condition also causes the vertebrae to rotate toward the concavity. The vertebral column develops a second or compensatory curve in the opposite direction to keep the head centered over the feet (see Fig. 8-2, *A*).

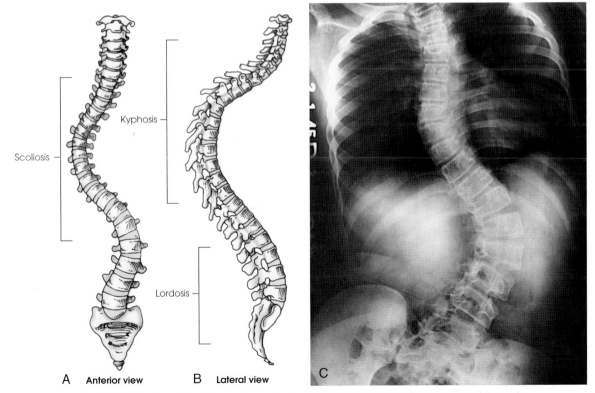

Fig. 8-2 **A,** Scoliosis, lateral curvature of spine. **B,** Kyphosis, increased convexity of thoracic spine, and lordosis, increased concavity of lumbar spine. **C,** PA thoracic and lumbar spine showing severe scoliosis.

Typical Vertebra

A typical vertebra is composed of two main parts—an anterior mass of bone called the *body* and a posterior ringlike portion called the *vertebral arch* (Figs. 8-3 and 8-4). The vertebral body and arch enclose a space called the *vertebral foramen*. In the articulated column, the vertebral foramina form the *vertebral canal.*

The body of the vertebra is approximately cylindric in shape and is composed largely of cancellous bony tissue covered by a layer of compact tissue. From the superior aspect, the posterior surface is flattened, and from the lateral aspect, the anterior and lateral surfaces are concave. The superior and inferior surfaces of the bodies are flattened and covered by a thin plate of *articular cartilage.*

In the articulated spine, the vertebral bodies are separated by *intervertebral disks.* These disks account for approximately one fourth of the length of the vertebral column. Each disk has a central mass of soft, pulpy, semigelatinous material called the *nucleus pulposus,* which is surrounded by an outer fibrocartilaginous disk called the *anulus fibrosus.* It is common for the pulpy nucleus to rupture or protrude into the vertebral canal, impinging on a spinal nerve. This condition is called *herniated nucleus pulposus* (HNP), or more commonly *slipped disk.* HNP most often occurs in the lumbar region as a result of improper body mechanics, and it can cause considerable discomfort and pain. HNP also occurs in the cervical spine as a result of trauma (i.e., whiplash injuries) or degeneration.

The vertebral arch (see Figs. 8-3 and 8-4) is formed by two *pedicles* and two *laminae* that support four articular processes, two transverse processes, and one spinous process. The pedicles are short, thick processes that project posteriorly, one from each side, from the superior and lateral parts of the posterior surface of the vertebral body. The superior and inferior surfaces of the pedicles, or roots, are concave. These concavities are called *vertebral notches.* By articulation with the vertebrae above and below, the notches form *intervertebral foramina* for the transmission of spinal nerves and blood vessels. The broad, flat *laminae* are directed posteriorly and medially from the pedicles.

The *transverse processes* project laterally and slightly posteriorly from the junction of the pedicles and laminae. The *spinous process* projects posteriorly and inferiorly from the junction of the laminae in the posterior midline. A congenital defect of the vertebral column in which the laminae fail to unite posteriorly at the midline is called *spina bifida.* In serious cases of spina bifida, the spinal cord may protrude from the affected individual's body.

Four articular processes, two superior and two inferior, arise from the junction of the pedicles and laminae to articulate with the vertebrae above and below (see Fig. 8-4). The articulating surfaces of the four articular processes are covered with fibrocartilage and are called *facets.* In a typical vertebra, each *superior articular process* has an articular facet on its posterior surface, and each *inferior articular process* has an articular facet on the anterior surface. The planes of the facets vary in direction in the different regions of the vertebral column and often vary within the same vertebra. The articulations between the articular processes of the vertebral arches are referred to as *zygapophyseal joints.* Some texts refer to these joints as *interarticular facet joints.*

The movable vertebrae, with the exception of the first and second cervical vertebrae, are similar in general structure. Each group has certain distinguishing characteristics, however, that must be considered in radiography of the vertebral column.

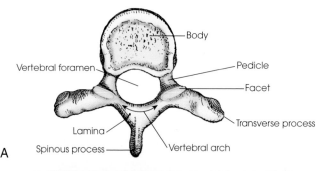

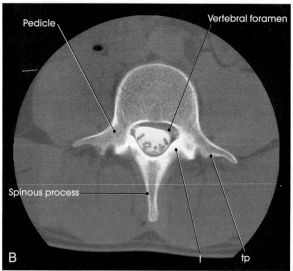

Fig. 8-3 A, Superior aspect of thoracic vertebra, showing structures common to all vertebral regions. **B,** Axial CT image of lumbar vertebra showing most of anatomy identified in **A**. Note spinal cord (*white*) within vertebral foramen. *l,* lamina; *tp,* transverse process.

(**B,** Modified from Kelley LL, Petersen CM: *Sectional anatomy for imaging professionals,* ed 2, St Louis, 2007, Mosby.)

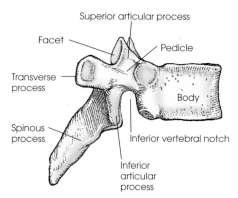

Fig. 8-4 Lateral aspect of thoracic vertebra, showing structures common to all vertebral regions.

Cervical Vertebrae

The first two cervical vertebrae are atypical in that they are structurally modified to join the skull. The seventh vertebra is also atypical and slightly modified to join the thoracic spine. Atypical and typical vertebrae are described in the following sections.

ATLAS

The *atlas,* the first cervical vertebra (C1), is a ringlike structure with no body and a very short spinous process (Fig. 8-5). The atlas consists of an *anterior arch,* a *posterior arch,* two *lateral masses,* and two transverse processes. The anterior and posterior arches extend between the lateral masses. The ring formed by the arches is divided into anterior and posterior portions by a ligament called the *transverse atlantal ligament.* The anterior portion of the ring receives the dens (odontoid process) of the axis, and the posterior portion transmits the proximal spinal cord.

The transverse processes of the atlas are longer than those of the other cervical vertebrae, and they project laterally and slightly inferiorly from the lateral masses. Each lateral mass bears a superior and an inferior articular process. The superior processes lie in a horizontal plane, are large and deeply concave, and are shaped to articulate with the occipital condyles of the occipital bone of the cranium.

AXIS

The *axis,* the second cervical vertebra (C2) (Figs. 8-6 and 8-7), has a strong conical process arising from the upper surface of its body. This process, called the *dens* or *odontoid process,* is received into the anterior portion of the atlantal ring to act as the pivot or body for the atlas. At each side of the dens on the superior surface of the vertebral body are the superior articular processes, which are adapted to join with the inferior articular processes of the atlas. These joints, which differ in position and direction from the other cervical zygapophyseal joints, are clearly visualized in an AP projection if the patient is properly positioned. The inferior articular processes of the axis have the same direction as the processes of the succeeding cervical vertebrae. The laminae of the axis are broad and thick. The spinous process is horizontal in position. Fig. 8-8 shows the relationship of C1 and C2 with the occipital condyles.

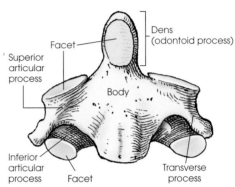

Fig. 8-6 Anterior aspect of axis (C2).

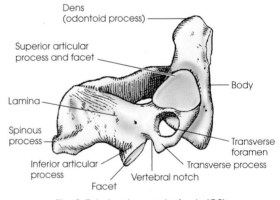

Fig. 8-7 Lateral aspect of axis (C2).

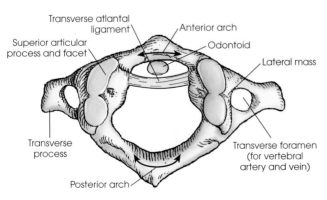

Fig. 8-5 Superior aspect of atlas (C1).

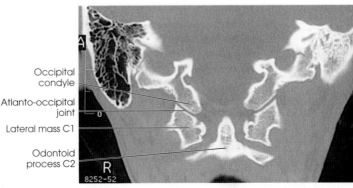

Fig. 8-8 Coronal MRI shows atlas, axis, and occipital bone of skull and their relationship.

(Courtesy Siemens Medical Systems, Iselin, NJ.)

SEVENTH VERTEBRA

The seventh cervical vertebra (C7), termed the *vertebra prominens,* has a long, prominent spinous process that projects almost horizontally to the posterior. The spinous process of this vertebra is easily palpable at the posterior base of the neck. It is convenient to use this process as a guide in localizing other vertebrae.

TYPICAL CERVICAL VERTEBRA

The *typical cervical vertebrae* (C3-6) have a small, transversely located, oblong body with slightly elongated anteroinferior borders (Fig. 8-9). The result is anteroposterior overlapping of the bodies in the articulated column. The transverse processes of the typical cervical vertebra arise partly from the sides of the body and partly from the vertebral arch. These processes are short and wide, are perforated by the *transverse foramina* for the transmission of the vertebral artery and vein, and present a deep concavity on their upper surfaces for the passage of the spinal nerves. All cervical vertebrae contain three foramina: the right and left transverse foramina and the vertebral foramen.

The pedicles of the typical cervical vertebra project laterally and posteriorly from the body, and their superior and inferior vertebral notches are nearly equal in depth. The laminae are narrow and thin. The spinous processes are short, have double pointed (bifid) tips, and are directed posteriorly and slightly inferiorly. Their palpable tips lie at the level of the interspace below the body of the vertebra from which they arise.

The superior and inferior articular processes are located posterior to the transverse processes at the point where the pedicles and laminae unite. Together the processes form short, thick columns of bone called *articular pillars.* The fibrocartilaginous articulating surfaces of the articular pillars contain facets. The zygapophyseal facet joints of the second through seventh cervical vertebrae lie at right angles to the midsagittal plane and are clearly shown in a lateral projection (Fig. 8-10, *A*).

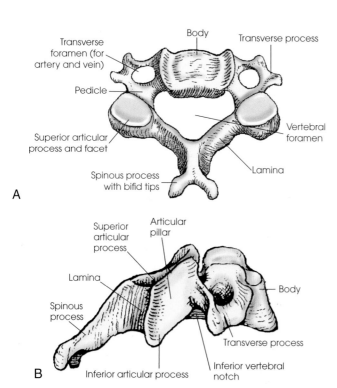

Fig. 8-9 A, Superior aspect of typical cervical vertebra. **B,** Lateral aspect of typical cervical vertebra.

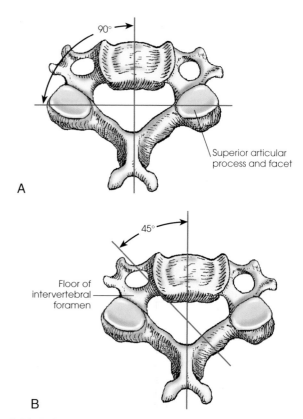

Fig. 8-10 A, Direction of cervical zygapophyseal joints. **B,** Direction of cervical intervertebral foramina.

The intervertebral foramina of the cervical region are directed anteriorly at a 45-degree angle from the midsagittal plane of the body (Fig. 8-11; see Fig. 8-10, *B*). The foramina are also directed at a 15-degree inferior angle to the horizontal plane of the body. Accurate radiographic demonstration of these foramina requires a 15-degree longitudinal angulation of the central ray and a 45-degree medial rotation of the patient (or a 45-degree medial angulation of the central ray). A lateral projection is necessary to show the cervical zygapophyseal joints. The positioning rotations required for showing the intervertebral foramina and zygapophyseal joints of the cervical spine are summarized in Table 8-1. A full view of the cervical spine is shown in Fig. 8-12 along with surrounding tissues.

TABLE 8-1

Positioning rotations needed to show intervertebral foramina and zygapophyseal joints

Area of spine	Intervertebral foramina	Zygapophyseal joint
Cervical spine	45 degrees oblique AP side up PA side down	Lateral _90°_
Thoracic spine	Lateral _90°_	70 degrees* AP side up PA side down
Lumbar spine	Lateral _90°_	30-60 degrees* AP side down PA side up

*From the anatomic position.

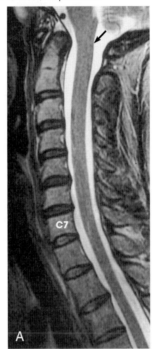

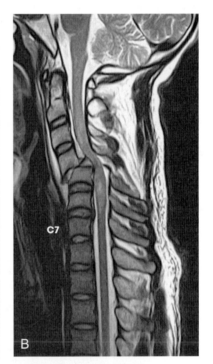

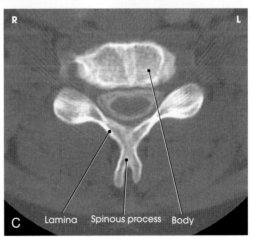

Fig. 8-12 A, MRI sagittal plane of cervical spine. Note position of spinal cord (*arrow*) in relation to vertebral bodies. **B,** MRI sagittal plane showing anterior displacement of C4 on C5. Narrowed spinal canal compresses spinal cord causing paralysis. **C,** Axial CT of typical cervical vertebra.

(**B,** Modified from Jackson SA, Thomas RM: *Cross-sectional imaging made easy,* New York, 2004, Churchill Livingstone; **C,** modified from Kelley LL, Petersen CM: *Sectional anatomy for imaging professionals,* ed 2, St Louis, 2007, Mosby.)

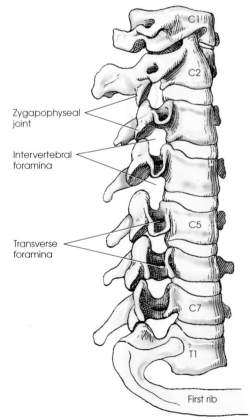

Fig. 8-11 Anterior oblique of cervical vertebrae, showing intervertebral transverse foramina and zygapophyseal joints.

Thoracic Vertebrae

The bodies of the thoracic vertebrae increase in size from the 1st to the 12th vertebrae. They also vary in form, with the superior thoracic bodies resembling cervical bodies and the inferior thoracic bodies resembling lumbar bodies. The bodies of the typical (third through ninth) thoracic vertebrae are approximately triangular in form (Figs. 8-13 and 8-14).

These vertebral bodies are deeper posteriorly than anteriorly, and their posterior surface is concave from side to side.

The posterolateral margins of each thoracic body have *costal facets* for articulation with the heads of the ribs (Fig. 8-15). The body of the first thoracic vertebra presents a whole costal facet near its superior border for articulation with the head of the first rib and presents a *demifacet*

(half-facet) on its inferior border for articulation with the head of the second rib. The bodies of the second through eighth thoracic vertebrae contain demifacets superiorly and inferiorly. The ninth thoracic vertebra has only a superior demifacet. Finally, the 10th, 11th, and 12th thoracic vertebral bodies have a single whole facet at the superior margin for articulation with the 11th and 12th ribs (Table 8-2).

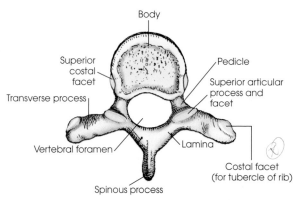

Fig. 8-13 Superior aspect of thoracic vertebra.

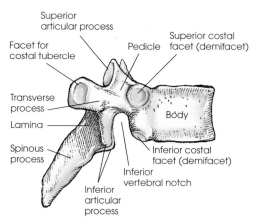

Fig. 8-14 Lateral aspect of thoracic vertebra.

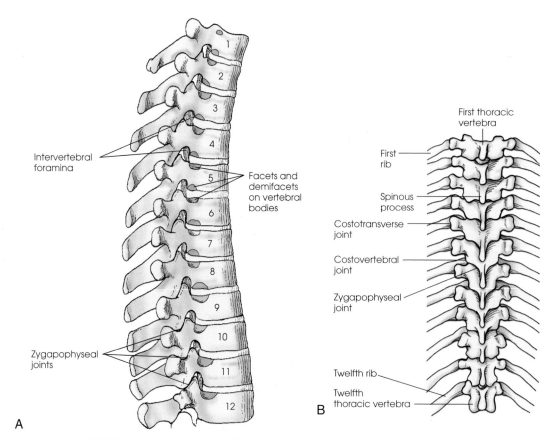

Fig. 8-15 Thoracic spine. **A,** Posterior oblique aspect showing zygapophyseal joints, intervertebral foramina, and facets and demifacets (see Table 8-2). **B,** Posterior aspect showing attachment of ribs and joints.

The transverse processes of the thoracic vertebrae project obliquely, laterally, and posteriorly. With the exception of the 11th and 12th pairs, each process has on the anterior surface of its extremity a small concave facet for articulation with the tubercle of a rib. The laminae are broad and thick, and they overlap the subjacent lamina. The spinous processes are long. From the fifth to the ninth vertebrae, the spinous processes project sharply inferiorly and overlap each other, but they are less vertical above and below this region. The palpable tip of each spinous process of the fifth to ninth thoracic vertebrae corresponds in position to the interspace *below* the vertebra from which it projects.

The zygapophyseal joints of the thoracic region (except the inferior articular processes of the 12th vertebra) angle anteriorly approximately 15 to 20 degrees to form an angle of 70 to 75 degrees (open anteriorly) to the midsagittal plane of the body (Fig. 8-16, *A*; see Fig. 8-15). To show the zygapophyseal joints of the thoracic region radiographically, the patient's body must be rotated 70 to 75 degrees from the anatomic position or 15 to 20 degrees from the lateral position.

The intervertebral foramina of the thoracic region are perpendicular to the midsagittal plane of the body (see Figs. 8-15 and 8-16, *B*). These foramina are clearly shown radiographically with the patient in a true lateral position (see Table 8-1). During inspiration, the ribs are elevated. The arms must also be raised enough to elevate the ribs, which otherwise cross the intervertebral foramina. A full view of the thoracic vertebrae is seen in Fig. 8-17 along with surrounding tissues.

TABLE 8-2
Costal facets and demifacets

Vertebrae	Vertebral border	Facet/demifacet*
T1	Superior	Whole facet
	Inferior	Demifacet
T2-T8	Superior	Demifacet
	Inferior	Demifacet
T9	Superior	Demifacet
	Inferior	None
T10-T12	Superior	Whole facet
	Inferior	None

*On *each side* of a vertebral body.

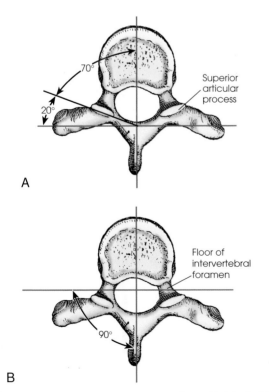

Superior articular process

Floor of intervertebral foramen

A

B

Fig. 8-16 A, Direction of thoracic zygapophyseal joints. **B,** Direction of thoracic intervertebral foramina.

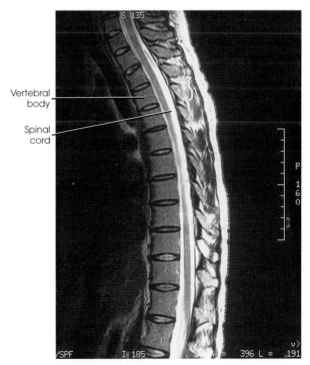

Vertebral body

Spinal cord

Fig. 8-17 MRI sagittal plane of thoracic vertebrae region showing vertebral bodies and relationship to spinal cord.

Lumbar Vertebrae

The lumbar vertebrae have large, bean-shaped bodies that increase in size from the first to the fifth vertebra in this region. The lumbar bodies are deeper anteriorly than posteriorly, and their superior and inferior surfaces are flattened or slightly concave (Fig. 8-18, A). At their posterior surface, these vertebrae are flattened anteriorly to posteriorly, and they are transversely concave. The anterior and lateral surfaces are concave from the top to the bottom (Fig. 8-18, B).

The transverse processes of lumbar vertebrae are smaller than those of the thoracic vertebrae. The superior three pairs are directed almost exactly laterally, whereas the inferior two pairs are inclined slightly superiorly. The lumbar pedicles are strong and are directed posteriorly; the laminae are thick. The spinous processes are large, thick, and blunt, and they have an almost horizontal projection posteriorly. The palpable tip of each spinous process corresponds in position with the interspace below the vertebra from which it projects. The *mamillary process* is a smoothly rounded projection on the back of each superior articular process. The *accessory process* is at the back of the root of the transverse process.

The body of the fifth lumbar segment is considerably deeper in front than behind, which gives it a wedge shape that adapts it for articulation with the sacrum. The intervertebral disk of this joint is also more wedge-shaped than the disks in the interspaces above the lumbar region. The spinous process of the fifth lumbar vertebra is smaller and shorter, and the transverse processes are much thicker than those of the upper lumbar vertebrae.

The laminae lie posterior to the pedicles and transverse processes. The part of the lamina between the superior and inferior articular processes is called the *pars interarticularis* (Fig. 8-19).

The zygapophyseal joints of the lumbar region (Figs. 8-20 and 8-21, A) are inclined posteriorly from the coronal plane, forming an average angle (open posteriorly) of 30 to 60 degrees to the midsagittal plane of the body.

The average angle increases from cephalad to caudad with L1-2 at 15 degrees, L2-3 at 30 degrees, and L3-4 through L5-S1 at 45 degrees. Table 8-3 shows, however, that these joint angles may vary widely at each level. Numerous upper joints have no angle, and many lower joints have an angle of 60 degrees or more. Although the customary 45-degree oblique body position shows most clinically significant lumbar zygapophyseal joints (L3 through S1), 25% of L1-2 and L2-3 joints are shown on an AP projection, and a small percentage of L4-5 and L5-S1 joints are seen on a lateral projection.

The intervertebral foramina of the lumbar region are situated at right angles to the midsagittal plane of the body except for the fifth, which turns slightly anteriorly (Fig. 8-21, B). The superior four pairs of foramina are shown radiographically with the patient in a true lateral position; the last pair requires slight obliquity of the body (see Table 8-1).

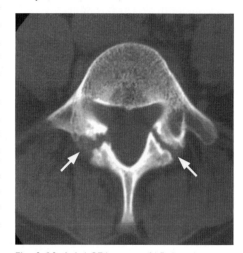

Fig. 8-19 Axial CT image of L5 showing fractures of right and left pars interarticularis (*arrows*).

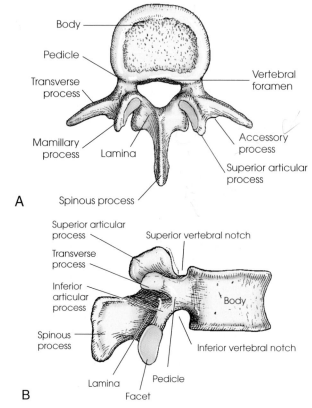

Fig. 8-18 A, Superior aspect of lumbar vertebra. **B,** Lateral aspect of lumbar vertebra.

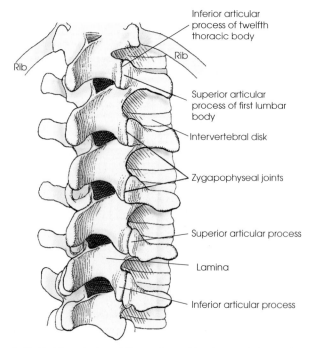

Fig. 8-20 Right posterior oblique view of lumbar vertebrae, showing zygapophyseal joints.

Spondylolysis is an acquired bony defect occurring in the pars interarticularis, the area of the lamina between the two articular processes. The defect may occur on one or both sides of the vertebra, resulting in a condition termed *spondylolisthesis*. This condition is characterized by the anterior displacement of one vertebra over another, generally the fifth lumbar over the sacrum. Spondylolisthesis almost exclusively involves the lumbar spine (Fig. 8-22).

Spondylolisthesis is of radiologic importance because oblique-position radiographs show the "neck" area of the "Scottie dog" (i.e., the pars interarticularis). (Oblique positions involving the lumbar spine, including the Scottie dog, are presented later in this chapter, starting with Fig. 8-95.) A full view of the lumbar vertebrae is seen in Fig. 8-23 along with surrounding tissues.

TABLE 8-3

Lumbar zygapophyseal joint angle*

Joint	Average angle (degrees)	Average range (degrees)	% at 0 degree[†]	% at 90 degrees[‡]
L1-L2	15	0-30	25	0
L2-L3	30	0-30	25	0
L3-L4	45	15-45	10	0
L4-L5	45	45-60	3	2
L5-S1	45	45-60	5	7

*In relation to the sagittal plane.
[†]Joint space oriented parallel to sagittal plane.
[‡]Joint space perpendicular to sagittal plane.
From Bogduk N, Twomey L: *Clinical anatomy of the lumbar spine*, ed 3, London, 1997, Churchill Livingstone.

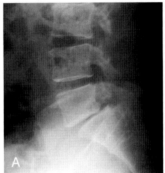
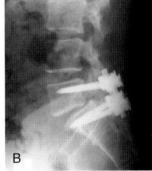

Fig. 8-22 Lateral lumbar spine showing spondylolisthesis. **A,** A 53-year-old man presenting with pain in the legs and difficulty standing for more than 5 minutes without pain. L4 is anteriorly displaced 20% over L5. **B,** Surgery performed to stabilize spondylolisthesis. The patient recovered fully from pain.

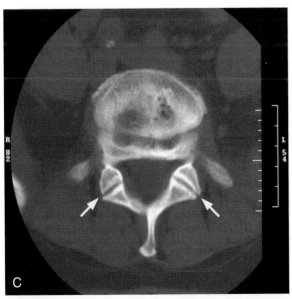

Fig. 8-21 A, Direction of lumbar zygapophyseal joints. **B,** Superior aspect showing orientation of lumbar intervertebral foramina. **C,** Axial CT image of lumbar spine showing angles of zygapophyseal joints (*arrows*).

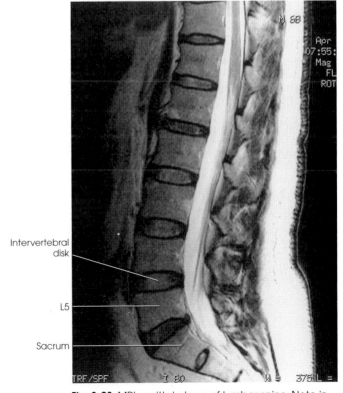

Fig. 8-23 MRI sagittal plane of lumbar spine. Note intervertebral disks between vertebral bodies.

Sacrum

The *sacrum* is formed by fusion of the five sacral vertebral segments into a curved, triangular bone (Figs. 8-24 and 8-25). The sacrum is wedged between the iliac bones of the pelvis, with its broad base directed obliquely, superiorly, and anteriorly and its apex directed posteriorly and inferiorly. Although the size and degree of curvature of the sacrum vary considerably in different patients, the bone is normally longer, narrower, more evenly curved, and more vertical in position in males than in females. The female sacrum is more acutely curved, with its greatest curvature in the lower half of the bone; it also lies in a more oblique plane, which results in a sharper angle at the junction of the lumbar and pelvic curves.

The superior portion of the first sacral segment remains distinct and resembles the vertebrae of the lumbar region (Fig. 8-26). The superior surface of the *base* of the sacrum corresponds in size and shape to the inferior surface of the last lumbar segment, with which it articulates to form the lumbosacral junction. The concavities on the upper surface of the pedicles of the first sacral segment and the corresponding concavities on the lower surface of the pedicles of the last lumbar segment form the last pair of intervertebral foramina. The *superior articular processes* of the first sacral segment articulate with the inferior articular processes of the last lumbar vertebra to form the last pair of zygapophyseal joints.

At its superior anterior margin, the base of the sacrum has a prominent ridge termed the *sacral promontory*. Directly behind the bodies of the sacral segments is the *sacral canal,* which is the continuation of the vertebral canal. The sacral canal is contained within the bone and transmits the sacral nerves. The anterior and posterior walls of the sacral canal are each perforated by four pairs of *pelvic sacral foramina* for the passage of the sacral nerves and blood vessels.

On each side of the sacral base is a large, winglike lateral mass called the *ala* (see Fig. 8-26, *B*). At the superoanterior part of the lateral surface of each ala is the *auricular surface,* a large articular process for articulation with similarly shaped processes on the iliac bones of the pelvis.

The inferior surface of the *apex* of the sacrum (Fig. 8-27) has an oval facet for articulation with the coccyx and the *sacral cornua,* two processes that project inferiorly from the posterolateral aspect of the last sacral segment to join the *coccygeal cornua.*

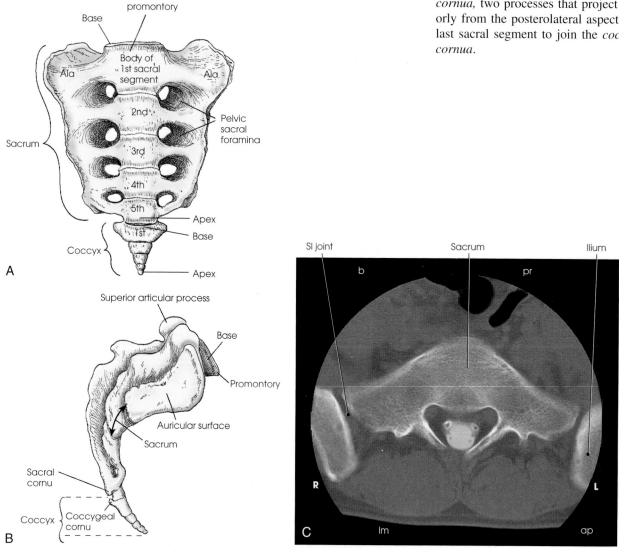

Fig. 8-24 A, Anterior aspect of sacrum and coccyx. **B,** Lateral aspect of sacrum and coccyx. **C,** Sagittal MRI scan of sacrum and coccyx.

Coccyx

The *coccyx* is composed of three to five (usually four) rudimentary *vertebrae* that have a tendency to fuse into one bone in the adult (see Fig. 8-24). The coccyx diminishes in size from its *base* inferiorly to its *apex*. From its articulation with the sacrum it curves inferiorly and anteriorly, often deviating from the midline of the body. The *coccygeal cornua* project superiorly from the posterolateral aspect of the first coccygeal segment to join the sacral cornua.

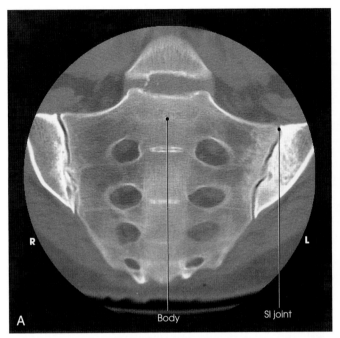

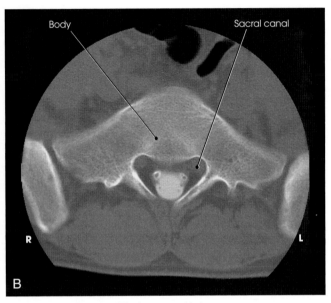

Fig. 8-25 A, Coronal CT of sacrum. Note sacroiliac (*SI*) joints. **B,** Axial CT of sacrum. Note angle of SI joints and sacral nerves in sacral canal.

(Modified from Kelley LL, Petersen CM: *Sectional anatomy for imaging professionals,* ed 2, St Louis, 2007, Mosby.)

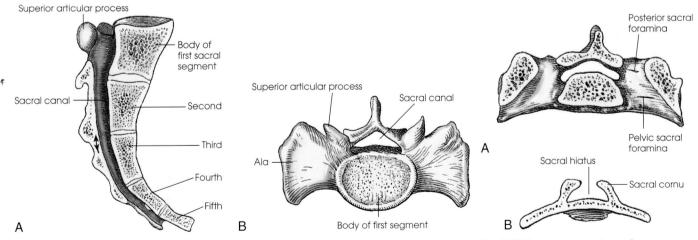

Fig. 8-26 A, Sagittal section of sacrum. **B,** Base of sacrum.

Fig. 8-27 Transverse sections of sacrum.
A, Section through superior sacral portion.
B, Section through inferior sacral portion.

Vertebral Articulations

The joints of the vertebral column are shown in Fig. 8-28 and summarized in Table 8-4. A detailed description follows.

The vertebral articulations consist of two types of joints: (1) *intervertebral* joints, which are between the two vertebral bodies and are *cartilaginous symphysis* joints that permit only slight movement of individual vertebrae but considerable motility for the column as a whole, and (2) *zygapophyseal* joints, which are between the articulation processes of the vertebral arches and are *synovial gliding* joints that permit free movement (see Fig. 8-20). The movements permitted in the vertebral column by the combined action of the joints are flexion, extension, lateral flexion, and rotation.

The articulations between the atlas and the occipital bone are *synovial ellipsoidal* joints and are called the *atlantooccipital articulations* (see Fig. 8-8). The anterior arch of the atlas rotates around the dens of the axis to form the *atlantoaxial* joint, which is a synovial gliding articulation and a *synovial pivot* articulation (see Table 8-4).

In the thoracic region, the heads of the ribs articulate with the bodies of the vertebrae to form the *costovertebral* joints, which are synovial gliding articulations. The tubercles of the ribs and the transverse processes of the thoracic vertebrae articulate to form *costotransverse* joints, which are also synovial gliding articulations (see Fig. 8-15).

The articulations between the sacrum and the two ilia—the sacroiliac joints—(see Fig. 8-25, *A*) are discussed in Chapter 7.

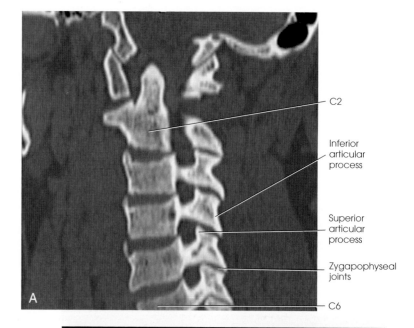

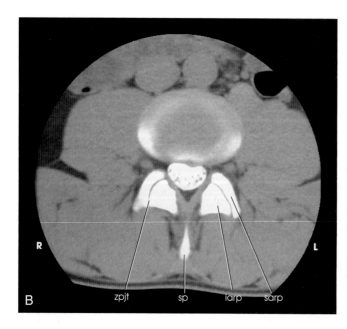

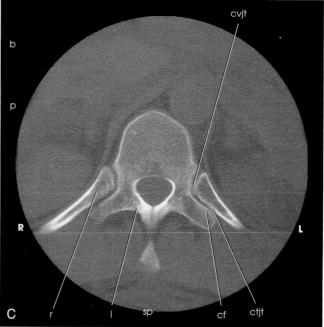

Fig. 8-28 Vertebral articulations. **A,** CT reformat of cervical spine showing zygapophyseal joints. **B,** CT scan of lumbar spine showing zygapophyseal joints. *iarp,* inferior articulating process; *sarp,* superior articulating process; *zpjt,* zygapophyseal joint. **C,** CT scan of thoracic vertebra. *cf,* costal facet; *ctjt,* costotransverse joint; *cvjt,* costovertebral joint; *l,* lamina; *r,* rib.

SUMMARY OF ANATOMY

Vertebral column (spine)
Vertebrae (24)
 Cervical (7)
 Thoracic (12)
 Lumbar (5)
 Sacral
 Coccygeal
True vertebrae
False vertebrae
Sacrum
Coccyx

Vertebral curvature
Curves
 Cervical
 Thoracic
 Lumbar
 Pelvic
Lordotic curve
Kyphotic curve
Lumbosacral angle
Primary curves
Secondary or compensatory curves

Typical vertebra
Body
Vertebral arch
Vertebral foramen
Vertebral canal
Articular cartilage plate
Intervertebral disks
Nucleus pulposus
Anulus fibrosus
Pedicles
Vertebral notches
Intervertebral foramina
Laminae
Transverse processes
Spinous process
Facets
Superior articular processes
Inferior articular processes
Zygapophyseal joints (interarticular facet joints)

Cervical vertebrae
Atlas (first)
 Anterior arch
 Posterior arch
 Lateral masses
 Transverse atlantal ligament
Axis (second)
 Dens (odontoid process)
Cervical (seventh)
 Vertebra prominens
Typical cervical vertebra
 Transverse foramina
 Articular pillars

Thoracic vertebrae
Costal facets
Demifacets

Lumbar vertebrae
Mamillary process
Accessory process
Pars interarticularis

Sacrum
Base
Superior articular processes
Sacral promontory
Sacral canal
Pelvic sacral foramina
Ala
Auricular surface
Apex
Sacral cornua

Coccyx
Base
Apex
Coccygeal cornua

Vertebral articulations
Atlantooccipital
Atlantoaxial
 Lateral (2)
 Medial (1—dens)
Costovertebral
Costotransverse
Intervertebral
Zygapophyseal

TABLE 8-4

Joints of the vertebral column

Joint	Structural classification		Movement
	Tissue	Type	
Atlantooccipital	Synovial	Ellipsoidal	Freely movable
Atlantoaxial			
Lateral (2)	Synovial	Gliding	Freely movable
Medial (1—dens)	Synovial	Pivot	Freely movable
Intervertebral	Cartilaginous	Symphysis	Slightly movable
Zygapophyseal	Synovial	Gliding	Freely movable
Costovertebral	Synovial	Gliding	Freely movable
Costotransverse	Synovial	Gliding	Freely movable

SUMMARY OF PATHOLOGY

Condition	Definition
Ankylosing spondylitis	Rheumatoid arthritis variant involving the sacroiliac joints and spine
Fracture	Disruption in the continuity of bone
Clay shoveler's	Avulsion fracture of the spinous process in the lower cervical and upper thoracic region
Compression	Fracture that causes compaction of bone and a decrease in length or width
Hangman's	Fracture of the anterior arch of C2 owing to hyperextension
Jefferson	Comminuted fracture of the ring of C1
Herniated nucleus pulposus	Rupture or prolapse of the nucleus pulposus into the spinal canal
Kyphosis	Abnormally increased convexity in the thoracic curvature
Lordosis	Abnormally increased concavity of the cervical and lumbar spine
Metastases	Transfer of a cancerous lesion from one area to another
Osteoarthritis or degenerative joint disease	Form of arthritis marked by progressive cartilage deterioration in synovial joints and vertebrae
Osteopetrosis	Increased density of atypically soft bone
Osteoporosis	Loss of bone density
Paget disease	Thick, soft bone marked by bowing and fractures
Scheuermann disease or adolescent kyphosis	Kyphosis with onset in adolescence
Scoliosis	Lateral deviation of the spine with possible vertebral rotation
Spina bifida	Failure of the posterior encasement of the spinal cord to close
Spondylolisthesis	Forward displacement of a vertebra over a lower vertebra, usually L5-S1
Spondylolysis	Breaking down of the vertebra
Subluxation	Incomplete or partial dislocation
Tumor	New tissue growth where cell proliferation is uncontrolled
Multiple myeloma	Malignant neoplasm of plasma cells involving the bone marrow and causing destruction of bone

EXPOSURE TECHNIQUE CHART ESSENTIAL PROJECTIONS

VERTEBRAL COLUMN

Part	cm	kVp*	tm	mA	mAs	AEC	SID	IR	Dose (mrad)†
Atlas and axis‡—AP	11	75	0.13	200s	26		40″	8 × 10 in	70
Dens‡—AP (Fuchs)	14	75		200s			40″	8 × 10 in	104
Cervical vertebrae—AP Axial‡	11	75		200s			40″	8 × 10 in	70
Cervical vertebrae—Lateral (Grandy)‡	11	75	0.23	200s	20	○○●	72″	24 × 30 cm	74
Cervical vertebrae—Hyperflexion and hyperextension‡	11	75	0.23	200s	20	○○●	72″	24 × 30 cm	74
Cervical intervertebral foramina—AP and PA axial oblique‡	11	75	0.1	200s	20		72″	8 × 10 in	74
Cervicothoracic region—lateral (swimmer's)‡	24	80	0.25	200s	50		40″	24 × 30 cm	430
Thoracic vertebrae—AP‡	21	80		200s		○○●	40″	35 × 43 cm	150
Thoracic vertebrae—lateral‡	33	80		200s		○○●	40″	35 × 43 cm	857
Lumbar vertebrae—AP‡	21	80		200s		○○●	40″	35 × 43 cm	159
Lumbar vertebrae—lateral‡	27	90		200s		○○●	40″	35 × 43 cm	916
Lumbar L5-S1—lateral‡	31	95		200s		○○●	40″	8 × 10 in	126
Zygapophyseal joints—AP oblique‡	23	85		200s		○○●	40″	30 × 35 cm	202
Lumbosacral junction and sacroiliac joints—AP axial‡	17	85		200s		○○●	40″	8 × 10 in	239
Sacroiliac joints—AP oblique‡	17	80		200s		○○●	40″	24 × 30 cm	250
Sacrum—AP axial‡	17	80		200s		○○●	40″	24 × 30 cm	156
Sacrum—lateral‡	31	90		200s		○○●	40″	24 × 30 cm	1135
Coccyx—AP axial‡	17	80		200s		○○●	40″	8 × 10 in	140
Coccyx—lateral‡	31	80	0.5	200s	100		40″	8 × 10 in	710
Thoracolumbar spine-scoliosis—PA (Frank and Ferguson)‡	23	90	0.2	200s	40		40″	35 × 43 cm	406

*kVp values are for a three-phase, 12-pulse generator or high frequency.
†Relative doses for comparison use. All doses are skin entrance for average adult at cm indicated.
‡Bucky, 16:1 grid. Screen-film speed 300 or equivalent CR.
s, small focal spot.

PROJECTIONS REMOVED

Because of significant advances in MRI, CT, and CT three-dimensional reconstruction, the following projections have been removed from this edition of the atlas. The projections eliminated may be reviewed in their entirety in the eleventh and all previous editions of this atlas.

Atlantooccipital articulations
• AP oblique

Dens
• AP axial oblique, Kasabach method

Pubic symphysis
• PA Chamberlain method

✦ AP PROJECTION
FUCHS METHOD

Fuchs[1] recommended the AP projection to show the dens when its upper half is not clearly shown in the open-mouth position. This patient position must not be attempted if fracture or degenerative disease of the upper cervical region is suspected.

Image receptor: 8 × 10 inch (18 × 24 cm) crosswise

Position of patient

• Place the patient in the supine position.
• Center the midsagittal plane of the body to the midline of the grid.
• Place the arms along the sides of the body.
• Place a support under the patient's knees for comfort.

[1]Fuchs AW: Cervical vertebrae (part 1), *Radiogr Clin Photogr* 16:2, 1940.

Position of part

• Place the IR in the Bucky tray, and center the IR to the level of the tips of the mastoid processes.
• Extend the chin until the tip of the chin and the tip of the mastoid process are vertical (Fig. 8-29).
• Adjust the head so that the midsagittal plane is perpendicular to the plane of the grid.
• *Shield gonads.*
• *Respiration:* Suspend.

Central ray

• Perpendicular to the midpoint of the IR; it enters the neck on the midsagittal plane just distal to the tip of the chin.

Collimation

• Adjust to 5 × 5 inches (13 × 13 cm) on the collimator.

Structures shown

The resulting image shows an AP projection of the dens lying within the circular foramen magnum (Fig. 8-30).

EVALUATION CRITERIA

The following should be clearly shown:
■ Evidence of proper collimation
■ Entire dens within the foramen magnum
■ Symmetry of the mandible, cranium, and vertebrae, indicating no rotation of the head or neck

PA PROJECTION
JUDD METHOD

Because of the difficulty in positioning the patient, especially a patient who has a potential fracture, this projection is no longer described in full. In addition, computed tomography (CT) is now used to evaluate the upper cervical area. This method is described in the tenth and previous editions.

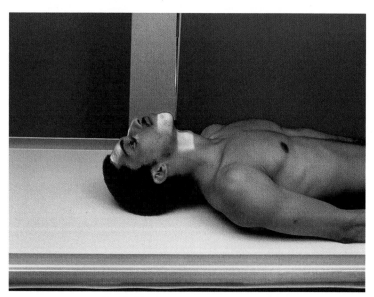

Fig. 8-29 AP dens: Fuchs method.

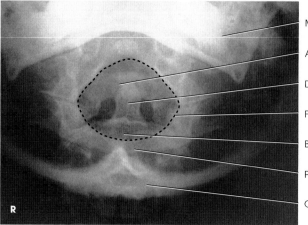

Mandible

Anterior arch of atlas

Dens

Foramen magnum

Body of axis

Posterior arch of C1

Occipital bone

Fig. 8-30 AP dens: Fuchs method.

♠ AP PROJECTION
Open-mouth

The open-mouth technique was described by Albers-Schönberg[1] in 1910 and by George[2] in 1919.

Image receptor: 8 × 10 inch (18 × 24 cm)

SID: A 30-inch (76-cm) SID is often used for this projection to increase the field of view of the odontoid area. See Chapter 1 for use of a 30-inch (76-cm) SID.

---

[1]Albers-Schönberg HE: *Die Röntgentechnik,* ed 3, Hamburg, 1910, Gräfe & Sillem.
[2]George AW: Method for more accurate study of injuries to the atlas and axis, *Boston Med Surg J* 181:395, 1919.

Position of patient
- Place the patient in the supine position.
- Center the midsagittal plane of the body to the midline of the grid.
- Place the patient's arms along the sides of the body, and adjust the shoulders to lie in the same horizontal plane.
- Place a support under the patient's knees for comfort.

Position of part
- Place the IR in the Bucky tray, and center the IR at the level of the axis.
- Adjust the patient's head so that the midsagittal plane is perpendicular to the plane of the table (Figs. 8-31 and 8-32).

- Select the exposure factors, and move the x-ray tube into position so that any minor change can be made quickly after the final adjustment of the patient's head. Although this position is not easy to hold, the patient is usually able to cooperate fully unless he or she is kept in the final, strained position too long.
- Have the patient open the mouth as wide as possible, and then adjust the head so that a line from the lower edge of the upper incisors to the tip of the mastoid process (occlusal plane) is perpendicular to the IR. A small support under the back of the head may be needed to facilitate opening of the mouth while proper alignment of the upper incisors and mastoid tips is maintained.
- *Shield gonads.*
- *Respiration:* Instruct the patient to keep the mouth wide open and to phonate "ah" softly during the exposure. This places the tongue in the floor of the mouth so that it is not projected on the atlas and axis and prevents movement of the mandible.

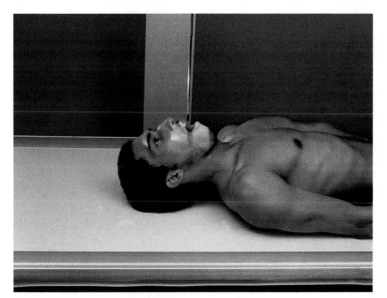

Fig. 8-31 AP atlas and axis.

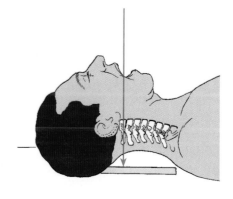

Fig. 8-32 Open-mouth spine alignment.

Atlas and Axis

Central ray

• Perpendicular to the center of the IR and entering the midpoint of the open mouth

Collimation

• Adjust to 5 × 5 inches (13 × 13 cm) on the collimator.

Structures shown

The image shows an AP projection of the atlas and axis through the open mouth (Figs. 8-33 and 8-34). If the patient has a deep head or a long mandible, the entire atlas is not shown. When the exactly superimposed shadows of the occlusal surface of the upper central incisors and the base of the skull are in line with those of the tips of the mastoid processes, the position cannot be improved. If the patient cannot open the mouth, tomography may be required (Fig. 8-35).

NOTE: If the upper teeth are projected over the dens, the neck is flexed too much toward the chest. If the base of the skull is projected over the dens, the neck is extended too much.

EVALUATION CRITERIA

The following should be clearly shown:
■ Evidence of proper collimation
■ Dens, atlas, axis, and articulations between the first and second cervical vertebrae
■ Entire articular surfaces of the atlas and axis (to check for lateral displacement)
■ Superimposed occlusal plane of the upper central incisors and the base of the skull
■ Mouth open wide
■ Shadow of the tongue not projected over the atlas and axis
■ Mandibular rami equidistant from dens

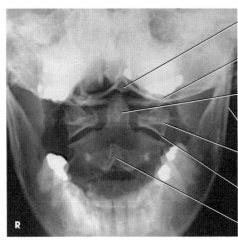

Occipital base

Occlusal surface of teeth

Dens (odontoid process)

Mandibular ramus

Lateral mass of atlas

Inferior articular process of atlas

Spinous process of axis

Fig. 8-33 Open-mouth atlas and axis.

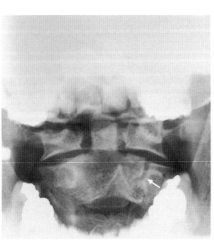

Fig. 8-34 Open-mouth atlas and axis, showing fracture of left lateral mass of axis (*arrow*).

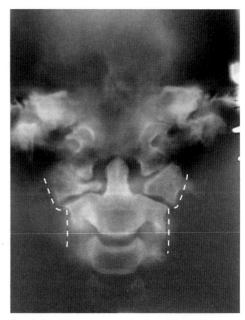

Fig. 8-35 AP upper cervical vertebrae tomogram of a patient who fell and landed on his head. A bursting-type Jefferson fracture caused outward displacement of both lateral masses of atlas. A tomogram is often necessary to show upper cervical area in trauma patients who cannot move their heads or open their mouths.

Atlas and Axis

LATERAL PROJECTION
R or L position

Image receptor: 8 × 10 inch (18 × 24 cm)

Position of patient
- Place the patient in the supine position.
- Place the arms along the sides of the body, and adjust the shoulders to lie in the same horizontal plane.
- Place a sponge or pad under the patient's head unless traumatic injury has been sustained, in which case the neck should not be moved.

Position of part
- With the IR in the vertical position and in contact with the upper neck, center it at the level of the atlantoaxial articulation (1 inch [2.5 cm] distal to the tip of the mastoid process).
- Adjust the IR so that it is parallel with the midsagittal plane of the neck, and then support the IR in position (Figs. 8-36 and 8-37).
- Extend the neck slightly so that the shadow of the mandibular rami does not overlap that of the spine.
- Adjust the head so that the midsagittal plane is perpendicular to the table.
- *Shield gonads.*
- *Respiration:* Suspend.

Central ray
- Perpendicular to a point 1 inch (2.5 cm) distal to the adjacent mastoid tip. A grid and close collimation should be used to minimize secondary radiation.

Structures shown
The resulting image shows a lateral projection of the atlas and axis. The atlanto-occipital articulations are also shown (Fig. 8-38).

EVALUATION CRITERIA
The following should be clearly shown:
- Upper cervical vertebrae
- Superimposed laminae of the axis and superimposed posterior arches of the atlas
- Neck extended so that the mandibular rami does not overlap the axis or atlas
- Nearly superimposed rami of the mandible

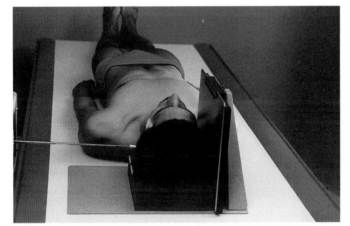

Fig. 8-36 Position for lateral atlas and axis.

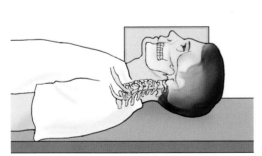

Horizontal CR to C4

Fig. 8-37 Side view as seen for centering central ray (*CR*).

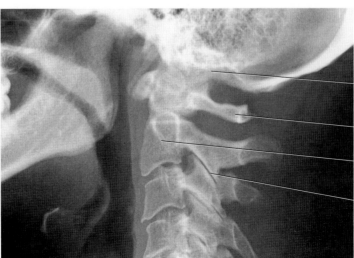

Atlantooccipital articulation

Posterior arch atlas

Body of axis

Zygapophyseal joint

Fig. 8-38 Lateral atlas and axis.

AP AXIAL PROJECTION

Image receptor: 8 × 10 inch (18 × 24 cm) lengthwise

Position of patient
- Place the patient in the supine or upright position with the back against the IR holder.
- Adjust the patient's shoulders to lie in the same horizontal plane to prevent rotation.

Position of part
- Center the midsagittal plane of the patient's body to the midline of the table or vertical grid device.
- Extend the chin enough so that the occlusal plane is perpendicular to the tabletop. This prevents superimposition of the mandible and mid-cervical vertebrae (Figs. 8-39 and 8-40).
- Center the IR at the level of C4.
- Adjust the head so that the midsagittal plane is in straight alignment and perpendicular to the IR.

- Provide support for the head of any patient who has a pronounced lordotic curvature. This support helps compensate for the curvature and reduce image distortion.
- *Shield gonads.*
- *Respiration:* Suspend.

Central ray
- Directed through C4 at an angle of 15 to 20 degrees cephalad. The central ray enters at or slightly inferior to the most prominent point of the thyroid cartilage.

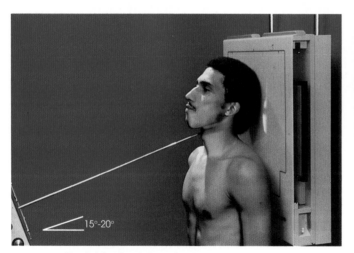

Fig. 8-39 AP axial cervical vertebrae: upright.

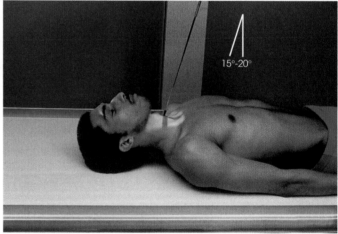

Fig. 8-40 AP axial cervical vertebrae: recumbent.

Collimation

- Adjust 10 inch (25 cm) lengthwise and 1 inch (2.5 cm) beyond the skin shadow on the sides.

Structures shown

The resulting image shows the lower five cervical bodies and the upper two or three thoracic bodies, the interpediculate spaces, the superimposed transverse and articular processes, and the intervertebral disk spaces (Fig. 8-41). This projection is also used to show the presence or absence of cervical ribs.

The following should be clearly shown:

- Evidence of proper collimation
- Area from superior portion of C3 to T2 and surrounding soft tissue
- Shadows of the mandible and occiput superimposed over the atlas and most of the axis
- Open intervertebral disk spaces
- Spinous processes equidistant to the pedicles and aligned with the midline of the cervical bodies
- Mandibular angles and mastoid processes equidistant to the vertebrae

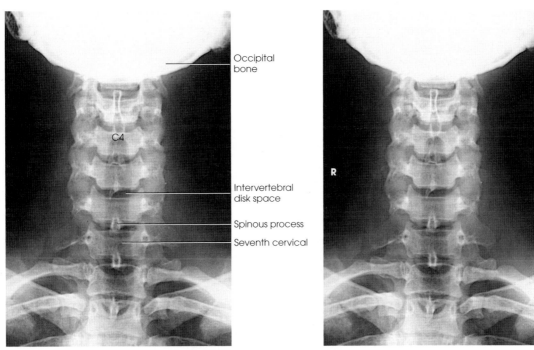

Occipital bone

C4

Intervertebral disk space

Spinous process

Seventh cervical

R

Fig. 8-41 AP axial cervical vertebrae.

LATERAL PROJECTION
GRANDY METHOD[1]
R or L position

Image receptor: 8 × 10 inch (18 × 24 cm) lengthwise

SID: A 60- to 72-inch (152- to 183-cm) SID is recommended because of the increased object-to-IR distance (OID). A longer distance helps show C7.

Position of patient

- Place the patient in a true lateral position, either seated or standing, before a vertical grid device. The long axis of the cervical vertebrae should be parallel to the plane of the IR.
- Have the patient sit or stand straight, and adjust the height of the IR so that it is centered at the level of C4. The top of the IR is about 1 inch (2.5 cm) above the external acoustic meatus (EAM).

[1]Grandy CC: A new method for making radiographs of the cervical vertebrae in the lateral position, *Radiology* 4:128, 1925.

Position of part

- Center the coronal plane that passes through the mastoid tips to the midline of the IR.
- Move the patient close enough to the vertical grid device to permit the adjacent shoulder to rest against the device for support (Fig. 8-42). (This projection may be performed without the use of a grid.)
- Rotate the shoulders anteriorly or posteriorly according to the natural kyphosis of the back: If the patient is round shouldered, rotate the shoulders anteriorly; otherwise, rotate them posteriorly.
- Adjust the shoulders to lie in the same horizontal plane, depress them as much as possible, and immobilize them by attaching one small sandbag to each *wrist*. The sandbags should be of equal weight.

- Be careful to ensure that the patient does not elevate the shoulder.
- Elevate the chin slightly, or have the patient protrude the mandible to prevent superimposition of the mandibular rami and the spine. At the same time and with the midsagittal plane of the head vertical, ask the patient to look steadily at one spot on the wall; this helps maintain the position of the head.
- *Shield gonads*.
- *Respiration*: Suspend respiration at the end of full expiration to obtain maximum depression of the shoulders.

NOTE: Refer to Chapter 13 in Volume 2 for details related to performing this projection on patients with suspected cervical spine trauma.

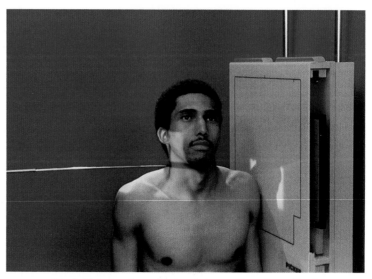

Fig. 8-42 Lateral cervical vertebrae: Grandy method.

Central ray

- Horizontal and perpendicular to C4. With such centering, the magnified outline of the shoulder *farthest* from the IR is projected below the lower cervical vertebrae.

Collimation

- Adjust to 8 × 10 inch (18 × 24 cm).

Structures shown

The image shows a lateral projection of the cervical bodies and their interspaces, the articular pillars, the lower five zygapophyseal joints, and the spinous processes (Figs. 8-43 and 8-44). Depending on how well the shoulders can be depressed, a good lateral projection must include C7; sometimes T1 and T2 can also be seen.

EVALUATION CRITERIA

The following should be clearly shown:
- Evidence of proper collimation
- All seven cervical vertebrae and at least one third of the T1 (otherwise a separate radiograph of the cervicothoracic region is recommended)
- Neck extended so that mandibular rami are not overlapping the atlas or axis
- Superimposed or nearly superimposed rami of the mandible
- No rotation or tilt of the cervical spine indicated by superimposed open zygapophyseal joints and intervertebral disk spaces
- Spinous processes shown in profile
- C4 in the center of the radiograph
- Bone and soft tissue detail

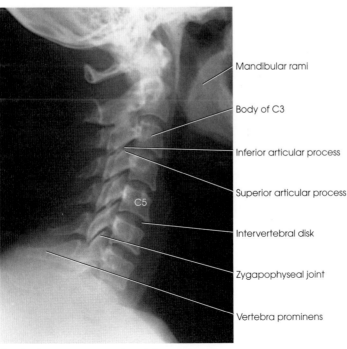

Mandibular rami

Body of C3

Inferior articular process

Superior articular process

Intervertebral disk

Zygapophyseal joint

Vertebra prominens

C5

Fig. 8-43 Lateral cervical vertebrae: Grandy method.

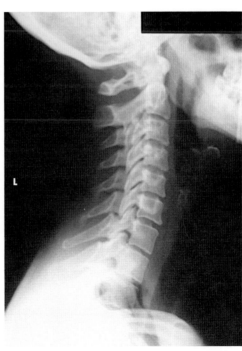

L

Fig. 8-44 Same projection as in Fig. 8-43 provides excellent visualization of all seven cervical vertebrae and T1.

LATERAL PROJECTION
R or L position
Hyperflexion and
hyperextension

NOTE: This procedure must not be attempted until cervical spine pathology or fracture has been ruled out.

Functional studies of the cervical vertebrae in the lateral position are performed to show normal AP movement or an absence of movement resulting from trauma or disease. The spinous processes are elevated and widely separated in the hyperflexion position and are depressed in close approximation in the hyperextension position.

Image receptor: 10 × 12 inch (24 × 30 cm) lengthwise

SID: A 60- to 72-inch (152- to 183-cm) SID is recommended because of the increased OID. A longer distance helps show C7.

Position of patient
- Place the patient in a true lateral position, either seated or standing, before a vertical grid device.
- Have the patient sit or stand straight, and adjust the height of the IR so that it is centered at the level of C4. The top of the IR is about 2 inches (5 cm) above the EAM.

Position of part
- Move the patient close enough to the vertical grid device to permit the adjacent shoulder to rest against the grid for support.
- Keep the midsagittal plane of the patient's head and neck parallel with the plane of the IR.
- Alternatively, perform the projection without using a grid.
  Hyperflexion
- Ask the patient to drop the head forward and then draw the chin as close as possible to the chest so that the cervical vertebrae are placed in a position of *hyperflexion* (forced flexion) for the first exposure (Fig. 8-45).
  Hyperextension
- Ask the patient to elevate the chin as much as possible so that the cervical vertebrae are placed in a position of *hyperextension* (forced extension) for the second exposure (Fig. 8-46).
- *Shield gonads.*
- *Respiration:* Suspend.

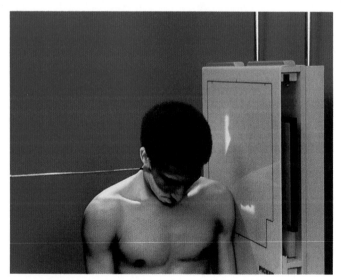

Fig. 8-45 Lateral cervical vertebrae: hyperflexion.

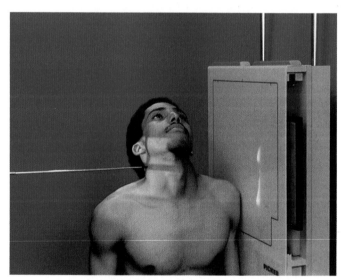

Fig. 8-46 Lateral cervical vertebrae: hyperextension.

Central ray

• Horizontal and perpendicular to C4

Collimation

• Adjust to 10 × 12 inches (24 × 30 cm) on the collimator.

Structures shown

The resulting images show the motility of the cervical spine when hyperflexed (Fig. 8-47) and hyperextended (Fig. 8-48). The intervertebral disks and the zygapophyseal joints are also shown.

NOTE: The radiologist evaluates the posterior aspect of vertebral bodies for intersegmental alignment.

The following should be clearly shown:
■ Evidence of proper collimation
   Hyperflexion
■ Body of the mandible almost vertical for hyperflexion in a normal patient
■ All seven spinous processes in profile
■ All seven cervical vertebrae in true lateral position
   Hyperextension
■ Body of the mandible almost horizontal in a normal patient
■ All seven cervical vertebrae in true lateral position

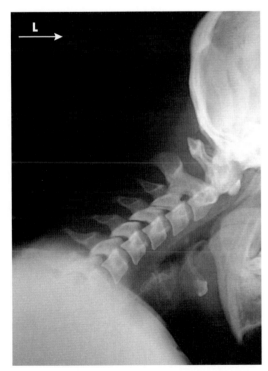

Fig. 8-47 Lateral cervical spine: hyperflexion. Note correct marking.

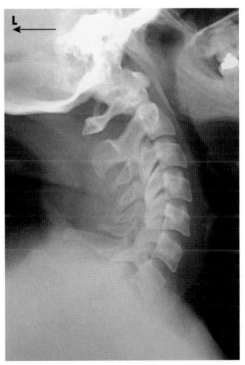

Fig. 8-48 Lateral cervical spine: hyperextension. Note correct marking.

♠ AP AXIAL OBLIQUE PROJECTION
RPO and LPO positions

Oblique projections for showing the cervical intervertebral foramina were first described by Barsóny and Koppenstein.[1,2] Both sides are examined for comparison.

[1]Barsóny T, Koppenstein E: Eine neue Method zur Röntgenuntersuchung der Halswirbelsäule, *Fortschr Roentgenstr* 35:593, 1926.
[2]Barsóny T, Koppenstein E: Beitrag zur Aufnahmetechnik der Halswirbelsäule; Darstellung der Foramina intervertebralia, *Röntgenpraxis* 1:245, 1929.

Image receptor: 8 × 10 inch (18 × 24 cm) lengthwise

SID: A 60- to 72-inch (152- to 183-cm) SID is recommended because of the increased OID.

Position of patient

- Place the patient in a supine or upright position facing the x-ray tube. The upright position (standing or seated) is preferable for the patient's comfort and makes it easier to position the patient.

Position of part

- Adjust the body (including the head) at a 45-degree angle, and center the cervical spine to the midline of the IR.
- Center the IR to the third cervical body (1 inch [2.5 cm] superior to the most prominent point of the thyroid cartilage) to compensate for the cephalic angulation of the central ray.

Upright position

- Ask the patient to sit or stand straight without strain and to rest the adjacent shoulder firmly against the vertical grid device for support.
- Ensure that the degree of body rotation is 45 degrees.
- While the patient looks straight ahead, elevate and, if needed, protrude the chin so that the mandible does not overlap the spine (Fig. 8-49). Turning the chin to the side causes slight rotation of the superior vertebrae and should be avoided.

Semisupine position

- Rotate the patient's head and body approximately 45 degrees.
- Center the cervical spine to the midline of the grid.
- Place suitable supports under the lower thorax and the elevated hip.
- Place a support under the patient's head, and adjust it so that the cervical column is horizontal.
- Check and adjust the 45-degree body rotation.
- Elevate the patient's chin and protrude the jaw as for the upright study (Fig. 8-50). Turning the chin to the side causes slight rotation of the superior vertebrae and should be avoided.
- *Shield gonads.*
- *Respiration:* Suspend.

NOTE: See p. 444 for Summary of Oblique Projections.

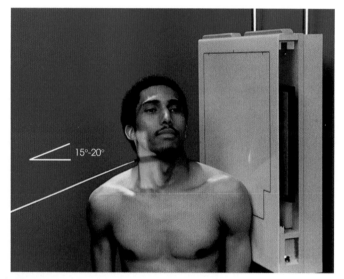

Fig. 8-49 Upright AP axial oblique right intervertebral foramina: LPO position.

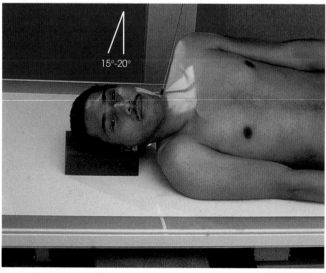

Fig. 8-50 Recumbent AP axial oblique left intervertebral foramina: RPO position.

Central ray

- Directed to C4 at a cephalad angle of 15 to 20 degrees so that the central ray coincides with the orientation of the foramina

Collimation

- Adjust to 8 × 10 inch (18 × 24 cm).

Structures shown

The resulting image shows the intervertebral foramina and pedicles *farthest* from the IR and an oblique projection of the bodies and other parts of the cervical vertebrae (Fig. 8-51). (See Summary of Oblique Projections, p. 444.)

(See Summary of Oblique Projections, p. 444.)

EVALUATION CRITERIA

The following should be clearly shown:

- Evidence of proper collimation
- Open intervertebral foramina *farthest* from the IR, from C2-3 to C7-T1
- Open intervertebral disk spaces
- Uniform size and contour of the foramina
- Elevated chin that does not overlap the atlas and axis
- Occipital bone not overlapping the axis
- C1-7 and T1

AP OBLIQUE PROJECTION
Hyperflexion and hyperextension

Boylston[1] suggested using functional studies of the cervical vertebrae in the oblique to show fractures of the articular processes and obscure dislocations and subluxations. When acute injury has been sustained, manipulation of the patient's head must be performed by a physician.

The patient is placed in a direct frontal body position facing the x-ray tube, with the shoulders held firmly against the grid device. The head is carefully rotated maximally to one side and kept in that position while the neck is flexed for the first exposure and extended for the second exposure. Both sides are examined for comparison.

[1]Boylston BF: Oblique roentgenographic views of the cervical spine in flexion and extension: an aid in the diagnosis of cervical subluxations and obscure dislocations, *J Bone Joint Surg Am* 39:1302, 1957.

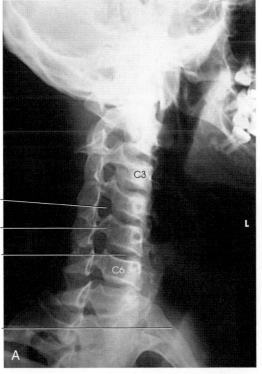
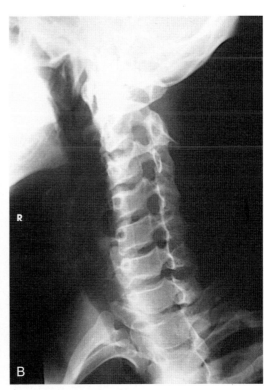

Intervertebral foramen C4-C5

Pedicle C5

C5-C6 Intervertebral disk space

First rib

C3

C6

R

L

A

B

Fig. 8-51 AP axial oblique intervertebral foramina. **A,** LPO position showing right side. **B,** RPO position showing left side.

▲ PA AXIAL OBLIQUE PROJECTION
RAO and LAO positions

Image receptor: 8 × 10 inch (18 × 24 cm) lengthwise

SID: A 60- to 72-inch (152- to 183-cm) SID is recommended because of the increased OID.

Position of patient
- Place the patient prone or upright with the back toward the x-ray tube. For the patient's comfort and accurate adjustment of the part, the standing or seated-upright position is preferred.

Position of part
- *Upright position:* Ask the patient to sit or stand straight with the arms by the side and rest the shoulder against the grid device. Rotate the patient's entire body to a 45-degree angle. Center the cervical spine to the midline of the grid device (Fig. 8-52).

- *Semiprone position:* Place the patient's body at an angle of 45 degrees and the cervical spine centered to the midline of the grid. Have the patient use the forearm and flexed knee of the elevated side to support the body and maintain the position (Figs. 8-53 and 8-54). Place a suitable support under the patient's head to position the long axis of the cervical column parallel with the IR.
- To allow for the caudal angulation of the central ray, center the IR at the level of C5 (1 inch [2.5 cm] caudal to the most prominent point of the thyroid cartilage).
- Adjust the position of the patient's head so that the midsagittal plane is aligned with the plane of the spine.
- Elevate and protrude the patient's chin just enough to prevent superimposition of the mandible with the upper cervical vertebrae. Turning the chin to the side causes rotation of the superior vertebrae and should be avoided. (The chin has to be turned slightly for the semi-prone position.)
- *Shield gonads.*
- *Respiration:* Suspend.

Central ray
- Directed to C4 at an angle of 15 to 20 degrees caudad so that it coincides with the orientation of the foramina

Collimation
- Adjust to 8 × 10 inches (18 × 24 cm) on the collimator.

Structures shown
The resulting image shows the intervertebral foramina and pedicles *closest* to the IR and an oblique projection of the bodies and other parts of the cervical column (Fig. 8-55). (See Summary of Oblique Projections, p. 444.)

EVALUATION CRITERIA

The following should be clearly shown:
- Evidence of proper collimation
- Open intervertebral foramina *closest* to the IR, from the first and second cervical vertebrae to the seventh cervical and first thoracic vertebrae
- Open intervertebral disk spaces
- Elevated chin and protruded jaw so that the angle of the mandible does not overlap the first and second cervical vertebrae
- Occipital bone not overlapping the axis
- All seven cervical and the first thoracic vertebrae

RESEARCH: This projection was researched and standardized by Laura Aaron, PhD, RT(R)(M)(QM).

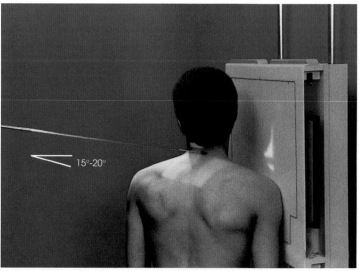

15°-20°

Fig. 8-52 PA axial oblique right intervertebral foramina: RAO position.

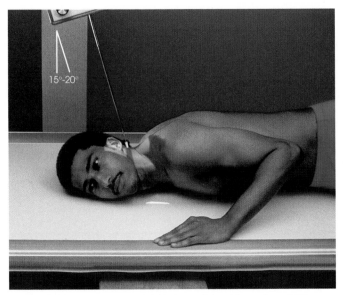

Fig. 8-53 PA axial oblique right intervertebral foramina: RAO position.

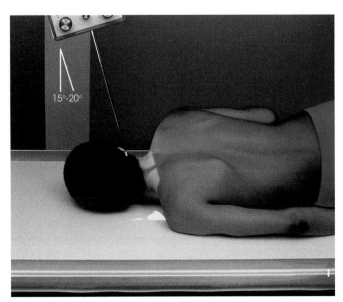

Fig. 8-54 PA axial oblique left intervertebral foramina: LAO position.

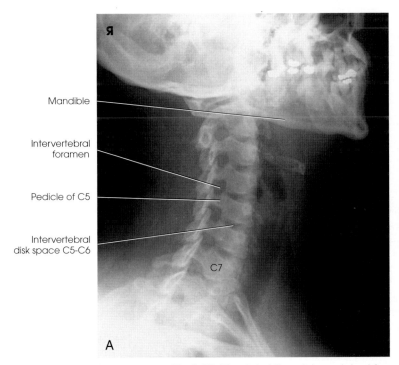

Mandible

Intervertebral foramen

Pedicle of C5

Intervertebral disk space C5-C6

C7

A

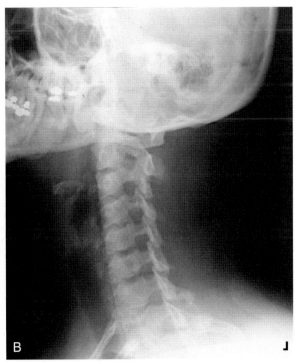

B

Fig. 8-55 PA axial oblique intervertebral foramina. **A,** RAO position showing right side. **B,** LAO position showing left side.

AP PROJECTION
OTTONELLO METHOD

With the Ottonello method, the mandibular shadow is blurred or obliterated by having the patient perform an even chewing motion of the mandible during the exposure. The patient's head must be rigidly immobilized to prevent movement of the vertebrae. The exposure time must be long enough to cover several complete excursions of the mandible. This projection is also referred to as the "wagging jaw."

Image receptor: 8 × 10 inch (18 × 24 cm) lengthwise

Position of patient
- Place the patient in the supine position.
- Center the midsagittal plane of the body to the midline of the grid.
- Place the patient's arms along the sides of the body, and adjust the shoulders to lie in the same horizontal plane.
- Place a support under the knees for the patient's comfort.

Position of part
- Adjust the patient's head so that the midsagittal plane is aligned with the lower body and is perpendicular to the table.
- Elevate the patient's chin enough to place the occlusal surface of the upper incisors and the mastoid tips in the same vertical plane.
- Immobilize the head, and have the patient practice opening and closing the mouth until the mandible can be moved smoothly without striking the teeth together (Fig. 8-56).
- Place the IR in a Bucky tray, and center the IR at the level of C4.
- To blur the mandible, use an exposure technique with a low milliamperage (mA) and long exposure time (minimum of 1 second).
- *Shield gonads.*
- *Respiration:* Suspend.

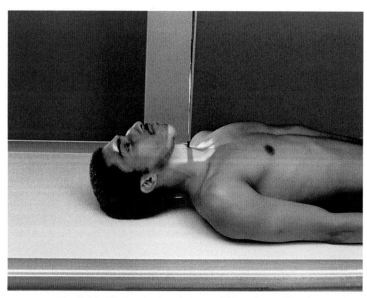

Fig. 8-56 AP cervical vertebrae: Ottonello method.

Cervical Vertebrae

Central ray

- Perpendicular to C4; the central ray enters at the most prominent point of the thyroid cartilage

Structures shown

The resulting image shows an AP projection of the entire cervical column, with the mandible blurred or obliterated (Figs. 8-57 and 8-58).

The following should be clearly shown:

- All seven cervical vertebrae
- Blurred mandible with resultant visualization of the underlying atlas and axis

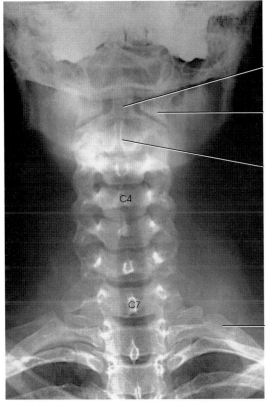

Fig. 8-57 AP cervical spine: Ottonello method with chewing motion of mandible and use of perpendicular central ray.

Dens

C1 lateral mass

Spinous process of C2

C4

C7

First rib

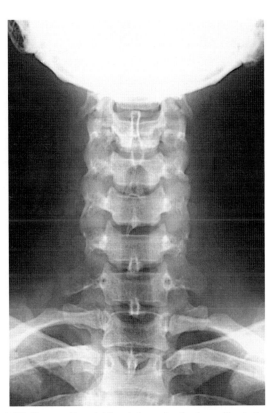

Fig. 8-58 Conventional AP axial cervical spine with stationary mandible and 15- to 20-degree cephalad angulation of central ray.

Vertebral Arch (Pillars)
AP AXIAL PROJECTION[1]

NOTE: The procedure must not be attempted until cervical spine pathology or fracture has been ruled out.

The vertebral arch projections, sometimes referred to as *pillar* or *lateral mass* projections, are used to show the posterior elements of the cervical vertebrae, the upper three or four thoracic vertebrae, the articular processes and their facets, the laminae, and the spinous processes. The central ray angulations that are employed project the vertebral arch elements free of the anteriorly situated vertebral bodies and transverse processes. When the central ray angulation is correct, the resultant image resembles a hemisection of the vertebrae. In addition to frontal plane delineation of the articular pillars and facets, vertebral arch projections are especially useful for showing the cervicothoracic spinous processes in patients with whiplash injury.[1]

Image receptor: 8 × 10 inch (18 × 24 cm) or 10 × 12 inch (24 × 30 cm)

Position of patient
- Adjust the patient in the supine position with the midsagittal plane of the body centered to the midline of the grid.
- Depress the patient's shoulders, and adjust them to lie in the same horizontal plane.

Position of part
- With the midsagittal plane of the head perpendicular to the table, *hyperextend* the patient's neck. The success of this projection depends on this hyperextension (Figs. 8-59 and 8-60).
- If the patient cannot tolerate hyperextension without undue discomfort, the oblique projection described in the next section is recommended.
- *Shield gonads.*
- *Respiration:* Suspend.

[1]Dorland P, Frémont J: Aspect radiologique normal du rachis postérieur cervicodorsal (vue postérieure ascendante), *Semaine Hop* 1457, 1957.

[1]Abel MS: Moderately severe whiplash injuries of the cervical spine and their roentgenologic diagnosis, *Clin Orthop* 12:189, 1958.

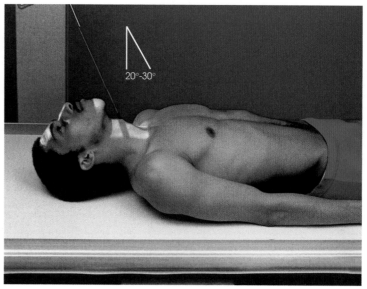

Fig. 8-59 AP axial vertebral arch.

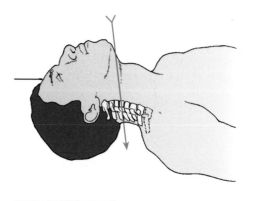

Fig. 8-60 AP axial vertebral arch.

Vertebral Column

Central ray

- Directed to C7 at an average angle of 25 degrees caudad (range 20 to 30 degrees). The central ray enters the neck in the region of the thyroid cartilage.
- The degree of the central ray angulation is determined by the cervical lordosis. The goal is to have the central ray coincide with the plane of the articular facets so that a greater angle is required when the cervical curve is accentuated, and a lesser angle is required when the curve is diminished.
- To reduce an accentuated cervical curve and place C3-7 in the same plane as T1-4, the originators[1] of this technique have suggested that a radiolucent wedge be placed under the patient's neck and shoulders, with the head extended over the edge of the wedge.

---

[1]Dorland P, Frémont J: Aspect radiologique normal du rachis postérieur cervicodorsal (vue postérieure ascendante), *Semaine Hop* 1457, 1957.

Structures shown

The resulting image shows the posterior portion of the cervical and upper thoracic vertebrae, including the articular and spinous processes (Fig. 8-61).

EVALUATION CRITERIA

The following should be clearly shown:
- Vertebral arch structures, especially the superior and inferior articulating processes (pillars), without overlapping of the vertebral bodies and transverse processes
- Articular processes
- Open zygapophyseal joints between the articular processes

NOTE: For a PA axial projection showing both sides on one IR, rest the patient's head on the table with the neck fully extended and the midsagittal plane of the head perpendicular to the table. Direct the central ray at an average angle of 40 degrees cephalad (range 35 to 45 degrees).

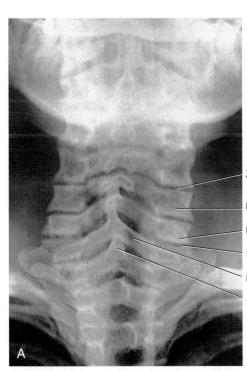

Zygapophyseal joint

Pillar or lateral mass

Inferior articular process

Superior articular process

Lamina

Spinous process

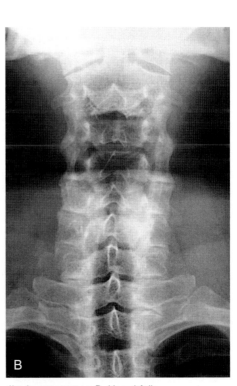

Fig. 8-61 AP axial. **A,** Central ray parallel with plateau of articular processes. **B,** Head fully extended but inadequate central ray angulation; central ray not parallel with zygapophyseal joints.

Vertebral Arch (Pillars)

AP AXIAL OBLIQUE PROJECTION

R and L head rotations[1]

These radiographic projections are used to show the vertebral arches or pillars when the patient cannot hyperextend the head for the AP or PA axial projection. Both sides are examined for comparison.

Image receptor: 8 × 10 inch (18 × 24 cm)

---

[1]Dorland P et al: Techniques d'examen radiologique de l'arc postérieur des vertebres cervicodorsales, *J Radiol* 39:509, 1958.

Position of patient
• Place the patient in the supine position.

Position of part
• Rotate the patient's head 45 to 50 degrees, turning the jaw away from the side of interest. A 45- to 50-degree rotation of the head usually shows the articular processes of C2-7 and T1. A rotation of 60 to 70 degrees is sometimes required to show the processes of C6 and T1-4 (Figs. 8-62 and 8-63).

• Position the IR so that the top edge is at the level of the mastoid tip.
• *Shield gonads.*
• *Respiration:* Suspend.

Central ray
• Directed to exit the spinous process of C7 at an average angle of 35 degrees caudad (range 30 to 40 degrees)

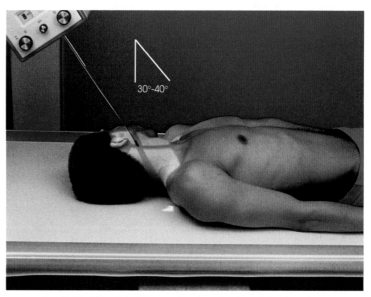

Fig. 8-62 AP axial oblique showing right vertebral arches.

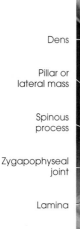
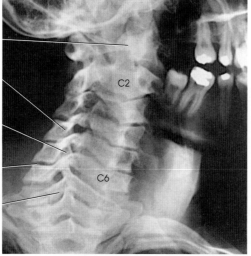
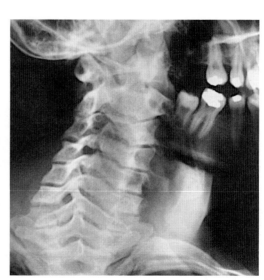

Fig. 8-63 AP axial oblique showing right vertebral arches.

✹ LATERAL PROJECTION
SWIMMER'S TECHNIQUE
R or L position

The *swimmer's technique* is performed when shoulder superimposition obscures C7 on a lateral cervical spine projection or when a lateral projection of the upper thoracic vertebra is needed. After reviewing the original publications of Twining[1] and Pawlow[2] and other pertinent publications,[3-5] the authors determined that the current technique descriptions are a combination of their recommendations. The following description identifies the historical origins and provides the authors' recommendations for the optimal positioning technique.

[1]Twining EW: Lateral view of the lung apices, *Br J Radiol* 10:123, 1937.
[2]Pawlow MK: Zur Frage über die seitliche Strahlenrichtung bei den Aufnahmen der unteren Hals und oberen Brustwirbel, *Rüntgenpraxis* 1:285, 1929.
[3]Bartsch GW: Radiography of the upper dorsal spine, *X-ray Tech* 10:135, 1938.
[4]Fletcher JC: Radiography of the upper thoracic vertebrae: lateral projection, *Radiogr Clin Photogr* 14:10, 1938.
[5]Monda LA: Modified Pawlow projection for the upper thoracic spine, *Radiol Technol* 68:117, 1996.

Image receptor: 10 × 12 inch (24 × 30 cm) lengthwise

Position of patient
- *Recumbent:* Place the patient in a lateral recumbent position with the head elevated on the patient's arm or other firm support (Fig. 8-64).
- *Upright:* Place the patient in a lateral position, either seated or standing, against a vertical grid device (Fig. 8-65).

Position of part
- Center the midcoronal plane of the body to the midline of the grid.
- Extend the arm closest to the IR above the head. If the patient is upright, flex the elbow and rest the forearm on the patient's head[1] (see Fig. 8-65). In addition, the humeral head can be moved anteriorly[2] (recommended) or posteriorly.[3]
- Position the arm away from the IR down along the patient's side, and depress the shoulder as much as possible.[1] In addition, the humeral head can be moved in the opposite direction to that of the other shoulder[2,3] (posterior recommended).

- Adjust the head and body in a true lateral position, with the midsagittal plane parallel to the plane of the IR. If the patient is recumbent, a support may be placed under the lower thorax.
- Center the IR at the level of the C7-T1 interspace, which is located 2 inches (5 cm) above the jugular notch.
- *Shield gonads.*
- *Respiration:* Suspend; or if patient can cooperate and can be immobilized, a breathing technique can be used to blur the lung anatomy.

Central ray
- Directed to the C7-T1 interspace: perpendicular[2] if the shoulder away from the IR is well depressed or at a caudal angle of 3 to 5 degrees[4] when the shoulder is immobile and cannot be depressed sufficiently.
- Monda[5] recommended angling 5 to 15 degrees cephalad to show better the intervertebral disk spaces when the spine is tilted because of broad shoulders or a nonelevated lower spine. The proper angle results in a central ray perpendicular to the long axis of the tilted spine.

NOTE: See Chapter 13 in Volume 2 for a description of positioning used for patients with suspected cervical spine trauma.

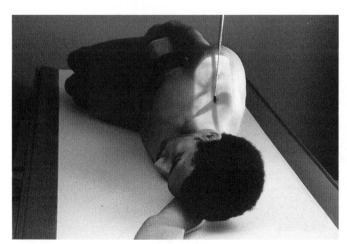

Fig. 8-64 Recumbent lateral cervicothoracic region: Pawlow method.

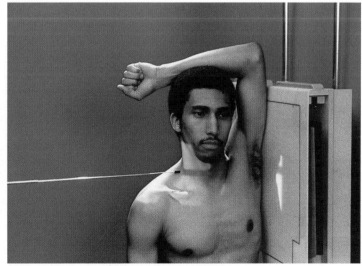

Fig. 8-65 Upright lateral cervicothoracic region: Twining method.

Collimation

- Close collimation is very important on this projection. Adjust collimator to 10 × 12 inches (24 × 30 cm).

◣ COMPENSATING FILTER

This projection should always be performed with the use of a compensating filter because of the extreme difference between the thin lower neck and the very thick upper thoracic region. With the use of a specially designed filter, the C7-T1 area can be shown on one image.

Structures shown

The image shows a lateral projection of the cervicothoracic vertebrae between the shoulders (Figs. 8-66 and 8-67).

EVALUATION CRITERIA

The following should be clearly shown:
- Evidence of proper collimation
- Lower cervical and upper thoracic vertebra, not appreciably rotated from lateral position
- Humeral heads minimally superimposed on vertebral column
- Adequate x-ray penetration through the shoulder region

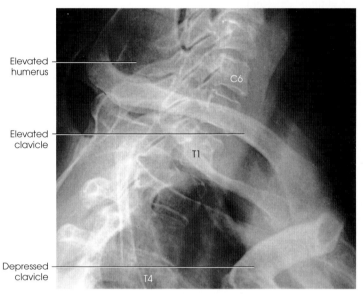

Fig. 8-66 Lateral cervicothoracic region: swimmer's technique with Ferlic filter.

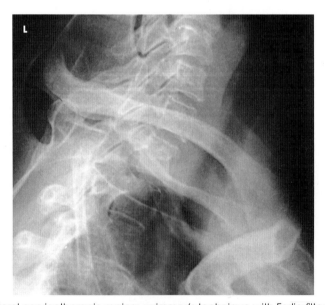

Fig. 8-67 Lateral cervicothoracic region: swimmer's technique with Ferlic filter showing bony structures.

♠ AP PROJECTION

Image receptor: 14 × 17 inch (35 × 43 cm) or 7 × 17 inch (18 × 43 cm) lengthwise

Position of patient
- Place the patient in the supine or upright position.
- Place the patient's arms along the sides of the body, and adjust the shoulders to lie in the same horizontal plane.
- If the patient is supine, let the head rest directly on the table or on a thin pillow to avoid accentuating the thoracic kyphosis.
- If the upright position is used, ask the patient to sit or stand up as straight as possible.

Position of part
- Center the midsagittal plane of the body to the midline of the grid.
- For the *supine position,* to reduce kyphosis, flex the patient's hips and knees to place the thighs in vertical position. Immobilize the feet with sandbags (Fig. 8-68).
- If the patient's limbs cannot be flexed, support the knees to relieve strain.
- For the *upright position,* have the patient stand so that the patient's weight is equally distributed on the feet to prevent rotation of the vertebral column.
- If the patient's lower limbs are of unequal length, place a support of the correct height under the foot of the shorter side.

- Place the superior edge of the IR 1½ to 2 inches (3.8 to 5 cm) above the shoulders on an average patient. This positions the IR so that T7 appears near the center of the image, and all the thoracic vertebrae are shown.
- *Shield gonads.*
- *Respiration:* The patient may be allowed to take shallow breaths during the exposure, or respiration is suspended at the end of full expiration.

Central ray
- Perpendicular to the IR. The center of the central ray should be approximately halfway between the jugular notch and the xiphoid process (see Fig. 8-68).
- Collimate closely to the spine.

Collimation
- Adjust to 7 × 17 inches (18 × 43 cm) on the collimator for a routine examination. When a full thorax image is requested, adjust to 14 × 17 inches (35 × 43 cm).

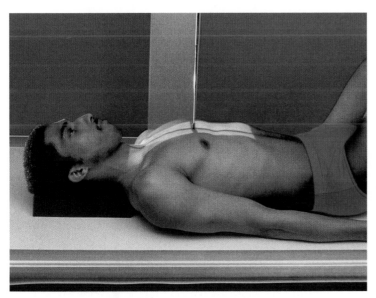

Fig. 8-68 AP thoracic vertebrae.

Thoracic Vertebrae

NOTE: As suggested by Fuchs,[1] a more uniform density of the thoracic vertebrae can be obtained if the "heel effect" of the tube is used (Figs. 8-69 and 8-70). With the tube positioned so that the cathode end is toward the feet, the greatest percentage of radiation goes through the thickest part of the thorax.

[1]Fuchs AW: Thoracic vertebrae, *Radiogr Clin Photogr* 17:2, 1941.

Structures shown

The image shows an AP projection of the thoracic bodies, intervertebral disk spaces, transverse processes, costovertebral articulations, and surrounding structures (see Fig. 8-69). In many radiology departments, a full 14 × 17 inch (35 × 43 cm) projection of the thoracic spine and chest is routinely performed, in particular for trauma patients. These larger field projections are typically done using a thoracic filter. With the larger field, the radiologist has a better view of the ribs, shoulder, diaphragm, and lungs (Fig. 8-70). The thoracic spine can be difficult to evaluate. CT is often used to see the vertebrae in detail (Fig. 8-71).

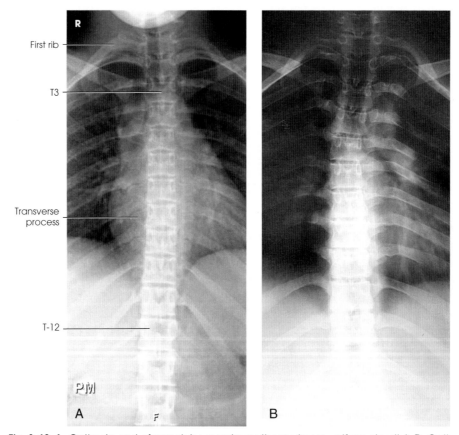

Fig. 8-69 A, Cathode end of x-ray tube over lower thorax (more uniform density). **B,** Cathode end of x-ray tube over upper thorax (nonuniform density).

Vertebral Column

Thoracic Vertebrae

◥ COMPENSATING FILTER

This projection can be improved significantly with the use of a compensating filter. Various wedge filters are available to assist in providing an even density of the entire thoracic spine on one image.

The following should be clearly shown:
- Evidence of proper collimation
- All 12 thoracic vertebrae
- All vertebrae shown with uniform density (or two radiographs can be taken for the upper and lower vertebrae)
- X-ray beam collimated to the thoracic spine as shown in Fig. 8-69, *A*

- Spinous processes at the midline of the vertebral bodies
- Vertebral column aligned to the middle of the radiograph
- Ribs, shoulders, lungs, and diaphragm if a 14 × 17 inch (35 × 43 cm) IR is used

RESEARCH: This projection was researched and standardized by Laura Aaron, PhD, RT(R)(M)(QM).

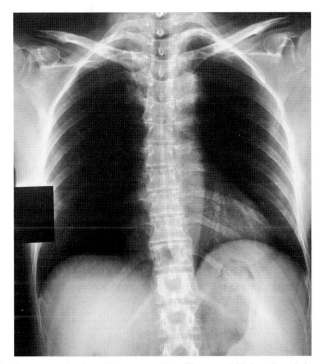

Fig. 8-70 Entire thorax projection. Compensating filter used. Note all vertebrae shown at same density.

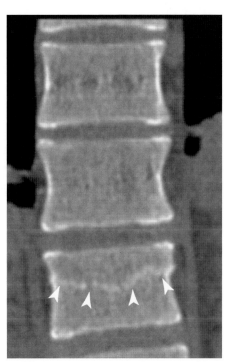

Fig. 8-71 CT thin-section scan thoracic spine shows unstable injury at T-5 after car accident. Arrows show various fractures.

⚕ LATERAL PROJECTION
R or L position

Image receptor: 14 × 17 inch (35 × 43 cm) or 7 × 17 inch (18 × 43 cm) lengthwise

Position of patient

- Place the patient in the lateral recumbent position. (*Note:* Oppenheimer[1] also suggests the use of the upright position.)
- If possible, use the left lateral position to place the heart closer to the IR, which minimizes overlapping of the vertebrae by the heart.
- Have the patient dressed in an open-backed gown so that the vertebral column can be exposed for adjustment of the position.

[1]Oppenheimer A: The apophyseal intervertebral articulations roentgenologically considered, *Radiology* 30:724, 1938.

Position of part

- Place a firm pillow under the patient's head to keep the long axis of the vertebral column horizontal.
- Flex the patient's hips and knees to a comfortable position.
- Place the superior edge of the IR 1½ to 2 inches (3.8 to 5 cm) above the relaxed shoulders. Center the posterior half of the thorax to the midline of the grid and at the level of T7 (Fig. 8-72). T7 is at the inferior angle of the scapulae.
- With the patient's knees exactly superimposed to prevent rotation of the pelvis, a small sandbag may be placed between the knees.
- Adjust the patient's arms at right angles to the long axis of the body to elevate the ribs enough to clear the intervertebral foramina.

- If the long axis of the vertebral column is not horizontal, elevate the lower or upper thoracic region with a radiolucent support (Fig. 8-73). This is the *preferred method.*
- *Shield gonads.*
- *Respiration:* The exposure can be made with the patient breathing normally to obliterate or diffuse the vascular markings and ribs or at the end of expiration.
- When the breathing technique is used, the patient should be instructed not to move. An increased exposure time (with a corresponding decrease in mA) can often improve visualization of the thoracic vertebrae.

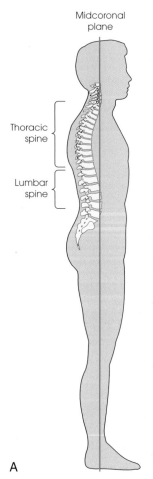
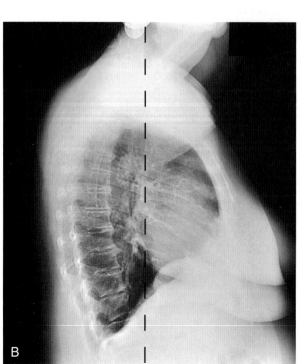

Fig. 8-72 A, Lateral view of body showing midcoronal plane. The plane divides the thorax in half, and thoracic vertebrae lie in posterior half. Centering for lateral thoracic vertebrae is on posterior half of thorax. **B,** Lateral chest showing entire thorax. Thoracic vertebrae are located in posterior half of thorax.

Central ray

- Perpendicular to the center of the IR at the level of T7 (inferior angles of the scapulae). The central ray enters the *posterior half* of the thorax.
- If the vertebral column is not elevated to a horizontal plane when the patient is in a recumbent position, angle the tube to direct the central ray perpendicular to the long axis of the thoracic column, and then center it at the level of T7. An average angle of 10 degrees cephalad is sufficient in most female patients; an average angle of 15 degrees is satisfactory in most male patients because of their greater shoulder width (Fig. 8-74; see Fig. 8-73). Fig. 8-75 shows positioning of the central ray for an upright lateral thoracic spine.

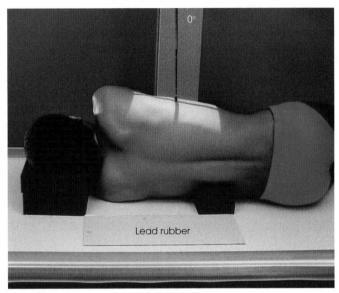

Fig. 8-73 Recumbent lateral thoracic spine. Support placed under lower thoracic region; perpendicular central ray. This is the preferred method of positioning.

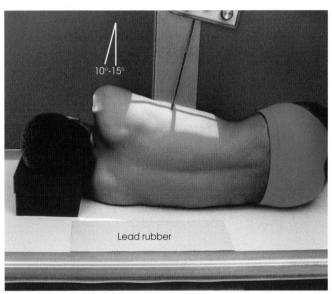

Fig. 8-74 No support under lower thoracic spine; central ray angled 10 to 15 degrees cephalad.

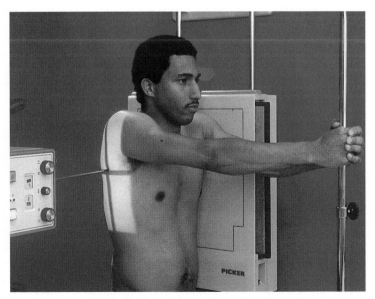

Fig. 8-75 Upright lateral thoracic spine.

Collimation

- Adjust to 7 × 17 inches (18 × 43 cm) on the collimator.

Improving radiographic quality

The quality of the radiographic image can be improved if a sheet of leaded rubber is placed on the table behind the patient (see Figs. 8-73 and 8-74). The lead absorbs the scatter radiation coming from the patient and prevents table scatter from affecting the image. Scatter radiation decreases the quality of the radiograph and blackens the spinous processes. More important with automatic exposure control (AEC), the scatter radiation coming from the patient is often sufficient to terminate the exposure prematurely. The resulting image may be underexposed because of the effect of the scatter radiation on the AEC device. For the same reason, close collimation is necessary for lateral spine radiographs; this is crucial when using digital radiography.

Structures shown

The resulting image is a lateral projection of the thoracic bodies that shows their interspaces, the intervertebral foramina, and the lower spinous processes. Because of the overlapping shoulders, the upper vertebrae may not be shown in this position (Figs. 8-76 and 8-77). If the upper thoracic area is the area of interest, a *swimmer's lateral* may be included with the examination. The younger the patient, the easier it is to show the upper thoracic bodies.

The following should be clearly shown:

- Evidence of proper collimation
- Vertebrae clearly seen through rib and lung shadows
- Twelve thoracic vertebrae centered on the IR. Superimposition of the shoulders on the upper vertebrae may cause underexposure in this area. The number of vertebrae visualized depends on the size and shape of the patient. T1 to T3 are not well visualized.
- Ribs superimposed posteriorly to indicate that the patient was not rotated
- Open intervertebral disk spaces
- Wide latitude of exposure
- X-ray beam tightly collated to reduce scatter radiation

RESEARCH: This projection was researched and standardized by Laura Aaron, PhD, RT(R)(M)(QM).

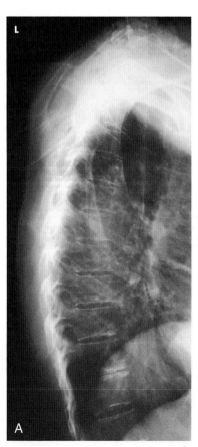 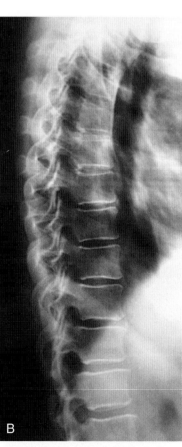

Fig. 8-76 Lateral thoracic spine. **A,** Suspended respiration with exposure of ½ second. **B,** Breathing technique with exposure of 1½ seconds. Note that lung's markings are blurred.

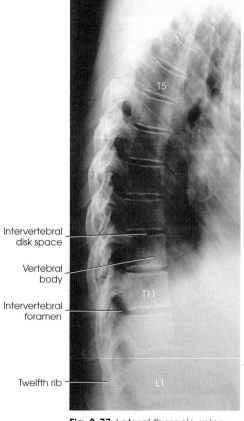

Intervertebral disk space

Vertebral body

Intervertebral foramen

Twelfth rib

T5

T11

L1

Fig. 8-77 Lateral thoracic spine with breathing technique.

AP OR PA OBLIQUE PROJECTION
RAO and LAO or RPO and LPO
Upright and recumbent positions

The thoracic zygapophyseal joints are examined using PA oblique projections as recommended by Oppenheimer[1] or using AP oblique projections as recommended by Fuchs.[2] The joints are well shown with either projection. AP obliques show the joints *farthest* from the IR, and PA obliques show the joints *closest* to the IR. Although the difference in OID between the two projections is not great, the same rotation technique is used bilaterally.

---

[1]Oppenheimer A: The apophyseal intervertebral articulations roentgenologically considered, *Radiology* 30:724, 1938.
[2]Fuchs AW: Thoracic vertebrae (part 2), *Radiogr Clin Photogr* 17:42, 1941.

Upright position

Image receptor: 14 × 17 inch (35 × 43 cm)

Position of patient
- Place the patient, standing or sitting upright, in a lateral position before a vertical grid.

Position of part
- Rotate the body 20 degrees anterior (PA oblique) or posterior (AP oblique) so that the coronal plane forms an angle of 70 degrees from the plane of the IR.
- Center the patient's vertebral column to the midline of the grid, and have the patient rest the adjacent shoulder firmly against it for support.
- Adjust the height of the IR 1½ to 2 inches (3.8 to 5 cm) above the shoulders to center the IR to T7.

- For the PA oblique, flex the elbow of the arm adjacent to the grid and rest the hand on the hip. For the AP oblique, the arm adjacent to the grid is brought forward to avoid superimposing the humerus on the upper thoracic vertebrae.
- For the PA oblique, have the patient grasp the side of the grid device with the outer hand (Fig. 8-78). For the AP oblique, have the patient place the outer hand on the hip.
- Adjust the patient's shoulders to lie in the same horizontal plane.
- Have the patient stand straight to place the long axis of the vertebral column parallel with the IR.
- The weight of the patient's body must be equally distributed on the feet, and the head must not be turned laterally.
- *Shield gonads.*
- *Respiration:* Suspend at the end of expiration.

NOTE: See p. 444 for Summary of Oblique Projections.

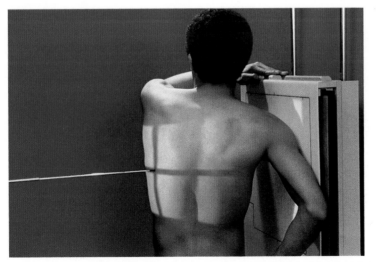
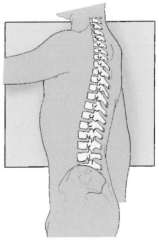

Fig. 8-78 PA oblique zygapophyseal joints: RAO for joints closest to film.

Recumbent position

Image receptor: 14 × 17 inch (35 × 43 cm) or 7 × 17 inch (18 × 43 cm)

Position of patient
- Place the patient in a lateral recumbent position.
- Elevate the head on a firm pillow so that its midsagittal plane is continuous with that of the vertebral column.
- Flex the patient's hips and knees to a comfortable position.

Position of part
- For anterior (PA oblique) rotation, place the lower arm behind the back and the upper arm forward with the hand on the table for support (Fig. 8-79).
- For posterior (AP oblique) rotation, adjust the lower arm at right angles to the long axis of the body, flex the elbow, and place the hand under or beside the head. Place the upper arm posteriorly and support it (Fig. 8-80).
- Rotate the body slightly, either anteriorly or posteriorly 20 degrees, so that the coronal plane forms an angle of 70 degrees with the horizontal.
- Center the vertebral column to the midline of the grid.
- Center the IR 1½ to 2 inches (3.8 to 5 cm) above the shoulders to center it at the level of T7.
- If needed, apply a compression band across the hips, but be careful not to change the position.
- *Shield gonads.*
- *Respiration:* Suspend at the end of expiration.

Central ray
- Perpendicular to the IR exiting or entering the level of T7

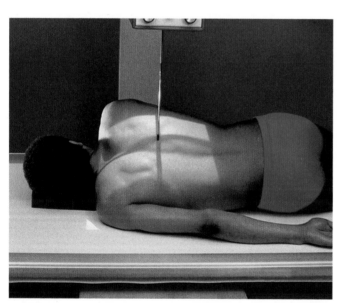

Fig. 8-79 PA oblique zygapophyseal joints: LAO for joints closest to film.

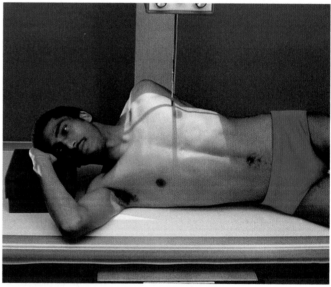

Fig. 8-80 AP oblique zygapophyseal joints: RPO for joints farthest from film.

Structures shown

The images show oblique projections of the zygapophyseal joints (*arrows* on Figs. 8-81 and 8-82). The number of joints shown depends on the thoracic curve. A greater degree of rotation from the lateral position is required to show the joints at the proximal and distal ends of the region in patients with an accentuated dorsal kyphosis. The inferior articular processes of T12, having an inclination of about 45 degrees, are not shown in this projection. (See Summary of Oblique Projections on p. 444.)

The following should be clearly shown:

- All 12 thoracic vertebrae
- Zygapophyseal joints closest to the IR on PA obliques and the joints farthest from the film on AP obliques
- Wide exposure latitude

NOTE: The AP oblique projection shows the cervicothoracic spinous processes well and is used for this purpose when the patient cannot be satisfactorily positioned for a direct lateral projection.

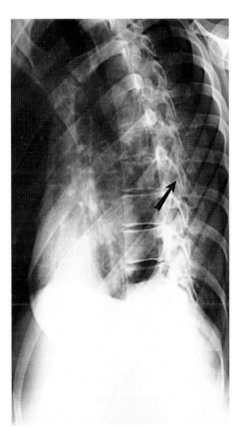

Fig. 8-81 Upright PA oblique zygapophyseal joints: LAO position. *Arrow* indicates articulation that is closest to IR.

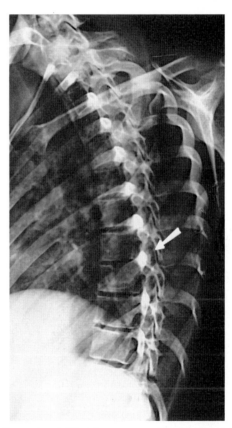

Fig. 8-82 Recumbent AP oblique zygapophyseal joints: RPO position. *Arrow* indicates articulation that is farthest from IR.

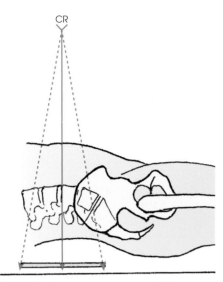

Fig. 8-83 Lumbar spine showing intervertebral disk spaces are not parallel; diverging central ray (*CR*).

♠ AP PROJECTION
PA PROJECTION (OPTIONAL)

If possible, gas and fecal material should be cleared from the intestinal tract for the examination of bones lying within the abdominal and pelvic regions. The urinary bladder should be emptied just before the examination to eliminate superimposition caused by the secondary radiation generated within a filled bladder.

An AP or PA projection may be used, but the AP projection is more commonly employed. The AP projection is generally used for recumbent examinations. The extended limb position accentuates the lordotic curve resulting in distortion of the bodies and poor delineation of the intervertebral disk spaces (Figs. 8-83 and 8-84). This curve can be reduced by flexing the patient's hips and knees enough to place the back in firm contact with the radiographic table (Figs. 8-85 and 8-86).

The PA projection places the intervertebral disk spaces at an angle closely paralleling the divergence of the beam of radiation (Fig. 8-87; see Fig. 8-84, *C*). This projection also reduces the dose to the patient.[1] For this reason, the PA projection is sometimes used for upright studies of the lumbar and lumbosacral spine.

---

[1]Heriard JB, Terry JA, Arnold AL: Achieving dose reduction in lumbar spine radiography, *Radiol Technol* 65:97, 1993.

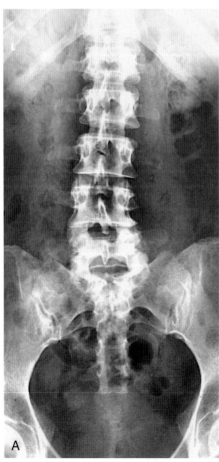

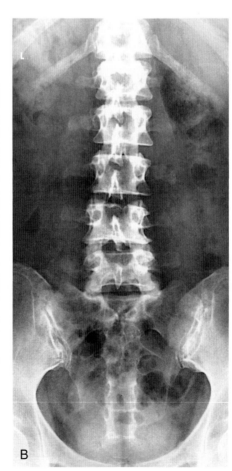

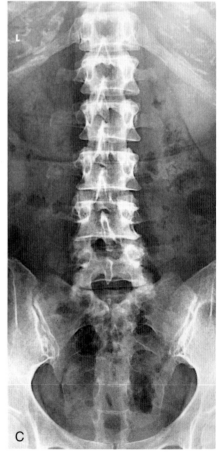

Fig. 8-84 Lumbar spine: AP and PA comparison on same patient. **A,** AP with limbs extended. **B,** AP with limbs flexed. **C,** PA.

Special positioning

- If a patient is having *severe* back pain, place a footboard on the radiographic table, and stand the table upright before beginning the examination.
- Have the patient stand on the footboard, and position the part for the projection.
- Turn the table to the horizontal position for the exposure and return it to the upright position for the next projection.
- Although this procedure takes a few minutes, the patient appreciates its ability to minimize the pain.

Image receptor: 14 × 17 inch (35 × 43 cm)

SID: 48 inches (122 cm) is suggested to reduce distortion and open the intervertebral joint spaces more completely.

Position of patient

- Examine the lumbar or lumbosacral spine with the patient recumbent.

Position of part

- Center the midsagittal plane of the patient's body to the midline of the grid.
- Adjust the patient's shoulders and hips to lie in the same horizontal plane.

- Flex the patient's elbows, and place the hands on the upper chest so that the forearms do not lie within the exposure field.
- A radiolucent support under the lower pelvic side can be used to reduce rotation when necessary.
- Reduce lumbar lordosis by flexing the patient's hips and knees enough to place the back in firm contact with table (see Fig. 8-86).
- To show the lumbar spine and sacrum, center the 14 × 17 inch (35 × 43 cm) IR at the level of the iliac crests (L4). Carefully palpate the crest of the ilium. It is possible to be misled by the contour of the heavy muscles and fatty tissue lying above the bone.
- To show the lumbar spine only, center the IR 1½ inches (3.8 cm) above the iliac crest (L3).
- *Shield gonads.*
- *Respiration:* Suspend at the end of expiration.

Central ray

- Perpendicular to the IR at the level of the iliac crests (L4) for a *lumbosacral* examination.

Collimation

- Adjust to 8 × 17 inches (18 × 43 cm) on the collimator for a routine examination and 14 × 17 inches (35 × 43 cm) when a full abdomen image is requested. Ensure that the sacroiliac joints are included.

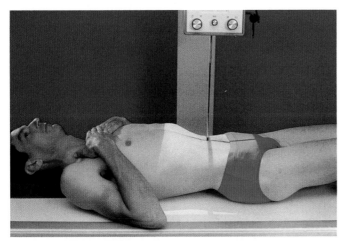

Fig. 8-85 AP lumbar spine with limbs extended, creating increased lordotic curve.

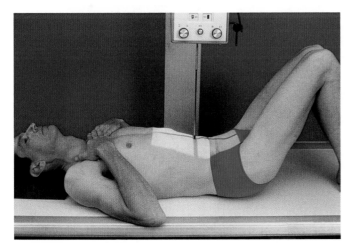

Fig. 8-86 AP lumbar spine with limbs flexed, decreasing lordotic curve.

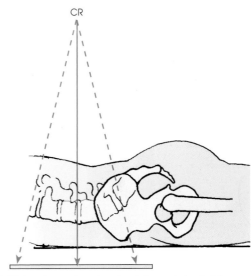

Fig. 8-87 Lumbar spine showing intervertebral disk spaces nearly parallel with divergent PA x-ray beam.

Structures shown, AP and PA

The image shows the lumbar bodies, intervertebral disk spaces, interpediculate spaces, laminae, and spinous and transverse processes (Fig. 8-88). When the larger IR is used, the images include one or two of the lower thoracic vertebrae, the sacrum coccyx, and the pelvic bones. Because of the angle at which the last lumbar segment joins the sacrum, this lumbosacral disk space is not shown well in the AP projection. The positions used for this purpose are described in the next several sections.

Many radiologists request or prefer that the AP projection be performed with the collimator open to the IR size. This projection provides additional information about the abdomen, in particular when the projection is done for trauma purposes. The larger field enables visualization of the liver, kidney, spleen, and psoas muscle margins along with air or gas patterns (see Fig. 8-88, *B*). CT and magnetic resonance imaging (MRI) are used often specifically to identify pathology (Fig. 8-89).

The following should be clearly shown:
- Evidence of proper collimation
- Area from the lower thoracic vertebrae to the sacrum
- X-ray beam collimated to the lateral margin of the psoas muscles
- No artifact across the mid-abdomen from any elastic in the patient's underclothing
- X-ray penetration of all vertebral structures
- Open intervertebral joints
- Sacroiliac joints equidistant from the vertebral column
- Symmetric vertebrae, with spinous processes centered to the bodies

RESEARCH: This projection was researched and standardized by Laura Aaron, PhD, RT(R)(M)(QM).

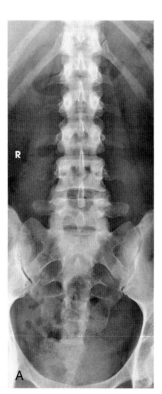
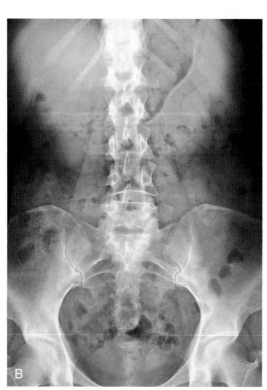
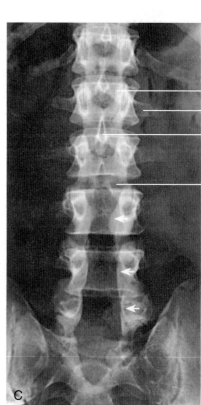

L1 vertebrae

Transverse process

L1 spinous process

L2-L3 intervertebral joint

Fig. 8-88 AP lumbosacral spine. **A,** Close collimation technique. **B,** Collimation opened to IR size 14 × 17 inch (35 × 43 cm) to show abdomen along with lumbar spine. **C,** AP lumbar spine showing spina bifida (*arrows*).

Vertebral Column

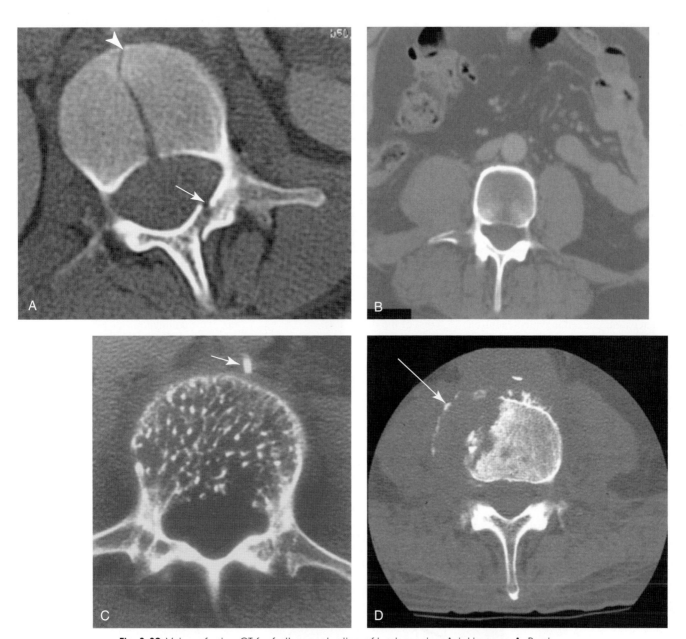

Fig. 8-89 Value of using CT for further evaluation of lumbar spine. Axial images. **A,** Burst fracture of L2. Fracture of vertebral body (*arrowhead*) and fracture of left lamina (*arrow*). **B,** Fracture of transverse process of L4. **C,** Hemangioma of L3 with no involvement of pedicles or laminae. *Arrow* points to catheter in common third artery for CT angiography. **D,** Osteomyelitis seen in L3. *Arrow* points to tuberculous abscess with paravertebral calcification in wall.

♠ LATERAL PROJECTION
R or L position

Image receptor: 14 × 17 inch (35 × 43 cm)

Position of patient
- For the lateral position, use the same body position (recumbent or upright) as for the AP or PA projection.
- Have the patient dressed in an open-backed gown so that the spine can be exposed for final adjustment of the position.

Position of part
- Ask the patient to turn onto the affected side and flex the hips and knees to a comfortable position.
- When examining a thin patient, adjust a suitable pad under the dependent hip to relieve pressure.

- Align the midcoronal plane of the body to the midline of the grid and ensure that it is vertical. On most patients, the long axis of the bodies of the lumbar spine is situated in the midcoronal plane (Fig. 8-90).
- With the patient's elbow flexed, adjust the dependent arm at right angles to the body.
- To prevent rotation, superimpose the knees exactly, and place a small sandbag between them.
- Place a suitable radiolucent support under the lower thorax, and adjust it so that the long axis of the spine is *horizontal* (Fig. 8-91, *A*). This is the *preferred method* of positioning the spine.
- When using a 14 × 17 inch (35 × 43 cm) IR, center it at the level of the crest of the ilium (L4).
- *Respiration:* Suspend at the end of expiration.

Central ray
- Perpendicular to the level of the crest of the ilium (L4) when using a 14 × 17 inch (35 × 43 cm) IR. The central ray enters the midcoronal plane (see Fig. 8-91, *A*).
- When the spine cannot be adjusted so that it is horizontal, angle the central ray caudad so that it is perpendicular to the long axis (see Fig. 8-91, *B*). The degree of central ray angulation depends on the angulation of the lumbar column and the breadth of the pelvis. In most instances, an average caudal angle of 5 degrees for men and 8 degrees for women with a wide pelvis is used.

Collimation
- Adjust to 8 × 17 inches (18 × 43 cm) on the collimator.

Structures shown
The image shows the lumbar bodies and their interspaces, the spinous processes, and the lumbosacral junction (Fig. 8-92). This projection gives a profile image of the intervertebral foramina of L1-4. The L5 intervertebral foramina (right and left) are not usually well visualized in this projection because of their oblique direction. Consequently, oblique projections are used for these foramina.

EVALUATION CRITERIA
The following should be clearly shown:
- Evidence of proper collimation
- Area from the lower thoracic vertebrae to the coccyx using 14 × 17 inch (35 × 43 cm) IR
- Open intervertebral disk spaces and intervertebral foramina
- Superimposed posterior margins of each vertebral body
- Vertebrae aligned down the middle of the image
- Nearly superimposed crests of the ilia when the x-ray beam is not angled
- Spinous processes in profile

RESEARCH: This projection was rewritten and standardized by Laura Aaron, PhD, RT(R)(M)(QM).

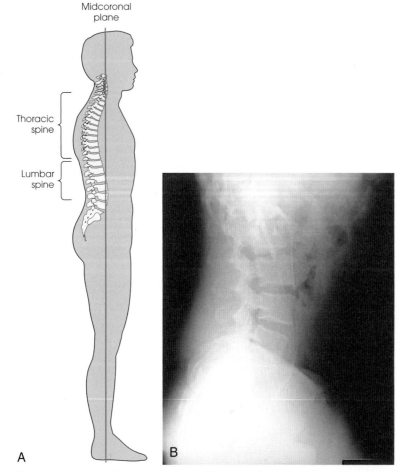

Midcoronal plane

Thoracic spine

Lumbar spine

A

B

Fig. 8-90 A, Lateral view of body showing midcoronal plane. The plane goes through lumbar bodies. **B,** Lateral abdomen showing lumbar bodies located near midcoronal plane.

Improving radiographic quality

The quality of the radiographic image can be improved if a sheet of leaded rubber is placed on the table behind the patient (see Fig. 8-91). The lead absorbs scatter radiation coming from the patient and prevents table scatter. Scatter radiation decreases the quality of the radiograph and blackens the spinous processes. More importantly, with AEC, scatter radiation coming from the patient is often sufficient to terminate the exposure prematurely. As a result, the image may be underexposed. For the same reason, close collimation is necessary for lateral spine radiographs. Scattered radiation control is crucial when using computed radiography.

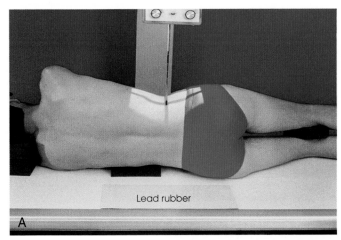 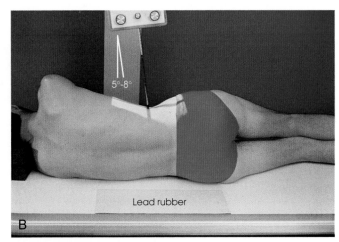

Fig. 8-91 Lateral lumbar spine. **A,** Horizontal spine and perpendicular central ray. This is the preferred method of positioning. **B,** Spine is angled and central ray directed caudad to be perpendicular to long axis of spine.

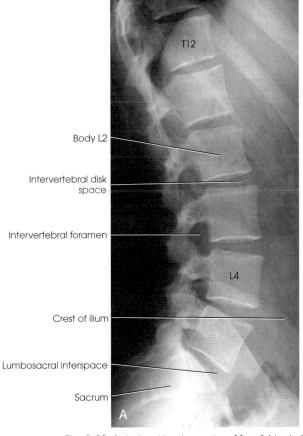 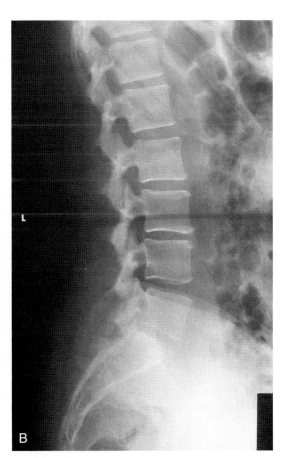

Fig. 8-92 **A,** Lateral lumbar spine, 11 × 14 inch (28 × 35 cm) IR. **B,** Lateral lumbosacral spine, 14 × 17 inch (35 × 43 cm) IR.

L5-S1 Lumbosacral Junction

♠ LATERAL PROJECTION
R or L position

Image receptor: 8 × 10 inch (18 × 24 cm)

Position of patient
- Examine the L5-S1 lumbosacral region with the patient in the lateral recumbent position.

Position of part
- With the patient in the recumbent position, adjust the pillow to place the midsagittal plane of the head in the same plane with the spine.
- Adjust the midcoronal plane of the body (passing through the hips and shoulders) so that it is perpendicular to the IR.
- Flex the patient's elbow, and adjust the dependent arm in a position at right angles to the body (Fig. 8-93, *A*).

- If possible, fully extend the patient's hips for this study.
- As described for the lateral projection, place a radiolucent support under the lower thorax and adjust it so that the long axis of the spine is *horizontal* (see Fig. 8-93, *A*). This is the *preferred method.*
- Superimpose the knees exactly, and place a support between them.
- *Shield gonads.*
- *Respiration:* Suspend.

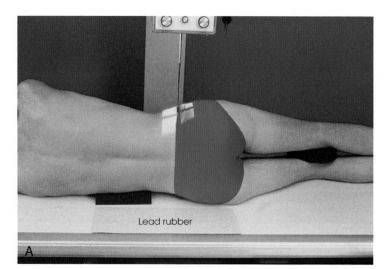

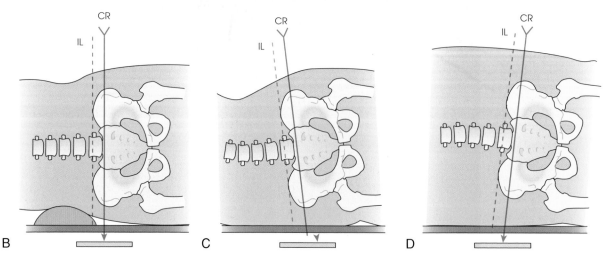

Fig. 8-93 A, Lateral L5-S1. **B,** Optimal L5-S1 joint position. Lower abdomen is blocked to place spine parallel with IR. Interiliac (*IL*) line is perpendicular, and central ray (*CR*) is perpendicular. **C,** Typical lumbar spine curvature. If blocking cannot be used, angle CR caudad and parallel to IL. **D,** Typical lumbar spine position in a patient with a large waist. IL shows that CR must be angled cephalad to open joint space.

(Modified from Francis C: Method improves consistency in L5-S1 joint space films, *Radiol Technol* 63:302, 1992.)

Central ray

- The elevated anterior superior iliac spine (ASIS) is easily palpated and found in all patients when lying on the side. The ASIS provides a standardized and accurate reference point from which to center the L5-S1 junction.
- Center on a coronal plane 2 inches (5 cm) posterior to ASIS and 1½ inches (3.8 cm) inferior to iliac crest.
- Center the IR to the central ray.
- Use close collimation.
- When the spine is not in the true horizontal position, the central ray is angled 5 degrees caudally for male patients and 8 degrees caudally for female patients.

- Francis[1] identified an alternative technique to show the open L5-S1 interspace when the spine is not horizontal:
  1. With the patient in the lateral position, locate both iliac crests.
  2. Draw an imaginary line between the two points (interiliac plane).
  3. Adjust central ray angulation to be parallel with the interiliac line (see Fig. 8-93, *B* to *D*).

Collimation

- Adjust to 6 × 8 inches (15 × 20 cm) on the collimator. This is a high-scatter projection. Close collimation is essential.

Structures shown

The resulting image shows a lateral projection of the lumbosacral junction, the lower one or two lumbar vertebrae, and the upper sacrum (Fig. 8-94).

---

[1]Francis C: Method improves consistency in L5-S1 joint space films, *Radiol Technol* 63:302, 1992.

The following should be clearly shown:
- Evidence of proper collimation
- Open lumbosacral intervertebral joint
- Collimated x-ray beam that includes all of L5 and the upper sacrum
- Lumbosacral joint in the center of the exposure area
- Crests of the ilia closely superimposing each other when the x-ray beam is not angled

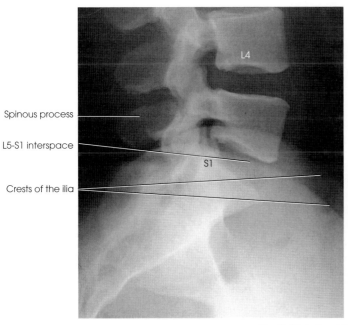

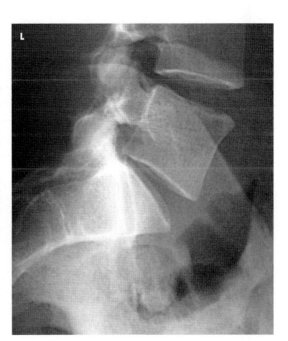

Spinous process

L5-S1 interspace

Crests of the ilia

L4

S1

L

Fig. 8-94 Lateral L5-S1.

♠ AP OBLIQUE PROJECTION
RPO and LPO positions

The plane of the zygapophyseal joints of the lumbar vertebrae forms an angle of 30 to 60 degrees to the midsagittal plane in most patients. The angulation varies from patient to patient, however, and from cephalad to caudad and side to side in the same patient (see Table 8-3). For comparison, radiographs are generally obtained from both sides.

Image receptor: 14 × 17 inch (35 × 43 cm) or 8 × 10 inch (18 × 24 cm) for the last zygapophyseal joint

Position of patient

- When oblique projections are indicated, they are generally performed immediately after the AP projection and in the same body position (recumbent or upright).

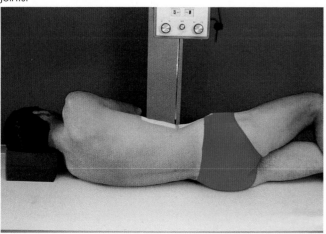

Fig. 8-95 AP oblique lumbar spine: RPO for right zygapophyseal joints.

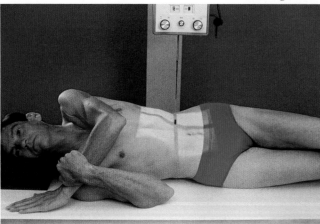

Fig. 8-96 AP oblique lumbar spine: LPO for left zygapophyseal joints.

Position of part

- Have the patient turn from the supine position toward the affected side approximately 45 degrees to show the joints *closest* to the IR (opposite the thoracic zygapophyseal joints).
- Adjust the patient's body so that the long axis of the patient is parallel with the long axis of the radiographic table.
- Center the patient's spine to the midline of the grid. In the oblique position, the lumbar spine lies in the longitudinal plane that passes 2 inches (5 cm) medial to the elevated ASIS.
- Ask the patient to place the arms in a comfortable position. A support may be placed under the elevated shoulder, hip, and knee to avoid patient motion (Figs. 8-95 and 8-96).
- Check the degree of body rotation, and make any necessary adjustments. An oblique body position 60 degrees from the plane of the IR may be needed to show the L5-S1 zygapophyseal joint and articular processes.
- *Shield gonads.*

- *Respiration:* Suspend at the end of expiration.

NOTE: Although the customary 45-degree oblique body position shows most L3-S1 zygapophyseal joint spaces, 25% of L1-2 and L2-3 joints are shown on an AP projection, and a small percentage of L4-5 and L5-S1 joints are seen on a lateral projection.

Central ray
Lumbar region
- Enter 2 inches (5 cm) medial to the elevated ASIS and 1½ inches (3.8 cm) above the iliac crest (L3).
Fifth zygapophyseal joint
- Enter 2 inches (5 cm) medial to the elevated ASIS and then up to a point midway between the iliac crest and the ASIS.
- Center the IR to the central ray.

Collimation
- 9 × 14 inches (23 × 35 cm) for 14 × 17 inches (35 × 43 cm) IR
- 8 × 10 inches (18 × 24 cm) for 8 × 10 inches (18 × 24 cm) IR

Structures shown
The resulting image shows an oblique projection of the lumbar or lumbosacral spine or both, showing the articular processes of the side closest to the IR. Both sides are examined for comparison (Figs. 8-97 and 8-98).

When the body is placed in a 45-degree oblique position and the lumbar spine is radiographed, the articular processes and the zygapophyseal joints are shown. When the patient has been properly positioned, images of the lumbar vertebrae have the appearance of Scottie dogs. Fig. 8-97 identifies the different structures that compose the Scottie dog. (See Summary of Oblique Projections, p. 444.)

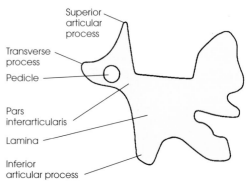

Superior articular process

Transverse process

Pedicle

Pars interarticularis

Lamina

Inferior articular process

Fig. 8-97 Parts of Scottie dog.

Zygapophyseal Joints

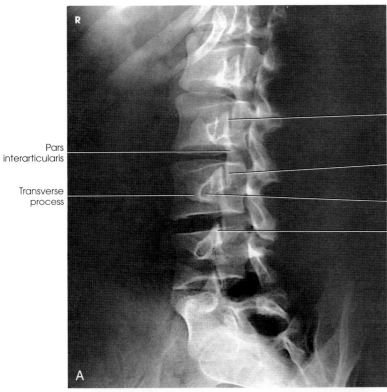

Zygapophyseal joint

Inferior articular process

Pedicle

Superior articular process

Pars interarticularis

Transverse process

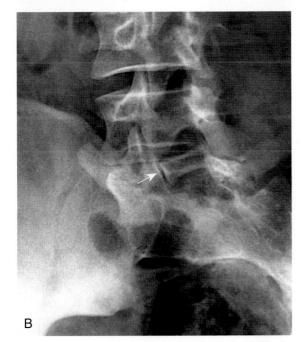

Fig. 8-98 A, AP oblique lumbar spine: RPO for right zygapophyseal joints. (Note Scottie dogs.) **B,** AP oblique lumbar spine: RPO showing L5-S1 zygapophyseal joint (*arrow*) using a 60-degree position.

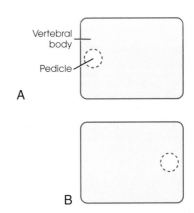

Vertebral body

Pedicle

Fig. 8-99 *Box* represents vertebral body, and *circle* represents pedicle. **A,** Pedicle is anterior on vertebral body, which means the patient is not rotated enough. **B,** Pedicle is posterior on vertebral body, which means the patient is rotated too much.

Zygapophyseal Joints

PA OBLIQUE PROJECTION
RAO and LAO positions

Image receptor: 14 × 17 inch (35 × 43 cm) lengthwise; 8 × 10 inch (18 × 24 cm) for last zygapophyseal joint

Position of patient
- Examine the patient in the upright or recumbent prone position. The recumbent position is generally used because it facilitates immobilization.
- Greater ease in positioning the patient and a resultant higher percentage of success in duplicating results make the semiprone position preferable to the semisupine position. The OID is increased, however, which can affect resolution.

Position of part
- The joints *farthest* from the IR are shown with the PA oblique projection (opposite thoracic zygapophyseal joints).

- From the prone position, have the patient turn to a semiprone position and support the body on the forearm and flexed knee.
- Align the body to center L3 to the midline of the grid (Fig. 8-100).
- Adjust the degree of body rotation to an angle of 45 degrees. An oblique body position 60 degrees from the plane of the IR may be needed to show the L5-S1 zygapophyseal joints and articular processes.
- Center the IR at the level of L3.
- To show the lumbosacral joint, position the patient as described previously but center L5.
- *Shield gonads.*
- *Respiration:* Suspend at the end of expiration.

Central ray
- Perpendicular to enter L3 (1 to 1½ inches [2.5 to 3.8 cm] above the crest of the ilium). The central ray enters the elevated side approximately 2 inches (5 cm) lateral to the palpable spinous process.

Structures shown
The image shows an oblique projection of the lumbar or lumbosacral vertebrae, showing the articular processes of the side farther from the IR (Figs. 8-101 to 8-103). The T12-L1 articulation between the 12th thoracic and 1st lumbar vertebrae, having the same direction as those in the lumbar region, is shown on the larger IR. The fifth lumbosacral joint is usually well shown in oblique positions (see Fig. 8-103).

When the body is placed in a 45-degree oblique position, and the lumbar spine is radiographed, the articular processes and zygapophyseal joints are shown. When the patient has been properly positioned, images of the lumbar vertebrae have the appearance of Scottie dogs. Fig. 8-101 identifies the different structures that compose the Scottie dog. (See Summary of Oblique Projections, p. 444.)

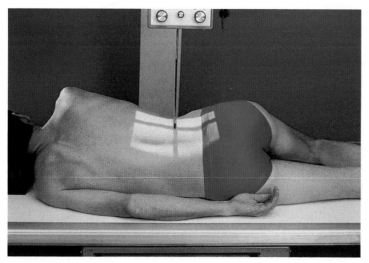

Fig. 8-100 PA oblique lumbar spine: LAO for right zygapophyseal joint.

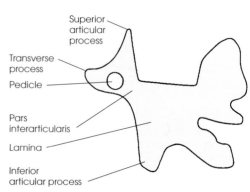

Superior articular process

Transverse process

Pedicle

Pars interarticularis

Lamina

Inferior articular process

Fig. 8-101 Parts of Scottie dog.

Zygapophyseal Joints

EVALUATION CRITERIA

The following should be clearly shown:

- Area from the lower thoracic vertebrae to the sacrum
- Zygapophyseal joints *farthest* from the IR
  - ☐ When the joint is not well seen, and the pedicle is quite anterior on the vertebral body, the patient is not rotated enough.
  - ☐ When the joint is not well seen, and the pedicle is quite posterior on the vertebral body, the patient is rotated too much.
- Vertebral column parallel with the tabletop so that the T12-L1 and L1-2 intervertebral joint spaces remain open

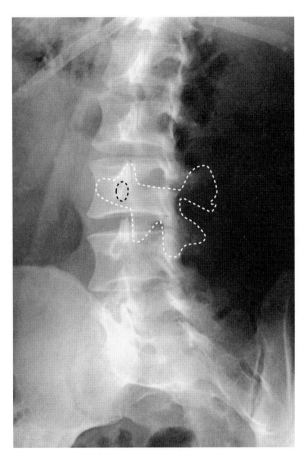

Fig. 8-102 PA oblique lumbar spine: LAO for right zygapophyseal joints. (Note Scottie dogs.)

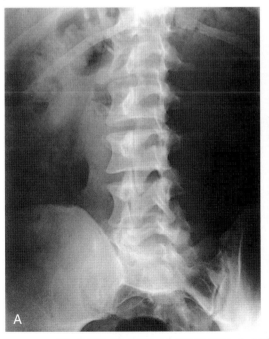 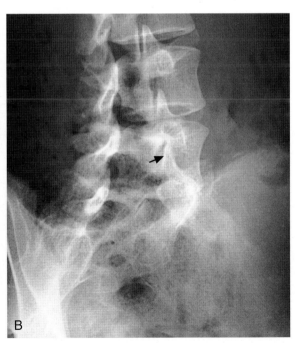

Fig. 8-103 PA oblique lumbar spine. **A,** LAO for right zygapophyseal joints. **B,** RAO for left L5 zygapophyseal joint (*arrow*).

♠ AP OR PA AXIAL PROJECTION
FERGUSON METHOD[1]

Image receptor: 8 × 10 inch (18 × 24 cm) or 10 × 12 inch (24 × 30 cm) lengthwise

[1]Ferguson AB: The clinical and roentgenographic interpretation of lumbosacral anomalies, *Radiology* 22:548, 1934.

Position of patient
- For the AP axial projection of the lumbosacral and sacroiliac joints, position the patient in the supine position.

Position of part
- With the patient supine and the midsagittal plane centered to the grid, extend the patient's lower limbs or abduct the thighs and adjust in the vertical position (Fig. 8-104).

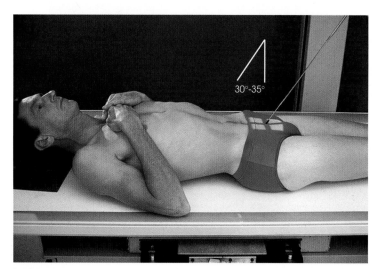

Fig. 8-104 AP axial lumbosacral junction and sacroiliac joints: Ferguson method.

- Ensure that the pelvis is not rotated.
- *Shield gonads.*
- *Respiration:* Suspend.

Central ray
- Ferguson originally recommended an angle of 45 degrees.
- Directed through the lumbosacral joint at an average angle of 30 to 35 degrees cephalad.[1] The central ray enters about 1½ inches (3.8 cm) superior to the pubic symphysis on the midsagittal plane (Fig. 8-105).
- An angulation of 30 degrees in male patients and 35 degrees in female patients is usually satisfactory. By noting the contour of the lower back, unusual accentuation or diminution of the lumbosacral angle can be estimated, and the central ray angulation can be varied accordingly.
- Center the IR to the central ray.

Collimation
- Adjust to 8 × 10 inches (18 × 24 cm) or 10 × 12 inches (24 × 30 cm) on the collimator.

Structures shown
The resulting image shows the lumbosacral joint and a symmetric image of both sacroiliac joints free of superimposition (Fig. 8-106).

[1]Lisbon E, Bloom RA: Anteroposterior angulated view, *Radiology* 149:315, 1983.

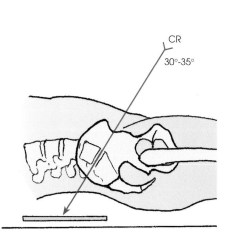

Fig. 8-105 AP axial sacroiliac joints: Ferguson method.

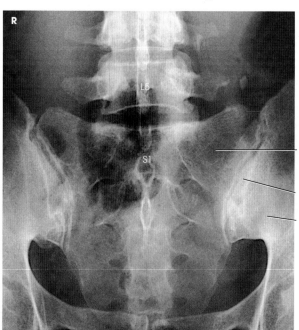

Fig. 8-106 AP axial lumbosacral junction and sacroiliac joints: Ferguson method.

Lumbosacral Junction and Sacroiliac Joints

The following should be clearly shown:
- Evidence of proper collimation
- Lumbosacral junction and sacrum
- Open intervertebral space between L5 and S1
- Both sacroiliac joints adequately penetrated

NOTE: The PA axial projection for the lumbosacral junction can be modified in accordance with the AP axial projection just described. With the patient in the prone position, the central ray is directed through the lumbosacral joint to the midpoint of the IR at an average angle of 35 degrees caudad. The central ray enters the spinous process of L4 (Figs. 8-107 and 8-108).

Meese[1] recommended the prone position for examinations of the sacroiliac joints because their obliquity places them in a position more nearly parallel with the divergence of the beam of radiation. The central ray is directed perpendicularly and is centered at the level of the ASIS. It enters the midline of the patient about 2 inches (5 cm) distal to the spinous process of L5 (Fig. 8-109).

---

[1]Meese T: Die dorso-ventrale Aufnahme der Sacro-iliacalgelenke, *Fortschr Roentgenstr* 85:601, 1956.

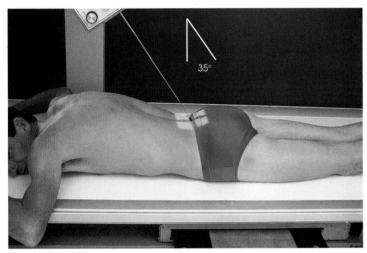

Fig. 8-107 PA axial lumbosacral junction and sacroiliac joints.

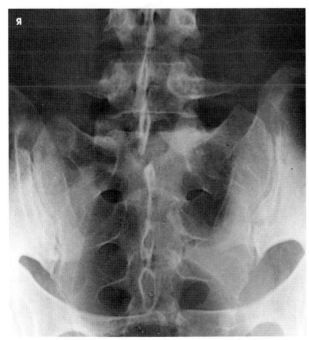

Fig. 8-108 PA axial lumbosacral junction and sacroiliac joints.

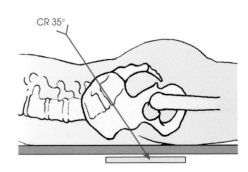

Fig. 8-109 PA bilateral sacroiliac joints.

AP OBLIQUE PROJECTION
RPO and LPO positions

Image receptor: 8 × 10 inch (18 × 24 cm) or 10 × 12 inch (24 × 30 cm) lengthwise. Both obliques are usually obtained for comparison.

Position of patient
- Place the patient in the supine position, and elevate the head on a firm pillow.

Position of part
- Use the LPO position to show the right joint and the RPO position to show the left joint. The side being examined is farther from the IR.
- Elevate the side under examination approximately 25 to 30 degrees, and support the shoulder, lower thorax, and upper thigh (Figs. 8-110 and 8-111).
- Adjust the patient's body so that its long axis is parallel with the long axis of the radiographic table.

- Align the body so that a sagittal plane passing 1 inch (2.5 cm) medial to the ASIS of the elevated side is centered to the midline of the grid.
- Check the rotation at several points along the back.
- Center the IR at the level of the ASIS.
- *Shield gonads.* Collimating close to the joint may shield the gonads in male patients. It may be difficult to use contact shielding in female patients.
- *Respiration:* Suspend.

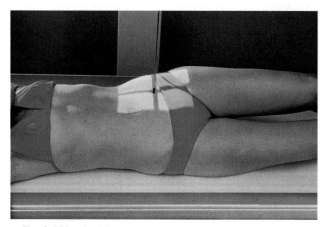

Fig. 8-110 AP oblique sacroiliac joint. RPO shows left joint.

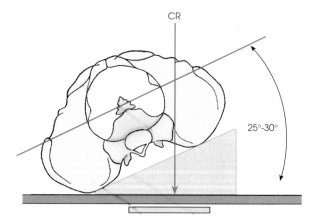

Fig. 8-111 Degree of obliquity required to show sacroiliac joint for AP projection.

Central ray

- Perpendicular to the center of the IR, entering 1 inch (2.5 cm) medial to the elevated ASIS

Collimation

- Adjust to 6 × 10 inches (15 × 24 cm) or 6 × 12 inches (15 × 30 cm) on the collimator.

Structures shown

The image shows the sacroiliac joint *farthest* from the IR and an oblique projection of the adjacent structures. Both sides are examined for comparison (Fig. 8-112). (See Summary of Oblique Projections, p. 444.)

The following should be clearly shown:
- Evidence of proper collimation
- Open sacroiliac joint space with minimal overlapping of the ilium and sacrum
- Joint centered on the radiograph

NOTE: An AP axial oblique can be obtained by positioning the patient as described. For the AP axial oblique, the central ray is directed at an angle of 20 to 25 degrees cephalad, entering 1 inch (2.5 cm) medial and 1½ inches (3.8 cm) distal to the elevated ASIS (Fig. 8-113).

NOTE: Brower and Kransdorf[1] summarized difficulties in imaging the sacroiliac joints because of patient positioning and variability.

---

[1]Brower AC, Kransdorf MJ: Evaluation of disorders of the sacroiliac joint, *Appl Radiol* 21:31, 1992.

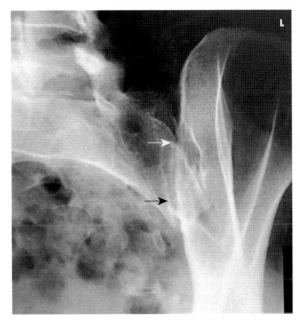

Fig. 8-112 AP oblique sacroiliac joint. RPO shows left joint (*arrows*).

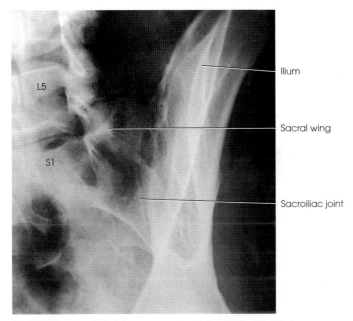

Fig. 8-113 AP axial oblique sacroiliac joint. RPO with 20-degree cephalad angulation shows left joint.

PA OBLIQUE PROJECTION
RAO and LAO positions

Image receptor: 8 × 10 inch (18 × 24 cm) or 10 × 12 inch (24 × 30 cm) lengthwise. Both obliques are usually obtained for comparison.

Position of patient
- Place the patient in a semiprone position.
- Use the RAO position to show the right joint and the LAO position to show the left joint. The side being examined is *closer* to the IR.
- Have the patient rest on the forearm and flexed knee of the elevated side.
- Place a small, firm pillow under the head.

Position of part
- Adjust the patient by rotating the side of interest toward the radiographic table until a body rotation of 25 to 30 degrees is achieved. The forearm and flexed knee usually furnish sufficient support for this position.
- Check the degree of rotation at several points along the anterior surface of the patient's body.
- Adjust the patient's body so that its long axis is parallel with the long axis of the table.

- Center the body so that a point 1 inch (2.5 cm) medial to the ASIS closest to the IR is centered to the grid (Figs. 8-114 and 8-115).
- Center the IR at the level of the ASIS.
- *Shield gonads.* Collimating close to the joint may shield the gonads in male patients. It may be difficult to use contact shielding in female patients.
- *Respiration:* Suspend.

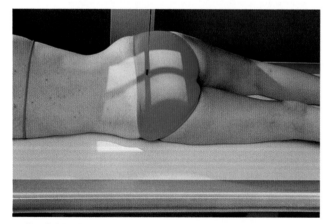

Fig. 8-114 PA oblique sacroiliac joint. LAO shows left joint.

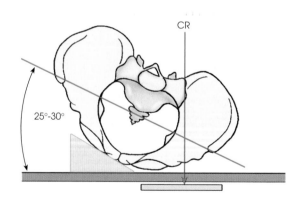

Fig. 8-115 Degree of obliquity required to show sacroiliac joint for PA projection.

Central ray

- Perpendicular to the IR and centered 1 inch (2.5 cm) medial to the ASIS closest to the IR

Structures shown

The resulting image shows the sacroiliac joint closest to the IR (Fig. 8-116). (See Summary of Oblique Projections, p. 444.)

The following should be clearly shown:

- Open sacroiliac joint space closest to the IR or minimal overlapping of the ilium and sacrum
- Joint centered on the radiograph

NOTE: A PA axial oblique can be obtained by positioning the patient as described previously. For the PA axial oblique, the central ray is directed 20 to 25 degrees caudad to enter the patient at the level of the transverse plane, pass 1½ inches (3.8 cm) distal to the L5 spinous process, and exit at the level of the ASIS (Fig. 8-117).

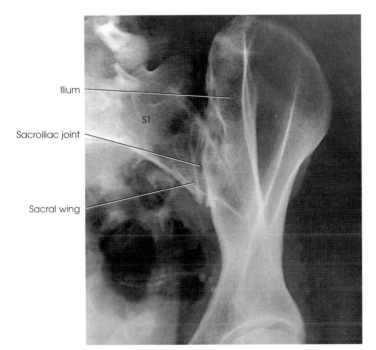

Fig. 8-116 PA oblique sacroiliac joint. LAO shows left joint.

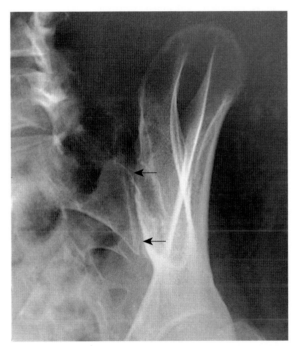

Fig. 8-117 PA axial oblique sacroiliac joint. LAO with 20-degree caudal central ray shows left joint (*arrows*).

♠ AP AND PA AXIAL PROJECTIONS

Because bowel content may interfere with the image, the colon should be free of gas and fecal material for examinations of the sacrum and coccyx. A physician's order for a bowel preparation may be needed. The urinary bladder should be emptied before the examination.

Image receptor: 10 × 12 inch (24 × 30 cm) for sacrum; 8 × 10 inch (18 × 24 cm) for coccyx

Position of patient

- Place the patient in the supine position for the AP axial projection of the sacrum and coccyx so that the bones are as close as possible to the IR. The supine position is most often used. The prone position can be used without appreciable loss of detail and is particularly appropriate for patients with a painful injury or destructive disease.

Position of part

- With the patient either supine or prone, center the midsagittal plane of the body to the midline of the table grid.
- Adjust the patient so that both ASIS are equidistant from the grid.
- Have the patient flex the elbows and place the arms in a comfortable, bilaterally symmetric position.
- When the supine position is used, place a support under the patient's knees.
- *Shield gonads* on men. Women cannot be shielded for this projection.
- *Respiration:* Suspend.

Central ray

Sacrum

- With the patient supine, direct the central ray 15 degrees cephalad and center it to a point 2 inches (5 cm) superior to the pubic symphysis (Figs. 8-118 to 8-120).
- With the patient prone, angle the central ray 15 degrees caudad and center it to the clearly visible sacral curve (Fig. 8-121).

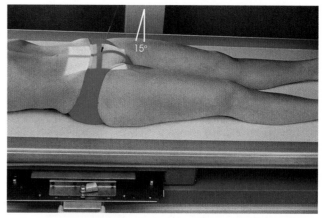

Fig. 8-118 AP axial sacrum.

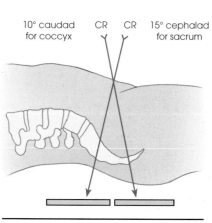

Fig. 8-119 CR angles for AP axial sacrum and coccyx.

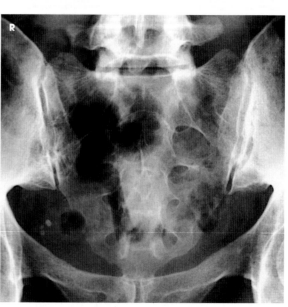

Fig. 8-120 AP axial sacrum.

Coccyx

- With the patient *supine,* direct the central ray 10 degrees caudad and center it to a point about 2 inches (5 cm) superior to the pubic symphysis (Figs. 8-122 and 8-123).
- With the patient *prone,* angle the central ray 10 degrees cephalad and center it to the easily palpable coccyx.
- Center the IR to the central ray.

Collimation

- *Sacrum:* 10 × 12 inches (24 × 30 cm)
- *Coccyx:* 8 × 10 inches (18 × 24 cm)

Structures shown

The resulting image shows the sacrum or coccyx free of superimposition (see Figs. 8-120, 8-121, and 8-123).

EVALUATION CRITERIA

The following should be clearly shown:
- Evidence of proper collimation
  ### Sacrum
- Sacrum free of foreshortening, with the sacral curvature straightened
- Pubic bones not overlapping the sacrum
- Short-scale contrast
- No rotation of the sacrum, as indicated by symmetric alae
- Sacrum centered and seen in its entirety

- Tight collimation evident to improve the radiographic contrast
- Fecal material not overlapping the sacrum
  ### Coccyx
- Coccygeal segments not superimposed
- Short-scale contrast on the radiograph
- No rotation
- Coccyx centered and seen in its entirety
- Tight collimation evident to improve the visibility

Radiation protection

- Because the ovaries lie within the exposure area, use close collimation for female patients to limit the irradiated area and the amount of scatter radiation.
- For male patients, use gonad shielding in addition to close collimation.

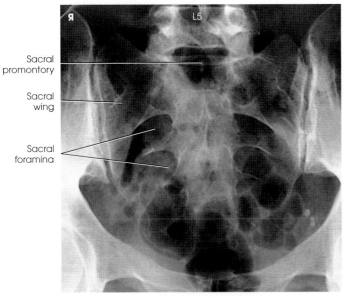

Sacral promontory

Sacral wing

Sacral foramina

Fig. 8-121 PA axial sacrum.

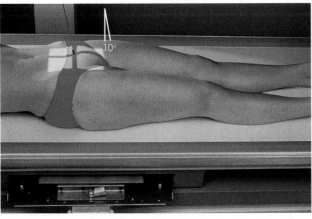

Fig. 8-122 AP axial coccyx.

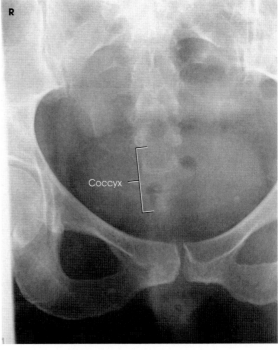

Coccyx

Fig. 8-123 AP axial coccyx.

Vertebral Column

✦ LATERAL PROJECTIONS
R or L position

Image receptor: 10 × 12 inch (24 × 30 cm) for sacrum; 8 × 10 inch (18 × 24 cm) lengthwise for coccyx

Position of patient
- Ask the patient to turn onto the indicated side and flex the hips and knees to a comfortable position.

Position of part
- Adjust the arms in a position at right angles to the body.
- Superimpose the knees, and if needed, place positioning sponges under and between the ankles and between the knees.
- Adjust a support under the body to place the long axis of the spine horizontal. The interiliac plane is perpendicular to the IR.
- Adjust the pelvis and shoulders so that the true lateral position is maintained (i.e., no rotation) (Figs. 8-124 and 8-125).
- To prepare for accurate positioning of the central ray, center the sacrum or coccyx to the midline of the grid.
- *Shield gonads.*
- *Respiration:* Suspend.

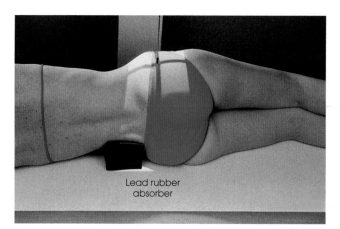

Fig. 8-124 Lateral sacrum.

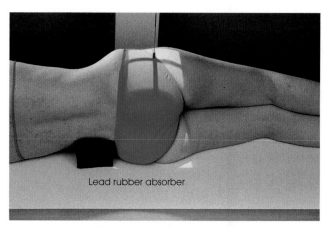

Fig. 8-125 Lateral coccyx.

Sacrum and Coccyx

Central ray

- The elevated ASIS is easily palpated and found on all patients when they are lying on their side and provides a standardized reference point from which to center the sacrum and coccyx (Fig. 8-126).

Sacrum

- Perpendicular and directed to the level of the ASIS and to a point 3½ inches (9 cm) posterior. This centering should work with most patients. The exact position of the sacrum depends on the pelvic curve.

Coccyx

- Perpendicular and directed toward a point 3½ inches (9 cm) posterior to the ASIS and 2 inches (5 cm) inferior. This centering should work for most patients. The exact position of the coccyx depends on the pelvic curve.
- Center the IR to the central ray.
- Use close collimation.

Collimation

- *Sacrum:* 10 × 12 inches (24 × 30 cm)
- *Coccyx:* 6 × 8 inches (15 × 20 cm)

Structures shown

The resulting image shows a lateral projection of the sacrum or coccyx (Figs. 8-127 and 8-128).

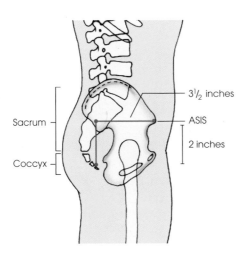

Fig. 8-126 Lateral sacrum, coccyx, and ilium (*dashed outline*) showing centering points. ASIS provides a standardized reference point for central ray positioning.

Improving radiographic quality

The quality of the radiograph can be improved if a sheet of leaded rubber is placed on the table behind the patient (see Figs. 8-124 and 8-125). The lead absorbs the scatter radiation coming from the patient. Scatter radiation decreases the quality of the radiograph. More importantly, with AEC the scatter radiation coming from the patient is often sufficient to terminate the exposure prematurely, resulting in an underexposed radiograph. For the same reason, close collimation is necessary for lateral sacrum and coccyx images. This is crucial when using CT.

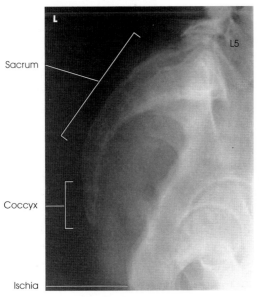

Fig. 8-127 Lateral sacrum.

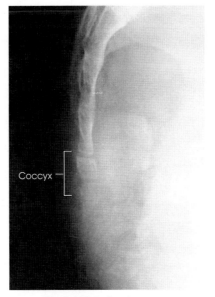

Fig. 8-128 Lateral coccyx.

Lumbar Intervertebral Disks

PA PROJECTION
WEIGHT-BEARING METHOD
R and L bending

Image receptor: 14 × 17 inch (35 × 43 cm) lengthwise

Position of patient
- Perform this examination with the patient in the standing position. Duncan and Hoen[1] recommended that the PA projection be used because in this direction the divergent rays are more nearly parallel with the intervertebral disk spaces.

[1]Duncan W, Hoen T: A new approach to the diagnosis of herniation of the intervertebral disc, *Surg Gynecol Obstet* 75:257, 1942.

Position of part
- With the patient facing the vertical grid device, adjust the height of the IR to be at the level of L3.
- Adjust the patient's pelvis for rotation by ensuring that the ASIS are equidistant from the IR.
- Center the midsagittal plane of the patient's body to the midline of the vertical grid device (Fig. 8-129).
- Let the patient's arms hang unsupported by the sides.
- Make one radiograph with the patient *bending* to the right and one with the patient *bending* to the left (Fig. 8-130).

- Have the patient lean directly lateral as far as possible without rotation and without lifting the foot. The degree of bending must not be forced, and the patient must not be supported in position.
- Ensure that the midsagittal plane of the lower lumbar column and sacrum remains centered to the grid device as the upper portion moves laterally.
- *Shield gonads.*
- *Respiration:* Suspend.

Central ray
- Directed perpendicular to L3 at an angle of 15 to 20 degrees caudad or projected through the L4-5 or L5-S1 interspaces, if these are the areas of interest
- Use close collimation.

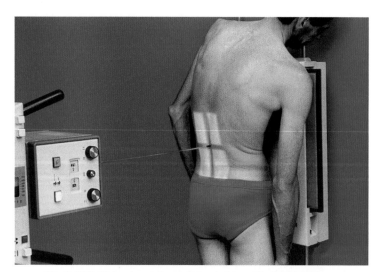

Fig. 8-129 PA lumbar intervertebral disks with right bending.

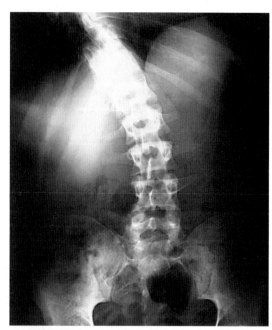

Fig. 8-130 PA lumbar radiograph. Note pelvis is straight, and only lumbar spine is bent.

Structures shown

The resulting images show bending PA projections of the lower thoracic region and the lumbar region for demonstration of the mobility of the intervertebral joints. In patients with disk protrusion, this type of examination is used to localize the involved joint as shown by limitation of motion at the site of the lesion (see Fig. 8-130).

EVALUATION CRITERIA

The following should be clearly shown:
- Area from the lower thoracic interspaces to all of the sacrum
- No rotation of the patient in the bending position
- Bending direction correctly identified on the image with appropriate lead markers

Radiation protection

The PA projection is recommended instead of the AP projection whenever the clinical information provided by the examination is not compromised. With the PA projection, the patient's gonad area and breast tissue receive significantly less radiation than when the AP projection is used. In addition, proper collimation reduces the radiation dose to the patient. Lead shielding material should be placed between the x-ray tube and a male patient's gonads to protect this area further from unnecessary radiation.

☀ PA AND LATERAL PROJECTIONS

FRANK ET AL. METHOD[1,2,3]

The method described has been endorsed by the American College of Radiology, the Academy of Orthopedic Physicians, and Center for Development and Radiation Health of the Department of Health and Human Services. Endorsement includes use of the PA projection, compensating filters, lateral breast protection, and non-use of graduated screens.

Scoliosis is an abnormal lateral curvature of the vertebral column with some associated rotation of the vertebral bodies at the curve. This condition may be caused by disease, surgery, or trauma, but it is frequently idiopathic. Scoliosis is commonly detected in the adolescent years. If not detected and treated, it may progress to the point of debilitation.

---

[1]Frank ED et al: Use of the posteroanterior projection: a method of reducing x-ray exposure to specific radiosensitive organs, *Radiol Technol* 54:343, 1983.
[2]Frank ED et al: A method of reducing x-ray exposure to specific radiosensitive organs, *Can J Radiol* 15(2):10, 1984.
[3]Gray JE, Stears JG, Frank ED: Shaped, lead-loaded filters for use in diagnostic radiology, *Radiology* 146(3):825, 1983.

Diagnosis and monitoring of scoliosis requires a series of radiographs that may include upright, supine, and bending studies. A typical scoliosis study might include the following projections:

- PA (or AP) upright
- PA (or AP) upright with lateral bending
- Lateral upright (with or without bending)
- PA (or AP) prone or supine

The PA (or AP) and lateral upright projections show the amount or degree of curvature that occurs with the force of gravity acting on the body (Fig. 8-131). Spinal fixation devices, such as Harrington rods, may also be evaluated. Bending studies are often used to differentiate between primary and compensatory curves. Primary curves do not change when the patient bends, whereas secondary curves do change with bending.

Because scoliosis is generally diagnosed and evaluated during the teenage years, proper radiographic techniques are important. Ideally, large film-screen systems and grids, such as 14 × 36 inches (35 × 90 cm), are used to show the entire spine with one exposure. The wide range of body part thicknesses and specific gravities in the thoracic and abdominal areas necessitates the use of compensating filters.

To expose the length of the 36-inch (90-cm) IR, a minimum 60-inch (152-cm) SID is used.

Digital Imaging

- The most recent advance in scoliosis radiography had been the introduction of computed radiography (CR) long imaging plates. The plate for scoliosis consists of two interlocked 14- × 17-inch (35- × 43-cm) cassettes in a 14- × 34-inch (34- × 86-cm) plate. The system contains special image stitching software that automatically merges the images together by aligning markers on the image. Image processing is applied to optimize the displayed image. One image will appear on the computer (Fig. 8-132, *A*).

Collimation

- Collimation is crucial because of the large area exposed. Adjust to 12 × 36 inches (30 × 91 cm). For the AP, adjust to 12 × 36 inches (30 × 91 cm) for the lateral. If curvature is severe, adjust to the full 14 × 36 inches (35 × 91 cm). Always check previous examination images to determine extent of curvature.

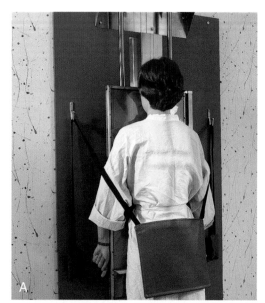 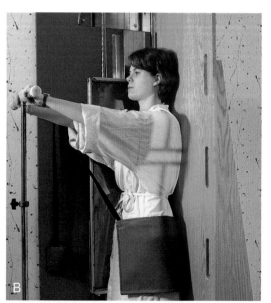

Fig. 8-131 Standing full spine radiography, using 14 × 36 inch (35 × 90 cm) IR. **A,** PA projection: Frank et al. method. **B,** Lateral projection.

RADIATION PROTECTION

In 1983, Frank et al.[1] described the use of the PA projection for radiography of scoliosis. Also in 1983, Frank and Kuntz[2] described a simple method of protecting the breasts during radiography of scoliosis. By 1986, the federal government had endorsed the use of these techniques in an article by Butler et al.[3]

Radiation protection is crucial. Collimation must be closely limited to irradiate only the thoracic and lumbar spine. The gonads should be shielded by placing a lead apron at the level of the ASIS between the patient and the x-ray tube. The breasts should be shielded with leaded rubber or leaded acrylic (Figs. 8-132 and 8-133), or the breast radiation exposure should be decreased by performing PA projections.

[1]Frank ED et al: Use of the posteroanterior projection: a method of reducing x-ray exposure to specific radiosensitive organs, *Radiol Technol* 54:343, 1983.
[2]Frank ED, Kuntz JI: A simple method of protecting the breasts during upright lateral radiography for spine deformities, *Radiol Technol* 55:532, 1983.
[3]Butler PF et al: Simple methods to reduce patient exposure during scoliosis radiography, *Radiol Technol* 57:411, 1986.

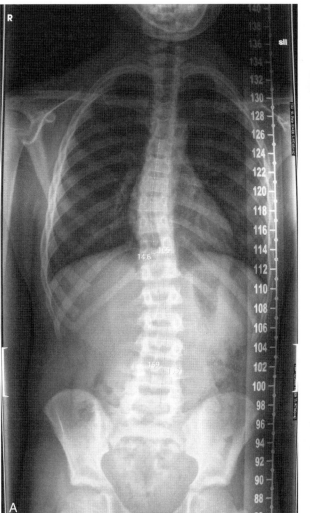
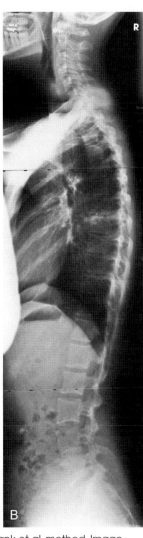

Fig. 8-132 Standing full-spine radiography. **A,** PA projection: Frank et al. method. Image was made using computed radiography (CR) plate, and computer software "stitched" the image together. **B,** Lateral projection. Note breast shielding.

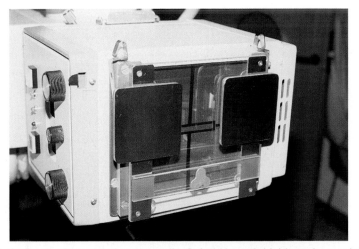

Fig. 8-133 Collimator face showing magnetically held breast shields and gonad shield.

(Courtesy Nuclear Associates, Carlyle, PA.)

⚜ PA PROJECTION
FERGUSON METHOD[1]

The patient should be positioned to obtain a PA projection (in lieu of the AP projection) to reduce radiation exposure[2] to selected radiosensitive organs. The decision whether to use a PA or AP projection is often determined by the physician or institutional policy.

Image receptor: 14 × 36 inch (35 × 90 cm) or 14 × 17 inch (35 × 43 cm) lengthwise

Position of patient

- For a PA projection, place the patient in a seated or standing position in front of a vertical grid device.
- Have the patient sit or stand straight, and then adjust the height of the IR to include about 1 inch (2.5 cm) of the iliac crests (Fig. 8-134).

---

[1]Ferguson AB: *Roentgen diagnosis of the extremities and spine,* New York, 1939, Harper & Row.
[2]Frank ED et al: Use of the posteroanterior projection: a method of reducing x-ray exposure to specific radiosensitive organs, *Radiol Technol* 54:343, 1983.

Position of part
First radiograph

- Adjust the patient in a normally seated or standing position to check the spinal curvature.
- Center the midsagittal plane of the patient's body to the midline of the grid.
- Allow the patient's arms to hang relaxed at the sides. If the patient is seated, flex the elbows and rest the hands on the lap (Fig. 8-135).
- Do not support the patient or use a compression band.
- *Shield gonads.*

Second radiograph

- Elevate the patient's hip or foot on the convex side of the primary curve approximately 3 or 4 inches (7.6 to 10.2 cm) by placing a block, a book, or sandbags under the buttock or foot (Fig. 8-136). Ferguson[1] specified that the elevation must be sufficient to make the patient expend some effort in maintaining the position.
- Do not support the patient in these positions.
- Do not employ a compression band.
- *Shield gonads.*
- *Respiration:* Suspend.

---

[1]Ferguson AB: *Roentgen diagnosis of the extremities and spine,* New York, 1939, Harper & Row.

- Obtain additional radiographs (if needed) with elevation of the hip on the side opposite the major or primary curve (Fig. 8-137) or with the patient in a recumbent position (Fig. 8-138).

Central ray
- Perpendicular to the midpoint of the IR

Collimation
- 12 × 36 inches (30 × 91 cm) for 14 × 36 inch (35 × 91 cm) IR
- 12 × 14 inches (30 × 35 cm) for 14 × 17 inch (35 × 43 cm) IR

Structures shown

The resulting images show PA projections of the thoracic and lumbar vertebrae, which are used for comparison to distinguish the deforming or primary curve from the compensatory curve in patients with scoliosis (see Figs. 8-135 to 8-138).

EVALUATION CRITERIA

The following should be clearly shown:
- Evidence of proper collimation
- Thoracic and lumbar vertebrae to include about 1 inch (2.5 cm) of the iliac crests
- Vertebral column aligned down the center of the radiograph
- Correct identification marker

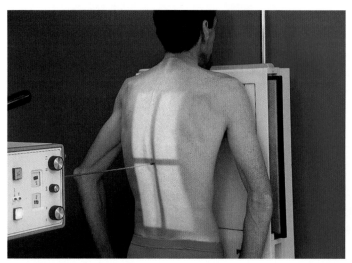

Fig. 8-134 PA thoracic and lumbar spine for scoliosis, upright.

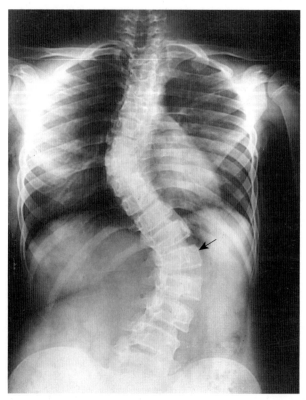

Fig. 8-135 PA thoracic and lumbar spine for scoliosis, upright, showing structural (major or primary) curve (*arrow*).

Vertebral Column

NOTE: Another widely used scoliosis series consists of four images of the thoracic and lumbar spine: a direct PA projection with the patient standing, a direct PA projection with the patient prone, and PA projections with alternate right and left lateral flexion in the prone position. The right and left bending positions are described in the next section. For the scoliosis series, 35 × 43 cm (14 × 17 inch) IRs are used and are placed to include about 1 inch (2.5 cm) of the crests of ilia.

NOTE: Young et al.[1] described their application of this scoliosis procedure in detail. They recommended the addition of a lateral position, made with the patient standing upright, to show spondylolisthesis or show exaggerated degrees of kyphosis or lordosis. Kittleson and Lim[2] described the Ferguson and the Cobb methods of measurement of scoliosis.

---

[1]Young LW et al: Roentgenology in scoliosis: contribution to evaluation and management, *Radiology* 97:778, 1970.
[2]Kittleson AC, Lim LW: Measurement of scoliosis, *AJR Am J Roentgenol* 108:775, 1970.

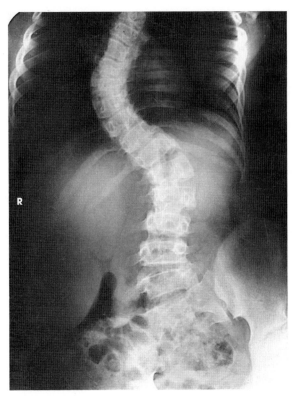

Fig. 8-136 PA thoracic and lumbar spine with left hip elevated.

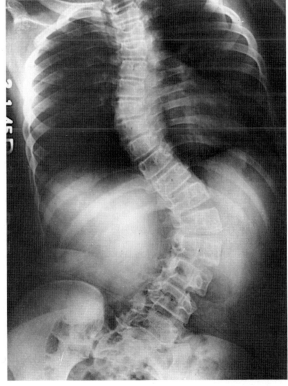

Fig. 8-137 PA thoracic and lumbar spine with right hip elevated.

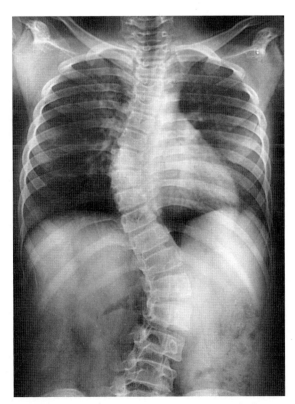

Fig. 8-138 PA thoracic and lumbar spine for scoliosis, prone.

AP PROJECTION
R and L bending

Image receptor: 10 × 12 inch (24 × 30 cm) or 14 × 17 inch (35 × 43 cm) lengthwise for each exposure

Position of patient

- Place the patient in the supine position, and center the midsagittal plane of the body to the midline of the grid.

Position of part

- Make the first radiograph with maximum right bending, and make the second radiograph with maximum left bending.
- To obtain equal bending force throughout the spine, cross the patient's leg on the opposite side to be flexed over the other leg. A right bending requires the left leg to be crossed over the right.
- Move both of the patient's heels toward the side that is flexed. Immobilize the heels with sandbags.
- Move the shoulders directly lateral as far as possible without rotating the pelvis (Fig. 8-139).
- After the patient is in position, apply a compression band to prevent movement.
- *Shield gonads.*
- *Respiration:* Suspend.

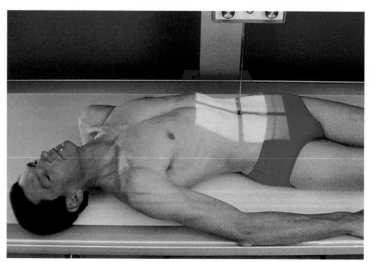

Fig. 8-139 AP lumbar spine, right bending.

Central ray

- Perpendicular to the level of the third lumbar vertebra, 1 to 1½ inches (2.5 to 3.8 cm) above the iliac crest on the midsagittal plane
- Center the IR to the central ray.

Structures shown

The resulting images show AP projections of the lumbar vertebrae, made in maximum right and left lateral flexion (Figs. 8-140 and 8-141). These studies are used in patients with early scoliosis to determine the presence of structural change when bending to the right and left. The studies are also used to localize a herniated disk as shown by limitation of motion at the site of the lesion and to show whether there is motion in the area of a spinal fusion. The latter examination is usually performed 6 months after the fusion operation.

The following should be clearly shown:

- Site of the spinal fusion centered and including the superior and inferior vertebrae
- No rotation of the pelvis (symmetric ilia)
- Bending directions correctly identified with appropriate lead markers
- Sufficient radiographic density to show the degree of movement when vertebrae are superimposed

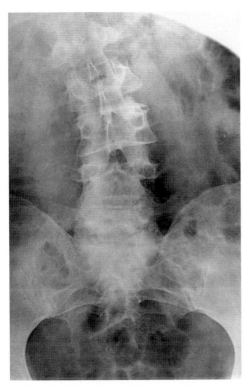

Fig. 8-140 AP lumbar spine, right bending spinal fusion series.

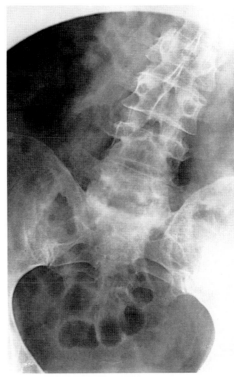

Fig. 8-141 AP lumbar spine, left bending spinal fusion series.

LATERAL PROJECTION
R or L position
Hyperflexion and hyperextension

Image receptor: 14 × 17 inch (35 × 43 cm) lengthwise for each exposure

Position of patient
- Adjust the patient in a lateral recumbent position.
- Center the midcoronal plane to the midline of the grid.

Position of part
- For the first radiograph, have the patient lean forward and draw the thighs up to flex the spine forcibly as much as possible (Fig. 8-142).

- For the second radiograph, have the patient lean the thorax backward and posteriorly extend the thighs and limbs as much as possible (Fig. 8-143).
- After the patient is in position, apply a compression band across the pelvis to prevent movement.
- Center the IR at the level of the spinal fusion.
- *Shield gonads.*
- *Respiration:* Suspend.

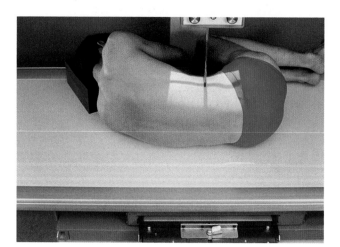

Fig. 8-142 Hyperflexion position.

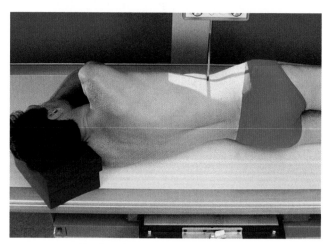

Fig. 8-143 Hyperextension position.

Lumbar Spine: Spinal Fusion

Central ray

- Perpendicular to the spinal fusion area or L3

Structures shown

The resulting images show two lateral projections of the spine made in hyperflexion (Fig. 8-144, *A*) and hyperextension (Fig. 8-144, *B*) to determine whether motion is present in the area of a spinal fusion or to localize a herniated disk as shown by limitation of motion at the site of the lesion.

The following should be clearly shown:

- Site of the spinal fusion in the center of the radiograph
- No rotation of the vertebral column (posterior margins of the vertebral bodies are superimposed)
- Hyperflexion and hyperextension identification markers correctly used for each respective projection

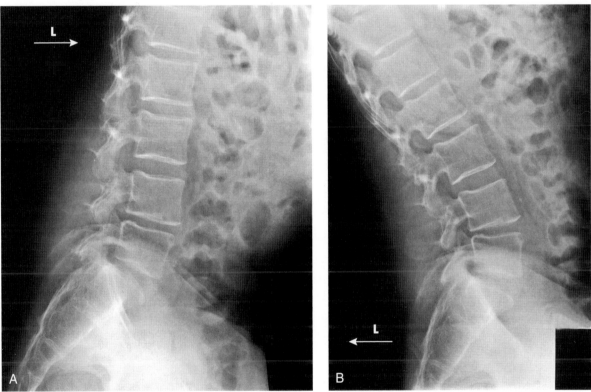

Fig. 8-144 A, Lateral with hyperflexion. **B,** Lateral with hyperextension. Note position of markers and accurate use of arrows.

SUMMARY OF OBLIQUE PROJECTIONS

CERVICAL OBLIQUES

Projection	Position—degrees	Structures shown	CR (degrees)
AP obliques	LPO—45	R: IFs (side up)	15-20
	RPO—45	L: IFs (side up)	15-20
PA obliques	LAO—45	L: IFs (side down)	15-20
	RAO—45	R: IFs (side down)	15-20

THORACIC OBLIQUES

Projection	Position—degrees	Structures shown	CR (degrees)
AP obliques	LPO—70	R: Z joints (joints up)	0
	RPO—70	L: Z joints (joints up)	0
PA obliques	LAO—70	L: Z joints (joints down)	0
	RAO—70	R: Z joints (joints down)	0

LUMBAR OBLIQUES

Projection	Position—degrees	Structures shown	CR (degrees)
AP obliques	LPO—45	L: Z joints (joints down)	0
	RPO—45	R: Z joints (joints down)	0
PA obliques	LAO—45	R: Z joints (joints up)	0
	RAO—45	L: Z joints (joints up)	0

SACROILIAC OBLIQUES

Projection	Position—degrees	Structures shown	CR (degrees)
AP obliques	LPO—25-30	R: SI joint (joint up)	0
	RPO—25-30	L: SI joint (joint up)	0
PA obliques	LAO—25-30	L: SI joint (joint down)	0
	RAO—25-30	R: SI joint (joint down)	0

IF, intervertebral foramina; *SI,* sacroiliac; *Z,* zygapophyseal.

9

BONY THORAX

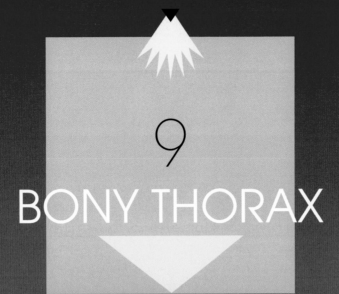

Posterior rib numbers

Anterior rib numbers

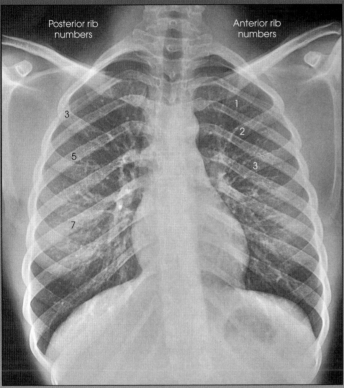

PROJECTIONS, POSITIONS, AND METHODS

Page	Essential	Anatomy	Projection	Position	Method
458	🌲	Sternum	PA oblique	RAO	
460		Sternum	PA oblique	Modified prone	MOORE
462	🌲	Sternum	Lateral	R or L upright	
464	🌲	Sternum	Lateral	R or L recumbent	
466	🌲	Sternoclavicular articulations	PA		
467	🌲	Sternoclavicular articulations	PA oblique	RAO or LAO	BODY ROTATION
468	🌲	Sternoclavicular articulations	PA oblique	RAO or LAO	CENTRAL RAY ANGULATION
474	🌲	Upper anterior ribs	PA		
476	🌲	Posterior ribs	AP		
478	🌲	Ribs: *axillary*	AP oblique	RPO or LPO	
480	🌲	Ribs: *axillary*	PA oblique	RAO or LAO	
482		Costal joints	AP axial		

The icons in the Essential column indicate projections that are frequently performed in the United States and Canada. Students should be competent in these projections.

Bony Thorax

The *bony thorax* supports the walls of the pleural cavity and diaphragm used in respiration. The thorax is constructed so that the volume of the thoracic cavity can be varied during respiration. The thorax also protects the heart and lungs.

The bony thorax is formed by the sternum, 12 pairs of ribs, and 12 thoracic vertebrae. The bony thorax protects the heart and lungs. Conical in shape, the bony thorax is narrower above than below, more wide than deep, and longer posteriorly than anteriorly.

Sternum

The *sternum,* or breastbone, is directed anteriorly and inferiorly and is centered over the midline of the anterior thorax (Figs. 9-1 to 9-3). A narrow, flat bone about 6 inches (15 cm) in length, the sternum consists of three parts: manubrium, body, and xiphoid process. The sternum supports the clavicles at the superior manubrial angles and provides attachment to the costal cartilages of the first seven pairs of ribs at the lateral borders.

The *manubrium,* the superior portion of the sternum, is quadrilateral in shape and is the widest portion of the sternum. At its center, the superior border of the manubrium has an easily palpable concavity termed the *jugular notch.* In the upright position, the jugular notch of the average person lies anterior to the interspace between the second and third thoracic vertebrae. The manubrium slants laterally and posteriorly on each side of the jugular notch, and an oval articular facet called

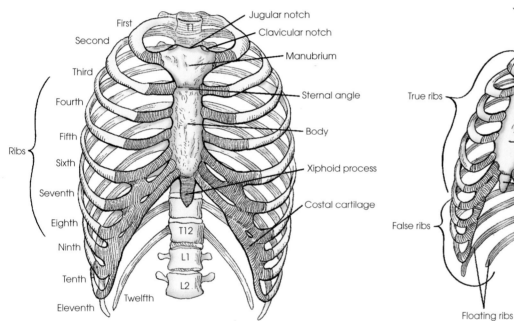

Fig. 9-1 Anterior aspect of bony thorax.

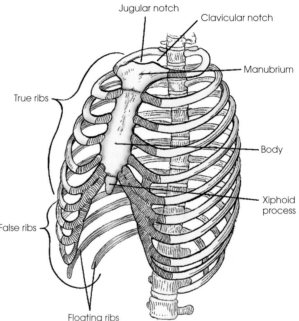

Fig. 9-2 Anterolateral oblique aspect of bony thorax.

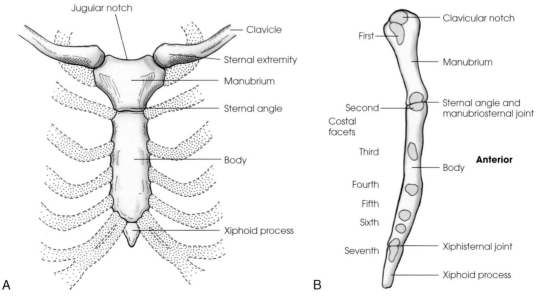

Fig. 9-3 A, Anterior aspect of sternum and sternoclavicular joints. **B,** Lateral sternum.

the *clavicular notch* articulates with the sternal extremity of the clavicle. On the lateral borders of the manubrium, immediately below the articular notches for the clavicles, are shallow depressions for the attachment of the cartilages of the first pair of ribs.

The *body* is the longest part of the sternum (4 inches [10.2 cm]) and is joined to the manubrium at the *sternal angle,* an obtuse angle that lies at the level of the junction of the second costal cartilage. The manubrium and the body contribute to the attachment of the second costal cartilage. The succeeding five pairs of costal cartilages are attached to the lateral borders of the body. The sternal angle is palpable; in the normally formed thorax, it lies anterior to the interspace between the fourth and fifth thoracic vertebrae when the body is upright.

The *xiphoid process,* the distal and smallest part of the sternum, is cartilaginous in early life and partially or completely ossifies, particularly the superior portion, in later life. The xiphoid process is variable in shape and often deviates from the midline of the body. In the normal thorax, the xiphoid process lies over the 10th thoracic vertebra and serves as a useful bony landmark for locating the superior portion of the liver and the inferior border of the heart.

Ribs

The 12 pairs of ribs are numbered consecutively from superiorly to inferiorly (Fig. 9-4; see Figs. 9-1 and 9-2). The rib number corresponds to the thoracic vertebra to which it attaches. Each rib is a long, narrow, curved bone with an anteriorly attached piece of hyaline cartilage, the *costal cartilage*. The costal cartilages of the first through seventh ribs attach directly to the sternum. The costal cartilages of the 8th through 10th ribs attach to the costal cartilage of the 7th rib. The ribs are situated in an oblique plane slanting anteriorly and inferiorly so that their anterior ends lie 3 to 5 inches (7.6 to 12.5 cm) below the level of their vertebral ends. The degree of obliquity gradually increases from the 1st to the 9th rib and then decreases to the 12th rib. The first seven ribs are called *true ribs* because they attach directly to the sternum. Ribs 8 to 12 are called *false ribs* because they do not attach directly to the sternum. The last two ribs (11th and 12th ribs) are often called *floating ribs* because they are attached only to the vertebrae. The spaces between the ribs are referred to as the *intercostal spaces*.

The number of ribs may be increased by the presence of cervical or lumbar ribs, or both. *Cervical ribs* articulate with the C7 vertebra but rarely attach to the sternum. Cervical ribs may be free or articulate or fuse with the first rib. Lumbar ribs are less common than cervical ribs. *Lumbar ribs* can lend confusion to images. They can confirm the identification of the vertebral level, or they can be erroneously interpreted as a fractured transverse process of the L1 vertebra.

Ribs vary in breadth and length. The first rib is the shortest and broadest; the breadth gradually decreases to the 12th rib, the narrowest rib. The length increases from the 1st to the 7th rib and then gradually decreases to the 12th rib.

A typical rib consists of a *head,* a flattened *neck,* a *tubercle,* and a *body* (Figs. 9-5 and 9-6). The ribs have *facets* on their heads for articulation with the vertebrae. The facet is divided on some ribs into superior and inferior portions for articulation with demifacets on the vertebral bodies. The tubercle also contains a facet for articulation with the transverse process of the vertebra. The 11th and 12th ribs do not have a neck or tubercular facets. The two ends of a rib are termed the *vertebral end* and the *sternal end*.

From the point of articulation with the vertebral body, the rib projects posteriorly at an oblique angle to the point of articulation with the transverse process. The rib turns laterally to the *angle* of the body, where the bone arches anteriorly, medially, and inferiorly in an oblique plane. Located along the inferior and internal border of each rib is the *costal groove,* which contains costal arteries, veins, and nerves. Trauma to the ribs can damage these neurovascular structures, causing pain and hemorrhage.

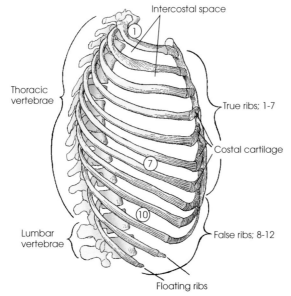

Fig. 9-4 Lateral aspect of bony thorax.

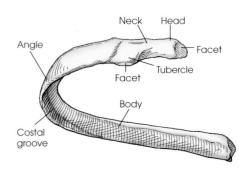

Fig. 9-5 Typical rib viewed from posterior.

Bony Thorax Articulations

The eight joints of the bony thorax are summarized in Table 9-1. A detailed description follows.

The *sternoclavicular* joints are the only points of articulation between the upper limbs and the trunk (see Fig. 9-3). Formed by the articulation between the sternal extremity of the clavicles and the clavicular notches of the manubrium, these *synovial gliding* joints permit free movement (the gliding of one surface on the other). A circular disk of fibrocartilage is interposed between the articular ends of the bones in each joint, and the joints are enclosed in articular capsules.

TABLE 9-1

Joints of the bony thorax

| Joint | Structural classification | | Movement |
	Tissue	Type	
Sternoclavicular	Synovial	Gliding	Freely movable
Costovertebral:			
1st-12th ribs	Synovial	Gliding	Freely movable
Costotransverse			
1st-10th ribs	Synovial	Gliding	Freely movable
Costochondral			
1st-10th ribs	Cartilaginous	Synchondroses	Immovable
Sternocostal			
1st rib	Cartilaginous	Synchondroses	Immovable
2nd-7th ribs	Synovial	Gliding	Freely movable
Interchondral			
6th-9th ribs	Synovial	Gliding	Freely movable
9th-10th ribs	Fibrous	Syndesmoses	Slightly movable
Manubriosternal	Cartilaginous	Symphysis	Slightly movable
Xiphisternal	Cartilaginous	Synchondroses	Immovable

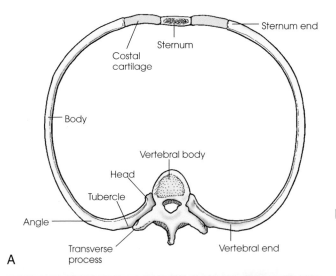

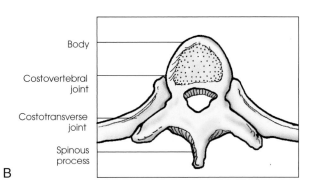

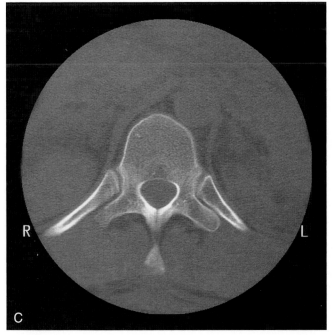

Fig. 9-6 A, Superior aspect of rib articulating with thoracic vertebra and sternum. **B,** Enlarged image of costovertebral and costotransverse articulations. **C,** MRI transverse image showing costovertebral and costotransverse articulations.

(**C,** From Kelley LL, Petersen CM: *Sectional anatomy for imaging professionals,* ed 2, St Louis, 2007, Mosby.)

Posteriorly, the head of a rib is closely bound to the demifacets of two adjacent vertebral bodies to form a synovial gliding articulation called the *costovertebral joint* (Fig. 9-7, *A*; see Fig. 9-6). The 1st, 10th, 11th, and 12th ribs each articulate with only one vertebral body.

The tubercle of a rib articulates with the anterior surface of the transverse process of the lower vertebra at the *costotransverse joint,* and the head of the rib articulates at the costovertebral joint. The head of the rib also articulates with the body of the same vertebra and articulates with the vertebra directly above. The costotransverse articulation is also a *synovial gliding* articulation. The articulations between the tubercles of the ribs and the transverse processes of the vertebrae permit only superior and inferior movements of the first six pairs. Greater freedom of movement is permitted in the succeeding four pairs.

Costochondral articulations are found between the anterior extremities of the ribs and the costal cartilages (see Fig. 9-7, *B*). These articulations are *cartilaginous synchondroses* and allow no movement. The articulations between the costal cartilages of the true ribs and the sternum are called *sternocostal* joints. The first pair of ribs, rigidly attached to the sternum, form the first sternocostal joint. This is a *cartilaginous synchondrosis* type of joint, which allows no movement. The second through seventh sternocostal joints are considered synovial gliding joints and are freely movable. *Interchondral* joints are found between the costal cartilages of the sixth and seventh, seventh and eighth, and eighth and ninth ribs (see Fig. 9-7, *C*). These interchondral joints are *synovial gliding* articulations. The interchondral articulation between the 9th and 10th ribs is a *fibrous syndesmosis* and is only slightly movable.

The *manubriosternal* joint is a *cartilaginous symphysis* joint, and the *xiphisternal* joints are *cartilaginous synchondrosis* joints that allow little or no movement (see Figs. 9-3, *B,* and 9-7, *B* and *C*).

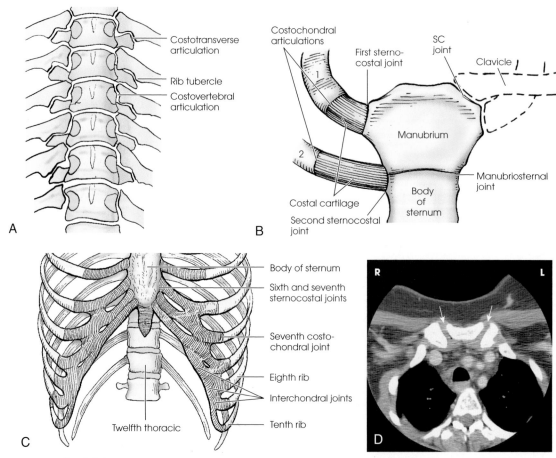

Fig. 9-7 Rib articulations. **A,** Anterior aspect of thoracic spine, showing costovertebral articulations. **B,** Anterior aspect of manubrium, sternum, and first two ribs, showing articulations. *SC,* sternoclavicular. **C,** Lower sternum and ribs, showing intercostal, costochondral, and sternocostal joints. **D,** CT cross-section image of upper thorax showing manubrium and angulation of sternoclavicular joints (*arrows*).

RESPIRATORY MOVEMENT

The normal oblique orientation of the ribs changes little during quiet respiratory movements; however, the degree of obliquity *decreases* with deep *inspiration* and *increases* with deep *expiration*. The first pair of ribs, which are rigidly attached to the manubrium, rotate at their vertebral ends and move with the sternum as one structure during respiratory movements.

On deep inspiration, the anterior ends of the ribs are carried anteriorly, superiorly, and laterally while the necks are rotated inferiorly (Fig. 9-8, *A*). On deep expiration, the anterior ends are carried inferiorly, posteriorly, and medially, while the necks are rotated superiorly (Fig. 9-8, *B*). The last two pairs of ribs are depressed and held in position by the action of the diaphragm when the anterior ends of the upper ribs are elevated during respiration.

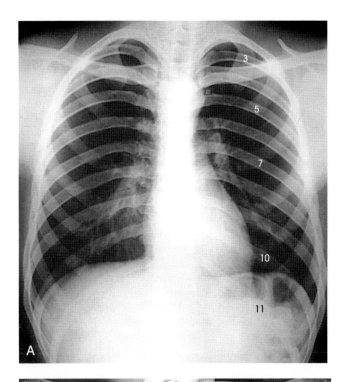

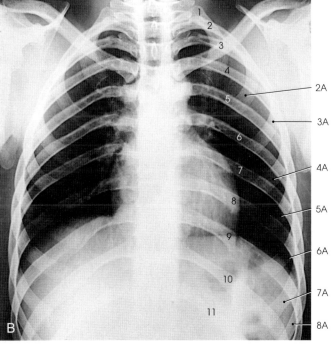

Fig. 9-8 Respiratory lung movement. **A,** Full inspiration with posterior ribs numbered. **B,** Full expiration with ribs numbered. Anterior ribs are labeled with *A*.

DIAPHRAGM

The ribs located above the diaphragm are best examined radiographically through the air-filled lungs, whereas the ribs situated below the diaphragm must be examined through the upper abdomen. Because of the difference in penetration required for the two regions, the position and respiratory excursion of the diaphragm play a large role in radiography of the ribs.

The position of the diaphragm varies with body habitus: It is at a higher level in hypersthenic patients and at a lower level in asthenic patients (Fig. 9-9). In sthenic patients of average size and shape, the right side of the diaphragm arches posteriorly from the level of about the 6th or 7th costal cartilage to the level of the 9th or 10th thoracic vertebra when the body is in the upright position. The left side of the diaphragm lies at a slightly lower level. Because of the oblique location of the ribs and the diaphragm, several pairs of ribs appear on radiographs to lie partly above and partly below the diaphragm.

The position of the diaphragm changes considerably with the body position, reaching its lowest level when the body is upright and its highest level when the body is supine. For this reason, it is desirable to place the patient in the upright position for examination of the ribs above the diaphragm and in a recumbent position for examination of the ribs below the diaphragm.

The respiratory movement of the diaphragm averages about 1½ inches (3.8 cm) between deep inspiration and deep expiration. The movement is less in hypersthenic patients and more in hyposthenic patients. Deeper inspiration or expiration and greater depression or elevation of the diaphragm are achieved on the second respiratory movement than on the first. This greater movement should be taken into consideration when the ribs that lie at the diaphragmatic level are examined.

When the body is placed in the supine position, the anterior ends of the ribs are displaced superiorly, laterally, and posteriorly. For this reason, the anterior ends of the ribs are less sharply visualized when the patient is radiographed in the supine position.

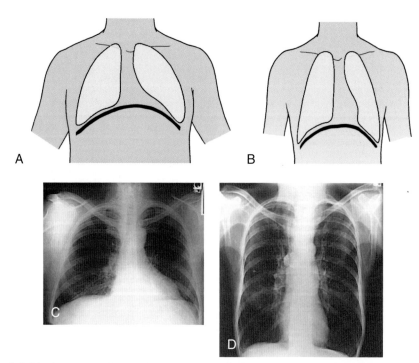

Fig. 9-9 Diaphragm position and body habitus. **A,** A hypersthenic patient has a diaphragm positioned higher. **B,** An asthenic patient has a diaphragm positioned lower. **C,** Chest radiograph of a hypersthenic patient. **D,** Chest radiograph of an asthenic patient. Note position of diaphragm on these extremely different body types.

BODY POSITION

Although in rib examinations it is desirable to take advantage of the effect that body position has on the position of the diaphragm, the effect is not of sufficient importance to justify subjecting a patient to a painful change from the upright position to the recumbent position or vice versa. Even minor rib injuries are painful, and slight movement frequently causes the patient considerable distress. Unless the change in position can be effected with a tilting radiographic table, patients with recent rib injury should be examined in the position in which they arrive in the radiology department. An ambulatory patient can be positioned for recumbent images with minimal discomfort by bringing the tilt table to the vertical position for each positioning change. The patient stands on the footboard, is comfortably adjusted, and is then lowered to the horizontal position.

TRAUMA PATIENTS

The first and usually the only requirement in the initial radiographic examination of a patient who has sustained severe trauma to the rib cage is to take AP and lateral projections of the chest. These projections are obtained not only to show the site and extent of rib injury, but also to investigate the possibility of injury to the underlying structures by depressed rib fractures. Patients are examined in the position in which they arrive, usually recumbent on a stretcher. The recumbent position is necessary to show the presence of air or fluid levels using the decubitus technique.

SUMMARY OF ANATOMY

Bony thorax	Ribs	Bony thorax articulations
Sternum	Costal cartilage	Sternoclavicular
Ribs (12)	True ribs	Costovertebral
Thoracic vertebrae (12)	False ribs	Costotransverse
	Floating ribs	Costochondral
Sternum	Cervical ribs	Sternocostal
Manubrium	Lumbar ribs	Interchondral
Jugular notch	Intercostal spaces	Manubriosternal
Clavicular notch	Head	Xiphisternal
Body	Neck	
Sternal angle	Tubercle	
Xiphoid process	Body	
	Facets	
	Vertebral end	
	Sternal end	
	Angle	
	Costal groove	

SUMMARY OF PATHOLOGY

Condition	Definition
Fracture	Disruption of the continuity of bone
Metastases	Transfer of a cancerous lesion from one area to another
Osteomyelitis	Inflammation of bone owing to a pyogenic infection
Osteopetrosis	Increased density of atypically soft bone
Osteoporosis	Loss of bone density
Paget disease	Thick, soft bone marked by bowing and fractures
Tumor	New tissue growth where cell proliferation is uncontrolled
Chondrosarcoma	Malignant tumor arising from cartilage cells
Multiple myeloma	Malignant neoplasm of plasma cells involving the bone marrow and causing destruction of bone

EXPOSURE TECHNIQUE CHART ESSENTIAL PROJECTIONS

BONY THORAX

Part	cm	kVp*	tm	mA	mAs	AEC	SID	IR	Dose†(mrad)
Sternum—*PA oblique*‡	20	65	0.22	200s	45		30″	24 × 30 cm	306
Sternum—*Lateral*‡	29	70	0.4	200s	80		72″	24 × 30 cm	710
Sternoclavicular articulations—*PA*‡	17	65		200s		○●○	40″	8 × 10 in	195
Sternoclavicular articulations—*PA oblique*‡	18	65	0.15	200s	30		40″	8 × 10 in	208
Upper anterior ribs—*PA*‡	21	70	0.16	200s	32		40″	35 × 43 cm	60
Posterior ribs—*AP upper*‡	21	70	0.16	200s	32		40″	35 × 43 cm	60
Posterior ribs—*AP lower*‡	21	70		200s		●●○	40″	35 × 43 cm	159
Ribs: axillary—*AP oblique*‡	23	70	0.16	200s	32		40″	35 × 43 cm	82
Ribs: axillary—*PA oblique*‡	23	70	0.16	200s	32		40″	35 × 43 cm	82

*kVp values are for a three-phase, 12-pulse generator or high frequency.
†Relative doses for comparison use. All doses are skin entrance for average adult at cm indicated.
‡Bucky, 16:1 grid. Screen-film speed 300 or equivalent CR.
s, Small focal spot.

Bony Thorax Articulations

Sternum

The position of the sternum with respect to the denser bony and soft tissue thoracic structures makes it a difficult structure to radiograph satisfactorily. Few problems are involved in obtaining a lateral projection, but because of the location of the sternum directly anterior to the thoracic spine, an AP or PA projection provides little useful diagnostic information. To separate the vertebrae and sternum, it is necessary to rotate the body from the prone position or to angle the central ray medially. The exact degree of required angulation depends on the depth of the chest, with deep chests requiring less angulation than shallow chests (Fig. 9-10 and Table 9-2).

Angulation of the body or the central ray to project the sternum to the right of the thoracic vertebrae clears the sternum of the vertebrae but superimposes it over the posterior ribs and the lung markings (Fig. 9-11). If the sternum is projected to the left of the thoracic vertebrae, it is also projected over the heart and other mediastinal structures (Fig. 9-12). The superimposition of the homogeneous density of the heart can be used to advantage (compare Figs. 9-11 and 9-12).

The pulmonary structures, particularly in elderly persons and heavy smokers, can cast confusing markings over the sternum, unless the motion of *shallow* breathing is used to eliminate them. If motion is desired, the exposure time should be long enough to cover several phases of shallow respiration (Figs. 9-13 and 9-14). The milliampere (mA) must be relatively low to achieve the desired milliampere-second (mAs).

If a female patient has large, pendulous breasts, they should be drawn to the sides and held in position with a wide bandage to prevent them from overlapping the sternum and to position the sternum closer to the image receptor (IR). This positioning is particularly important in the lateral projection, in which the breast can obscure the inferior portion of the sternum.

Radiation Protection

Protection of the patient from unnecessary radiation is a professional responsibility of the radiographer (see Chapter 1 for specific guidelines). In this chapter, the *Shield gonads* statement indicates that the patient is to be protected from unnecessary radiation by restricting the radiation beam using proper collimation. In addition, the placement of lead shielding between the gonads and the radiation source is appropriate when the clinical objectives of the examination are not compromised.

TABLE 9-2

Sternum: thickness and central ray angulation

Depth of thorax (cm)	Depth of tube angulation
15	22
16.5	21
18	20
19.5	19
21	18
22.5	17
24	16
25.5	15
27	14
28.5	13
30	12

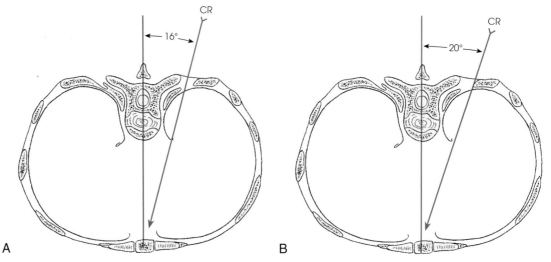

Fig. 9-10 A, Drawing of 24-cm chest. **B,** Drawing of 18-cm chest. *CR,* central ray.

Bony Thorax

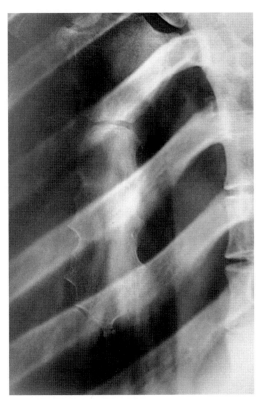

Fig. 9-11 PA oblique sternum, LAO position.

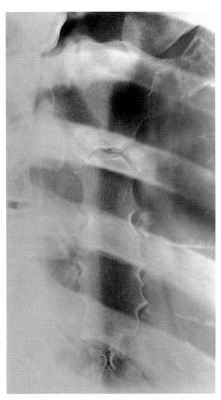

Fig. 9-12 PA oblique sternum, RAO position.

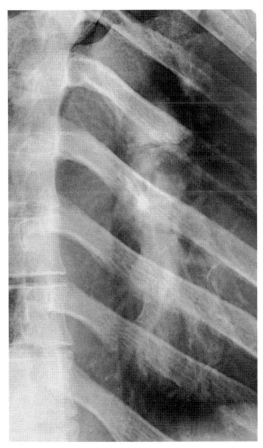

Fig. 9-13 Suspended respiration.

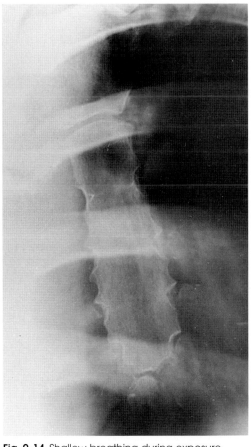

Fig. 9-14 Shallow breathing during exposure.

⚜ PA OBLIQUE PROJECTION
RAO position

Image receptor: 10 × 12 inch (24 × 30 cm) lengthwise

NOTE: This position may be difficult to perform on trauma patients. Use an upright position if necessary or possible.

SID: A 30-inch (76-cm) source-to-IR distance (SID) is recommended to blur the posterior ribs. See page 31, Chapter 1, for use of a 30-inch (76-cm) SID.

Position of patient
- With the patient prone, adjust the body into RAO position to use the heart for contrast as previously described.
- Have the patient support the body on the forearm and flexed knee.

Position of part
- Adjust the elevation of the left shoulder and hip so that the thorax is rotated just enough to prevent superimposition of the vertebrae and sternum.
- Estimate the amount of rotation with sufficient accuracy by placing one hand on the patient's sternum and the other hand on the thoracic vertebrae to act as guides while adjusting the degree of obliquity. The average rotation is about 15 to 20 degrees (Fig. 9-15).

- Align the patient's body so that the long axis of the sternum is centered to the midline of the grid.
- Place the top of the IR about 1½ inches (3.8 cm) above the jugular notch.
- *Shield gonads.*
- *Respiration:* When breathing motion is to be used, instruct the patient to take slow, shallow breaths during the exposure. When a short exposure time is to be used, instruct the patient to suspend breathing at the end of expiration to obtain a more uniform density.

NOTE: On trauma patients, obtain this projection with the patient supine, and use the LPO position and AP oblique projection.

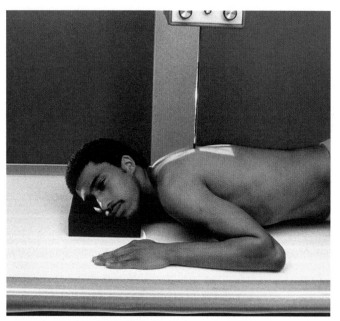
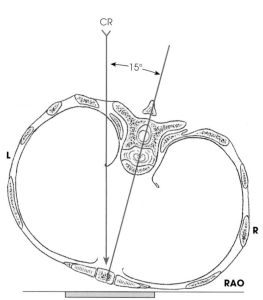

Fig. 9-15 PA oblique sternum, RAO position. Line drawing is an axial view (from feet upward). *CR,* central ray.

Central ray

- Perpendicular to IR. The central ray enters the *elevated side* of the posterior thorax at the level of T7 and approximately 1 inch (2.5 cm) lateral to the midsagittal plane.

Collimation

- Adjust to 10 × 12 inches (24 × 30 cm) on the collimator.

Structures shown

This image shows a slightly oblique projection of the sternum (Fig. 9-16). The detail depends largely on the technical procedure employed. If breathing motion is used, the pulmonary markings are obliterated.

The following should be clearly shown:

- Evidence of proper collimation
- Entire sternum from jugular notch to tip of xiphoid process
- Reasonably good visibility of the sternum through the thorax, including blurred pulmonary markings if a breathing technique was used
- Minimally rotated sternum and thorax, as shown by the following:
  - Sternum projected just free of superimposition from vertebral column
  - Minimally obliqued vertebrae to prevent excessive rotation of the sternum
  - Lateral portion of manubrium and sternoclavicular joint free of superimposition by the vertebrae
- Sternum projected over the heart

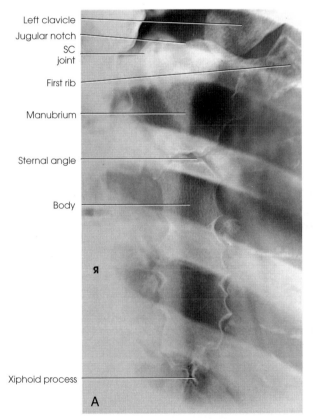

Left clavicle
Jugular notch
SC joint
First rib
Manubrium
Sternal angle
Body
Xiphoid process

A

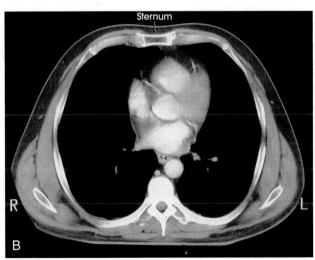

Sternum

R   L

B

Fig. 9-16 A, PA oblique sternum, RAO position. *SC,* sternoclavicular. **B,** CT is often used today to image the sternum. Image shows sternum in axial plane.

(**B,** Modified from Kelley LL, Petersen CM: *Sectional anatomy for imaging professionals,* ed 2, St Louis, 2007, Mosby.)

PA OBLIQUE PROJECTION
MOORE METHOD
Modified prone position

Image receptor: 10 × 12 inch (24 × 30 cm) lengthwise

SID: A 30-inch (76-cm) SID is recommended. This short distance assists in blurring the posterior ribs.

Radiography of the sternum can be difficult to perform on an ambulatory patient who is having acute pain. The alternative positioning method described by Moore[1] employs a modified prone position that makes it possible to produce a high-quality sternum image in a more comfortable manner for the patient.

[1]Moore TF: An alternative to the standard radiographic position for the sternum, *Radiol Technol* 60:133, 1988.

Position of patient
- Before positioning the patient, place the IR crosswise in the Bucky tray. Place the x-ray tube at a 30-inch (76-cm) SID, angle it 25 degrees, and direct the central ray to the center of the IR. The x-ray tube is positioned over the patient's right side.
- Place a marker on the tabletop near the patient's head to indicate the exact center of the IR.
- Have the patient stand at the side of the radiographic table directly in front of the Bucky tray.
- Ask the patient to bend at the waist, and place the sternum in the center of the table directly over the previously positioned IR.

Position of part
- Place the patient's arms above the shoulders and the palms down on the table. The arms act as a support for the side of the head (Fig. 9-17).
- Ensure that the patient is in a true prone position and that the mid-sternal area is at the center of the radiographic table.
- *Shield gonads.*
- *Respiration:* A shallow breathing technique produces the best results. Instruct the patient to take slow, shallow breaths during the exposure. A low mA setting and an exposure time of 1 to 3 seconds is recommended. When a low mA setting and long exposure time cannot be employed, instruct the patient to suspend respiration at the end of expiration to obtain a more uniform density.

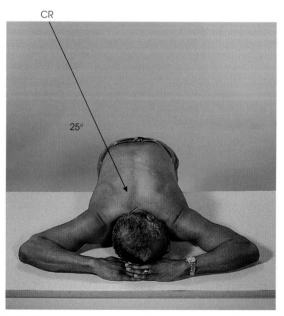

Fig. 9-17 PA oblique projection: Moore method. *CR,* central ray.

Central ray

- The central ray is already angled 25 degrees and centered to the IR. If patient positioning is accurate, the central ray enters at the level of T7 and approximately 2 inches (5 cm) to the right of the spine. This angulation places the sternum over the lung to maintain maximum contrast of the sternum.
- The x-ray tube angulation can be adjusted for extremely large or small patients. Large patients require *less* angulation, and thin patients require *more* angulation than the standard 25-degree angle.

Structures shown

This image shows a slightly oblique projection of the sternum (Fig. 9-18). The degree of detail shown depends largely on the technique used. If a breathing technique is used, the pulmonary markings are obliterated.

EVALUATION CRITERIA

The following should be clearly shown:

- Entire sternum from the jugular notch to the tip of the xiphoid process
- Reasonably good visibility of the sternum through the thorax
- Blurred pulmonary markings if a breathing technique was used
- Blurred posterior ribs if a reduced SID was used
- Sternum projected free of superimposition from the vertebral column

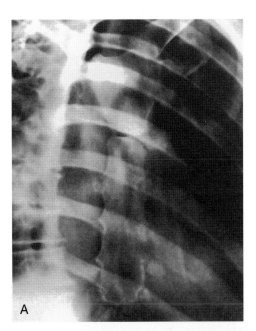

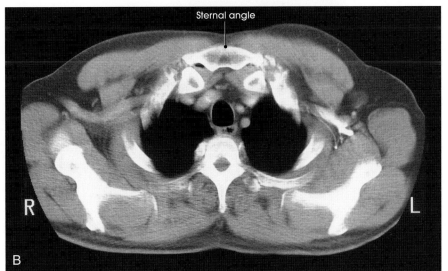

Fig. 9-18 A, PA oblique projection: Moore method. **B,** CT image shows sternal angle in axial plane.

(**B,** Modified from Kelley LL, Petersen CM: *Sectional anatomy for imaging professionals,* ed 2, St Louis, 2007, Mosby.)

Bony Thorax

✹ LATERAL PROJECTION
R or L position
Upright

Image receptor: 10 × 12 inch (24 × 30 cm) lengthwise

SID: Use a 72-inch (183-cm) SID to reduce magnification and distortion of the sternum.

Position of patient
- Place the patient in a lateral position, either seated or standing, before a vertical grid device.

Position of part
- Have the patient sit or stand straight.
- Rotate the shoulders posteriorly, and have the patient lock the hands behind the back.
- Center the sternum to the midline of the grid.
- Being careful to keep the midsagittal plane of the body vertical, place the patient close enough to the grid so that the shoulder can be rested firmly against it.

- Adjust the patient in a true lateral position so that the broad surface of the sternum is perpendicular to the plane of the IR (Fig. 9-19).
- Large breasts on female patients should be drawn to the sides and held in position with a wide bandage so that their shadows do not obscure the lower portion of the sternum.
- Adjust the height of the IR so that its upper border is 1½ inches (3.8 cm) above the jugular notch.
- For a direct lateral projection of just the sternoclavicular region, center vertically placed 8 × 10 inch (18 × 24 cm) IR at the level of the jugular notch.
- *Shield gonads.*
- *Respiration:* Suspended deep inspiration. This provides sharper contrast between the posterior surface of the sternum and the adjacent structures.

Central ray
- Perpendicular to the center of the IR and entering the lateral border of the mid-sternum

Collimation
- Adjust to 10 × 12 inches (24 × 30 cm) on the collimator.

Structures shown
A lateral image of the entire length of the sternum shows the superimposed sternoclavicular joints and medial ends of the clavicles (Fig. 9-20, *A*). A lateral projection of only the sternoclavicular region is shown in Fig. 9-20, *B*.

EVALUATION CRITERIA
The following should be clearly shown:
- Evidence of proper collimation
- Sternum in its entirety
- Manubrium free of superimposition by the soft tissue of the shoulders
- Sternum free of superimposition by the ribs
- Lower portion of the sternum unobscured by the breasts of a female patient (a second radiograph with increased penetration may be necessary)

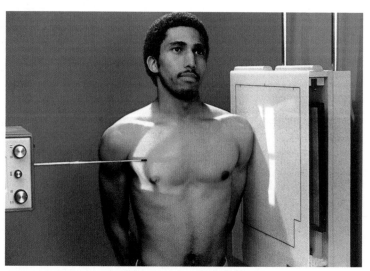

Fig. 9-19 Lateral sternum.

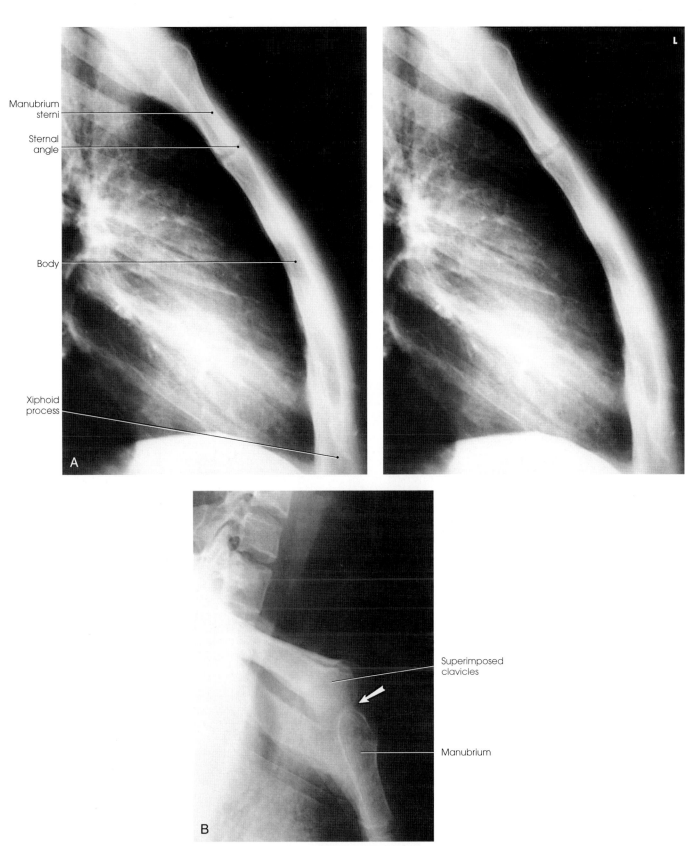

Manubrium
sterni

Sternal
angle

Body

Xiphoid
process

A

L

B

Superimposed
clavicles

Manubrium

Fig. 9-20 A, Lateral sternum. **B,** Lateral sternoclavicular joint (*arrow*).

⚜ LATERAL PROJECTION
R or L position
Recumbent

Image receptor: 10 × 12 inch (24 × 30 cm) lengthwise

SID: A 72-inch (180-cm) SID is preferred. If this distance cannot be obtained with the overhead tube, the maximum allowed distance should be obtained.

Position of patient

- Place the patient in the lateral recumbent position.
- Flex the patient's hips and knees to a comfortable position.

Position of part

- Extend the patient's arms over the head to prevent them from overlapping the sternum.
- Rest the patient's head on the arms or on a pillow (Fig. 9-21, *A*).
- Place a support under the lower thoracic region to position the long axis of the sternum horizontally.
- Adjust the rotation of the patient's body so that the broad surface of the sternum is perpendicular to the plane of the IR.
- Center the sternum to the midline of the grid.

- Apply a compression band across the hips for immobilization, if necessary.
- Adjust the height of the IR so that its upper border is 1½ inches (3.8 cm) above the jugular notch.
- *Shield gonads.*
- *Respiration:* Suspend at the end of deep inspiration to obtain high contrast between the posterior surface of the sternum and the adjacent structures.

NOTE: Use the dorsal decubitus position for examination of a patient with severe injury. In this situation, a grid-front IR or stationary grid should be used (Fig. 9-21, *B*). SID of 72 inches (180 cm) can be used for this position.

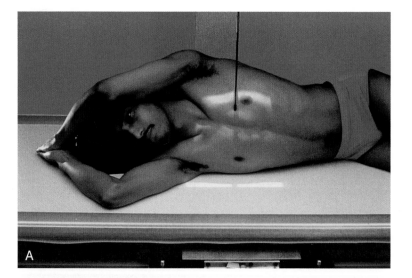

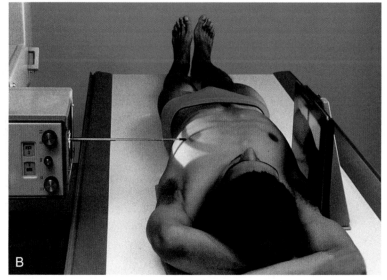

Fig. 9-21 A, Lateral sternum. **B,** Dorsal decubitus position for lateral sternum.

Central ray

- Perpendicular to the center of the IR and entering the lateral border of the mid-sternum

Collimation

- Adjust to 10 × 12 inches (24 × 30 cm) on the collimator.

Structures shown

The lateral aspect of the entire length of the sternum is shown (Fig. 9-22).

The following should be clearly shown:
- Evidence of proper collimation
- Lateral image of the sternum in its entirety
- Sternum free of superimposition by the soft tissues of the shoulders or arms
- Sternum free of superimposition by the ribs
- Inferior portion of the sternum unobscured by the breasts of a female patient (a second radiograph with increased penetration may be necessary)

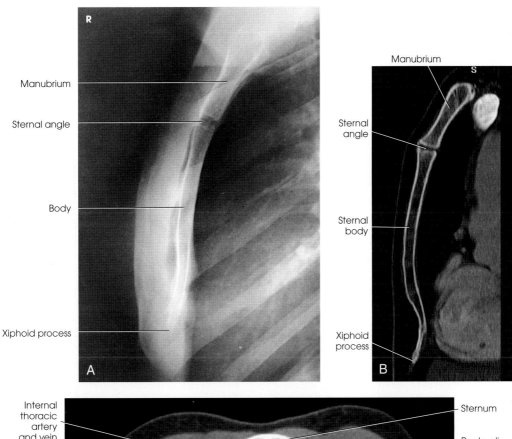

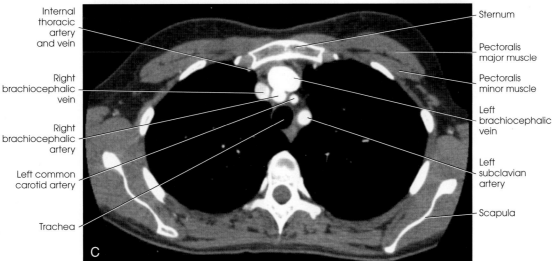

Fig. 9-22 A, Lateral sternum. **B,** Sagittal CT reformat of sternum. **C,** Axial CT scan of chest showing sternum in relation to surrounding organs.

(**B** and **C,** From Kelley LL, Petersen CM: *Sectional anatomy for imaging professionals,* ed 2, St Louis, 2007, Mosby.)

Sternoclavicular Articulations

☀ PA PROJECTION

NOTE: This position may be difficult to perform on trauma patients. Use the upright position if the patient is able.

Image receptor: 8 × 10 inch (18 × 24 cm) crosswise

Position of patient
- Place the patient in the prone position.
- Center the midsagittal plane of the patient's body to the midline of the grid.
- Adapt the same procedure for use with a patient who is standing or seated upright.

Position of part
- Center the IR at the level of the spinous process of the third thoracic vertebra, which lies posterior to the jugular notch.
- Place the patient's arms along the sides of the body with the palms facing upward.
- Adjust the shoulders to lie in the same transverse plane.
- For a bilateral examination, rest the patient's head on the chin and adjust it so that the midsagittal plane is vertical.

- For a unilateral projection, ask the patient to turn the head to face the affected side and rest the cheek on the table (Fig. 9-23). Turning the head rotates the spine slightly away from the side being examined and provides better visualization of the lateral portion of the manubrium.
- *Shield gonads.*
- *Respiration:* Suspend at the end of expiration to obtain a more uniform density.

Central ray
- Perpendicular to the center of the IR and entering T3

Collimation
- Adjust to 6 × 8 inches (15 × 20 cm) on the collimator.

Structures shown
A PA projection shows the sternoclavicular joints and the medial portions of the clavicles (Figs. 9-24 and 9-25).

EVALUATION CRITERIA
The following should be clearly shown:
- Evidence of proper collimation
- Both sternoclavicular joints and the medial ends of the clavicles
- Sternoclavicular joints through the superimposing vertebral and rib shadows
- No rotation present on a bilateral examination; slight rotation present on a unilateral examination

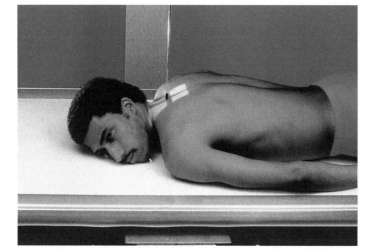

Fig. 9-23 Unilateral examination to show left sternoclavicular articulation.

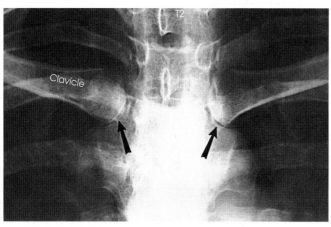

Fig. 9-24 Bilateral sternoclavicular joints (*arrows*).

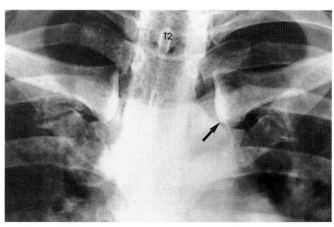

Fig. 9-25 Unilateral sternoclavicular joint (*arrow*).

⚕ PA OBLIQUE PROJECTION
BODY ROTATION METHOD
RAO or LAO position

NOTE: This position may be difficult in trauma patients. Use the upright position if the patient is able.

Image receptor: 8 × 10 inch (18 × 24 cm) crosswise

Position of patient
- Place the patient in a prone or seated-upright position.

Position of part
- Keeping the affected side adjacent to the IR, position the patient at enough of an oblique angle to project the vertebrae well behind the sternoclavicular joint closest to the IR. The angle is usually about 10 to 15 degrees.
- Adjust the patient's position to center the joint to the midline of the grid.
- Adjust the shoulders to lie in the same transverse plane (Fig. 9-26, *A* and *B*).
- *Shield gonads.*
- *Respiration:* Suspend at the end of expiration to obtain a more uniform density.

Central ray
- Perpendicular to the sternoclavicular joint closest to the IR. The central ray enters at the level of T2-3 (about 3 inches [7.6 cm] distal to the vertebral prominens) and 1 to 2 inches (2.5 to 5 cm) lateral from the midsagittal plane. If the central ray enters the right side, the left sternoclavicular joint is shown, and vice versa (see Fig. 9-26, *B*).
- Center the IR to the central ray.

Collimation
- Adjust to 6 × 8 inches (15 × 20 cm) on the collimator.

Structures shown
A slightly oblique image of the sternoclavicular joint is shown (see Fig. 9-26, *C*).

EVALUATION CRITERIA
The following should be clearly shown:
- Evidence of proper collimation
- Sternoclavicular joint of interest in the center of the radiograph, with the manubrium and the medial end of the clavicle included
- Open sternoclavicular joint space
- Sternoclavicular joint of interest immediately adjacent to the vertebral column with minimal obliquity
- Reasonably good visibility of the sternoclavicular joint through the superimposing rib and lung fields

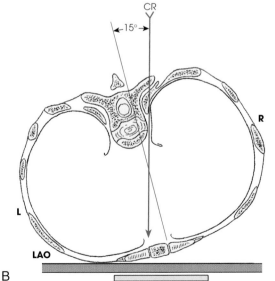

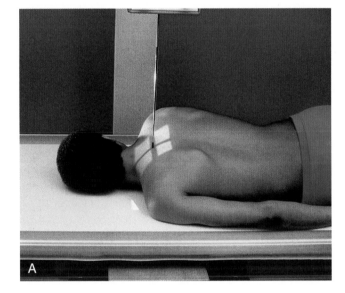

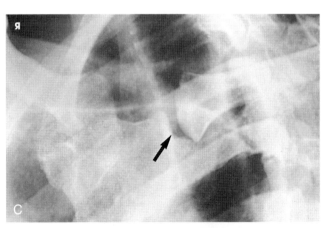

Fig. 9-26 A, PA oblique sternoclavicular joint, LAO position: Body rotation method. **B,** Axial view (from feet upward) of central ray position in relation to spine and sternoclavicular joint. **C,** PA oblique sternoclavicular joint, LAO position. The joint closest to IR is shown (*arrow*). *CR,* central ray.

PA OBLIQUE PROJECTION
CENTRAL RAY ANGULATION
METHOD
Non-Bucky

Image receptor: 8 × 10 inch (18 × 24 cm) crosswise

NOTE: For this projection, the joint is closer to the IR, and less distortion is obtained than when the previously described body rotation method is used. A grid IR placed on the tabletop also enables the joint to be projected with minimal distortion. Also, this position may be difficult to perform on trauma patients. Use the upright position if the patient is able.

Position of patient
- Place the patient in the prone position on a grid IR positioned directly under the upper chest.
- Center the grid to the level of the sternoclavicular joints.
- To avoid grid cutoff, place the grid on the radiographic table with its long axis running *perpendicular* to the long axis of the table.

Position of part
- Extend the patient's arms along the sides of the body with the palms of the hands facing upward.
- Adjust the shoulders to lie in the same transverse plane.
- Ask the patient to rest the head on the chin or to rotate the chin toward the side of the joint being radiographed (Fig. 9-27).

Central ray
- From the side opposite that is being examined, direct to the midpoint of the IR at an angle of 15 degrees toward the midsagittal plane. A small angle is satisfactory in examinations of sternoclavicular articulations because only a slight anteroposterior overlapping of the vertebrae and these joints occurs.
- The central ray should enter at the level of T2-3 (about 3 inches [7.6 cm] distal to the vertebral prominens) and 1 to 2 inches (2.5 to 5 cm) lateral to the midsagittal plane. If the central ray enters the left side, the right side is shown and vice versa.

Collimation
- Adjust to 6 × 8 inches (15 × 20 cm) on the collimator.

Structures shown
A slightly oblique image of the sternoclavicular joint is shown (Figs. 9-28 and 9-29).

EVALUATION CRITERIA
The following should be clearly shown:
- Evidence of proper collimation
- Sternoclavicular joint of interest in the center of the radiograph, with the manubrium and the medial end of the clavicle included
- Open sternoclavicular joint space
- Sternoclavicular joint of interest immediately adjacent to the vertebral column with minimal obliquity
- Reasonably good visibility of the sternoclavicular joint through the superimposing rib and lung fields

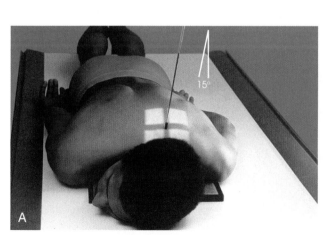

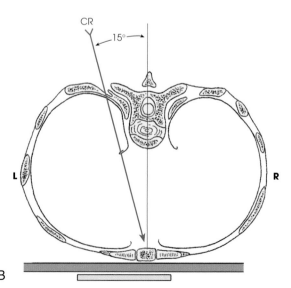

Fig. 9-27 A, PA oblique sternoclavicular joint: Central ray (*CR*) angulation method. CR enters left side to show right joint. **B,** Axial view (from feet upward) of CR position in relation to spine and sternoclavicular joint.

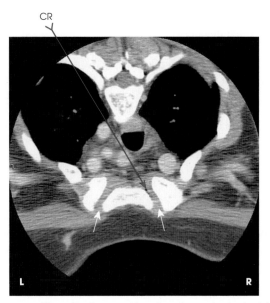

Fig. 9-28 CT axial image with patient prone, showing sternoclavicular joints (*white arrows*) and path of central ray (*CR*). View is from feet looking upward.

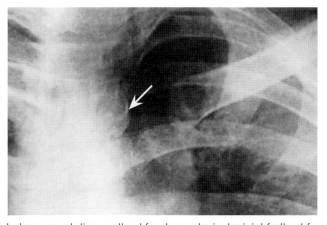

Fig. 9-29 Central ray angulation method for sternoclavicular joint farthest from x-ray tube (*arrow*).

(From Kurzbauer R: The lateral projection in the roentgenography of the sternoclavicular articulation, *AJR Am J Roentgenol* 56:104, 1946.)

Ribs

In radiography of the ribs, an IR 14 × 17 inches (35 × 43 cm) should be used to identify the ribs involved and to determine the extent of trauma or pathologic condition. An IR 11 × 14 inches (28 × 36 cm) is often used with smaller patients. Projections can be made in recumbent and upright positions. If the area in question involves the first and last ribs, additional images may be required to show the affected area better (Fig. 9-30).

After the lesion is localized, the next step is to determine (1) the position required to place the affected rib region parallel with the plane of the IR and (2) whether the radiograph should be made to include the ribs above or below the diaphragm.

The anterior portion of the ribs, usually referred to simply as the *anterior ribs,* is often examined with the patient facing the IR for a PA projection (Fig. 9-31). The posterior portion of the ribs, or the *posterior ribs,* is more commonly radiographed with the patient facing the x-ray tube in the same manner as for an AP projection (Fig. 9-32).

The axillary portion of the ribs is best shown using an oblique projection. Because the lateral projection results in superimposition of the two sides, it is generally used only when fluid or air levels are evaluated after rib fractures.

When the ribs superimposed over the heart are involved, the body must be rotated to obtain a projection of the ribs free of the heart, or the radiographic exposure must be increased to compensate for the density of the heart. Although the anterior and posterior ends are superimposed, the left ribs are cleared of the heart when the LAO position (Fig. 9-33) or RPO position (Fig. 9-34) is used. These two body positions place the right-sided ribs parallel with the plane of the IR and are reversed to obtain comparable projections of the left-sided ribs. Technical factors that result in a short-scale radiograph are often used (about 70 kVp).

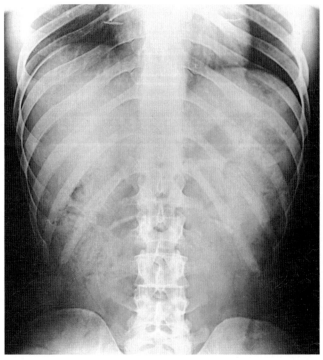

Fig. 9-30 AP lower ribs.

Bony Thorax

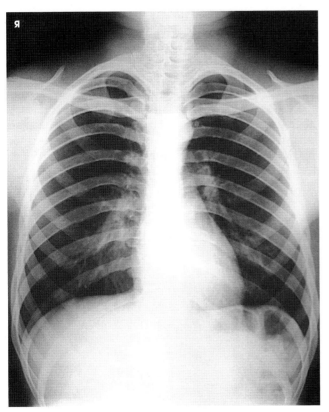

Fig. 9-31 PA ribs.

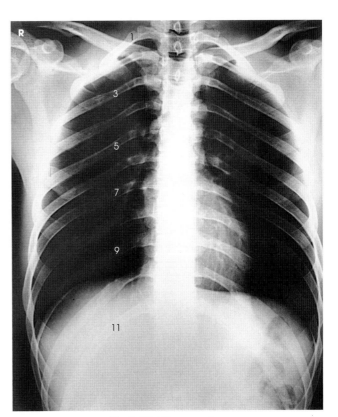

Fig. 9-32 AP upper ribs.

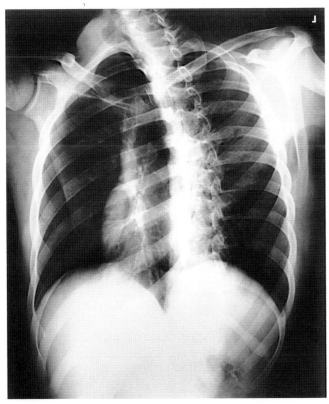

Fig. 9-33 PA oblique ribs, LAO position.

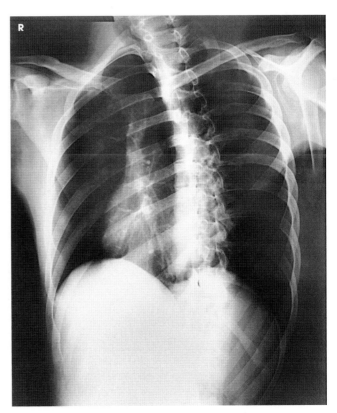

Fig. 9-34 AP oblique ribs, RPO position.

RESPIRATION

In radiography of the ribs, the patient is usually examined with respiration suspended in either full inspiration or expiration. Occasionally, shallow breathing may be used to obliterate lung markings. If this technique is used, breathing must be shallow enough to ensure that the ribs are not elevated or depressed as described in the anatomy portion of this chapter. Examples of shallow breathing and suspended respiration are compared in Figs. 9-35 and 9-36.

Rib fractures can cause a great deal of pain and hemorrhage because of the closely related neurovascular structures. This situation commonly makes it difficult for the patient to breathe deeply for the required radiograph. Deeper inspiration is attained if the patient fully understands the importance of expanding the lungs and if the exposure is made after the patient takes the second deep breath.

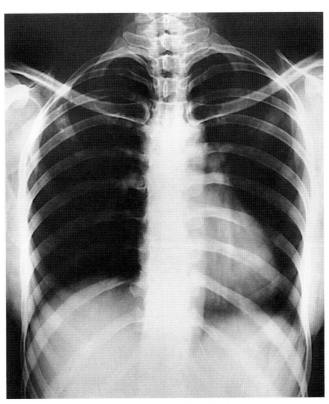

Fig. 9-35 Shallow breathing technique.

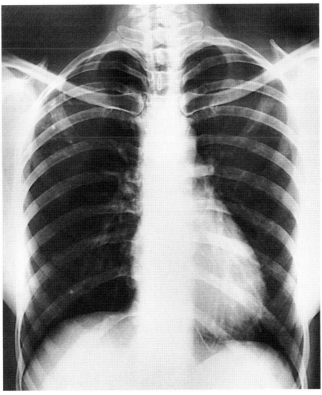

Fig. 9-36 Suspended respiration technique.

PA PROJECTION

Image receptor: 14 × 17 inch (35 × 43 cm) lengthwise

Position of patient

- Position the patient either upright or recumbent for a PA projection.
- Because the diaphragm descends to its lowest level in the upright position, use the standing or seated-upright position for projections of the upper ribs when the patient's condition permits (Fig. 9-37). The upright position is also valuable for showing fluid levels in the chest.

Position of part

- Center the midsagittal plane of the patient's body to the midline of the grid.
- To include the upper ribs, adjust the IR position to project approximately 1½ inches (3.8 cm) above the upper border of the shoulders.
- Rest the patient's hands against the hips with the palms turned outward to rotate the scapulae away from the rib cage.
- Adjust the shoulders to lie in the same transverse plane.
- If the patient is prone, rest the head on the chin and adjust the midsagittal plane to be vertical (Fig. 9-38).

- To image affected ribs unilaterally, use 11 × 14 inch (28 × 35 cm) collimator size for contrast improvement.
- For hypersthenic patients with wide rib cages, include the entire lateral surface of the affected rib area on the radiograph. This may require moving the patient laterally to include all of the affected ribs.
- *Shield gonads.*
- *Respiration:* Suspend at full inspiration to depress the diaphragm as much as possible.

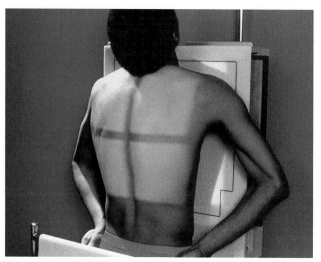

Fig. 9-37 PA ribs, upright position.

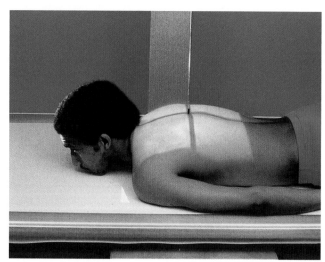

Fig. 9-38 PA ribs, recumbent position.

Central ray
- Perpendicular to the center of IR. If the IR is positioned correctly, the central ray is at the level of T7.
- A useful option for showing the seventh, eighth, and ninth ribs is to angle the x-ray tube about 10 to 15 degrees caudad. This angulation aids in projecting the diaphragm below that of the affected ribs.

Collimation
- Adjust to 14 × 17 inches (35 × 43 cm) on the collimator.

Structures shown
PA projection best shows the anterior ribs above the diaphragm (Figs. 9-39 and 9-40). The posterior ribs are seen. The anterior ribs are shown with greater detail, however, because they lie closer to the IR.

EVALUATION CRITERIA
The following should be clearly shown:
- Evidence of proper collimation
- First through ninth ribs in their entirety, with the posterior portions lying above the diaphragm
- First through seventh anterior ribs from both sides, in their entirety and above the diaphragm
- In a unilateral examination, ribs from the opposite side possibly not included in their entirety.
- Ribs visible through the lungs with sufficient contrast

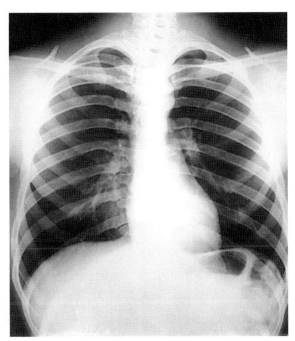

Fig. 9-39 PA ribs, normal centering.

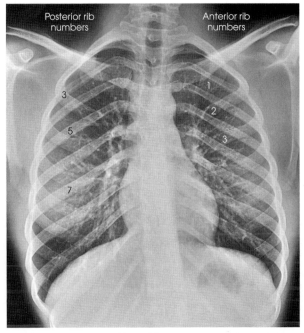

Fig. 9-40 PA ribs, with 10- to 15-degree caudal angulation.

⚘ AP PROJECTION

Image receptor: 14 × 17 inch (35 × 43 cm)

Position of patient

- Have the patient face the x-ray tube in either an upright or a recumbent position.
- When the patient's condition permits, use the upright position to image ribs above the diaphragm and the supine position to image ribs below the diaphragm to permit gravity to assist in moving the patient's diaphragm.

Position of part

- Center the midsagittal plane of the patient's body to the midline of the grid.

Ribs above diaphragm

- Place the IR lengthwise 1½ inches (3.8 cm) above the upper border of the *relaxed* shoulders.
- Rest the patient's hands, palms outward, against the hips. This position moves the scapula off the ribs. Alternatively, extend the arms to the vertical position with the hands under the head (Fig. 9-41).
- Adjust the patient's shoulders to lie in the same transverse plane, and rotate them forward to draw the scapulae away from the rib cage.
- *Shield gonads.*
- *Respiration:* Suspend at *full inspiration* to *depress* the diaphragm.

Ribs below diaphragm

- Place the IR crosswise in the Bucky tray with the lower edge positioned at the level of the iliac crests. This positioning ensures inclusion of the lower ribs because of the divergent x-rays.
- Adjust the patient's shoulders to lie in the same transverse plane.
- Place the patient's arms in a comfortable position (Fig. 9-42).
- *Shield gonads.*
- *Respiration:* Suspend at *full expiration* to *elevate* the diaphragm.

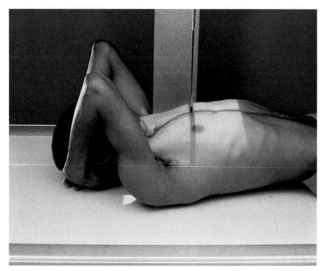

Fig. 9-41 AP ribs above diaphragm.

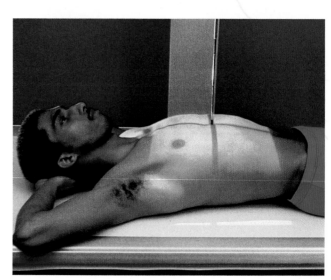

Fig. 9-42 AP ribs below diaphragm.

Central ray

• Perpendicular to the center of the IR

NOTE: Refer to the Exposure Technique Chart on p. 455 for the different exposure settings for the upper and lower rib projections.

Collimation

• Adjust to 14 × 17 inches (35 × 43 cm) on the collimator. If smaller IR is used, collimate to the smaller size.

Structures shown

AP projection best shows the posterior ribs above or below the diaphragm, according to the region examined (Figs. 9-43 and 9-44). The anterior ribs are seen. The posterior ribs are shown with greater detail, however, because they lie closer to the IR.

EVALUATION CRITERIA

The following should be clearly shown:

■ Evidence of proper collimation
■ For ribs above the diaphragm, 1st through 10th posterior ribs from both sides in their entirety
■ For ribs below the diaphragm, 8th through 12th posterior ribs on both sides in their entirety
■ Ribs visible through the lungs or abdomen
■ In a unilateral examination, ribs from the opposite side possibly not included in their entirety

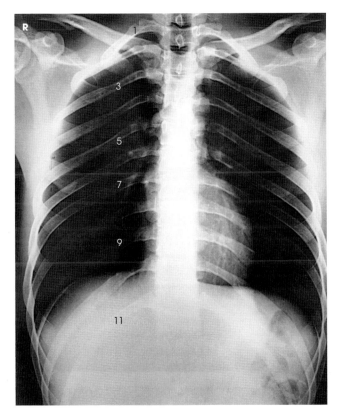

Fig. 9-43 AP ribs above diaphragm.

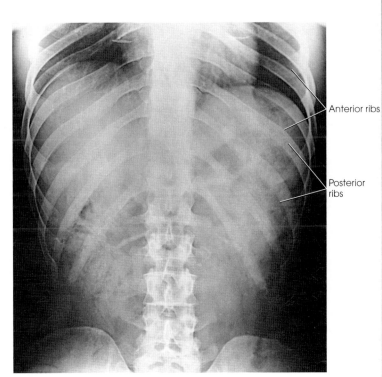

Fig. 9-44 AP lower ribs.

Axillary
♠ AP OBLIQUE PROJECTION
RPO or LPO position

Image receptor: 14 × 17 inch (35 × 43 cm)

Position of patient
- Examine the patient in the upright or recumbent position.
- Unless contraindicated by the patient's condition, use the upright position to image ribs above the diaphragm, and use the recumbent position to image ribs below the diaphragm. Gravity assists by moving the diaphragm.

Position of part
- Position the patient's body for a 45-degree AP oblique projection using the RPO or LPO position. Place the *affected* side closest to the IR.
- Center the affected side on a longitudinal plane drawn midway between the midsagittal plane and the lateral surface of the body.
- Position this plane to the midline of the grid.
- If the patient is in the recumbent position, support the elevated hip.
- Abduct the arm of the affected side, and elevate it to carry the scapula away from the rib cage.

- Rest the patient's hand on the head if the upright position is used (Fig. 9-45), or place the hand under or above the head if the recumbent position is used (Fig. 9-46).
- Abduct the opposite limb with the hand on the hip.
- Center the IR with the top 1½ inches (3.8 cm) above the upper border of the relaxed shoulder to image ribs above the diaphragm or with the lower edge of the IR at the level of the iliac crest to image ribs below the diaphragm.
- *Shield gonads.*
- *Respiration:* Suspend at the end of *deep expiration* for ribs *below* the diaphragm and at the end of *full inspiration* for ribs *above* the diaphragm.

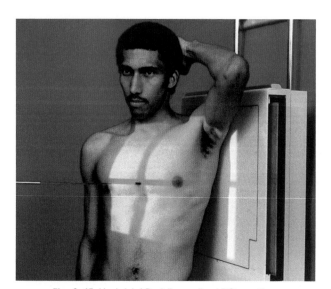

Fig. 9-45 Upright AP oblique ribs, LPO position.

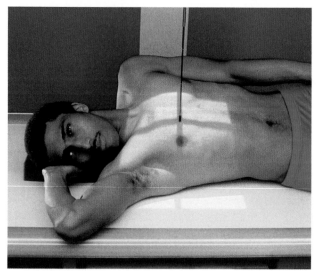

Fig. 9-46 Recumbent AP oblique ribs, RPO position.

Central ray
- Perpendicular to the center of IR
- Closest to IR

Collimation
- Adjust to 14 × 17 inches (35 × 43 cm) on the collimator. If a smaller IR is used, collimate to the smaller size.

Structures shown
In these images, the axillary portion of the ribs closest to the IR are projected free of superimposition (Fig. 9-47). The posterior ribs closest to the IR are also well shown.

The following should be clearly shown:
- Evidence of proper collimation
- Approximately twice as much distance between the vertebral column and the lateral border of the ribs on the affected side as is present on the unaffected side
- Axillary portion of the ribs free of superimposition
- First through 10th ribs visible above the diaphragm for upper ribs
- Eighth through 12th ribs visible below the diaphragm for lower ribs
- Ribs visible through the lungs or abdomen according to region examined

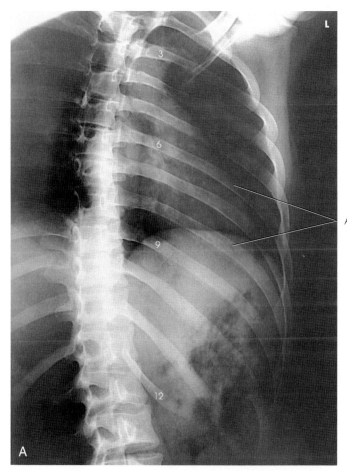

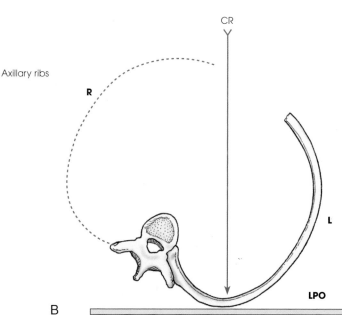

Fig. 9-47 A, AP oblique ribs. LPO position shows left-side ribs. **B,** Axial view (from feet upward) of ribs and central ray (*CR*), LPO position.

Axillary
▲ PA OBLIQUE PROJECTION
RAO or LAO position

Image receptor: 14 × 17 inch (35 × 43 cm)

Position of patient
- Examine the patient in the upright or recumbent position.
- Unless contraindicated by the patient's condition, use the upright position to image ribs above the diaphragm, and use the recumbent position to image ribs below the diaphragm. Gravity assists by moving the diaphragm.

Position of part
- Position the body for a 45-degree PA oblique projection using the RAO or LAO position. Place the affected side away from the IR (Fig. 9-48).
- If the recumbent position is used, have the patient rest on the forearm and flexed knee of the elevated side (Fig. 9-49).
- Align the body so that a longitudinal plane drawn midway between the midline and the lateral surface of the body side up is centered to the midline of the grid.

- Center IR with the top 1½ inches (3.8 cm) above the upper border of the shoulder to image ribs above the diaphragm or with the lower edge of IR at the level of the iliac crest to image ribs below the diaphragm.
- *Shield gonads.*
- *Respiration:* Suspend at the end of *full expiration* for ribs *below* the diaphragm and at the end of *full inspiration* for ribs *above* the diaphragm.

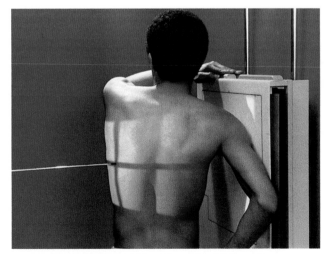

Fig. 9-48 Upright PA oblique ribs, RAO position.

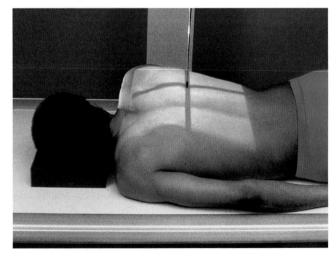

Fig. 9-49 Recumbent PA oblique ribs, LAO position.

Central ray
• Perpendicular to center of IR

Collimation
• Adjust to 14 × 17 inches (35 × 43 cm) on the collimator. If a smaller IR is used, collimate to the smaller size.

Structures shown
In these images, the axillary portion of the ribs farthest from the IR is projected free of bony superimposition (Fig. 9-50). The anterior ribs farthest from the IR are also shown.

EVALUATION CRITERIA
The following should be clearly shown:
■ Evidence of proper collimation
■ Approximately twice as much distance between the vertebral column and the lateral border of the ribs on the affected side as is present on the unaffected side
■ Axillary portion of the ribs free of superimposition
■ First through 10th ribs visible above the diaphragm for upper ribs
■ Eighth through 12th ribs visible below the diaphragm for lower ribs
■ Ribs visible through the lungs or abdomen according to the region examined

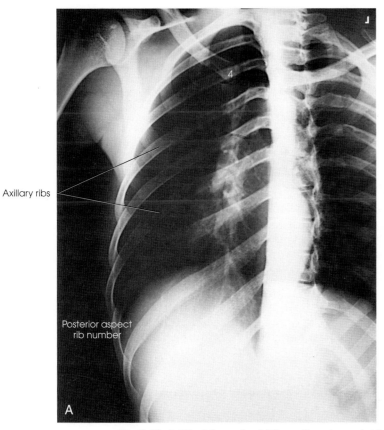

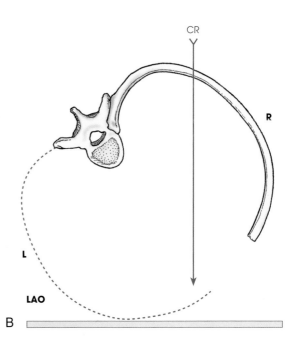

Fig. 9-50 A, PA oblique ribs. LAO position shows right-side ribs. PA projection radiograph is placed in the anatomic position for display. **B,** Axial view (from feet upward) of ribs and central ray (*CR*) with the patient in LAO position.

AP AXIAL PROJECTION

This projection is recommended to show the costal joints in patients with rheumatoid spondylitis.

Image receptor: 11 × 14 inch (28 × 35 cm) lengthwise

Position of patient

- Place the patient in the supine position.
- Have the patient's head rest directly on the radiographic table to avoid accentuating the dorsal kyphosis.

Position of part

- Center the midsagittal plane to the midline of the grid.
- If the patient has pronounced dorsal kyphosis, extend the arms over the head; otherwise, place the arms along the sides of the body.
- Adjust the patient's shoulders to lie in the same transverse plane (Fig. 9-51).
- With the IR in the Bucky tray, adjust its position so that the midpoint of the IR coincides with the central ray.

- Apply compression across the thorax, if necessary.
- *Shield gonads.*
- *Respiration:* Suspend at the end of full inspiration because the lung markings are less prominent at this phase of breathing.

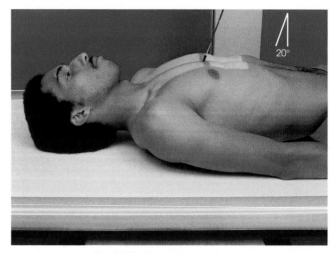

Fig. 9-51 AP axial costal joints.

Bony Thorax

Central ray

- Directed 20 degrees cephalad and entering the midline about 2 inches (5 cm) above the xiphoid process
- Increase the angulation of the central ray slightly (5 to 10 degrees) when examining patients who have pronounced dorsal kyphosis.

Structures shown

The costovertebral and costotransverse joints are shown (Fig. 9-52).

EVALUATION CRITERIA

Open costovertebral and costotransverse joints should be clearly shown.

NOTE: In large-boned patients, the two sides may need to be examined separately to show the costovertebral joints. These projections are obtained by alternately rotating the body approximately 10 degrees medially; the elevated side is shown best.

In their studies of the costal joints (costovertebral and costotransverse), Hohmann and Gasteiger[1] found that the central ray generally must be angled 30 degrees cephalad in the average patient. The central ray angulation is increased to 35 to 40 degrees when accentuated kyphosis is present. In patients with severe curvature of the spine, the pelvis is also elevated on a suitable support. For localized studies, the central ray may be centered to T4 for the upper area and to T8 for the lower area.

[1]Hohmann D, Gasteiger W: Roentgen diagnosis of the costovertebral joints, *Fortschr Roentgenstr* 112:783, 1970 (in German); Abstract, *Radiology* 98:481, 1971.

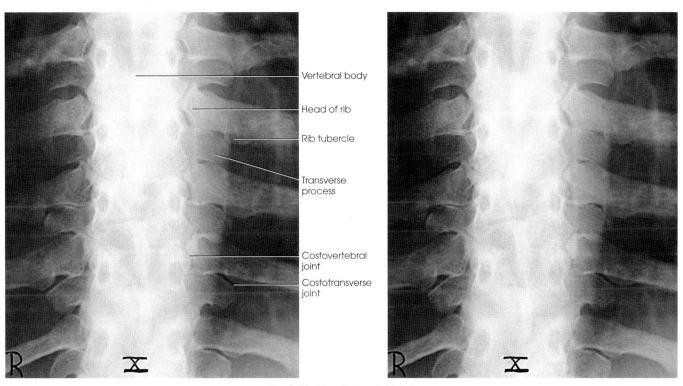

Vertebral body

Head of rib

Rib tubercle

Transverse process

Costovertebral joint

Costotransverse joint

Fig. 9-52 AP axial costal joints.

10

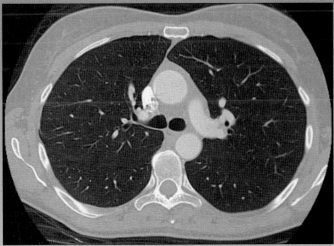

THORACIC VISCERA

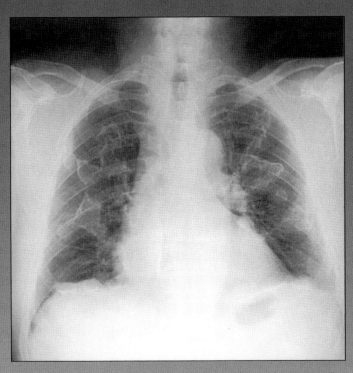

SUMMARY OF PROJECTIONS

PROJECTIONS, POSITIONS, AND METHODS

Page	Essential	Anatomy	Projection	Position	Method
500		Trachea	AP		
502		Trachea and superior mediastinum	Lateral	R or L	
504	⚕	Chest: *lungs and heart*	PA		
508	⚕	Chest: *lungs and heart*	Lateral	R or L	
512	⚕	Chest: *lungs and heart*	PA oblique	RAO and LAO	
516	⚕	Chest: *lungs and heart*	AP oblique	RPO and LPO	
518	⚕	Chest	AP		
520	⚕	Pulmonary apices	AP axial	Lordotic	LINDBLOM
522		Pulmonary apices	PA axial		
523		Pulmonary apices	AP axial		
524	⚕	Lungs and pleurae	AP or PA	R or L lateral decubitus	
526	⚕	Lungs and pleurae	Lateral	R or L, ventral or dorsal decubitus	

Icons in the Essential column indicate projections frequently performed in the United States and Canada. Students should be competent in these projections.

Body Habitus

The general shape of the human body, or the *body habitus,* determines the size, shape, position, and movement of the internal organs. Fig. 10-1 outlines the general shape of the thorax in the four types of body habitus and how each appears on radiographs of the thoracic area.

Thoracic Cavity

The *thoracic cavity* is bounded by the walls of the thorax and extends from the *superior thoracic aperture,* where structures enter the thorax, to the *inferior thoracic aperture*. The *diaphragm* separates the thoracic cavity from the abdominal cavity. The anatomic structures that pass from the thorax to the abdomen go through openings in the diaphragm (Fig. 10-2).

The thoracic cavity contains the *lungs* and *heart;* organs of the *respiratory, cardiovascular,* and *lymphatic* systems; the *inferior portion of the esophagus;* and the *thymus gland*. Within the cavity are three separate chambers: a single *pericardial cavity* and the *right* and *left pleural cavities*. These cavities are lined by shiny, slippery, and delicate *serous membranes*. The space between the two pleural cavities is called the *mediastinum*. This area contains all the thoracic structures except the lungs and pleurae.

Respiratory System

The *respiratory system* consists of the pharynx (described in Chapter 15 in Volume 2), trachea, bronchi, and two lungs. The air passages of these organs communicate with the exterior through the pharynx, mouth, and nose, each of which, in addition to other described functions, is considered a part of the respiratory system.

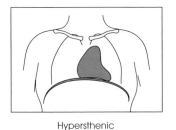
Hypersthenic

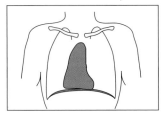
Sthenic

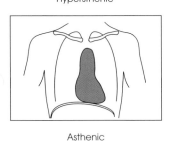
Asthenic

Hyposthenic

Fig. 10-1 Four types of body habitus. Note general shape of thorax, size and shape of lungs, and position of heart. Knowledge of this anatomy is helpful to position accurately for projections of the thorax.

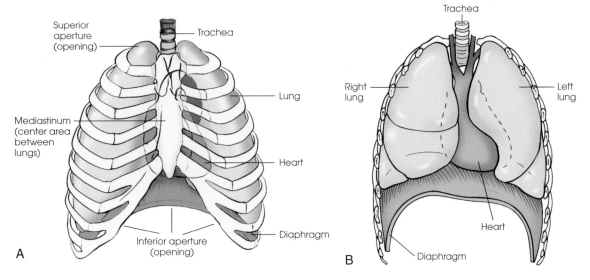

Fig. 10-2 A, Thoracic cavity. **B,** Thoracic cavity with anterior ribs removed.

TRACHEA

The *trachea* is a fibrous, muscular tube with 16 to 20 C-shaped cartilaginous rings embedded in its walls for greater rigidity (Fig. 10-3, *A*). It measures approximately ½ inch (1.3 cm) in diameter and 4½ inches (11 cm) in length, and its posterior aspect is flat. The cartilaginous rings are incomplete posteriorly and extend around the anterior two thirds of the tube. The trachea lies in the midline of the body, anterior to the esophagus in the neck. In the thorax, the trachea is shifted slightly to the right of the midline as a result of the arching of the aorta. The trachea follows the curve of the vertebral column and extends from its junction with the larynx at the level of the sixth cervical vertebra in-feriorly through the mediastinum to about the level of the space between the fourth and fifth thoracic vertebrae. The last tracheal cartilage is elongated and has a hooklike process, the *carina*, which extends posteriorly on its inferior surface. At the carina, the trachea divides, or bifurcates, into two lesser tubes—the primary bronchi. One of these bronchi enters the right lung, and the other enters the left lung.

The *primary bronchi* slant obliquely inferiorly to their entrance into the lungs, where they branch out to form the right and left bronchial branches (Fig. 10-3, *B*). The *right primary bronchus* is shorter, wider, and more vertical than the *left primary bronchus*. Because of the more ver-tical position and greater diameter of the right main bronchus, foreign bodies entering the trachea are more likely to pass into the right bronchus than the left bronchus.

After entering the lung, each primary bronchus divides, sending branches to each lobe of the lung: three to the right lung and two to the left lung. These *secondary bronchi* divide further and decrease in caliber. The bronchi continue dividing into *tertiary bronchi*, then to smaller *bronchioles*, and end in minute tubes called the *terminal bronchioles* (see Fig. 10-3). The extensive branching of the trachea is commonly referred to as the *bronchial tree* because it resembles a tree trunk (see box).

SUBDIVISIONS OF THE BRONCHIAL TREE

Trachea
  Primary bronchi
    Secondary bronchi
      Tertiary bronchi
        Bronchioles
          Terminal bronchioles

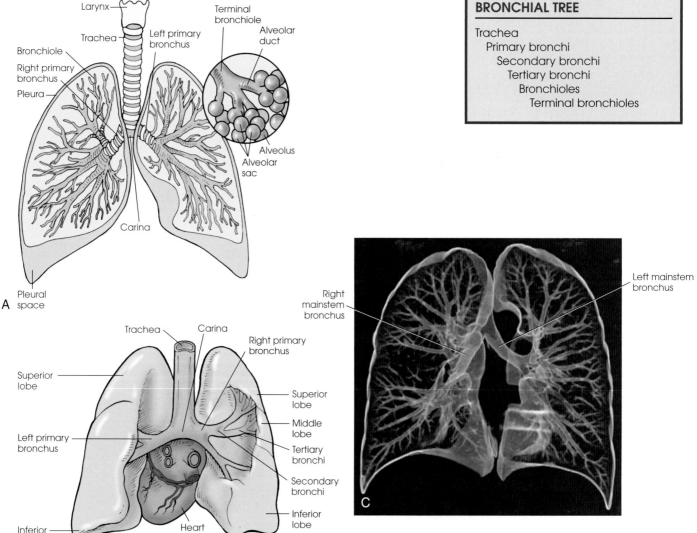

Fig. 10-3 A, Anterior aspect of respiratory system. **B,** Posterior aspect of heart, lungs, trachea, and bronchial trees. **C,** Coronal, three-dimensional CT image of central and peripheral airways.

(**C,** From Kelley LL, Petersen CM: *Sectional anatomy for imaging professionals,* ed 2, St Louis, 2007, Mosby.)

ALVEOLI

The terminal bronchioles communicate with *alveolar ducts*. Each duct ends in several *alveolar sacs*. The walls of the alveolar sacs are lined with *alveoli* (see Fig. 10-3, *A*). Each lung contains millions of alveoli. Oxygen and carbon dioxide are exchanged by diffusion within the walls of the alveoli.

LUNGS

The *lungs* are the organs of respiration (Fig. 10-4). They are the mechanism for introducing oxygen into the blood and removing carbon dioxide from the blood. The lungs are composed of a light, spongy, highly elastic substance, the *parenchyma,* and they are covered by a layer of serous membrane. Each lung presents a rounded *apex* that reaches above the level of the clavicles into the root of the neck and a broad *base* that, resting on the obliquely placed diaphragm, reaches lower in back and at the sides than in front. The right lung is about 1 inch (2.5 cm) shorter than the left lung because of the large space occupied by the liver, and it is broader than the left lung because of the position

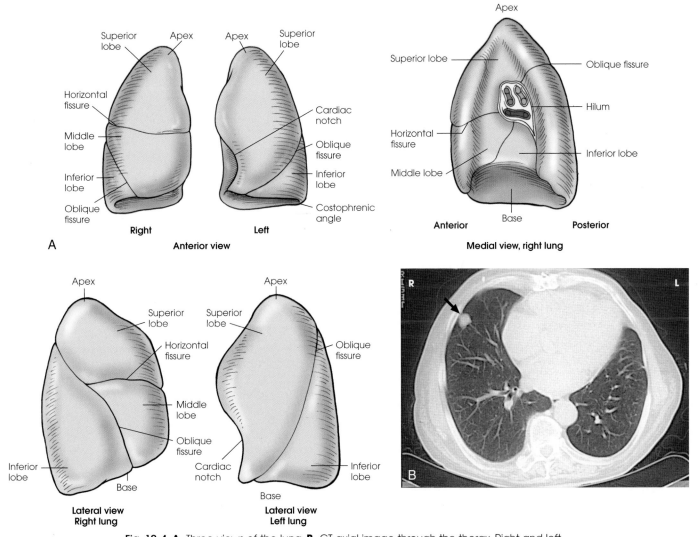

Fig. 10-4 A, Three views of the lung. **B,** CT axial image through the thorax. Right and left lungs are shown in actual position within thorax and in relation to heart. Note nodule in right anterior lung (*arrow*).

(**B,** Courtesy Siemens Medical Systems, Iselin, NJ.)

of the heart. The lateral surface of each lung conforms with the shape of the chest wall. The inferior surface of the lung is concave, fitting over the diaphragm, and the lateral margins are thin. During respiration, the lungs move inferiorly for inspiration and superiorly for expiration (Fig. 10-5). During inspiration, the lateral margins descend into the deep recesses of the parietal pleura. In radiology, this recess is called the *costophrenic angle* (see Fig. 10-5, *B*). The mediastinal surface is concave with a depression, called the *hilum,* that accommodates the bronchi, pulmonary blood vessels, lymph vessels, and nerves. The inferior mediastinal surface of the left lung contains a concavity called the *cardiac notch*. This notch conforms to the shape of the heart.

Each lung is enclosed in a double-walled, serous membrane sac called the *pleura* (see Fig. 10-3, *A*). The inner layer of the pleural sac, called the *visceral pleura,* closely adheres to the surface of the lung, extends into the interlobar fissures, and is contiguous with the outer layer at the hilum. The outer layer, called the *parietal pleura,* lines the wall of the thoracic cavity occupied by the lung and closely adheres to the upper surface of the diaphragm. The two layers are moistened by serous fluid so that they move easily on each other. The serous fluid prevents friction between the lungs and chest walls during respiration. The space between the two pleural walls is called the *pleural cavity*. Although the space is termed a cavity, the layers are actually in close contact.

Each lung is divided into *lobes* by deep fissures. The fissures lie in an oblique plane inferiorly and anteriorly from above, so that the lobes overlap each other in the AP direction. The *oblique fissures* divide the lungs into *superior* and *inferior lobes*. The superior lobes lie above and are anterior to the inferior lobes. The right superior lobe is divided further by a *horizontal fissure,* creating a *right middle lobe* (see Fig. 10-4). The left lung has no horizontal fissure and no middle lobe. The portion of the left lobe that corresponds in position to the right middle lobe is called the *lingula*. The lingula is a tongue-shaped process on the anteromedial border of the left lung. It fills the space between the chest wall and the heart.

Each of the five lobes divides into *bronchopulmonary segments* and subdivides into smaller units called *primary lobules*. The primary lobule is the anatomic unit of lung structure and consists of a terminal bronchiole with its expanded alveolar duct and alveolar sac.

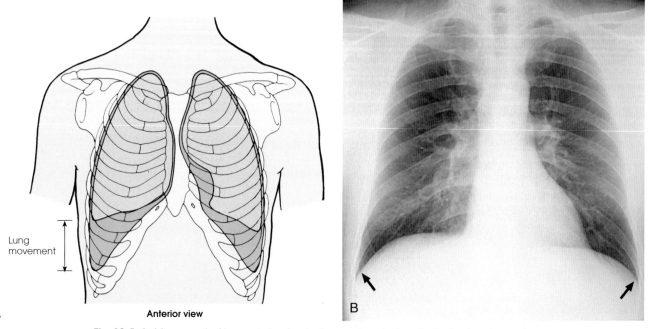

Lung movement

A   **Anterior view**   B

Fig. 10-5 A, Movement of lungs during inspiration and expiration. **B,** Costophrenic angles shown (*arrows*) on PA projection of chest.

Mediastinum

The *mediastinum* is the area of the thorax bounded by the sternum anteriorly, the spine posteriorly, and the lungs laterally (Fig. 10-6). The structures associated with the mediastinum are as follows:

- Heart
- Great vessels
- Trachea
- Esophagus
- Thymus
- Lymphatics
- Nerves
- Fibrous tissue
- Fat

The *esophagus* is the part of the digestive canal that connects the pharynx with the stomach. It is a narrow, musculomembranous tube about 9 inches (23 cm) in length. Following the curves of the vertebral column, the esophagus descends through the posterior part of the mediastinum and then runs anteriorly to pass through the esophageal hiatus of the diaphragm.

The esophagus lies just in front of the vertebral column, with its anterior surface in close relation to the trachea, aortic arch, and heart. This makes the esophagus valuable in certain heart examinations. When the esophagus is filled with barium sulfate, the posterior border of the heart and aorta are outlined well in lateral and oblique projections (Fig. 10-7). Frontal, oblique, and lateral images are often used in examinations of the esophagus. Radiography of the esophagus is discussed later in this chapter.

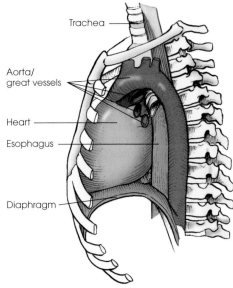

Fig. 10-6 Lateral view of mediastinum, identifying main structures.

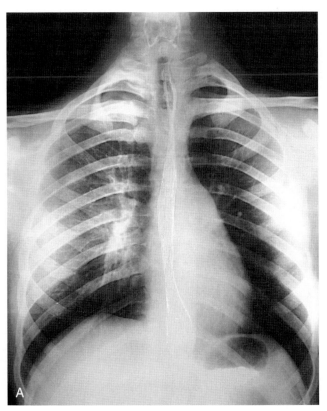

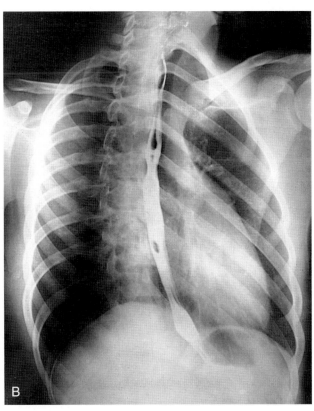

Fig. 10-7 A, PA projection of esophagus with barium sulfate coating its walls. **B,** PA oblique projection with barium-filled esophagus (RAO position).

491

The *thymus gland* is the primary control organ of the lymphatic system. It is responsible for producing the hormone *thymosin*, which plays a crucial role in the development and maturation of the immune system. The thymus consists of two pyramid-shaped lobes that lie in the lower neck and superior mediastinum, anterior to the trachea and great vessels of the heart and posterior to the manubrium. The thymus reaches its maximum size at puberty and then gradually undergoes atrophy until it almost disappears (Fig. 10-8).

In older individuals, lymphatic tissue is replaced by fat. At its maximum development, the thymus rests on the pericardium and reaches as high as the thyroid gland. When the thymus is enlarged in infants and young children, it can press on the retrothymic organs, displacing them posteriorly and causing respiratory disturbances. A radiographic examination may be made in the AP and lateral projections. For optimal image contrast, exposures should be made at the end of full inspiration.

COMPUTED TOMOGRAPHY

At the present time, computed tomography (CT) is used almost exclusively to image the anatomic areas of the thorax including the thymus gland. CT is excellent at showing all thoracic structures (Fig. 10-9).

SUMMARY OF ANATOMY

Body habitus	Pericardial	Bronchial tree	Right middle
Sthenic	cavity		lobe
Asthenic	Pleural cavities	**Alveoli**	Interlobar fissures
Hyposthenic	Serous	Alveolar duct	Oblique
Hypersthenic	membranes	Alveolar sac	fissures (2)
	Mediastinum	Alveoli	Horizontal
Thoracic cavity			fissure
Superior thoracic	**Respiratory**	**Lungs**	Lingula
aperture	**system**	Parenchyma	Bronchopulmo-
Inferior thoracic	Pharynx	Apex	nary segments
aperture	Trachea	Base	Primary lobules
Diaphragm	Carina	Costophrenic	
Thoracic viscera	Primary bronchi	angles	**Mediastinum**
Lungs	Right primary	Hilum	Heart
Heart	bronchus	Cardiac notch	Great vessels
Respiratory	Left primary	Pleura	Trachea
system	bronchus	Visceral pleura	Esophagus
Cardiac	Secondary	Parietal pleura	Thymus
system	bronchi	Serous fluid	Lymphatics
Lymphatic	Tertiary	Pleural cavity	Nerves
system	bronchi	Lobes	Fibrous tissue
Inferior	Bronchioles	Superior lobes	Fat
esophagus	Terminal	Inferior lobes	
Thymus gland	bronchioles		

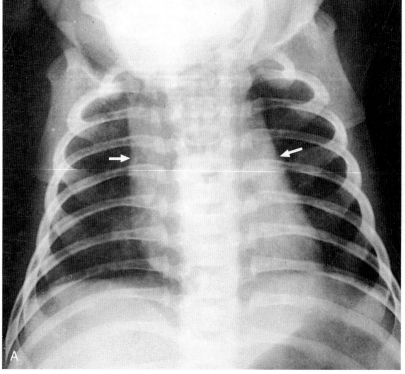

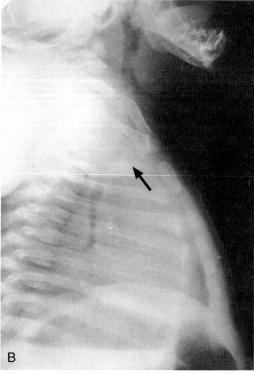

Fig. 10-8 A, PA chest radiograph showing mediastinal enlargement caused by hypertrophy of thymus (*arrows*). **B,** Lateral chest radiograph showing enlarged thymus (*arrow*).

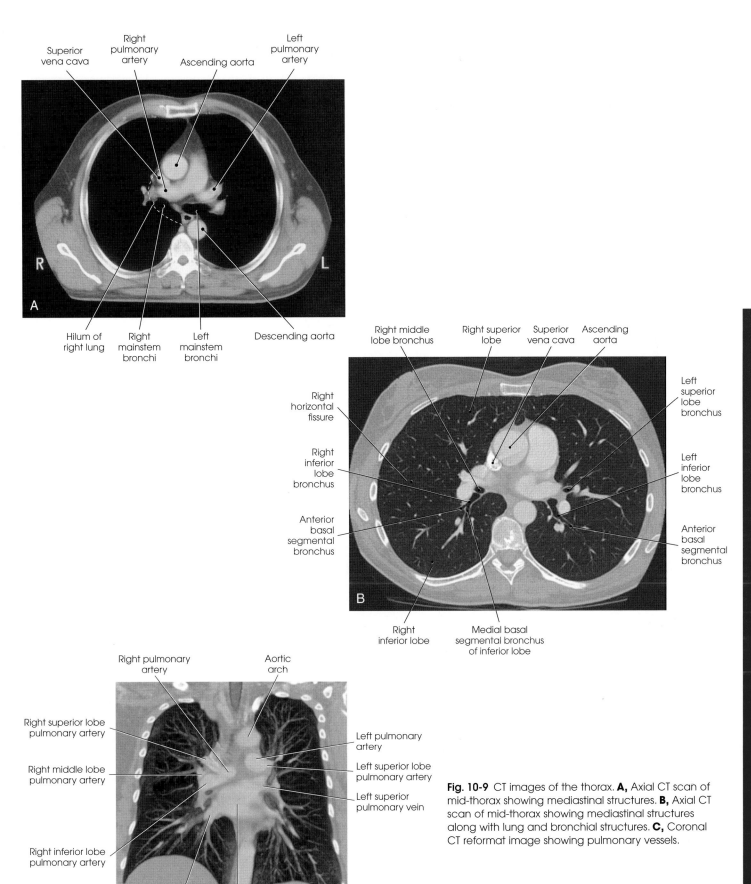

Superior vena cava

Right pulmonary artery

Ascending aorta

Left pulmonary artery

R

L

A

Hilum of right lung

Right mainstem bronchi

Left mainstem bronchi

Descending aorta

Right middle lobe bronchus

Right superior lobe

Superior vena cava

Ascending aorta

Right horizontal fissure

Left superior lobe bronchus

Right inferior lobe bronchus

Left inferior lobe bronchus

Anterior basal segmental bronchus

Anterior basal segmental bronchus

B

Right inferior lobe

Medial basal segmental bronchus of inferior lobe

Right pulmonary artery

Aortic arch

Right superior lobe pulmonary artery

Left pulmonary artery

Right middle lobe pulmonary artery

Left superior lobe pulmonary artery

Left superior pulmonary vein

Right inferior lobe pulmonary artery

C

Right inferior pulmonary vein

Left atrium

Fig. 10-9 CT images of the thorax. **A,** Axial CT scan of mid-thorax showing mediastinal structures. **B,** Axial CT scan of mid-thorax showing mediastinal structures along with lung and bronchial structures. **C,** Coronal CT reformat image showing pulmonary vessels.

SUMMARY OF PATHOLOGY

Condition	Definition
Aspiration/foreign body	Inspiration of a foreign material into the airway
Atelectasis	Collapse of all or part of the lung
Bronchiectasis	Chronic dilation of the bronchi and bronchioles associated with secondary infection
Bronchitis	Inflammation of the bronchi
Chronic obstructive pulmonary disease	Chronic condition of persistent obstruction of bronchial airflow
Cystic fibrosis	Disorder associated with widespread dysfunction of the exocrine glands, abnormal secretion of sweat and saliva, and accumulation of thick mucus in the lungs
Emphysema	Destructive and obstructive airway changes leading to an increased volume of air in the lungs
Epiglottitis	Inflammation of the epiglottis
Fungal disease	Inflammation of the lung caused by a fungal organism
Histoplasmosis	Infection caused by the yeastlike organism *Histoplasma capsulatum*
Granulomatous disease	Condition of the lung marked by formation of granulomas
Sarcoidosis	Condition of unknown origin often associated with pulmonary fibrosis
Tuberculosis	Chronic infection of the lung caused by the tubercle bacillus
Hyaline membrane disease or respiratory distress syndrome	Underaeration of the lungs caused by lack of surfactant
Metastases	Transfer of a cancerous lesion from one area to another
Pleural effusion	Collection of fluid in the pleural cavity
Pneumoconiosis	Lung diseases resulting from inhalation of industrial substances
Anthracosis or coal miner's lung or black lung	Inflammation caused by inhalation of coal dust (anthracite)
Asbestosis	Inflammation caused by inhalation of asbestos
Silicosis	Inflammation caused by inhalation of silicon dioxide
Pneumonia	Acute infection in the lung parenchyma
Aspiration	Pneumonia caused by aspiration of foreign particles
Interstitial or viral or pneumonitis	Pneumonia caused by a virus and involving the alveolar walls and interstitial structures
Lobar or bacterial	Pneumonia involving the alveoli of an entire lobe without involving the bronchi
Lobular or bronchopneumonia	Pneumonia involving the bronchi and scattered throughout the lung
Pneumothorax	Accumulation of air in the pleural cavity resulting in collapse of the lung
Pulmonary edema	Replacement of air with fluid in the lung interstitium and alveoli
Tumor	New tissue growth where cell proliferation is uncontrolled

EXPOSURE TECHNIQUE CHART ESSENTIAL PROJECTIONS

THORACIC VISCERA

Part	cm	kVp*	tm	mA	mAs	AEC	SID	IR	Dose† (mrad)
Chest: Lungs and heart—*PA*‡	22	110	[illegible]	300s		●● ○	72″	35 × 43 cm	16
Chest: Lungs and heart—*PA lateral*‡	33	1[illegible]	[illegible]	300s		○○ ●	72″	35 × 43 cm	41
Chest: Lungs and heart—*PA obliques*‡	25	[illegible]	[illegible]	[illegible]		●● ○	72″	35 × 43 cm	33
Chest: Lungs and heart—*AP*§	[illegible]	[illegible]	[illegible]	[illegible]s	2.4		40″	35 × 43 cm	8
Pulmonary apices—*PA axial*‡	[illegible]	[illegible]	[illegible]	300s		●● ○	72″	35 × 43 cm	24
Lungs and pleurae—*Lateral decubitus*‡	22	[illegible]	[illegible]	300s	3		72″	35 × 43 cm	22
Lungs and pleurae—*Dorsal/ventral decubitus*‡	33	125	0.02	300s	6		72″	35 × 43 cm	41

*kVp values are for a three-phase, 12-pulse generator or high frequency.
†Relative doses for comparison use. All doses are skin entrance for average adult at cm indicated.
‡Bucky, 16:1 grid. Screen-film speed 300.
§Tabletop, standard IR. Screen-film speed 300 or equivalent CR.
s, Small focal spot.

General Positioning Considerations

For radiography of the heart and lungs, the patient is placed in an *upright position* whenever possible to prevent engorgement of the pulmonary vessels and to allow gravity to depress the diaphragm. Of equal importance, the upright position shows air and fluid levels. In the recumbent position, gravitational force causes the abdominal viscera and diaphragm to move superiorly; it compresses the thoracic viscera, which prevents full expansion of the lungs. Although the difference in diaphragm movement is not great in hyposthenic individuals, it is marked in hypersthenic individuals. Figs. 10-10 and 10-11 illustrate the effect of body position in the same patient. The left lateral chest position (Fig. 10-12) is most commonly employed because it places the heart closer to the IR, resulting in a less magnified heart image. Left and right lateral chest images are compared in Figs. 10-12 and 10-13.

A *slight amount of rotation* from the PA or lateral projections causes considerable distortion of the heart shadow. To prevent this distortion, the body must be carefully positioned and immobilized.

PA CRITERIA

For PA projections, procedures are as follows:
- Instruct the patient to sit or stand upright. If the standing position is used, the weight of the body must be equally distributed on the feet.
- Position the patient's head upright, facing directly forward.
- Have the patient depress the shoulders and hold them in contact with the grid device to carry the clavicles below the lung apices. Except in the presence of an upper thoracic scoliosis, a faulty body position can be detected by the asymmetric appearance of the sternoclavicular joints. Compare the clavicular margins in Figs. 10-14 and 10-15.

LATERAL CRITERIA

For lateral projections, procedures are as follows:
- Place the side of interest against the IR holder.
- Have the patient stand so that the weight is equally distributed on the feet. The patient should not lean toward or away from the IR holder.
- Raise the patient's arms to prevent the soft tissue of the arms from superimposing the lung fields.
- Instruct the patient to face straight ahead and raise the chin.
- To determine rotation, examine the posterior aspects of the ribs. Radiographs without rotation show superimposed posterior ribs (see Figs. 10-12 and 10-13).

OBLIQUE CRITERIA

In oblique projections, the patient rotates the hips with the thorax and points the feet directly forward. The shoulders should lie in the same transverse plane on all radiographs.

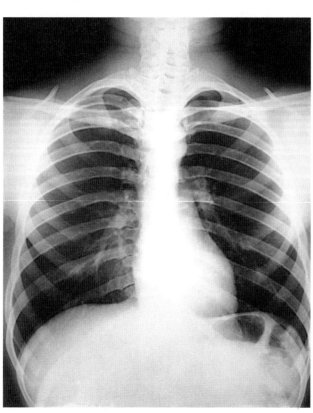

Fig. 10-10 Upright chest radiograph.

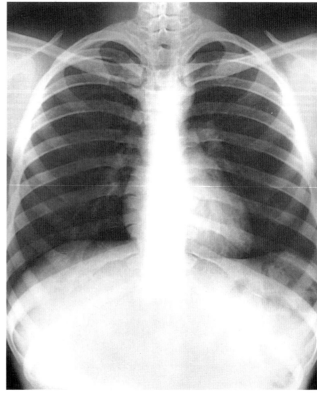

Fig. 10-11 Prone chest radiograph.

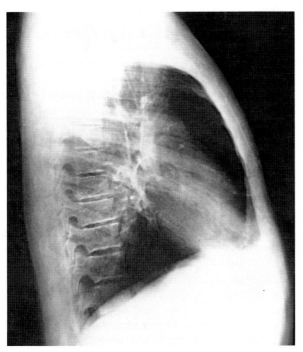

Fig. 10-12 Left lateral chest.

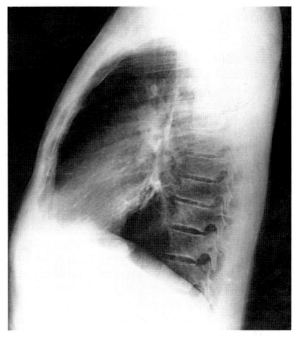

Fig. 10-13 Right lateral chest.

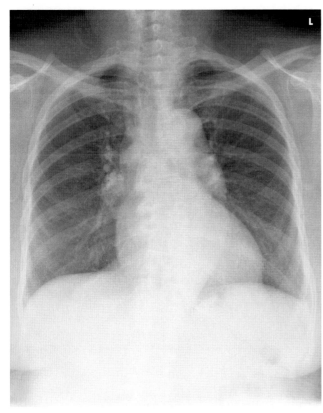

Fig. 10-14 PA chest without rotation.

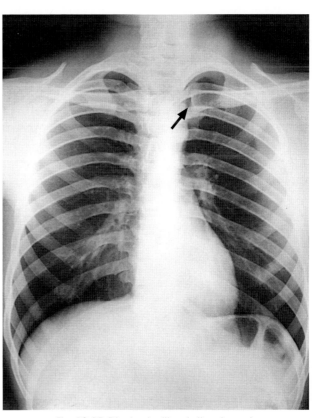

Fig. 10-15 PA chest with rotation (*arrow*).

Breathing Instructions

During *normal inspiration,* the costal muscles pull the anterior ribs superiorly and laterally, the shoulders rise, and the thorax expands from front to back and from side to side. These changes in the height and AP dimension of the thorax must be considered when positioning the patient.

Deep inspiration causes the diaphragm to move inferiorly, resulting in elongation of the heart. Radiographs of the heart should be obtained at the end of normal inspiration to prevent distortion. More air is inhaled during the second breath (and without strain) than during the first breath.

When *pneumothorax* (gas or air in the pleural cavity) is suspected, one exposure is often made at the end of full inspiration and another at the end of full expiration to show small amounts of free air in the pleural cavity that might be obscured on the inspiration exposure (Figs. 10-16 and 10-17). Inspiration and expiration radiographs are also used to show the movement of the diaphragm, the occasional presence of a foreign body, and atelectasis (absence of air).

Technical Procedure

The projections required to show the thoracic viscera adequately are usually requested by the attending physician and are determined by the clinical history of the patient. The PA projection of the chest is the most common projection and is used in all lung and heart examinations. Right and left oblique and lateral projections are also employed as required to supplement the PA projection. It is often necessary to improvise variations of the basic positions to project a localized area free of superimposed structures.

The exposure factors and accessories employed in examining the thoracic viscera depend on the radiographic characteristics of the individual patient's pathologic condition. Normally, chest radiography uses a high kilovolt (peak) (kVp) to penetrate and show all thoracic anatomy on the radiograph. The kVp can be lowered if exposures are made without a grid.

If the selected kVp is too low, the radiographic contrast may be too high, resulting in few shades of gray. The lung fields may appear properly penetrated on such a radiograph, but the mediastinum appears underexposed. If the selected kVp is too high, the contrast may be too low, and the finer lung markings are not shown. Adequate kVp penetrates the mediastinum and shows a faint shadow of the spine. Whenever possible, a minimum source-to-IR distance (SID) of 72 inches (183 cm) should be used to minimize magnification of the heart and to obtain greater recorded detail of the delicate lung structures (Fig. 10-18). A 120-inch (305-cm) SID is commonly used in radiography of the chest.

A grid technique is recommended for opaque areas within the lung fields and to show the lung structure through thickened pleural membranes (Figs. 10-19 and 10-20). This technique produces an image with higher contrast.

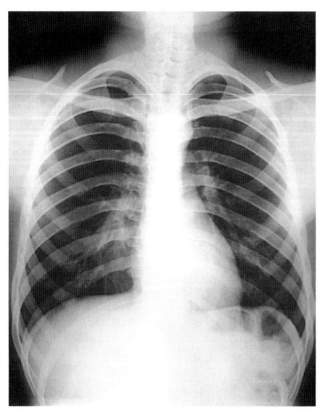

Fig. 10-16 PA chest during inspiration.

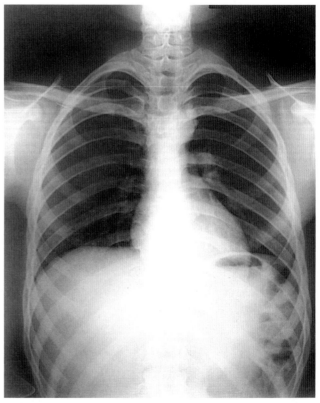

Fig. 10-17 PA chest during expiration.

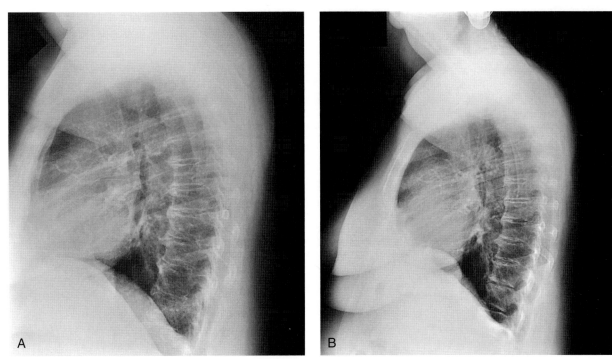

Fig. 10-18 A, Lateral chest radiograph performed at 44-inch (112-cm) SID. **B,** Radiograph in the same patient performed at 72-inch (183-cm) SID. Note decreased magnification and greater recorded detail of lung structures.

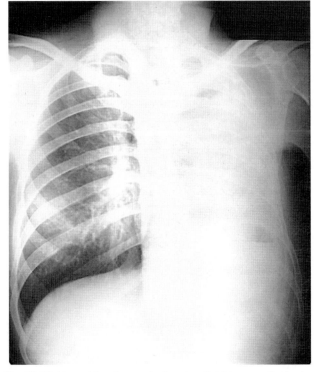

Fig. 10-19 Nongrid radiograph showing fluid-type pathologic condition in same patient as in Fig. 10-20.

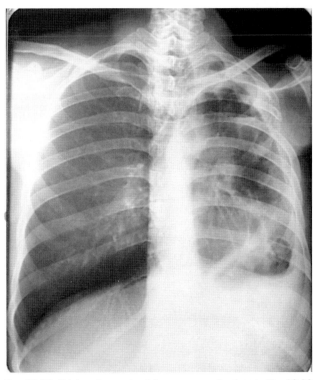

Fig. 10-20 Grid radiograph of the same patient as in Fig. 10-19.

Radiation Protection

Protection of the patient from unnecessary radiation is the professional responsibility of the radiographer (see Chapter 1 for specific guidelines). In this chapter, the *Shield gonads* statement indicates that the patient is to be protected from unnecessary radiation by restricting the radiation beam using proper collimation. In addition, the placement of lead shielding between the gonads and the radiation source is appropriate when the clinical objectives of the examination are not compromised. An example of a properly placed lead shield is shown in Fig. 10-25.

AP PROJECTION

When preparing to radiograph the trachea for the AP projection, use a grid technique to minimize scatter radiation because the kVp must be high enough to penetrate the sternum and the cervical vertebrae.

Image receptor: 10 × 12 inch (24 × 30 cm) lengthwise

Position of patient
- Examine the patient in either the supine or the upright position.

Position of part
- Center the midsagittal plane of the body to the midline of the grid.
- Adjust the patient's shoulders to lie in the same transverse plane.
- Extend the patient's neck slightly, and adjust it so that the midsagittal plane is perpendicular to the plane of the IR (Fig. 10-21).
- Center the IR at the level of the manubrium.
- Collimate closely to the neck.
- *Shield gonads.*
- *Respiration:* Instruct the patient to inhale slowly *during* the exposure to ensure that the trachea is filled with air.

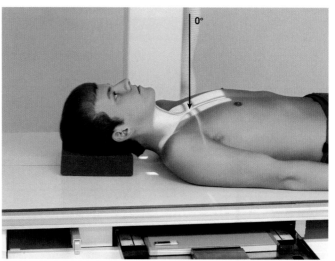

Fig. 10-21 AP trachea.

(The new positioning photographs in this chapter were submitted by Scott Slinkard, a radiography student at the Southeast Hospital College of Nursing & Health Sciences in Cape Girardeau, Missouri. The model in the photos is Tyler Glueck, also a student in the same program. The authors thank these students for their contribution to *Merrill's.*)

Trachea

Central ray

- Perpendicular through the manubrium to the center of the IR

Structures shown

AP projection shows the outline of the air-filled trachea. Under normal conditions, the trachea is superimposed on the shadow of the cervical vertebrae (Fig. 10-22).

The following should be clearly shown:
- Area from the mid-cervical to the mid-thoracic region
- Air-filled trachea
- No rotation

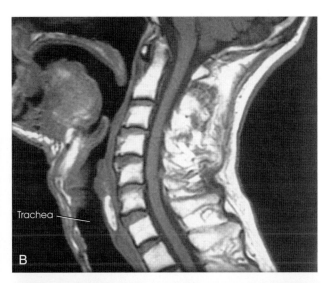

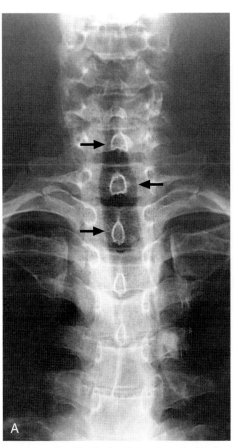

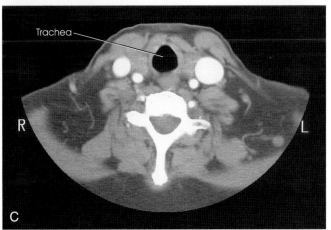

Fig. 10-22 A, AP trachea during inspiration showing air-filled trachea (*arrows*). CT and MRI are often used to evaluate the trachea and surrounding tissues. **B,** Sagittal MRI of neck. **C,** Axial CT of neck.

(**B** and **C,** Modified from Kelley LL, Petersen CM: *Sectional anatomy for imaging professionals,* ed 2, St Louis, 2007, Mosby.)

LATERAL PROJECTION
R or L position

Image receptor: 10 × 12 inch (24 × 30 cm) lengthwise

Position of patient

- Place the patient in a lateral position, either seated or standing, before a vertical grid device. If the standing position is used, the weight of the patient's body must be equally distributed on the feet.

Position of part

- Instruct the patient to clasp the hands behind the body and rotate the shoulders posteriorly as far as possible (Fig. 10-23). This position keeps the superimposed shadows of the arms from obscuring the structures of the superior mediastinum. If necessary, immobilize the arms in this position with a wide bandage.
- Adjust the patient's position to center the trachea to the midline of the IR. The trachea lies in the coronal plane that passes approximately midway between the jugular notch and the midcoronal plane.
- Adjust the height of the IR so that the upper border is at or above the level of the laryngeal prominence.
- Readjust the position of the body, being careful to have the midsagittal plane vertical and parallel with the plane of the IR.
- Extend the neck slightly.
- *Shield gonads.*
- *Respiration:* Make the exposure during slow inspiration to ensure that the trachea is filled with air.

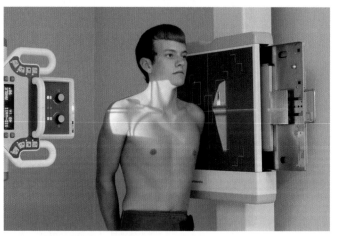

Fig. 10-23 Lateral trachea and superior mediastinum.

Central ray

- Horizontal through a point midway between the jugular notch and the mid-coronal plane (Fig. 10-24, *A*) and through a point 4 to 5 inches (10.2 to 12.7 cm) lower to show the superior mediastinum (Fig. 10-24, *B*)

Structures shown

A lateral projection shows the air-filled trachea and the regions of the thyroid and thymus glands. This projection, first described by Eiselberg and Sgalitzer,[1] is used extensively to show retrosternal extensions of the thyroid gland, thymic enlargement in infants (in the recumbent position), and the opacified pharynx and upper esophagus and an outline of the trachea and bronchi. It is also used to locate foreign bodies.

[1]Eiselberg A, Sgalitzer DM: X-ray examination of the trachea and the bronchi, *Surg Gynecol Obstet* 47:53, 1928.

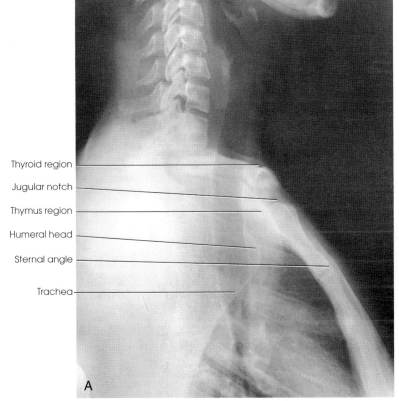

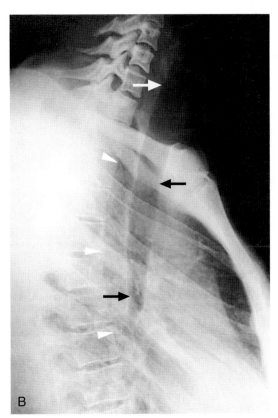

Thyroid region
Jugular notch
Thymus region
Humeral head
Sternal angle
Trachea

Fig. 10-24 A, Lateral superior mediastinum. **B,** Thoracic mediastinum with air-filled trachea (*arrows*) and esophagus (*arrowheads*).

Lungs and Heart
♠ PA PROJECTION

Image receptor: 14 × 17 inch (35 × 43 cm) lengthwise, or crosswise for hypersthenic patients

SID: Minimum SID of 72 inches (183 cm) is recommended to decrease magnification of the heart and increase recorded detail of the thoracic structures.

Position of patient

- If possible, always examine patients in the upright position, either standing or seated, so that the diaphragm is at its lowest position, and air or fluid levels are seen. Engorgement of the pulmonary vessels is also avoided.

Position of part

- Place the patient, with arms hanging at sides, before a vertical grid device.
- Adjust the height of the IR so that its upper border is about 1½ to 2 inches (3.8 to 5 cm) above the relaxed shoulders.
- Center the midsagittal plane of the patient's body to the midline of the IR.

- Have the patient stand straight, with the weight of the body equally distributed on the feet.
- Extend the patient's chin upward or over the top of the grid device, and adjust the head so that the midsagittal plane is vertical.
- Ask the patient to flex the elbows and to rest the *backs of the hands* low on the hips, below the level of the costophrenic angles. Depress the shoulders and adjust to lie in the same transverse plane. These movements will position the clavicles below the apices of the lungs.
- Rotate the shoulders forward so that both touch the vertical grid device. This movement will rotate the scapula outward and laterally to remove them from the lungs (Figs. 10-25 and 10-26).

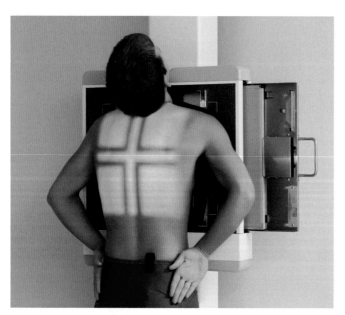

Fig. 10-25 Patient positioned for PA chest.

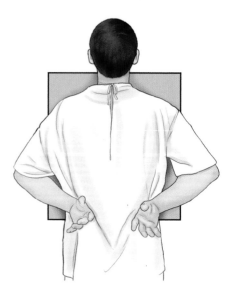

Fig. 10-26 PA chest showing correct position of hands if the patient is able.

- If an immobilization band is used, be careful not to rotate the body when applying the band. The least amount of rotation results in considerable distortion of the heart shadow.
- If a female patient's breasts are large enough to be superimposed over the lower part of the lung fields, especially the costophrenic angles, ask the patient to pull the breasts upward and laterally. This is especially important when ruling out the presence of fluid. Have the patient hold the breasts in place by leaning against the IR holder (Figs. 10-27 and 10-28).
- *Shield gonads:* Place a lead shield between the x-ray tube and the patient's pelvis (see Fig. 10-25).

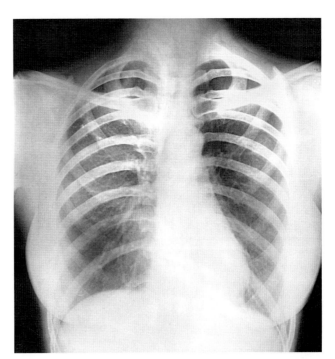

Fig. 10-27 Breasts superimposed over lower lungs.

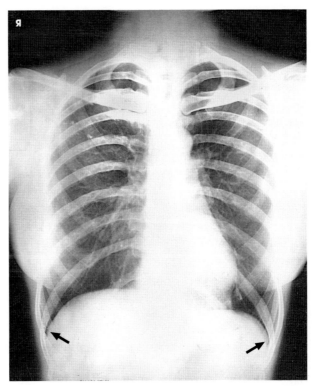

Fig. 10-28 Correct placement of breasts. Costophrenic angles are clearly seen (*arrows*).

■ *Respiration:* Full inspiration. The exposure is made after the *second* full inspiration to ensure maximum expansion of the lungs. The lungs expand transversely, anteroposteriorly, and vertically, with vertical being the greatest dimension.

■ For certain conditions, such as pneumothorax and the presence of a foreign body, radiographs are sometimes made at the end of full inspiration and expiration (Figs. 10-29 to 10-31). Pneumothorax is shown more clearly on expiration because collapse of the lung is accentuated.

Central ray

• Perpendicular to the center of the IR. The central ray should enter at the level of T7 (inferior angle of the scapula).

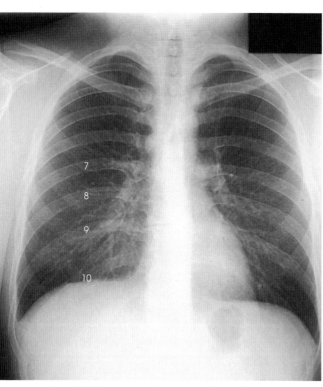

Fig. 10-29 Inspiration (posterior rib numbers).

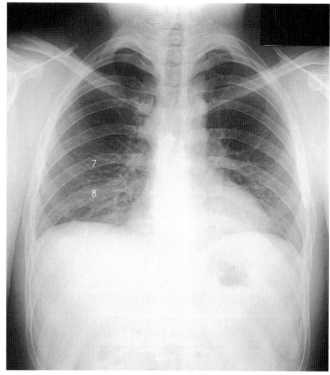

Fig. 10-30 Expiration in the same patient as in Fig. 10-29 (posterior rib numbers).

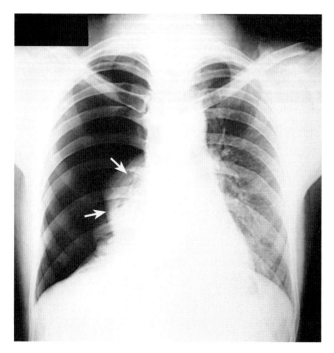

Fig. 10-31 PA chest during expiration. The patient had blunt trauma to the right chest. Left side is normal. Pneumothorax is seen on entire right side, and totally collapsed lung is seen near hilum (*arrows*).

Collimation

- Adjust to 14 × 17 inches (35 × 43 cm) on the collimator.

Structures shown

PA projection of the thoracic viscera shows the air-filled trachea, the lungs, the diaphragmatic domes, the heart and aortic knob, and, if enlarged laterally, the thyroid or thymus gland (Fig. 10-32). The vascular markings are much more prominent on the projection made at the end of expiration. The bronchial tree is shown from an oblique angle. The esophagus is well shown when it is filled with a barium sulfate suspension.

EVALUATION CRITERIA

The following should be clearly shown:
- Evidence of proper collimation
- Entire lung fields from the apices to the costophrenic angles
- No rotation; sternal ends of the clavicles equidistant from the vertebral column
- Trachea visible in the midline
- Scapulae projected outside the lung fields
- Ten posterior ribs visible above the diaphragm
- Sharp outlines of heart and diaphragm
- Faint shadow of the ribs and superior thoracic vertebrae visible through the heart shadow
- Lung markings visible from the hilum to the periphery of the lung
- With inspiration and expiration chest images, diaphragm shown on expiration at a higher level so that at least one less rib is seen within the lung field

NOTE: Inferior lobes of both lungs should be carefully checked for adequate penetration on women with large, pendulous breasts.

Cardiac studies with barium

PA chest radiographs are often obtained with the patient swallowing a bolus of barium sulfate to outline the posterior heart and aorta. The barium used in cardiac examinations should be thicker than the barium used for the stomach so that the contrast medium descends more slowly and adheres to the esophageal walls. The patient should hold the barium in the mouth until just before the exposure is made. Then the patient takes a deep breath and swallows the bolus of barium; the exposure is made at this time (see Fig. 10-7).

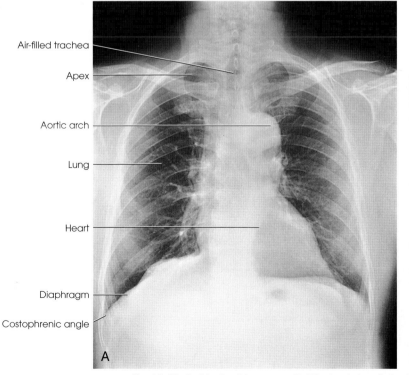

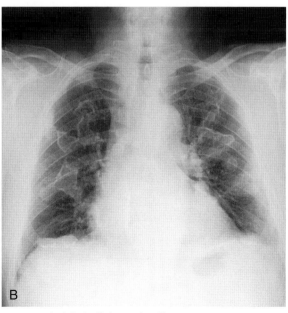

Fig. 10-32 A, PA chest in a man. **B,** PA chest showing pneumoconiosis in both lungs (multiple, irregular-shaped white areas are built-up coal dust).

Lungs and Heart

⚑ LATERAL PROJECTION

R or L position

Image receptor: 14 × 17 inch (35 × 43 cm) lengthwise

SID: Minimum SID of 72 inches (183 cm) is recommended to decrease magnification of the heart and increase recorded detail of the thoracic structures.

Position of patient

- If possible, always examine the patient in the upright position, either standing or seated, so that the diaphragm is at its lowest position, and air and fluid levels can be seen. Engorgement of the pulmonary vessels is also avoided.
- Turn the patient to a true lateral position, with arms by the sides.
- To show the heart and left lung, use the left lateral position with the patient's left side against the IR.
- Use the right lateral position to show the right lung best.

Position of part

- Adjust the position of the patient so that the midsagittal plane of the body is parallel with the IR and the adjacent shoulder is touching the grid device.
- Center the thorax to the grid; the midcoronal plane should be perpendicular and centered to the midline of the grid.
- Have the patient extend the arms directly upward, flex the elbows, and with the forearms resting on the elbows, hold the arms in position (Figs. 10-33 and 10-34).
- Place an intravenous catheter stand in front of an unsteady patient. Have the patient extend the arms and grasp the stand as high as possible for support.
- Adjust the height of the IR so that the upper border is about 1½ to 2 inches (3.8 to 5 cm) above the shoulders.

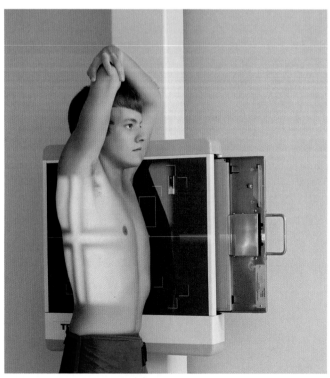

Fig. 10-33 Lateral chest.

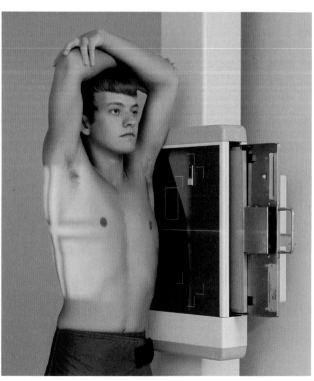

Fig. 10-34 Lateral chest.

- Recheck the position of the body; the midsagittal plane must be vertical. Depending on the width of the shoulders, the lower part of the thorax and hips may be a greater distance from the IR, but this body position is necessary for a true lateral projection. Having the patient *lean* against the grid device (foreshortening) results in distortion of all thoracic structures (Fig. 10-35). *Forward bending* also results in distorted structural outlines (Fig. 10-36).

- *Shield gonads.*
- *Respiration:* Full inspiration. The exposure is made after the *second* full inspiration to ensure maximum expansion of the lungs.

Central ray
- Perpendicular to the center of the IR. The central ray enters the patient on the midcoronal plane at the level of T7 or the inferior aspect of the scapula.

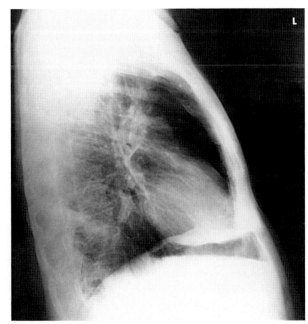

Fig. 10-35 Foreshortening.

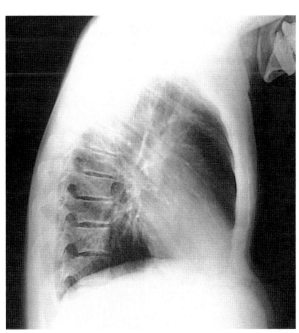

Fig. 10-36 Forward bending.

Collimation

- Adjust to 14 × 17 inches (35 × 43 cm) on the collimator.

Structures shown

The preliminary left lateral chest position is used to show the heart, the aorta, and left-sided pulmonary lesions (Figs. 10-37 and 10-38). The right lateral chest position is used to show right-sided pulmonary lesions (Fig. 10-39). These lateral projections are employed extensively to show the interlobar fissures, to differentiate the lobes, and to localize pulmonary lesions.

EVALUATION CRITERIA

The following should be clearly shown:
- Evidence of proper collimation
- Superimposition of the ribs posterior to the vertebral column
- Arm or its soft tissues not overlapping the superior lung field
- Long axis of the lung fields shown in vertical position, without forward or backward leaning
- Lateral sternum with no rotation
- Costophrenic angles and the lower apices of the lungs
- Penetration of the lung fields and heart
- Open thoracic intervertebral spaces and intervertebral foramina except in patients with scoliosis
- Sharp outlines of heart and diaphragm
- Hilum in the approximate center of the radiograph

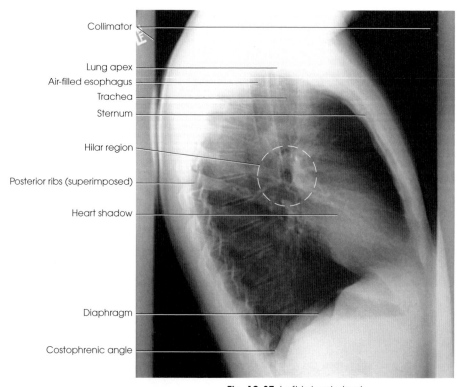

Fig. 10-37 Left lateral chest.

Collimator

Lung apex
Air-filled esophagus
Trachea
Sternum

Hilar region

Posterior ribs (superimposed)

Heart shadow

Diaphragm

Costophrenic angle

Cardiac studies with barium

The left lateral position is traditionally used during cardiac studies with barium. The procedure is the same as described for the PA chest projection (see p. 508).

(see p. 508)

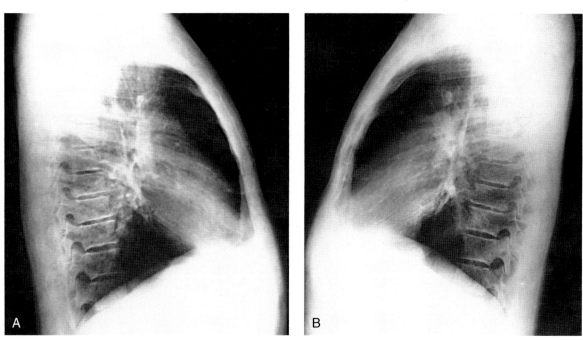

Fig. 10-38 A, Left lateral chest. **B,** Right lateral chest on same patient as in **A**. Note the size of the heart shadows.

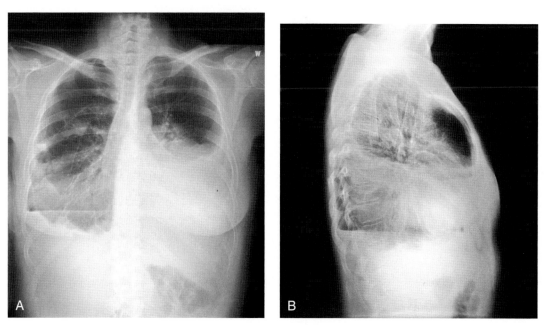

Fig. 10-39 A, PA chest. **B,** Lateral chest on same patient as in **A**. The importance of two projections is seen on this patient with multiple chest pathologies, including fluid, air-fluid level, pneumothorax, and enlarged heart.

Lungs and Heart
♠ PA OBLIQUE PROJECTION
RAO and LAO positions

Image receptor: 14 × 17 inch (35 × 43 cm) lengthwise

SID: Minimum SID of 72 inches (183 cm) is recommended to decrease magnification of the heart and to increase recorded detail of the thoracic structures.

Position of patient
- Maintain the patient in the position (standing or seated upright) used for the PA projection.
- Instruct the patient to let the arms hang free.
- Have the patient turn approximately 45 degrees toward the left side for LAO position and approximately 45 degrees toward the right side for RAO position.

- Ask the patient to stand or sit straight. If the standing position is used, the weight of the patient's body must be equally distributed on the feet to prevent unwanted rotation.
- For PA oblique projections, the side of interest is generally the side *farther* from the IR; however, the lung closest to the IR is also imaged.
- The top of the IR should be placed about 1½ to 2 inches (3.8 to 5 cm) above the vertebral prominens because the top of the shoulders may not be on the same plane.

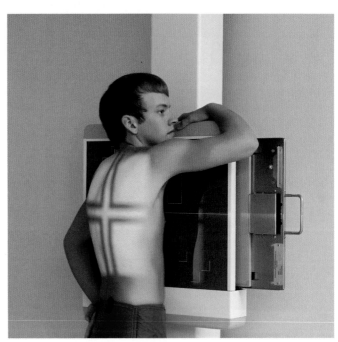

Fig. 10-40 PA oblique chest, LAO position.

Position of part

LAO position

- Rotate the patient 45 degrees to place the left shoulder in contact with the grid device, and center the thorax to the IR. Ensure that the right and left sides of the body are positioned to the IR.
- Instruct the patient to place the left hand on the hip with the palm outward.
- Have the patient raise the right arm to shoulder level and grasp the top of the vertical grid device for support.

- Adjust the patient's shoulders to lie in the same horizontal plane, and instruct the patient not to rotate the head (Fig. 10-40).
- Use a 55- to 60-degree oblique position when the examination is performed for a *cardiac series*. This projection is usually performed with barium contrast medium. The patient swallows the barium just before the exposure.
- *Shield gonads.*
- *Respiration:* Full inspiration. The exposure is made after the *second* full inspiration to ensure maximum expansion of the lungs.

RAO position

- Reverse the previously described position, placing the patient's right shoulder in contact with the grid device, the right hand on the hip, and the left hand on the top of the vertical grid device (Figs. 10-41 and 10-42).
- *Shield gonads.*
- *Respiration:* Full inspiration. The exposure is made after the second full inspiration to ensure maximum expansion of the lungs.

Central ray

- Perpendicular to the center of the IR. The central ray should be at the level of T7.

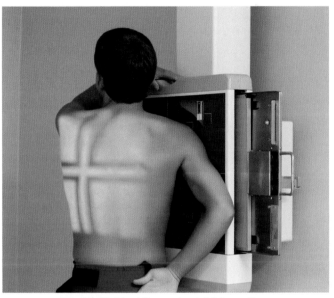

Fig. 10-41 PA oblique chest, RAO position.

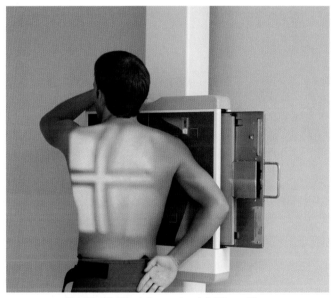

Fig. 10-42 PA oblique chest, RAO position.

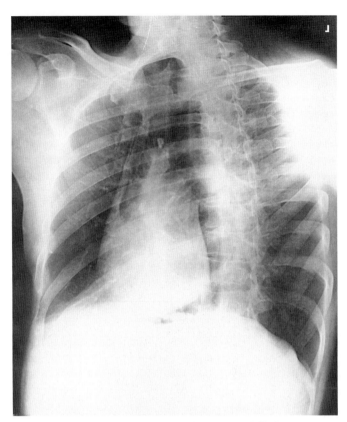

Fig. 10-43 PA oblique chest, LAO position at 45 degrees.

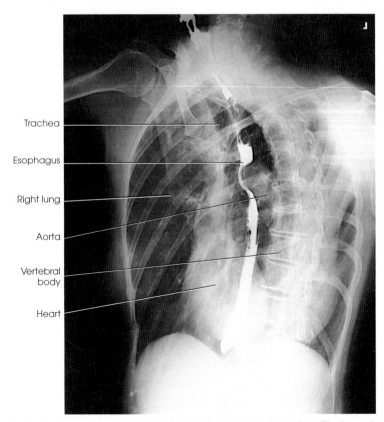

Trachea

Esophagus

Right lung

Aorta

Vertebral body

Heart

Fig. 10-44 PA oblique chest. LAO position is 60 degrees with barium-filled esophagus.

Collimation

- Adjust to 14 × 17 inches (35 × 43 cm) on the collimator.

Structures shown

LAO position The maximum area of the right lung field (side farther from the IR) is shown along with the thoracic viscera. The anterior portion of the left lung is superimposed by the spine (Figs. 10-43 and 10-44). Also shown are the trachea and its bifurcation (the carina) and the entire right branch of the bronchial tree. The heart, the descending aorta (lying just in front of the spinae), and the arch of the aorta are also presented.

RAO position The maximum area of the left lung field (side farther from the IR) is shown along with the thoracic viscera. The anterior portion of the right lung is superimposed by the spine (Figs. 10-45 and 10-46). Also shown are the trachea and the entire left branch of the bronchial tree. This position gives the best image of the left atrium, the anterior portion of the apex of the left ventricle, and the right retrocardiac space. When filled with barium, the esophagus is shown clearly in the RAO and LAO positions (see Fig. 10-46).

NOTE: The radiographs in this section, similar to the radiographs throughout this text, are printed as though the reader is looking at the patient's anterior body surface (see Chapter 1).

EVALUATION CRITERIA

The following should be clearly shown:
- Evidence of proper collimation
- Both lungs in their entirety
- Trachea filled with air
- Visible identification markers
- Heart and mediastinal structures within the lung field of the elevated side in oblique images of 45 degrees
- Maximum area of the right lung on LAO
- Maximum area of the left lung on RAO

Barium studies

RAO and LAO positions are routinely used during cardiac studies with barium. Follow the same procedure described in the PA chest section (see p. 507).

NOTE: A slight oblique position has been found to be of particular value in the study of pulmonary diseases. The patient is turned only slightly (10 to 20 degrees) from the RAO or LAO body position. This slight degree of obliquity rotates the superior segment of the respective lower lobe from behind the hilum and displays the medial part of the right middle lobe or the lingula of the left upper lobe free from the hilum. These areas are not clearly shown in the standard "cardiac oblique" of 45- to 60-degree rotation, largely because of superimposition of the spine.

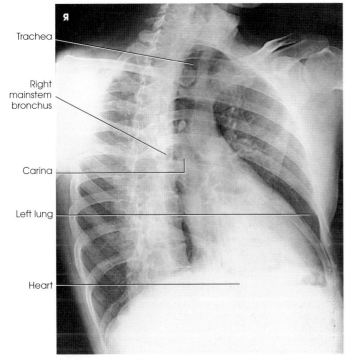

Trachea

Right mainstem bronchus

Carina

Left lung

Heart

Fig. 10-45 PA oblique chest, RAO position at 45 degrees.

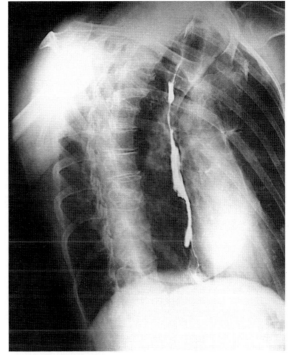

Fig. 10-46 PA oblique chest, RAO position at 60 degrees. Note barium in esophagus.

Lungs and Heart
✶ AP OBLIQUE PROJECTION
RPO and LPO positions

RPO and LPO positions are used when the patient is too ill to be turned to the prone position and sometimes as supplementary positions in the investigation of specific lesions. These positions are also used with the recumbent patient in contrast studies of the heart and great vessels.

One point the radiographer must bear in mind is that *RPO corresponds to the LAO position and LPO corresponds to the RAO position.* For AP oblique projections, the side of interest is generally the side closest to the IR. The resulting image shows the greatest area of the lung closest to the IR. The lung farthest from the IR is also imaged, and diagnostic information is often obtained for that side.

Image receptor: 14 × 17 inch (35 × 43 cm) lengthwise

SID: Minimum SID of 72 inches (183 cm) is recommended to decrease magnification of the heart and increase recorded detail of the thoracic structures.

Position of patient

- With the patient supine or facing the x-ray tube, either upright or recumbent, adjust the IR so that the upper border of the IR is about 1½ to 2 inches (3.8 to 5 cm) above the vertebral prominens or about 5 inches (12.7 cm) above the jugular notch.

Position of part

- Rotate the patient toward the correct side, adjust the body at a 45-degree angle, and center the thorax to the grid.
- If the patient is recumbent, support the elevated hip and arm. Ensure that both sides of the chest are positioned to the IR.
- Flex the patient's elbows and place the hands on the hips with the palms facing outward, or pronate the hands beside the hips. The arm closer to the IR may be raised as long as the shoulder is rotated anteriorly.
- Adjust the shoulders to lie in the same transverse plane in a position of forward rotation (Figs. 10-47 and 10-48).
- *Shield gonads.*
- *Respiration:* Full inspiration. The exposure is made after the *second* full inspiration to ensure maximum expansion of the lungs.

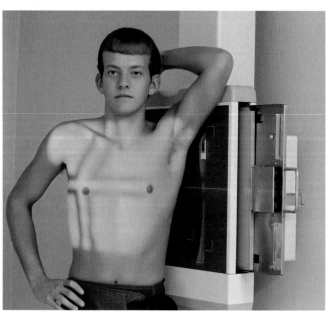

Fig. 10-47 Upright AP oblique chest, LPO position.

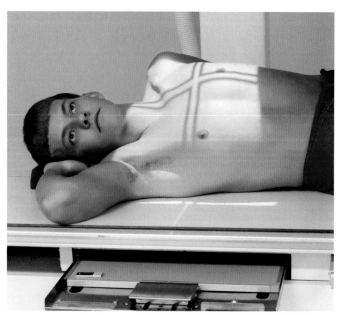

Fig. 10-48 Recumbent AP oblique chest, RPO position.

Central ray

- Perpendicular to the center of the IR at a level 3 inches (7.6 cm) below the jugular notch (central ray exits at T7)

Collimation

- Adjust to 14 × 17 inches (35 × 43 cm) on the collimator.

Structures shown

This radiograph presents an AP oblique projection of the thoracic viscera similar to the corresponding PA oblique projection (Fig. 10-49). The RPO position is comparable to the LAO position. The lung field of the elevated side usually appears shorter, however, because of magnification of the diaphragm. The heart and great vessels also cast magnified shadows as a result of being farther from the IR.

EVALUATION CRITERIA

The following should be clearly shown:

- Evidence of proper collimation
- Both lungs in their entirety
- Trachea filled with air
- Visible identification markers
- Lung fields and mediastinal structures
- Maximum area of the left lung on LPO
- Maximum area of the right lung on RPO

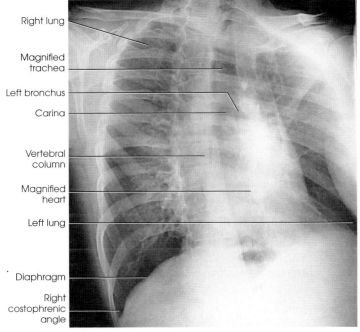
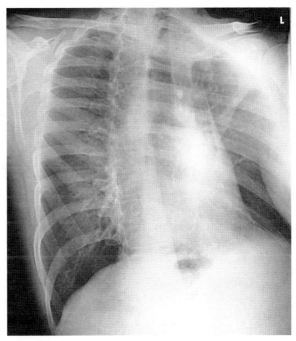

Right lung

Magnified trachea

Left bronchus

Carina

Vertebral column

Magnified heart

Left lung

Diaphragm

Right costophrenic angle

Fig. 10-49 AP oblique chest, LPO position.

⚶ AP PROJECTION*

The supine position is used when the patient is too ill to be turned to the prone position. It is sometimes used as a supplementary projection in the investigation of certain pulmonary lesions.

Image receptor: 14 × 17 inch (35 × 43 cm) lengthwise

SID: SID of 72 inches (183 cm) or 60 inches (150 cm) is recommended if it can be attained using the equipment available.

---

*See Chapter 28, Volume 3, for a full description of mobile AP.

Position of patient
• Place the patient in the supine or upright position with the back against the grid.

Position of part
• Center the midsagittal plane of the chest to the IR.
• Adjust the IR so that the upper border is approximately 1½ to 2 inches (3.8 to 5 cm) above the relaxed shoulders.
• If possible, flex the patient's elbows, pronate the hands, and place the hands on the hips to draw the scapulae laterally. (This maneuver is often impossible, however, because of the condition of the patient.)

• Adjust the shoulders to lie in the same transverse plane (Fig. 10-50).
• *Shield gonads.*
• *Respiration:* Full inspiration. The exposure is made after the *second* full inspiration to ensure maximum expansion of the lungs.

Central ray
• Perpendicular to the long axis of the sternum and the center of the IR. The central ray should enter about 3 inches (7.6 cm) below the jugular notch.

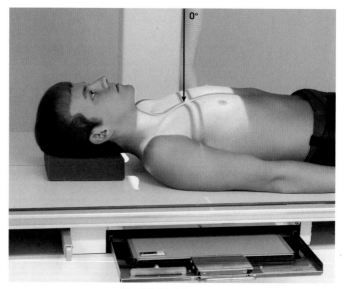

Fig. 10-50 AP chest.

Chest

Collimation

- Adjust to 14 × 17 inches (35 × 43 cm) on the collimator.

Structures shown

An AP projection of the thoracic viscera (Fig. 10-51) shows an image similar to the PA projection (Fig. 10-52). Being farther from the IR, the heart and great vessels are magnified and engorged, and the lung fields appear shorter because abdominal compression moves the diaphragm to a higher level. The clavicles are projected higher, and the ribs assume a more horizontal appearance.

EVALUATION CRITERIA

The following should be clearly shown:

- Evidence of proper collimation
- Medial portion of the clavicles equidistant from the vertebral column
- Trachea visible in the midline
- Clavicles lying more horizontal and obscuring more of the apices than in the PA projection
- Equal distance from the vertebral column to the lateral border of the ribs on each side
- Faint image of the ribs and thoracic vertebrae visible through the heart shadow
- Entire lung fields, from the apices to the costophrenic angles
- Pleural vascular markings visible from the hilar regions to the periphery of the lungs

NOTE: Resnick[1] recommended an angled AP projection to free the basal portions of the lung fields from superimposition by the anterior diaphragmatic, abdominal, and cardiac structures. He reported that this projection also differentiates middle lobe and lingular processes from lower lobe disease. For this projection, the patient may be either upright or supine, and the central ray is directed to the mid-sternal region at an angle of 30 degrees caudad. Resnick stated that a more suitable angulation may be chosen based on the preliminary films.

[1]Resnick D: The angulated basal view: a new method for evaluation of lower lobe pulmonary disease, *Radiology* 96:204, 1970.

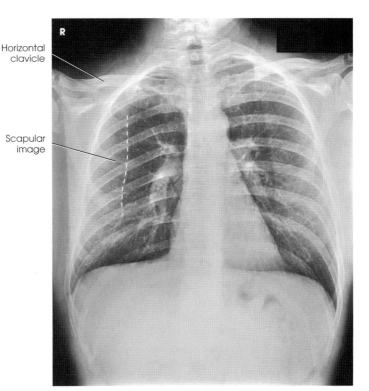

Horizontal clavicle

Scapular image

Fig. 10-51 AP chest.

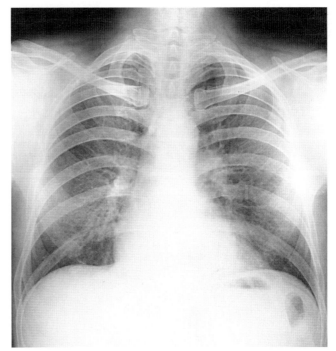

Fig. 10-52 PA chest.

Chest

♠ AP AXIAL PROJECTION
LINDBLOM METHOD
Lordotic position

Image receptor: 14 × 17 inch (35 × 43 cm) lengthwise

SID: Minimum SID of 72 inches (183 cm) is recommended to decrease magnification of the heart and to increase recorded detail of the thoracic structures.

Position of patient
- Place the patient in the upright position, facing the x-ray tube and standing approximately 1 ft (30.5 cm) in front of the vertical grid device.

Position of part
- Adjust the height of the IR so that the upper margin is about 3 inches (7.6 cm) above the upper border of the shoulders when the patient is adjusted in the lordotic position.

Lordotic position
- Adjust the patient for the AP axial projection, with the coronal plane of the thorax 15 to 20 degrees from vertical and the midsagittal plane centered to the midline of the grid (Fig. 10-53).

Oblique lordotic positions—LPO or RPO
- Rotate the patient's body approximately 30 degrees away from the position used for the AP projection, with the affected side toward and centered to the grid (Fig. 10-54).
- With either of the preceding positions, have the patient flex the elbows and place the hands, palms out, on the hips.
- Have the patient lean backward in a position of extreme lordosis and rest the shoulders against the vertical grid device.
- *Shield gonads.*
- *Respiration:* Full inspiration. The exposure is made after the *second* full inspiration to ensure maximum expansion of the lungs.

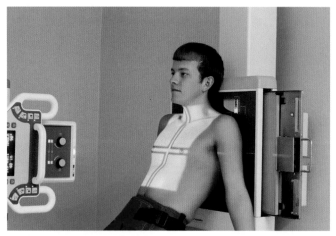

Fig. 10-53 AP axial pulmonary apices, lordotic position.

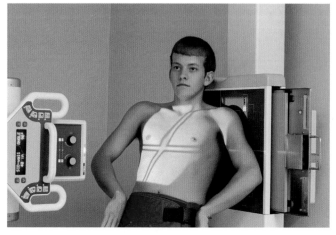

Fig. 10-54 AP axial oblique pulmonary apices, LPO lordotic position.

Thoracic Viscera

Pulmonary Apices

Central ray
- Perpendicular to the center of the IR at the level of the midsternum

Collimation
- Adjust to 14 × 17 inches (35 × 43 cm) on the collimator.

Structures shown
AP axial (Fig. 10-55) and AP axial oblique (Fig. 10-56) images of the lungs show the apices and conditions such as interlobar effusions.

EVALUATION CRITERIA
The following should be clearly shown:
- Evidence of proper collimation
  Lordotic position
- Clavicles lying superior to the apices
- Sternal ends of the clavicles equidistant from the vertebral column
- Apices and lungs in their entirety
- Clavicles lying horizontally with their medial ends overlapping only the first or second ribs
- Ribs distorted with their anterior and posterior portions superimposed
  Oblique lordotic position
- Dependent apex and lung of the affected side in its entirety

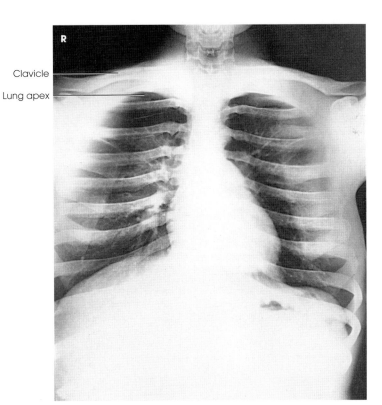

Fig. 10-55 AP axial pulmonary apices, lordotic position.

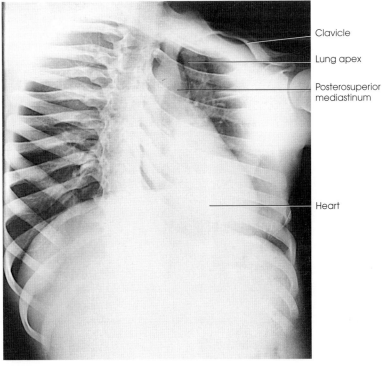

Fig. 10-56 AP axial oblique pulmonary apices, LPO lordotic position.

PA AXIAL PROJECTION

Image receptor: 10 × 12 inch (24 × 30 cm) or 11 × 14 inch (28 × 35 cm) crosswise

SID: Minimum SID of 72 inches (183 cm) is recommended to decrease magnification of the heart and to increase recorded detail of the thoracic structures.

Position of patient

- Position the patient seated or standing before a vertical grid device. If the patient is standing, the weight of the body must be equally distributed on the feet.

Position of part

- Adjust the height of the IR so that it is centered at the level of the jugular notch.
- Center the midsagittal plane of the patient's body to the midline of the IR, and rest the chin against the grid device.
- Adjust the patient's head so that the midsagittal plane is vertical, and then flex the elbows and place the hands, palms out, on the hips.
- Depress the patient's shoulders, rotate them forward, and adjust them to lie in the same transverse plane.
- Instruct the patient to keep the shoulders in contact with the grid device to move the scapulae from the lung fields (Fig. 10-57).
- *Shield gonads.*
- *Respiration:* Make the exposure at the end of *full inspiration* or as an option, at *full expiration*. The clavicles are elevated by inspiration and depressed by expiration; the apices move little, if at all, during either phase of respiration.

Central ray

Inspiration

- Directed 10 to 15 degrees cephalad through T3 to the center of the IR

Expiration (optional)

- Directed perpendicular to the plane of the IR and centered at the level of T3

Structures shown

The apices are projected above the shadows of the clavicles in the PA axial and PA projections (Fig. 10-58).

EVALUATION CRITERIA

The following should be clearly shown:

- Apices in their entirety
- Only the superior lung region adjacent to the apices
- Clavicles lying below the apices
- Medial portion of the clavicles equidistant from the vertebral column

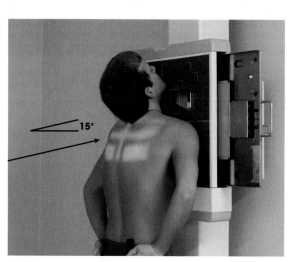

Fig. 10-57 PA axial pulmonary apices (inspiration).

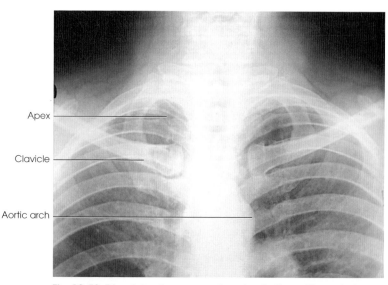

Fig. 10-58 PA axial pulmonary apices, inspiration with central ray angled.

Apex

Clavicle

Aortic arch

Thoracic Viscera

AP AXIAL PROJECTION

Image receptor: 10 × 12 inch (24 × 30 cm) or 11 × 14 inch (28 × 35 cm) crosswise

NOTE: This projection is recommended when the patient cannot be positioned for the lordotic position.

SID: Minimum SID of 72 inches (183 cm) is recommended to decrease magnification of the heart and to increase recorded detail of the thoracic structures.

Position of patient

• Examine the patient in the upright or supine position.

Position of part

• Center the IR to the midsagittal plane at the level of T2, and adjust the patient's body so that it is not rotated.

• Flex the patient's elbows and place the hands on the hips with the palms out, or pronate the hands beside the hips.
• Place the shoulders back against the grid and adjust them to lie in the same transverse plane (Fig. 10-59).
• *Shield gonads*.
• *Respiration:* Expose at the end of *full inspiration*.

Central ray

• Directed at an angle of 15 or 20 degrees cephalad to the center of the IR and entering the manubrium

Collimation

• Adjust to 14 × 17 inches (35 × 43 cm) on the collimator.

Structures shown

AP axial projection shows the apices lying below the clavicles (Fig. 10-60).

The following should be clearly shown:
■ Clavicles lying superior to the apices
■ Sternal ends of the clavicles equidistant from the vertebral column
■ Apices in their entirety
■ Superior lung region adjacent to the apices
■ Clavicles lying horizontally with their medial ends overlapping only the first or second ribs
■ Ribs distorted, with their anterior and posterior portions superimposed

NOTE: The AP axial projection is used in preference to the PA axial projection in hypersthenic patients and patients whose clavicles occupy a high position. The AP axial projection makes it possible to separate the apical and clavicular shadows without undue distortion of the apices.

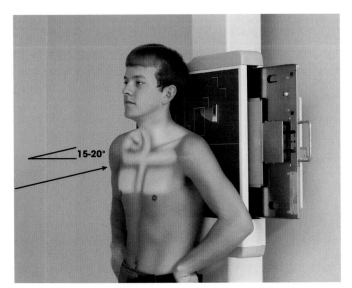

Fig. 10-59 AP axial pulmonary apices.

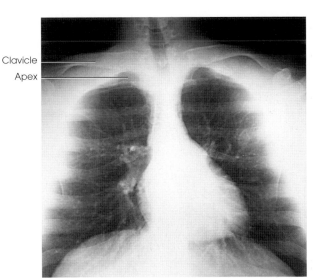

Clavicle
Apex

Fig. 10-60 AP axial pulmonary apices.

Pulmonary Apices

🦅 AP OR PA PROJECTION*
R or L lateral decubitus positions

Image receptor: 14 × 17 inch (35 × 43 cm) lengthwise

Position of patient
- Place the patient in a lateral decubitus position, lying on either the affected or the unaffected side, as indicated by the existing condition. A small amount of fluid in the pleural cavity is usually best shown with the patient lying on the affected side. With this positioning, the mediastinal shadows and the fluid do not overlap. A small amount of free air in the pleural cavity is generally best shown with the patient lying on the unaffected side.
- *Exercise care* to ensure that the patient does not fall off the cart. If a cart is used, *lock all wheels* securely in position.
- Achieve the best visualization by allowing the patient to remain in the position for *5 minutes before the exposure.* This allows fluid to settle and air to rise.

---

*See Chapter 28 for mobile description of the decubitus position.

Position of part
- If the patient is lying on the affected side, elevate the body 5 to 8 cm (2 to 3 inches) on a suitable platform or a firm pad.
- Extend the arms well above the head, and adjust the thorax in a true lateral position (Fig. 10-61).
- Place the anterior or posterior surface of the chest against a vertical grid device.
- Adjust the IR so that it extends approximately 1½ to 2 inches (3.8 to 5 cm) beyond the shoulders.
- *Shield gonads.*
- *Respiration:* Full inspiration. The exposure is made after the *second* full inspiration to ensure maximum expansion of the lungs.

Central ray
- *Horizontal* and perpendicular to the center of the IR at a level 3 inches (7.6 cm) below the jugular notch for AP and T7 for PA

Collimation
- Adjust to 14 × 17 inches (35 × 43 cm) on the collimator.

Structures shown
AP or PA projection obtained using the lateral decubitus position shows the change in fluid position and reveals any previously obscured pulmonary areas or, in the case of suspected pneumothorax, the presence of any free air (Figs. 10-62 to 10-64).

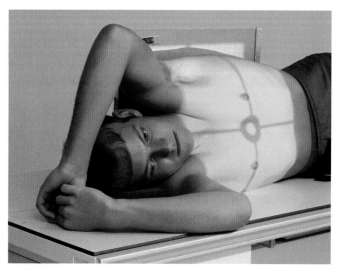

Fig. 10-61 AP projection, right lateral decubitus position. Side up is the affected side, so no table pad was used. This projection would demonstrate free air rising up to the left side.

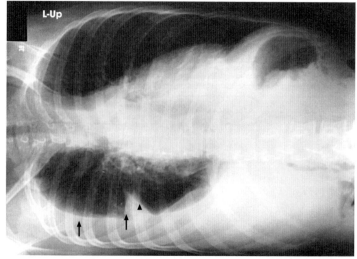

Fig. 10-62 AP projection, right lateral decubitus position, showing a fluid level (*arrows*) on the side that is down. Note the fluid in the lung fissure (*arrowhead*). Note correct marker placement, with the upper side of the patient indicated.

Lungs and Pleurae

EVALUATION CRITERIA

The following should be clearly shown:
- Evidence of proper collimation
- No rotation of the patient from a true frontal position, as evidenced by the clavicles being equidistant from the spine
- Affected side in its entirety
- Apices
- Proper identification visible to indicate that decubitus was performed
- Patient's arms not visible in the field of interest

NOTE: An exposure made with the patient leaning directly laterally from the upright PA position is sometimes useful for showing fluid levels in pulmonary cavities. Ekimsky[1] recommended this position, with the patient leaning laterally 45 degrees, to show small pleural effusions. He reported that the inclined position is simpler to perform than the decubitus position and is equally satisfactory.

---

[1]Ekimsky B: Comparative study of lateral decubitus views and those with lateral body inclination in small pleural effusions, *Vestn Rentgenol Radiol* 41:43, 1966. (In Russian.) Abstract: *Radiology* 87:1135, 1966.

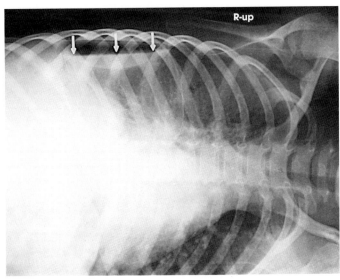

Fig. 10-63 AP projection, left lateral decubitus position, in same patient as in Fig. 10-64. *Arrows* indicate air-fluid level (air on the side up). Note correct marker placement, with upper side of the patient indicated.

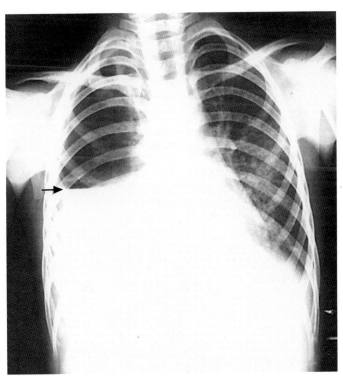

Fig. 10-64 Upright PA chest. *Arrow* indicates air-fluid level.

⬥ LATERAL PROJECTION
R or L position
Ventral or dorsal decubitus position

Image receptor: 14 × 17 inch (35 × 43 cm) lengthwise

Position of patient
- With the patient in a prone or supine position, elevate the thorax 2 to 3 inches (5 to 7.6 cm) on folded sheets or a firm pad, centering the thorax to the grid.
- Achieve the best visualization by allowing the patient to remain in the position for *5 minutes before the exposure.* This allows fluid to settle and air to rise.

Position of part
- Adjust the body in a true prone or supine position, and extend the arms well above the head.
- Place the affected side against a vertical grid device, and adjust it so that the top of the IR extends to the level of the thyroid cartilage (Fig. 10-65).
- *Shield gonads.*
- *Respiration:* Full inspiration. The exposure is made after the *second* full inspiration to ensure maximum expansion of the lungs.

Central ray
- *Horizontal* and centered to the IR. The central ray enters at the level of the midcoronal plane and 3 to 4 inches (7.6 to 10.2 cm) below the jugular notch for the dorsal decubitus and at T7 for the ventral decubitus.

Collimation
- Adjust to 14 × 17 inches (35 × 43 cm) on the collimator.

Structures shown
A lateral projection in the decubitus position shows a change in the position of fluid and reveals pulmonary areas that are obscured by the fluid in standard projections (Figs. 10-66 and 10-67).

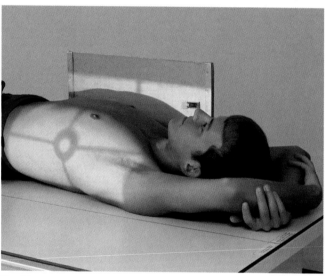

Fig. 10-65 Right lateral projection, dorsal decubitus position. Side up is the affected side, so no table pad was used. This projection would demonstrate free air rising up to the anterior chest.

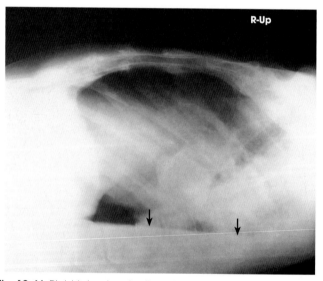

Fig. 10-66 Right lateral projection, dorsal decubitus position. *Arrows* indicate air-fluid level. Note correct marker placement, with upper side of the patient indicated.

EVALUATION CRITERIA

The following should be clearly shown:

- Evidence of proper collimation
- Entire lung fields, including the anterior and posterior surfaces
- No rotation of the thorax from a true lateral position
- Upper lung field not obscured by the arms
- Proper marker identification visible to indicate the decubitus was performed
- T7 in the center of the IR

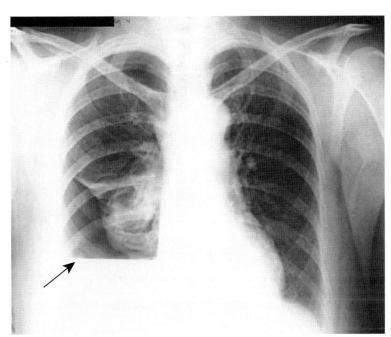

Fig. 10-67 Upright PA chest in same patient as in Fig. 10-66. Note right lung fluid level (*arrow*).

ADDENDUM A

SUMMARY OF ABBREVIATIONS, VOLUME ONE

AC	acromioclavicular	IP†	interphalangeal (hand and foot)	PIP	proximal interphalangeal (hand and foot)
AEC	automatic exposure control	IR	image receptor		
AP	anteroposterior	kVp	kilovolt peak	R	right
ARRT	American Registry of Radiologic Technologists	L	left	RA	radiologist assistant
		LAO	left anterior oblique	RAO	right anterior oblique
ASIS	anterior superior iliac spine	LLQ	left lower quadrant	RLQ	right lower quadrant
ASRT	American Society of Radiologic Technologists	LPO	left posterior oblique	RPA	radiology practitioner assistant
		LUQ	left upper quadrant	RPO	right posterior oblique
CAMRT	Canadian Association of Medical Radiation Technologists	mA	milliamperage	RUQ	right upper quadrant
		mAs	milliampere second	SC	sternoclavicular
CDC	Centers for Disease Control and Prevention	MC	metacarpal	SI	sacroiliac
		MCP	metacarpophalangeal	SID	source–to–image receptor (IR) distance
cm	centimeter	MMD	mean marrow dose		
CMC	carpometacarpal	MRI	magnetic resonance imaging	SMV	submentovertical
CR*	central ray	MTP	metatarsophalangeal	SSD	source-to-skin distance
CR*	computed radiography	NCRP	National Council on Radiation Protection	TEA	top ear attachment
CT	computed tomography			TMT	tarsometatarsal
DIP	distal interphalangeal (hand and foot)	OD	optical density	US	ultrasound
		OID	object-to-image receptor (IR) distance	VSM	verticosubmental
DR	direct digital radiography				
EAM	external acoustic meatus	OML	orbitomeatal line		
HNP	herniated nucleus pulposus	OR	operating room		
IOML	infraorbitomeatal line	PA	posteroanterior		
IP†	image plate				

*Note: CR has two different meanings.
†Note: IP has two different meanings.

Tammy Cutis, MS, RT(R), contributed the abbreviations box for each chapter in this edition.

INDEX

C

C3-C7 cervical vertebrae, **1:**370, 370f
Cadaveric
    images, **3:**257–258, 257f
    sections, **3:**240
Calcaneocuboid articulations, **1:**236–239,
        236f–238f, 236t
Calcaneus, **1:**271–275, 271f–275f
Calcification, **2:**391
Calculus, **2:**64
Caldwell method, **2:**296–299, **2:**334–335, **2:**372–
        373, **3:**252, 252f, 297f–299f, 334f–335f,
        372f–373f
Calibration, cross, **3:**463
Cameras
    gamma, **3:**388
    scintillation, **3:**388
Camp-Coventry method, **1:**308–309, 308f–309f
CAMRT. *See* Canadian Association of Medical
        Radiation Technologists (CAMRT).
Canadian Association of Medical Radiation
        Technologists (CAMRT), **1:**2, 85, 529
Canal
    alimentary. *See* Alimentary canal (digestive
        system).
    carpal, **1:**146–147, 146f–147f
Cancers
    adenomas, pituitary, **2:**284
    breast. *See* Mammography.
    carcinomas, **2:**111
    chondrosarcomas, **1:**182, 240, 454
    classification, tumor-node-metastasis (TNM),
        3:471, 471t
    epidemiology, **3:**469–470, 470t
    metastases. *See* Metastases.
    multiple myelomas, **1:**335, **2:**284, 454
    risk factors, external *vs.* internal, **3:**470–472,
        470t
    sarcomas, Ewing, **1:**240, **3:**115
    tissue origins, **3:**471, 471t
    tumors. *See* Tumors.
Captured lesions, **2:**432–433, 433f
Carbon (^{11}C), **3:**390–391
Carcinomas, **2:**111
Cardiac and vascular radiography, **3:**19–100
    anatomy, **3:**20–25, 20f–21f, 23f, 25f, 50–53,
        50f–53f
    angiography
        cerebral, **3:**50–56, 50f–56f
        digital substraction (DSA), **3:**27–38, 27f–38f
    aortography, **3:**38–39, 38f–39
    arteriography, **3:**40–43, 40f–43f
    catheterization, cardiac, **3:**75–97, 76t–77t,
        79f–83f, 82t, 85f–97f, 87t
    future trends, **3:**37
    historical development, **3:**26
    indications, **3:**26
    interventional, **3:**62–100. *See also* Interventional
        radiography.
    projections
        anterior circulation, **3:**57–60, 57f–60f
        aortic arch angiograms, **3:**57, 57f
        AP axial, **3:**60, 60f
        AP axial oblique, transorbital, **3:**60, 60f
        AP axial, supraorbital, **3:**58, 58f
        biplane oblique, simultaneous, **3:**57, 57f
        circulation, posterior, **3:**60–61, 60f–61f
        cranial vessels, **3:**57, 57f
        lateral, **3:**57, 57f, 60–61, 60f

Cardiac and vascular radiography—*cont'd*
    radiation protection, **3:**37
    resources, **3:**34n, 50n, 54n, 100
    terminology, **3:**26, 98–99
    venography, **3:**44–49, 44f–49f
Cardiac notch, **1:**490
Cardiopulmonary resuscitation (CPR), **2:**458
Cardiovascular system disorders, **3:**159–160
Carpal
    bones, **1:**102
    bridge, **1:**145, 145f
    canal, **1:**146–147, 146f–147f
    sulcus, **1:**102, 102f
    tunnel, **1:**102
Carpometacarpal (CMC) articulations
    anatomy, **1:**105–107, 105f–107f, 105t, 529
    first, **1:**118–120, 118f–120f
    projections, **1:**118–120, 118f–120f
Catheterization, cardiac, **3:**75–97, 76t–77t, 79f–83f,
        82t, 85f–97f, 87t
Cauda equina, **3:**279, 279f
Caudad, **1:**85
Caudocranial (CC) projections, **2:**398–399,
        398f–399f, 404–407, 405f–407f. *See also*
        Mammography.
    cleavage, **2:**426–427, 426f–427f
    exaggerated (XCCL), **2:**424–425, 424f–425f
    full breast, **2:**434–435, 434f–435f
    roll, lateral, **2:**428–429, 428f–429f
    roll, medial, **2:**428–429, 428f–429f
Causton method, **1:**242b
Cavities, body, **1:**68–69, 68f–69f
    abdominopelvic, **2:**85, 85f
    glenoid, **1:**188–191, 188f–191f, 205–206,
        205f–206f
    inferior thoracic, **1:**487, 487f
    left pleural, **1:**487, 487f
    medullary, **1:**76
    oral, **2:**59–70
    pelvic, **1:**332, 332f, 332t
    thoracic, **1:**68–69, 68f–69f
CC projections. *See* Caudocranial (CC)
        projections.
CDC. *See* Centers for Disease Control and
        Prevention (CDC).
Celiac disease, **2:**111
Centers for Disease Control and Prevention (CDC),
        1:16, **2:**230, 458, 529
Centimeters (cm), **1:**529
Central, **1:**85
Central nervous system (CNS), **3:**1–18
    anatomy, **3:**2–4
        brain, 2f, **3:**2
        divisions, **3:**2
        meninges, **3:**3
        spinal cord, **3:**3, 3f
        ventricular system, **3:**4, 4f
    computed tomography (CT), **3:**10–12, 10f–11f
    diskography, provocative, **3:**16–17, 17f
    examinations, plain radiographic, **3:**5
    magnetic resonance imaging (MRI), **3:**12–13,
        12f–13f
    myelography, **3:**6–9, 6f–9f
    pain management, interventional, **3:**16–17, 17f
    procedures
        interventional, **3:**14–16, 14f–17f
        vascular, **3:**14–16, 14f–17f
    resources, **3:**18
    terminology, **3:**18

Central rays (CRs)
    angulation method, **1:**468–469, 468f–469f
    directions, **1:**31
    terminology, **1:**529, **2:**458
Cephalad, **1:**85
Cerebellum, **3:**242–243
Cerebral spinal fluid (CSF), **3:**242–243
Cerebral vascular accidents (CVAs), **2:**458
Cervical intervertebral foramina, **1:**392–398,
        392f–398f
Cervical spine, **1:**370, **2:**33, **3:**192–193, 33f,
        192f–193f, 370f, 370t
Cervical vertebrae, **1:**369–373f, 369f–373f
    C3-C6, **1:**370, 370f
    C7, **1:**370, 370f
    projections, **1:**386–391, **1:**398–400, 386f–391f,
        398f–400f
Cervicothoracic regions, **1:**401–402, 401f–402f
CF. *See* Cystic fibrosis (CF).
Chamberlain method, **1:**382b
Charts
    exposure. *See also* Exposure.
        abdomen, **2:**87
        abdomen projections, **2:**87
        bony thorax, **1:**455
        digestive system (alimentary canal), **2:**110
        fundamentals, **1:**38–41, 39f–41f
        limbs, lower, **1:**241
        limbs, upper, **1:**108
        pelvis and upper femora, **1:**335
        shoulder girdle, **1:**182
        sinuses, paranasal, **2:**366
        skull, **2:**285
        thoracic viscera, **1:**495
        urinary system, **2:**191
        vertebral column, **1:**381
    phototimer technique, full-field digital
            mammography (FFDM), **2:**391
Chassard-Lapiné method, **2:**171, 171f
Chest projections
    chest-lungs-heart, **1:**504–520, 504f–520f
    mobile radiography, **3:**178–181, 178f–181f
    pediatric, **3:**118–121, 118f–121f. *See also*
            Pediatric populations.
CHF. *See* Congestive heart failure (CHF).
Children, radiographic procedures, **3:**101–148
    abdominal radiography, **3:**136–137, 136f. *See*
            also Abdomen.
    approaches, **3:**104–107, 106f
    chest radiography, **3:**118–121, 118f–121f
    comparisons
        advanced modalities, **3:**142–146, 143f,
                145f–146f
        assessments, **3:**122t
        protocols, **3:**130t
    densitometry, bone, **3:**460, 460f. *See also*
            Densitometry, bone.
    environments, **3:**101–103, 102f–103f
    examinations
        common, **3:**118–138
        unique, **3:**139–141, 139f–140f
    gastrointestinal (GI) procedures, **3:**137–138,
            137f–138f
    genitourinary procedures, **3:**137–138,
            137f–138f
    hip radiography, **3:**123–125, 123f–125f
    immobilization, **3:**117
    limb radiography, **3:**132–135, 132f
    pathology summaries, **3:**115

Index

Index

Index

Index

Index

Index

Index

Index

Index

Index

Index

Index

Index